ESSENTIAL
HERBAL
WISDOM

About the Author

Nancy Arrowsmith was born in 1950 in Oxford, England. She has lived in various areas of the United States, and also in Italy and the Lower Austrian countryside near the Bohemian border. Her home is now in Arizona, near the Mexican border. Her book *A Field Guide to the Little People* was first published in 1977, and has attained cult status since then with translations into several languages. She founded and edited Germany's first organic gardening magazine, and has been internationally active in the preservation of vegetable heirloom varieties. She has published extensively in German, and has lectured widely to a variety of audiences. Her interest in herbs recently led to a formal study of Chinese medicine, and she is now a licensed acupuncturist in the state of Arizona.

To Write to the Author

If you wish to contact the author or would like more information about this book, please write to the author in care of Llewellyn Worldwide and we will forward your request. Both the author and publisher appreciate hearing from you and learning of your enjoyment of this book and how it has helped you. Llewellyn Worldwide cannot guarantee that every letter written to the author can be answered, but all will be forwarded. Please write to:

Nancy Arrowsmith
% Llewellyn Worldwide
2143 Wooddale Drive, Dept. 978-0-7387-1488-2
Woodbury, MN 55125-2989, U.S.A.
Please enclose a self-addressed stamped envelope for reply,
or $1.00 to cover costs. If outside U.S.A., enclose international postal reply coupon.

Many of Llewellyn's authors have websites with additional information and resources. For more information, please visit our website at http://www.llewellyn.com.

Note: The author and publisher of this book are not responsible in any manner whatsoever for any injury that may occur through following the instructions contained herein. The recipes and remedies in this book are not meant to diagnose, treat, prescribe, or substitute for consultation with a licensed health care professional. They are not for commercial use or profit. New herbal recipes should always be taken in small amounts to allow the body to adjust and to test for possible allergic reactions.

NANCY ARROWSMITH

ESSENTIAL
HERBAL
WISDOM

A COMPLETE EXPLORATION
OF 50 REMARKABLE HERBS

Llewellyn Publications
Woodbury, Minnesota

First U.S. Edition
First Printing, 2009
Originally published in Germany as *Herbarium Magicum* by Allegria, an imprint of Ullstein Buchverlage GmbH, Berlin, 2007.

Book design by Steffani Sawyer
Cover design by Kevin R. Brown

Interior illustrations are used with permission from Dover publications (see page 561 for more details).

Llewellyn is a registered trademark of Llewellyn Worldwide, Ltd.

Arrowsmith, Nancy, 1950–
   [Herbarium Magicum. English]
   Essential herbal wisdom : a complete exploration of 50 remarkable herbs / Nancy Arrowsmith.—
1st U.S. ed.
       p. cm.
   Originally published: Herbarium Magicum. Germany: Allegria, 2007.
   Includes bibliographical references.
   ISBN 978-0-7387-1488-2
   1. Herbs. I. Title.
   SB351.H5A7713 2009
   635'.7—dc22
                            2008036942

Llewellyn Worldwide does not participate in, endorse, or have any authority or responsibility concerning private business transactions between our authors and the public.
   All mail addressed to the author is forwarded but the publisher cannot, unless specifically instructed by the author, give out an address or phone number.
   Any Internet references contained in this work are current at publication time, but the publisher cannot guarantee that a specific location will continue to be maintained. Please refer to the publisher's website for links to authors' websites and other sources.

Llewellyn Publications
A Division of Llewellyn Worldwide, Ltd.
2143 Wooddale Drive, Dept. 978-0-7387-1488-2
Woodbury, MN 55125-2989, U.S.A.
www.llewellyn.com

Printed in the United States of America

 Printed in the United States of America on recycled paper comprised of 15 percent post-consumer waste.

Dedicated to my father,
although herbs never were
his cup of tea.

Acknowledgments

A book that has been this long in the making—since the 1970s—has certainly been influenced by many people. When I started out, I was working in a shop in Munich, Germany, selling herbs. My gratitude goes to Wilhelm Lindig and his wife Elfriede, and to Gisela who taught me how to handle and to know herbs. They generously transmitted much of their practical knowledge to me. Wilhelm Lindig learned the trade from his father, and was such a master of his field that people came from all over Germany to visit his shop. I also thank the customers who came in and asked all those ingenious questions that kept me scurrying back to my books.

In the days before the Internet, most research had to be done in libraries. The librarians of the Bavarian Staatsbibliothek in Munich already knew me from my first book, and were as forthcoming as ever. I continued my research in the British Library in London. It was here that I met true British understatement. Sometime I couldn't avoid cracking up at some of the outrageous recipes in old books, and would burst out laughing. Instead of scolding me for making noise, someone would come over and say, "You must have found something quite amusing!?" But the most wonderful library was the one I found hidden behind the Herbarium in the Kensington Museum of Natural History. All the old, original herbals could be found here, and it was so little frequented that I often had several librarians waiting on me. The library was in one of the turreted towers of the building, and it felt like the proverbial ivory tower. I would have loved to have stayed there for much longer than I did. Later, I made use of the facilities of the Nationalbibliothek in Vienna, and, of course, did a lot of fact-checking on the Web. From my experience doing that, I would suggest that readers type in the botanical names instead of the plants' folk names to get a list of more serious sites. There is now a surprising amount of well-researched literature available on the Web.

When I first started this book, I thought it would be a simple work of compilation and grossly underestimated the time it would take for me to become proficient and knowledgeable in various areas of herbalism. It is not enough to simply copy recipes and hope that they are right. If the author does not have the practical knowledge of how to use herbs, then the herbal turns out to be like so many others of its kind, simply a rehashing of the experience of others. I don't know when it became obvious to me that my knowledge was very limited—probably after endless batches of poorly-dyed wool, partial poisoning after smoking the house with garden sage, or culinary experiments such as rendering badger fat or making jellies that no one would eat, and creating cosmetic creams that separated and refused to come together. My editors (of the first edition of this book, published in Germany in 2007) urged me just to finish it, but I was stubborn and wanted to really know what I was writing about. It is to their great credit that they showed exemplary patience despite prolonged delays, and never let an evil word fall.

As it is, two decades of acting as editor-in-chief of an organic gardening magazine—along with work building up a seed-saving organization, gardening, cooking, maintaining rare plants and animal breeds, and experiencing all facets of country living—have gone into the creation of this book. I feel I have some practical basis in the various areas of knowledge I have written about, although I am sure mistakes have still sneaked in here and there. For these, I apologize, and hope that they will be pointed out to me so that I can correct them in any future editions.

The readers of the gardening magazine, members of the seed-saving organization, and many organic farmers and gardeners asked me a lot of questions and told me about their experiences. For these I am very appreciative, since they taught me many things I would not otherwise have known. Extensive lecturing and attendance at meetings in both the Old World and the New, especially in Eastern Europe, helped me to see how people interacted with herbs in different cultures. Through my cooperation with many seed-saving organizations and gene banks, along with exchange programs with foreign scientists, I was able to gain insights into more formal areas of scientific endeavor.

After many years of publishing in German, I returned to the United States in 1999 and had to come to terms with a world that had certainly changed since I last lived here. It was also a challenge to begin writing exclusively in English again. My special thanks go to Donna Chesner, who remained confident about my knowledge and abilities when I had almost lost my own confidence in them. Neither the German nor the English edition of this book would have been possible without the concentrated and generous efforts of many friends and colleagues, including my agents, Nina Arrowsmith and Vito von Eichborn. Michael Goerden and Patricia Holland-Moritz at Ullstein Verlag orchestrated the harmonious cooperation with Sarah Heidelberger and Michael Korth that led to the German edition. Carrie Obry at Llewellyn paved the way for the American edition, helping me to focus my efforts on a very different reading public, and Sandy Sullivan painstakingly edited the English text.

Other, no less heartfelt, acknowledgments go to:

- my mother, grandmother, and grandfather, who passed on their gardening knowledge and enthusiasm
- my sister, who keeps asking questions
- Michael, who lived through the many years of this book with me
- Nina, who taught me to see plants with a child's eye and later helped me with her professional expertise
- the gardeners, farmers, and herbalists who live with their herbs
- the many I have not listed who helped me in more ways than I can name. It is their generosity that continues to move and inspire me.

At the beginning of Time, God and the Devil were at odds, even more so then than nowadays. If God set out to create something, then the Devil wanted to destroy it.

One day God decided to make Man and formed him out of clay, taking great care to smooth down his skin. Because the clay was not yet firm, God had to let the figure dry overnight.

That evening the Devil decided to go for an evening walk. He was delighted when he saw the clay figure, and even more delighted when he found out that God had made it. He picked up a stick and tore at the wet clay, poking holes in it until there were more holes than smooth surfaces. The Devil laughed at his good work and went to bed feeling very pleased with himself.

When God came to look at his work early the next morning, he was heartbroken. What had been a well-formed, handsome man was now just a crumbled mass of clay. God looked around for something to repair the clay figure, and, not finding anything better, tore up clumps of herbs and stuffed them into the holes. After he had filled out the figure, he smoothed wet clay over the grasses and dried clay. The results were not as good as the day before, but the clay dried fast and God was soon able to breathe life into a flawed, but healthy man and see that his work was good.

Since then, the plants that God used to repair his man of clay have served Mankind as healing herbs. They continue to save men and women from the Devil's troublemaking.

—An old Bulgarian folktale, from Oskar Dähnhardt's *Natursagen*

CONTENTS

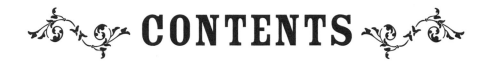

Lunar Herbs

INTRODUCTION

Plants and herbs are all-sensitive—as people with "green thumbs" well know. Herbs react to light, sound, and thought waves; to mineral content in the soil; to other plants in their vicinity; to moisture, magnetic forces, attention, love, and hate. They adapt with almost incredible rapidity (in evolutionary terms) to their surroundings. Plants are beings of amazing complexity that we have only begun to understand and appreciate ... they are imbued with all the magic and intricacy of life.

In this book, I attempt to show just how deeply rooted herbs are in our lives. They have been part of European culture for thousands of years, and of Eastern culture even longer. Herbs were gathered in North, Central, and South America, as well as in Africa and Australia, long before the arrival of European settlers. Many European herbs (such as plantain) made their way to the New World and subsequently naturalized themselves. Because my experience with herbs has mostly been in Europe (and I have gained a wealth of information about them from European herbalists, gardeners, and farmers), I have written in this book about common, cosmopolitan herbs that can be found in both Europe and North America. Of course, this is at the cost of omitting extremely interesting and versatile herbs from other parts of the world.

Herbs that furnished a good deal of the medicine, food, and even intoxicants of rural societies were once held in great veneration. Many cultures thought that plants, especially herbs, were inhabited by sprites and elves. In some areas, herbs still hold a special position as the "little people" of the plant world, small in size but great in power, the mundane yet magically gifted inhabitants of our planet.

While we often reject this view as superstitious, it is nonetheless my firm belief that there is some truth in it. Western culture has confined our approach to herbs to the material plane, and to practical utilization; we have suffered loss from the narrowness of this vision. We only know of herbs as aromatic and healing plants that give food aroma and enhance its nutritional value, or cure diseases. In our hurry to control all aspects of nature, we usually limit our interest in herbs to one active ingredient, forgetting the other elements.

It is counterproductive to handle plants and herbs with gross impartiality and insensitivity—growing them in monoculture, force-feeding them with artificial fertilizers, and harvesting them without a thought for the phases of the moon, solar influence, astrological signs, the moisture content of the air, the sunniness of the harvest weather, or the hour of harvest. Too often, herbs are harvested in the wild without regard for species conservation and then "popped" indiscriminately as capsules. *All* ancient accounts of herbal lore stress the fact that herbs are only to be picked at certain times and under certain planetary influences:

- when they are in full bloom
- in the morning
- at night
- under the influence of Leo, Scorpio, or Cancer
- during the winter
- not with the bare hand or with iron
- using silver, gold, or copper digging tools
- not by direct human touch (i.e., not without a tool, glove, etc.)

There must be a reason for these injunctions. They have been passed down to us from a time more in tune with the energies and patterns of nature, which recognized the interdependence of living and inanimate beings. While some of these admonitions cannot be easily followed in our day and age, can we take it upon ourselves to fully dismiss the knowledge of our forefathers and foremothers as "simple superstition"?

The uses to which herbs are put today are almost unlimited. As the famed English herbalist John Gerard wrote in the late sixteenth century,

> nothing can be confected, either delicate for the taste, dainty for the smell, pleasant for sight, wholesome for body, conservative or restorative for health, but it borroweth the rellish of an herb, the savor of a flour, the colour of a leafe, the juice of a plant, or the decoction of a root.[1]

Herbs are used as vermifuges, emmenagogues, diuretics, emollients, sudorifics, and styptics. They are expectorant, depurative, cathartic, stomachic, antispasmodic, rubefacient, laxative, or carminative in nature. They act as febrifuges, aphrodisiacs, vul-

---

1. Introduction, *Gerard's Herball* [1597]: *The essence thereof distilled by Marcus Woodward from the edition of Th. Johnson, 1636.* Ed. Marcus Woodward (London: Gerald How, 1927).

neraries, deobstruents, purgatives, antiseptics, or poisons, and are administered in the form of extracts, tinctures, pills, smelling salts, teas, salves, dusting powders, eye or ear drops, cough syrups, lozenges, electuaries, juices, powders, and as baths, poultices, compresses, liniments, plasters, bandages, hot pillows, pessaries, or suppositories. They flavor medicinal wines, beers, and distilled spirits, tonics, bitters, cordials, essential oils, inhalant mixtures, or are taken as snuff.

They are employed as cosmetic aids, used as toothbrushes, added to massage oils, soaps, cleansing mixtures, astringent waters, herbal vinegars, perfumes, face creams, freckle removers, shampoos, hair lighteners, mouth washes, and douches. Herbs are strewn and garlanded in rooms to freshen and perfume the air. They are used as water purifiers, air fresheners and incense, potpourri and herbal cushions, germicides and disinfectants. Herbs can kill or drive away moths, flies, rats, mice, fleas, vermin, and large animals. They attract cats and are used as medicines by veterinarians. They serve as dyes and scouring pads. Their fibers are made into rope, cloth, and paper; their fronds and stems are employed as bedstraw; their roots are used as teething rings and amulets; their fruits as rattles and toys; and their flowering stems as torches. Their leaves and stems furnish firewood, mulch, fertilizer, insecticides, or animal fodder.

Herbs are also used as oracles, as symbols in art and literature, as hallucinogens, narcotics and intoxicants, stimulants and sedatives. They are consumed as food preservatives and seasonings, pickles, preserves, candies, mustards, jellies, sauces, jams, and salads. Herbs are added to juices, syrups, and honey, and they are drunk as tea and coffee substitutes. Oil can be pressed from them, or they can be preserved in vinegar. The leaves are cooked as spinach and the roots, stems, and flower buds eaten as vegetables. Last but not least, they can be enjoyed solely for their unique aroma and appearance.

Despite the length of this work, and the amount of research involved in putting it together, I still believe that it is almost impossible to do more than touch upon all aspects of the different herbs in one book. However, I have attempted to treat each area of herbal knowledge as legitimate and equally valuable, which should help to present a fuller and broader vision of herbs, and uncover a rich compendium of knowledge that is practical as well as traditional.

The number of herbs still employed in medicine, cosmetics, and the kitchen is very large. A conservative estimate, counting only the most common, would include at least a thousand, and there are more than 500 that deserve to be included in any basic herbal (not counting the lesser-known herbs of other continents). Because of the limited space available in one book, I have limited the number of herbs instead of limiting the information offered for each herb. Trees, shrubs, and primarily culinary or highly toxic plants have been excluded, categorically. The herbs listed have been chosen for the multitude of their applications and for the number of historical references to them. They are not *just* medicinal or culinary or cosmetic herbs, but plants with a history of magical powers—herbs used in soothsaying or bread baking, herbs with their roots deep in our human consciousness.

On this note, I would like to wish the merely curious fascinating reading, beginners a meaningful adventure into knowledge, and experts encouragement for further study.

My wild field catalogue of flowers
Grow in my rhymes as thick as showers
Tedious and long as they may be
To some, they never weary me
The wood and mead and field of grain
I coud hunt oer and oer again
And talk to every blossom wild
Fond as a parent to a child
And cull them in my childish joy
By swarms and swarms and never cloy.

—JOHN CLARE, THE SHEPHERD'S CALENDAR, "MAY"

Mon: Closed
Tu: 12:00 pm - 8:00 pm
W: 12:00 pm - 8:00 pm
Thu: 10:00 am - 5:00 pm
Fri: Closed
Sat: 10:00 am - 5:00 pm
Sun: Closed

Customer ID: **********3511

Items that you checked out

Title: Down to a science! / adapted by
       Alexandra West.
ID: 39041109839968
Due: Thursday, December 26, 2019

Title:
 Essential herbal wisdom : a complete
 exploration of 50 remarkable herbs /
 Nancy Arrowsmith.
ID: 39041080411191
Due: Thursday, December 26, 2019

Title:
 The princess in black / Shannon Hale &
 Dean Hale ; illustrated by LeUyen Pham.
ID: 39041095412838
Due: Thursday, December 26, 2019

Total items: 3
Account balance: $0.00
12/5/2019 2:22 PM
Hold requests: 0
Ready for pickup: 0

Thank you for using the 3M™ SelfCheck
System.

3M™ SelfCheck System
WELCOME TO EXPRESS CHECKOUT
Pacifica Sharp Park Library
650-355-5196

Mon   Closed
Tu   12:00 pm - 8:00 pm
W   12:00 pm - 8:00 pm
Thu   10:00 am - 5:00 pm
Fri   Closed
Sat   10:00 am - 5:00 pm
Sun   Closed

Customer ID: ***********3511

Items that you checked out

Title: Down to a science! / adapted by
Alexandra West
ID 39041109839988
Due: Thursday, December 26, 2019

Title:
Essential herbal wisdom : a complete
exploration of 50 remarkable herbs /
Nancy Arrowsmith
ID 39041080411191
Due: Thursday, December 26, 2019

Title:
The princess in black / Shannon Hale &
Dean Hale ; illustrated by LeUyen Pham
ID 39041085412838
Due: Thursday, December 26, 2019

Total items: 3
Account balance: $0.00
12/12/2019 2:22 PM
Hold requests: 0
Ready for pickup: 0

Thank you for using the 3M™ SelfCheck
System.

We are at the parsley and the rue.

—TRADITIONAL ENGLISH SAYING

PEARLS OF HERBAL WISDOM

The Classification of Herbs

Carl Linnaeus, often heralded as the "Father of Taxonomy," founded our modern method of botanical classification in the last half of the eighteenth century. His system distinguishes plants by their determining external characteristics, dividing them into families, genera, and species according to their means of reproduction, number of leaves or petals, size of seeds, etc. This system enables scientists to classify newly discovered plants easily and accurately, but it does have one drawback. Because of its complexity and the foreign nomenclature used, it denies many laymen access. Without taking a course in botanical Latin, the uninitiated have few means of systematically approaching or naming plants found during a walk or in the garden.

Folk botanists have traditionally taken an eminently practical approach to the classification of herbs. If a plant grows, looks, or smells unusual, it is given a nickname to describe these characteristics. "Dog" or "sow" plants are common weeds, and graphic names such as piss-a-bed or goutweed are used to remind us of the medicinal effects of the plant on man and beast. Because of the numerous folk names developed by folk healers and herbalists, I have included as many as possible, in numerous languages, in each herb chapter. This way, it is easier to trace the plant's most consistent uses and discover new applications. I have also given the etymological derivations for the herb's names, in order to help dispel some of the mystery surrounding the plant's nomenclature.

Above and beyond this, I have employed an unorthodox method of classification in dividing the plants into sacred, solar, and lunar herbs. This will, I hope, serve to simplify categorization for beginners and allow herb enthusiasts to discover new aspects of the herbs they thought they knew so well.

Indeed there is a woundy luck in names, sirs,
And a main mystery, an' a man knew where to vind it.

—BEN JOHNSON, *A TALE OF A TUB*, IV.II

Names and Naming

In scientific circles, the use of the word "plant" (the generic term for members of the vegetable kingdom) has been mainly restricted, since 1550, to denote smaller plants and herbs; it is only rarely applied to trees and shrubs. In the seventeenth century, physician and botanist William Coles defined the word more widely: "By Plants I meane whatsoever the Superficies of the Earth doth put forth, if it be enbued with a vegetative Soule, and that onely."[2]

The word "herb" is derived from the Old French *erbe* and the Latin *herba*, which originally meant grass or grasses. In this book, "herb" is used to designate all those plants used in the preparation of food or medicine, or for their scent, flavor, or other useful properties. The term is occasionally combined with a proper name to form herb names, as in Herb Robert, Herb Bennet, etc.

The word "grass" originally had the same meaning as "herb," but has come to refer mostly to those plants pertaining to the botanical family **Poaceae** or **Gramineae**. The old meaning is preserved in common herb names such as lemon grass, goose grass, scurvy grass, etc.

An archaic term, "wort," is often used in herb names, although the word itself has long gone out of normal use. St. John's wort, figwort, pennywort, elfwort, and mugwort are all herbs. The Old English word léac or *leek* is employed in the same manner (as in houseleek). "Wood" is sometimes used to designate a woody herb, as in southernwood and wormwood.

"Weeds" are commonly assumed to be harmful plants of no value whatsoever. But many useful herbs still bear the name "weed"—duckweed, hawkweed, and seaweed, for example. And many plants of great value to humans are classified as weeds, the best example being nettles. Perhaps it would be best, in view of these considerations, to adopt a more charitable definition of the word "weed": a weed is a plant whose virtues we do not know or fully appreciate.

The Botanical Identification of Herbs

The plant descriptions given in this book are often sketchy due to the book's extensive nature. Therefore, a word of warning! If there is a golden rule associated with herb gathering, it is this: **if in doubt, do not pick the herb**. A good rule of thumb to follow when gathering herbs is to go out and identify the plant, physically, three separate times before picking it. This is not overcautious advice, since many wild herbs, especially the confusing members of the **Apiaceae (Umbelliferae)** family, can be poisonous. Local variations within a species can also be disconcerting, and it is wise to check a local botanical

---

2.   Coles, *Adam in Eden, or Nature's Paradise* (London: J. Streater, 1657).

guide for final identification before harvesting. Herbs found in the Alpine forests will not be identical to the same herbs found in the Colorado Rockies or the Scottish moors. Another cause of confusion is the many folk names that are assigned indiscriminately to plants. In many of these cases, it is easier to learn the correct botanical nomenclature than to torture yourself with misleading folk names.

A good precaution is to learn to identify all the poisonous plants in your neighborhood before progressing to the edible plants. It is easier to avoid picking the ten or twenty poisonous plants than it is to learn to identify hundreds of edible, healing plants, along with their many subspecies and variations.

Science when well digested is nothing but good sense and reason.

—STANISLAUS, KING OF POLAND, *MAXIMS*, NO. 43

A Solar and Lunar Method of Classification

My personal experience with herbs, along with the knowledge I have gleaned from old herbals and folk literature, has suggested a simple system of herbal classification. As mentioned previously, I've categorized the herbs in this book according to how each herb is directly influenced by the sun and the moon—the two most powerful heavenly bodies.[3] This is a highly subjective division, but it can form a basis for further insights into the nature of herbs.

Lunar herbs, strongly influenced by the movement and phases of the moon, tend to be leafy and fleshy and grow close to the ground. Muted colors of red, blue, white, and green predominate. These herbs are primarily tonic in their medicinal action. The effects are often more gradual, and they must often be taken regularly over several days or weeks for their restorative properties to unfold.

Among Solar herbs, bright yellow, orange, and green colors predominate. These tend to grow upward, with thin spiky leaves, and are strongly influenced by the solstices and movements of the sun. Solar herbs have mostly bitter or sharply aromatic medicinal properties.

There are a very small number of herbs that seem to balance, in equal measure, the principles of solar and lunar; these have been considered sacred in many countries. Fern and mistletoe are two of these sacred herbs, and are credited with unusual healing properties.

My solar/lunar classification system evolved from the system often used in the old herbals, in which some plants were considered male, and plants with different characteristics within the same species were considered female. For example, red blossoming

---

3. Please note that I have twice (within the Solar Herbs section) included a lunar herb with its solar equivalent: Hollyhock is solar, marshmallow lunar; Marjoram is solar, organy lunar.

yarrows were male, and white-blossoming yarrows were female. The division between the sun and the moon, male and female, and solar and lunar seems self-evident from a passive study and observation of nature. One of the first parallels drawn by children and members of "primitive" societies is the parallel between man and woman on the one hand, and the sun and the moon on the other. The sun's power is direct, warming, strong, and penetrating, with an easily foreseeable daily and yearly increase and decrease, like a man's vigor. The moon is always changing, waxing and waning like a woman's womb with child, growing full and then ebbing. These two opposite poles of authority—solar and lunar, male and female, yin and yang—extend their influence to all living things, down to the smallest herbs.

The Greek theory of the four humors divided people and diseases into four distinct groups, closely related to the four elements and the four temperatures (hot, cold, moist, dry). The humors were considered to be opposing pairs rather than a cycle, as is the case in Chinese medicine. Similar to the Chinese system, each humor was related to a season, to an element, and to temperature, moisture, or dryness. Diseases were classified as being hot, cold, moist, or dry to a certain degree and treated accordingly, either by giving herbs and medicines that counteracted that specific humor (such as cold and dry herbs to treat a moist fever), or by purging and bleeding the victim to try to reduce the influence of the offending humor. One of the seminal books of Western medicine, Robert Burton's *The Anatomy of Melancholy*, written in 1621, spends a thousand pages documenting the learned discussions of the time for the treatment of just one humor, melancholy.

The complex classification system of the four humors was then modified and simplified until herbs in herbals came to be grouped simply as male or female. It seems incongruous that the four humors has been mostly forgotten today—few people even know how important it once was in the history of Western medicines. Rudolf Steiner tried to reinstate it in his philosophy of anthroposophy, and Hildegard Medicine (based on the teachings of the medieval abbess Hildegard von Bingen) still makes use of it, but there is little popular understanding of how herbs can be male or female in their natures.

Season

Herbs definitely have their seasons. The most easily recognizable are those related to the reproductive process: germination, budding, blossoming, seeding, hibernation, and death. These seasons are closely related to the temporal seasons. But herbs also follow other natural patterns and seasonal rhythms. They are extremely sensitive to the movements of the moon, the sun, and the stars. The fact that the growth of herbs waxes and wanes with the moon and the lunar cycle was once considered self-evident. Astrological influences were also studied to determine the best sowing, planting, and harvesting procedures. A glimpse into almost any herbal written before the eighteenth century will support this. The procedures used to discover optimal magical, astrological, and botanical seasons of plants were often amazingly complex, as were the rituals used to gather the herbs. These teachings have since fallen into disrepute, although not in some rural areas where the ancient traditions still live on. There, plants are still sown "by the signs," and locals instinctively know the best time to harvest.

Given that the growth of plants corresponds to the waxing and the waning of the moon, most plants have more sap and more juice during the three days before the full moon. This should be taken into account when gathering herbs: oily, juicy, or fleshy plants you plan to use immediately should be gathered shortly before the full moon. If they are to be dried, however, these same plants should be gathered while the moon is on the wane. This helps to avoid spoilage during the drying process. Basket makers and carpenters know that dry, fibrous, or brittle plants will be suppler before the full moon. Leaf growth is greater before the full moon, and root growth after the full moon. There is also often a change in the weather around the time of the full moon. Most plants have a growth spurt during the May full moon, and the fall harvest moon once told farmers when to harvest various crops.

The sun influences all plants. Aside from the fact that herbs are traditionally considered most potent at the time of the solstices (mugwort and St. John's wort at the summer solstice, mistletoe at the winter solstice), plants respond directly to the rising and setting of the sun. Many flowers close in the evening with the sun, only to reopen at the first rays of dawn. Heliotropic plants such as the sunflower follow the sun in its travels across the sky, twisting around to catch the last rays with their heads. Indeed, most plants grow toward sunlight, craning their necks to get at the light. Ivy, however, turns away from direct light. All this has a practical bearing on herb harvesting: leafy and flowering parts should always be collected in the morning, just after the plants have awakened and the dew has dried. They are then under the beneficial influence of the sun, and at their freshest and strongest.

Herbal harvests should, if at all possible, be attuned to natural seasonal influences, and lunar and solar influences should also be taken into account. In most cases, leaves should be gathered when the plants are blooming or shortly before they blossom. Flowers are generally cut in the bloom and sometimes in the bud. Seeds and nuts are harvested at maturity. Roots are dug in the evening or early morning, and in fall or early spring when the juices return to the roots, or have not yet surged upward into the leafy parts.

Herbs should be gathered in quantities sufficient to last one year—and one year only, with a few exceptions. New, fresh plants will usually have grown to maturity during that year and can be gathered anew. One-year-old dried herbs usually have little medicinal value and should be disposed of quickly. Large amounts of leftover herbs can be boiled down with water and used as a cosmetic, as refreshing bath additives, or as warming foot and hand baths, or they can be thrown onto the compost heap. If larger amounts are needed for the winter, tinctures, oils, or salves can be prepared from the herbs while they are still fresh. Roots often keep longer than fresh plant parts.

> *To everything there is a season, and a time to every purpose under the heaven:*
> *A time to be born and a time to die, a time to plant,*
> *and a time to pluck up that which is planted, A time to kill, and a time to heal ...*
>
> —*ECCLESIASTES 3:1–3*

Place

An old Austrian peasant saying claims that the herbs needed to cure the major diseases of people living in a house will be found growing within a few yards of that house. This may seem fanciful, but there is a kernel of truth in it. It has something to do with the universal nature of the plants that grow near human habitations. Certain climactic situations and soil types will produce plants with the medicinal properties needed to treat the diseases caused by those same situations. For example, goutweed usually grows in damp places, where joint complaints are a widespread problem. Red, white, and yellow dead nettles proliferate where urinary problems or chronic infections abound. Nettles thrive where animals are raised and meat is a principal part of the human diet; nettles are a healthy addition to such diets. Pulmonary herbs often grow in places where allergies are a big problem. And so on. Plants are often trying to tell us something about the situation we are living in, and can point out remedies to the sensitive herbalist.

The strength, aroma, and taste of herbs vary considerably from place to place and from season to season. The nature of the soil, the sun, the precipitation or shade available, the altitude, the latitude, and the presence or absence of certain plant neighbors all exert their influence. As a result, the active ingredients of plants grown in different places may vary surprisingly. Mountain plants tend to be more potent, and wild plants are usually stronger in flavor than cultivated herbs. Plants that receive more sun tend to be sturdier and have higher ethereal oil contents. Herbs grown in the dark or the damp are often medicinally worthless. Plants grown in small, tight places near city air and exhaust fumes should not be used for cookery, medicine, or cosmetics. Observation and experience teaches the herbalist about the conditions needed to produce optimal results for each herb. Until one has fully mastered the secrets of a plant's growing preferences and its varying strengths, I advise picking several examples of the same species, from different areas and growing conditions, and mixing them well. This will avoid, for example, subjecting a patient to large fluctuations in the medicinal potency of the drug.

*Every clime, every country, and more than that, every private place, hath his proper remedies
growing in it, peculiar almost to the domineering and most frequent maladies of it.*

—Robert Burton, *The Anatomy of Melancholy*

Gathering Herbs

In those cultures attuned to nature and observant of her practices, herb gathering has been elevated to a high art, complete with rituals, spells, preparatory exercises, incantations, and rules. The ritual of praying to a plant before harvesting it was once widespread, but is now practiced only by the most "primitive" rural societies, those who are deeply religious in their relationship to nature. (These prayers were supposed to placate the resident spirit of the plant or convince it to sacrifice itself for the benefit of man, woman, child, or animal.) In other times and places, herb gathering has been accorded a much humbler position, and simply used to fulfill immediate material needs. In our day and age, it has all too often devolved to systematic rape of natural resources for short-term material gain.

It is now common knowledge that wild plants are part of an ecological whole, and that human beings should not unnecessarily disturb this ecological balance. Endangered species are often protected by law. Above and beyond these injunctions, care should be taken to leave enough plants in the wild to ensure the reproduction and survival of each and every species. According to the British Conservation of Wild Creatures and Wild Plants Act, it is illegal for unauthorized persons (i.e., those without permission of the owner or in possession of the land) to uproot *any* wild plant. It is strictly forbidden to destroy, uproot, or pick endangered rare species in most countries. Endangered species are usually listed in a book prepared for each country. In the Americas, rare stands of wild medicinal plants are often plundered and then sold to foreign markets, with disastrous effects on herb populations. Because of decreasing populations of herbs in the wild, most healing herbs are now being cultivated to ensure constant supplies for herbalists.

Here are some further practical hints to bear in mind while gathering wild and cultivated plants:

- The blossoming, distribution, and maturing times of herbs can vary widely according to altitude, latitude, the exposure of the gathering area, the microclimate, and the weather conditions prevalent that year. It is possible to harvest the same herb for several weeks or even months in different locations.

- Roots are usually dug with a fork, spade, or shovel. The flowering herb is picked or cut well above the ground by hand or with a knife or scissors. Leaves and flowering tops are cut cleanly or picked by hand. Seeds are usually gathered by hand or with the help of combs.

- A separate container should be used for each herb species, to avoid confusing or mixing them with each other.

- Herbs should be gathered in clean baskets or cloth or paper sacks, not in metal or plastic containers. Plastic bags will cause the fresh herb to sweat, wilt, and mildew, and metal may result in undesirable chemical reactions.

- Diseased, insect-infested, or discolored plants are best left alone. Herbs that discolor during the drying process should also be discarded.

- Leave standing at least a third of the wild plants found in any specific area, and at the very least three plants in one place, in order to ensure a new crop the next year. Herbs found growing singly or in twos should never be picked.

- Roots should only be gathered if the plant is common. Stands should be disturbed as little as possible. Never rip out or disturb roots when gathering flowers, leaves, or flowering tops.

- Herbs should not be pressed or packed down in baskets, but given enough air to breathe and spread out immediately after gathering in thin layers in airy rooms to dry. Most herbs are dried indoors, out of the direct sun.

- Be sure to process the herbs quickly after gathering them, drying them if needed, stripping the leaves from the stems, picking seeds, etc. Many herbs are spoiled irreparably if allowed to wilt into a soggy mess before the gatherer gets around to tincturing or drying them.

- In damp climates, make sure the herbs dry quickly to avoid mildew and spoilage. In hot, dry climates, never gather plants that are wilting in the midday sun, but gather them early in the morning after the night's moisture has evaporated.

So mays't thou live, till like ripe fruit thou dropt'
Into thy mother's lap, or be with ease Gather'd, not harshly pluck'd …

—John Milton, *Paradise Lost*, XI

Drying Herbs

The most widely practiced method of preserving fresh herbs for winter use is to dry them. All herbs should be dried as quickly as possible (but not in the direct sun), to prevent spoilage on the one hand and the loss of active ingredients on the other. The following points should be kept in mind when drying herbs:

- Strongly aromatic plants and herbs with volatile oils should, if at all possible, be dried in the shade without the help of artificial heat. If the climate is damp, artificial heat may be necessary to retain active ingredients.

- Flowers, leaves, flowering plants, small fruits, and seeds can be spread thinly on clean cloth or paper and dried in warm, shady, and airy attics or in warm rooms on high shelves.

- Another possibility is to spread them on racks or on a cloth hung up by its four ends over a warm stove or over a heating source that gives off steady heat.

- Yet another method is to bunch the herbs together in *small* bundles, and hang them upside down in a warm, airy room. The bundles must be checked regularly to prevent mildew and discoloring.

- Large roots can be cut into slices, threaded loosely onto a string, and hung over a slow oven or another heating source in a warm and airy room.

- Smaller roots can be split lengthwise and hung on strings like clothespins to dry.

- Large fruits, seeds, fleshy leaves, and sappy roots often have to be dried with the help of artificial heat to prevent spoilage. They can be dried (at the lowest setting!) in a dehydrator, on a rack above a warm oven, or very slowly in an open, lukewarm oven.

- In damp climates, it is better to dry herbs with artificial heat than to run the risk of mildew. In drier areas, spreading the plant parts thinly on racks in the shade is usually all that is needed.

- Discolored or diseased parts of the dried herbs should then be discarded, large stems removed, flowers and leaves sorted, leaves crumbled or shredded, and the roots cut or diced for storage.

I have lived long enough: my way of life / Is fall'n into the sear, the yellow leaf ...

—William Shakespeare, *Macbeth*, V.iii

Storing Herbs

There are few sights as pleasing and as reassuring as full larder shelves and bins filled with vegetables, pickles, preserves, jars, and bottles. Herbs keep well, and can be stored in a surprisingly small space. Fresh herbal juices, infusions, or teas can be kept for a day in the refrigerator or in a thermos bottle. Naturally conserved lotions, ointments, oils, and creams retain their freshness for several weeks or months if prepared with the freshest ingredients. They can usually be frozen. Most dried herbs keep well for a year in dry, cool conditions, well away from direct heat, sun, or damp. They need to breathe, and air should usually be allowed to circulate in their storage containers. In dry climates, cloth or paper containers are excellent, but in damp climates, the herbs need to be dried completely and protected from the damp in glass, ceramic, or enameled jars. Plastic or metal containers should be avoided. Herbs with volatile essential oils (kitchen herbs) and herbs that absorb water out of the atmosphere (hygroscopic herbs) keep best in airtight glasses and jars. Syrups, salves, jellies, preserves, oils, alcoholic extracts, tinctures, and other prepared mixtures may be stored for several years in tightly-closing or sealed sterile jars. Some preparations, such as St. John's wort oil, must be stored in dark containers. As a general rule, it is easiest to store all herbal preparations in dark containers. All storage containers should be checked regularly for possible spoilage and infestation by moths, insects, rodents, or molds.

Plant seeds will retain their viability, according to species, for a few days to several decades. Dry, cool, and dark storage conditions are ideal. In damp climates, seeds can be dried with the aid of silica gel and then stored in closed containers in a cool place, refrigerator, or freezer. In drier climates, the seeds are dried to 2–8 percent humidity, and then stored in closed containers in a refrigerator or freezer. Never freeze moist seeds, or the water in the seeds will expand during the freezing process and they will be ruined. Moist seeds quickly lose their ability to germinate.

In a house where there is plenty, supper is soon cooked.

—Miguel de Cervantes Saavedra, *Don Quixote*

Household Applications

Although housework is often considered drudgery, the knowledge of small skills, the discipline of routine, the familiarity of a light knowing touch, and the pleasures of sweet odors, rich viands, and cleansing herbs can make it into a lighter task. Sachets, potpourri, and bowls of scented herbs can help to sweeten and brighten a room, and moth-repelling mixtures will discourage moths and scent linens. Bunches of herbs hung on a string can even transform a sterile modern kitchen into a comforting place. Herbs can be used directly as cleansing solutions or added to other household mixtures. Dyes can be processed from them, soaps made from them, or beer brewed from them. They are extremely versatile household helpers, and it is a pleasant art to gradually appreciate their many household properties and to master their manifold applications.

Some respite to husbands the weather may send,
But housewives' affairs have never an end.

—Thomas Tusser, *Book of Housewifery*

Herbal Dyeing

Although dyeing is usually done with chemical products, many flowers, herbs, and shrubs are also well suited for this purpose. Plant dyes were once widespread, but are now becoming so rare that their value has risen proportionately. They produce warm, comforting tones in an astounding array of colors and nuances. The principal goal when dyeing with natural materials is to achieve a relatively fast color with the help of a mordant (from the Latin *mordere*, meaning "to bite"), which prepares the fibers to absorb color. Wool will take on color more readily and reliably than cloth. When using natural materials, keep in mind that the resulting color may be totally different from the color of the dyeing bath. Results vary widely according to the mordant and the strength of the dye, the hardness or alkalinity of the water, and the potency of the herb used. The intensity of the desired shade can be regulated by increasing the amount of the dye material used, by letting the wool draw longer in the dye bath, or by dyeing a second or third time. Easily available natural mordants are wood-ash solutions, stale wine, sorrel roots, willow or oak bark, washing soda, salt, vinegar, and powdered oak galls. The chemical substances alum, oxalic acid, bichromate of potash, copper or ferrous sulphate, and stannous chloride or tannic acid—although more drastic—are usually preferred as mordants because of the relative precision possible through exact measurement.

Here is a short list of the steps to be followed when dyeing wool for the first time:

- Wet 1 lb. of wool, squeeze, but do not wring dry, and set aside. Dissolve 3–4 oz. of alum and 1 oz. of cream of tartar in a little boiling water, and combine with 4 gallons of softened water in a large, covered, enameled or stainless steel pot. This container should be used solely for dyeing. Immerse the wool until completely covered with the warm liquid. Cover the pot, and heat the contents slowly. Simmer for 1 hour. Cool until lukewarm, then take out the wool. Gently squeeze dry, and roll in a towel. Some people prefer to let the wool cool in the mixture overnight and only remove it in the morning.

- Place at least 1 lb. of dyeing material (the rule of thumb is 1 lb. of dyeing material for each 2 lb. of wool, although this will vary with more or less concentrated dyeing material) in at least 4 gallons of softened, cold water, without the wool. Cover and let soak. Flowers usually only have to be soaked for 1 hour, but leaves should be left overnight. Woody stems may have to be heated and soaked for a week, reheating every day (if you do not heat the dye material every day or two, mold begins to form). Some dyestuffs must be fermented with either washing soda or ammonia to produce fast colors. Strain out the leaves and other residue carefully.

- Heat the dye bath to 140° F for heat-sensitive colors such as red or blue (madder, cleavers, indigo) or to the boiling point for strong browns and oranges. Cool until warm, and then add the wool, immersing it completely. Stir carefully a few times. Cover the pot, and simmer slowly until the desired tone is obtained.

- Take the pot from the stove, and either remove the wool or let it cool in the dye bath overnight. Intense colors can be obtained by insulating the tightly closed container in a hay box (a wooden box insulated with hay to keep the temperature constant) or under a comforter until cool. Rinse the wool in softened water until it stops "bleeding" and then hang it up to dry. Some dyers add ammonia, vinegar, or salt to the first rinse water to help "set" the colors. Some plants, such as yarrow, are very sensitive to ammonia, and the entire dyeing solution will change color dramatically the minute ammonia is added.

After a first few attempts with alum, experimentation with other mordants can begin. Samples of the different dye experiments should be saved, with a few notes on the methods and amounts used and their effectiveness. Since it is very difficult, if not impossible, to match colors precisely while working with natural ingredients, all the wool needed for one project must be dyed at one time. The great variety of shades and tones that can be produced and the unpredictability of results is one of the great challenges of dyeing with natural materials. What greater joy than suddenly, unexpectedly discovering a totally new color that can be produced from a familiar plant found growing in masses around the house?

Yellows, browns, golds, and greens are relatively easy to obtain with a wide variety of dye materials. The colors red and blue, as well as black, are much more difficult to produce. That is why plants such as madder, woad, and indigo have assumed such importance over the centuries. Madder roots produce deep red and purplish red colors as well as shades of pink and orange. Woad and indigo are used to prepare blue, green, and even black dyes. Another very useful dye plant is weld, which produces fast and clear yellow shades.

There are many other plants of interest to the dyer. Walnut hulls, oak leaves, horse chestnuts, tea leaves, and lichens will all produce browns without a mordant. The composite flowers (marigolds, tansy, daisies, yellow chamomile, etc.) all dye yellow, as do the flowering tops of lady's bedstraw. The roots of lady's bedstraw and cleavers dye, according to the mordant used, pink, orange, or red. Hollyhock flowers are reported to produce a pale blue color that, unfortunately, is not too fast. Yarrow dyes wool yellow and green. Nettles and marjoram impart a lighter green shade.

She is not afraid of snow for her household: for all her household are clothed with scarlet.
She maketh herself coverings of tapestry; her clothing is silk and purple.

—*PROVERBS 31:21–22*

Culinary Virtues

Because of their manifold uses in the kitchen, herbs play a far greater role in our daily diet than many of us would think. They are employed as culinary seasonings and added to fast as well as "slow" foods. They are important in sauce-making, beer-brewing, wine-making, bread-baking, garnishing, pickling, and candying, and are ingredients in syrups, vinegar, and salads. They are prepared as vegetables and side dishes and added to an astonishing variety of dishes as seasonings.

Before the invention of modern techniques of food preservation, herbs were even more widely used. Recipes handed down from the Middle Ages call for extravagantly lavish quantities of seasoning herbs. Purifying and disinfectant herbs were added to food to prevent diseases and to keep the food from spoiling without refrigeration. The practice of eating a heavily-spiced dessert, named *krude*, after every meal was widespread, so much so that pharmacists came to be known as *krudener*, or *krude*-seller. To this day, the Dutch name for herb is *kruid*, and the German, *kräuter*. In India, herbal chewing mixtures are still served after most meals to aid digestion.

The extent to which herbs are used in cookery varies greatly from country to country. As a rule, food is more heavily spiced in warmer, southern climates, and cooks are more restrained in their use of herbs in northern climates. Spices and herbs tend to grow more abundantly in the south, and foods can be preserved with herbs in warm climates. Lavish spicing is used as a digestive stimulus for heavy foods in hot weather, and also helps to provoke cooling perspiration.

In cookery, the term *à l'Anglaise*, or "in the English fashion," denotes dishes prepared with fresh, natural ingredients and with as few seasonings as possible. Germany, a northern country, contents itself with just a few cooking herbs and spices, among them parsley, dill, marjoram, juniper berries, coriander, caraway, and anise seeds. French cooking places great emphasis on fresh green herbs such as chervil, thyme, tarragon, parsley, laurel leaves, and garlic, while the Italian cooks of the south use all of these herbs and also the more pungent oregano, basil, rosemary, sage, and chili pepper. Spanish and South American cuisines make extensive use of chili, as well as cilantro, cumin, and garlic.

However, when herbs are used as seasonings, cooks often give little or no thought to their possible medicinal and nutritional effects. They forget that these may be considerable, and preventive medicine practiced in the kitchen is often more valuable than emergency medicine. Diet is probably the single most important contributing factor toward good health. Many diseases can be prevented, alleviated, and, in many cases, even cured through the wise use of diet. It is widely known that certain foods are harmful for those with allergies or heart trouble, and that sugar can be poison to diabetics. But few know that seasoning with lemon balm can hearten those with circulatory disorders, and that diabetics should season with savory and drink bean hull tea.

These diseases cannot be cured with herbal seasonings alone, but the wise use of herbs in the kitchen can help to prevent the disorder from ever becoming a serious problem, or can bring the patient one step further on the way to health. As the ninth-century herbal *The School of Salernum* so aptly puts it,

> Good dyet is a perfect way of curing:
> And worthy much regard and health assuring.
> A King that cannot rule him in his dyet,
> Will hardly rule his Realme in peace and quiet.[4]

Most culinary herbs aid the digestive process. Savory has a particularly beneficial effect on the gall bladder. Fennel, dill, anise, coriander, and caraway seeds make foods less "windy." Thyme, rosemary, and sage, as well as onions and garlic, have pronounced antiseptic properties and can help to ward off influenza and colds. Nettles contain much more readily available iron than spinach, and the iodine content of watercress is unusually high.

Fresh green herbs are usually added toward the end of the cooking process to preserve their fresh color, aroma, and taste. As usual, there are exceptions to this rule—for example, laurel leaves, which should be cooked with food to release their aroma. Most herbs combine well with each other, although there are some that do not harmonize. Lovage, for example, does not always mix well with other herbs, just as it does not grow companionably with other herbs in the garden.

A sensitive hand is needed to blend herbs well in cookery. As a general rule of thumb, start with herb mixes or single herbs, and season gently until you are more secure with the ins and outs of herbal compatibility. The merely skillful cook knows the best combinations of the herbs present on the kitchen shelf, and which herb can be best used with each food. The worthy cook appreciates the culinary virtues of each herb, and knows how to use them with zest, temperance, and restraint.

> *Cookery means the knowledge of Medea*
> *and of Circe and of Helen and of the Queen of Sheba.*
> *It means the knowledge of all herbs and fruits and balms and spices,*
> *and all that is healing and sweet in the fields and groves …*

—JOHN RUSKIN

Cosmetic Properties

The ancient Greeks correctly defined the true nature of the cosmetic art many centuries ago: it helps to make its users more worldly, and therefore quickens their knowl-

---

4. John Harrington, trans., *The School of Salernum* (Salerno, Italy: Ente Provinciale per il Turismo, 1953), 50.

edge of the world and helps attune them with the cosmos. This worldliness—both sacred and profane—was practiced with the help of herbal and vegetable substances, mineral and animal products. The main emphasis was on the liberal use of scents, oils, and perfumes. The original meaning of the word "perfume" was "to smoke the body thoroughly with scents, fumes, and pleasant odors," often herbal in origin.

In the sixteenth century, John Gerard gave voice to another truth about the cosmetic industry and the fickleness of human nature. In his words, "Far fetched and deare bought is best for ladies."[5] Women (and men) still prefer to buy exorbitantly expensive creams to embellish themselves, although simple, inexpensive products such as whole wheat flour, buttermilk, yogurt, eggs, avocados, pomegranates, herbs, vegetable oils, wine, and honey can be just as effective.

Herbs can be mixed with other ingredients or used alone as cleansing lotions, astringent waters, prepared creams, steaming mixtures, hair rinses, mouth washes, perfumes, and bath additives. Their action can be abrasive, soothing, cleansing, deodorant, drying, healing, styptic, softening, stimulating, moisturizing, astringent, tonic, scenting, or toning. The herbs most commonly used in cosmetics are chamomile, sage, peppermint, thyme, colt's foot, mallow, marigolds, lavender, lady's mantle, comfrey, rosemary, violets, and roses. It is also possible, under the supervision of a qualified herbalist, to take cosmetic herbs internally (as in a spring cure).

Much speaks for the use of natural or herbal ingredients as cosmetic aids. They are readily available, inexpensive, relatively easy to prepare, and, since they contain no chemical preservatives and no strong, unnecessary perfumes, are therefore less likely to irritate the skin or cause allergic reactions. A reliable book on natural cosmetics, one that lists the most important natural ingredients and their properties, is a helpful tool for beginners.

Here are a few practical suggestions for those who are eager to experiment with natural cosmetics:

- In order to ensure success, fresh or freshly dried ingredients must be used. Natural ingredients lose their strength, and may even damage the skin, if they are old, stale or rancid.

- It is best to mix small amounts of herbs, just enough for a few weeks, to avoid waste. Natural ingredients and freshly pressed oils spoil easily, and must be discarded if they smell rancid. It is possible to freeze some salves and lotions for later use.

- Mixed cosmetic preparations, teas, and lotions can be kept for a limited time in the refrigerator.

---

5. *Gerard's Herball* [1597]: *The essence thereof distilled by Marcus Woodward from the edition of Th. Johnson, 1636.* Ed. Marcus Woodward (London: Gerald How, 1927), 109.

- Herbal lotions will keep longer if the active ingredients are extracted in alcohol or in oil and then diluted as needed.

- Natural preservatives such as myrrh, benzoic tincture, or borax can be added to creams and mixtures to help preserve them.

- Mixed creams may separate into oil and water components, but can usually be brought back to their original consistency by stirring, shaking, or using a blender or electric mixer. Some experimentation is needed to make consistently smooth creams and salves. The rule of thumb is to first melt the wax, and only then add the oil. The best method is to get somebody with experience to teach you. Many books on the subject do not, unfortunately, offer much practical help.

> *Gentlewomen, imagine not that I undertake this Treatise to create in you*
> *the least self-conceit or extravagant opinion of your Merits, by putting into your hands*
> *an opportunity to render your selves more beautiful, if possibly it may be, but to preserve*
> *what you have, at least from the ruins of time, or any unfortunate accident; for neatness on*
> *this side [of] the Region of Pride is to be observed in that as well as in Apparel;*
> *nay in a cleanly observance, even Health itself is concerned.*
> —JOHN SHIRLEY, *THE ACCOMPLISHED LADIES RICH CLOSET OF RARITIES*

Strewing, Garlanding, and Festooning

One of the most pleasant and delightful ways of using herbs has, to our great loss, been almost forgotten during the last few centuries. One often reads of herbs strewn in banquet halls and kings and queens walking on carpets of rose blossoms, but who today has had the overwhelming joy of walking barefoot across a room cushioned with sweet-scented herbs?

This old custom had a very mundane origin. When floors were made of stamped earth, cold stone, or rough-planked wood, they were often strewn with absorbent materials such as sawdust to simplify the cleaning process. Rushes were thrown down on more festive holidays, adding a sweet note, clean and fresh, to the room. On very high occasions such as weddings and banquets, the most fragrant flowers and herbs were picked to throw at the feet of those celebrating there. Sir Isaac Newton observed that "at bride-ales the house and chambers were wont to be strowed with these odoriferous and sweet herbes to signifie that in wedlocke all pensive saleness and tow'ring cheer, all wrangling, strife, jarring, variance and discorde ought to be utterly excluded and abandoned."[6]

---

6. Newton, qtd. in E. and M. A. Radford, *Encyclopaedia of Superstitions* (London: Rider, 1947), 48.

The ancient Romans were so lavish in strewing herbs at banquets that they used to steep their wine with them, and gave their guests floral washing waters and herbal garlands to drive away the noxious effects of wine fumes:

> The use of flowry Crowns and Garlands is of no slender Antiquity, and higher than I conceive you apprehend it. For, beside the old Greeks and Romans, the Aegyptians made use hereof; who, beside the bravery of their Garlands, had little Birds upon them to peck at their Heads and Brows, and so to keep them from sleeping at their Festival compotations.[7]

Not only were guests wreathed in garlands, but lovers, poets, and victors were also honored with them.

In later centuries, people preferred to perfume their food with strong floral and herbal essences rather than strewing the dining room with odiferous herbs. Our times have grown particularly stingy. Even the parsimonious practice of hanging a bunch of sweet-smelling herbs from the ceiling has fallen away. But, despite our present frugality, I am convinced that herbs will be strewn, and flowers worn in buttonholes again. For example, we can bring the invigorating air of mountainous regions into our houses—in the fragrances of organy, wild thyme, horse and water mint, sage, juniper, fir, pine, and larch needles. With a few herbal pillows here, some potpourri there, a lighted aroma lamp in the hallway, we can trigger memories of mountain holidays.

> *Some others were again as seriously imploy'd*
> *In Strewing of those hearbs, at Bridalls us'd that be;*
> *Which every where they throwe with bountious hands and free*
> *The healthfull Balme and Mint, from their full laps doe fly,*
> *The sent-full Camomill, the verdurous Costmary.*
> *They hot Muscado oft with milder Maudlin cast:*
> *Strong Tansey, Fennell coole, they prodigally waste:*
> *Cleere Isop, and therewith the comfortable Thyme,*
> *Germander with the rest, each thing then in her prime:*
> *As well of wholesome hearbs, as every pleasant flower,*
> *Which Nature here produc't, to fit this happy houre.*
> *Amongst these strewing kinds, some other wilde that growe,*
> *As Burnet, all abroad, and Meadow-wort they throwe."*

—MICHAEL DRAYTON, *POLY-OLBION*, SONG XV

---

7. Sir Thomas Browne, "Of Garlands," *The Works of Sir Thomas Browne*, vol. 3 (London: Faber & Faber, 1965), 49.

Uses in Husbandry

The husbandman is husband to the soil and is held in bond to the house, as the word "husband" (from the Old Norse and Old English, meaning "house-bound") suggests. It is said that a housewife's work never ends, but the husbandman (or steward) only gains respite from his fields in winter or because of bad weather, and seldom is far from his animals and housebound tasks. Although the husbandman's existence is usually associated with hard labor and drudgery, it can also offer joys and rewards. The rewards can be of an aesthetic nature:

> Hence it is, that Emperours, Princes, Heroes, and Persons of the most glorious Qualifications, have trod on their Sceptres, fleighted their Thrones, cast away their Purples, and laid aside all other Exuberancies of State, to Court their Mother Earth in her own Dressings; Such Beauties there are to be discerned in Flowers, such Curiosities of Features to be found in Plants.[8]

Or, they can be practical:

> I have found out these certaine and approved Cures; wherein if every good Horse-lover, or Husbandman, will but acquaint his Knowledge with a few hearbes and common weeds, he shall be sure in every Field, Pasture, Meadow or Land furrow; nay, almost by every high-way side or blind ditch to finde that which shall preserve and keepe his Horse from all sodaine extremities.[9]

Seeing how many people are keeping horses these days, and how high veterinarians' costs can be, this argument should carry as much weight today. Last but not least, there are the social advantages of good husbandry:

> Is it not much more rational for parents to be employed in teaching their children how to cultivate a garden, to feed and rear animals, to make bread, beer, bacon, butter, and cheese, and to be able to do these things for themselves, or for others, than to leave them to prowl about the lanes and commons, or to mope at the heels of some crafty, sleek-headed pretended saint...?[10]

In any case, there is much room for much experimentation with herbal preparations for animals—in the barn, in the dairy, or for sale. Veterinary herbalists are almost unknown in our day and age, although animals do respond well to herbal treatment. Gourmet foods such as bakery products, or fresh cheese flavored with herbs, are sure to enjoy a

---

8. William Coles, introduction to *Adam in Eden, or Nature's Paradise* (London: J. Streater, 1657).

9. Gervase Markham, *Cheape and Good Husbandry* (1614), facsimile (New York: Da Capo Press, 1969), 18.

10. William Cobbett, *Cottage Economy* (London: P. Davies, 1926), 9.

renaissance. Farmer's markets and tourism profit from this development, not to speak of the positive effects on the health of the consumers. Hitherto forgotten crops such as hemp, spelt, and einkorn are being reintroduced, and there is also renewed interest in oil plants as well as in the use of herbs in beekeeping and small animal husbandry.

He [the husbandman] equalled the riches of kings in the happiness of his mind;
and returning home in the late evening, loaded his board with feasts unbought.

—VIRGIL'S GEORGICS, BK. IV

Gardening Hints

Gardening is a gentle art when practiced with skill, one befitting the attention of refined and cultured peoples everywhere. Not only can gardeners exercise despotic power over their small plot, but they can also train and discipline themselves through the ordered and benevolent use of that power.

While the scope of this book is too large to go into great detail on the cultivation, especially on a commercial basis, of each herb listed, I do offer general guidance for each plant. Keep in mind that herbs are particular in their choice of soils, the amount of moisture and sunlight they demand, and the plant neighbors, fertilizers, and chemical treatment they will tolerate. Because most herbs are used or eaten fresh, it is highly desirable to avoid putting toxic sprays or chemical fertilizers on them while they are growing. Organic gardening makes perfect sense for herbs.

Also remember, when planting your garden, that herbs tend to be more quarrelsome than vegetables. The ability to design an herb garden in a way that successfully takes into account all the plants' likes and dislikes is an art in itself. Rue and sweet basil, for instance, cannot live next to each other without ruining each other's lives. On the other hand, sage and rosemary can be good neighbors. Lovage and wormwood are poor companions. A little chamomile will stimulate grain growth in a field, but too much chamomile will overpower the grain. Although the idea of a small garden devoted exclusively to herbs is an attractive one, the prospective herb gardener should also consider the possibility of planting the herbs beside other vegetables and herbs in order to aid their growth and increase the health of both companions. In old European convent gardens and vineyards, herbs are often planted at the end of vegetable rows.

The single most difficult gardening task associated with herbs is getting them to germinate. Once established, herbs are usually easy to propagate from plant division, from cuttings, or simply by allowing the plants to go to seed. The novice home gardener may want to buy his or her first plants from a nursery, and then learn to propagate them. Another method is to sow the often-miniscule seeds a few at a time in sterilized, weed-free potting mixture in individual peat pots. Most seeds can be covered lightly with fine soil and placed in a warm place indoors. Keep the soil moist, but not wet. Some seeds will demand special treatment, such as the presence of light to trigger germination (arnica), or a period of frost before germination (sweet cicely). Thin the seedlings after they emerge to allow one sturdy plant per pot. Harden the plants off, gradually, in a sheltered place outdoors, and then plant them (peat pot and all) in their final position in the garden, being sure to bury the edges of the pot below the surface of the earth. They will grow vigorously, and transplantation shock should be minimal. Water well until they are established, but then ease off on the watering: most herbs actually prefer dry conditions and little fertilizer. Some herbs (such as hyssop or chives) should be replanted regularly to avoid depleting the soil, while others (such as catnip or horehound) will spring up repeatedly in the same place if they find it to their liking. Cuttings are generally taken in August, or again in the spring.

Many gardeners think that it will harm their plants to harvest them and are much too careful when it comes to cutting herbs. As a general rule, healthy plants will respond positively to harvesting if it is not too drastic, or does not take place too late in the year. Leafy herbs such as basil or savory will be forced to grow outward if the tops are nipped off. Plants that tend to woodiness, such as lavender, thyme, or winter savory, must be cut back in order to stimulate more growth in the lower parts of the plants. This will prevent the stalks from becoming too tough. Herbs should not be cut back as a last-gasp procedure in late fall, but in summer so that they can grow new leaves before winter frosts. If the plant is damaged right before the frost, it may succumb to the cold. In very hot, dry climates, pruned plants may dry out. It is always wise to save a little seed of your favorite herbs, in case a winter frost does kill them. Annual herbs, such as basil, will have to be re-sown every year.

A garden is like those pernicious machineries which catch a man's coat-skirt or his hand, and draw in his arm, his leg, and his whole body to irresistible destruction.

—RALPH WALDO EMERSON, *CONDUCT OF LIFE: WEALTH*

Seed Saving

The diversity of our cultivated plants is just as endangered as the diversity of our wild plants, if not more so. Because of this far-reaching genetic erosion, it is important to save that herb Grandma brought over from the old country, and also to save her recipes and her herbal lore. It is fairly easy to save seeds from herbs, and it is good to practice on them before moving on to saving seeds from vegetables, flowers, or grains.

Not only does it make sense to garden organically in the herb garden, but it is also highly advisable to save seeds from the varieties that do particularly well or propagate them with cuttings. Contrary to popular belief, there is an astounding variety available of the most common herbs. Thyme, for example, comes in a bewildering assortment of horticultural forms: variegated, golden-leaved, caraway-scented, lemon thyme, orange thyme, etc. Even wild mother-of-thyme will vary dramatically from one place to another, and include lemon-scented variants. Basil comes in all shapes, sizes, and odors, as does mint. The gardener who starts collecting these rarities may soon find the herbs taking over the garden! There is also substantial variation in the degree of cold-hardiness or drought-sensitivity between different plants. If these properties are to be maintained, and even better plants selected over the years, they will have to be propagated.

In folk tradition, herbs were always passed on from one garden to another, and were considered more potent if stolen or if the owner looked the other way when a neighbor dug out a plant. A more modern form of exchanging herbs is through garden fairs, garden and seed-saving exchanges, and across the garden fence. It is surprising how far some herbs travel this way. Despite stringent customs restrictions, most immigrants to the United States have managed to bring seeds of their favorite herbs with them, and they are now thriving in the new country. But many of these herbs and the traditions connected with them have not been passed on. These plants, and the knowledge about them, are acutely endangered if we do not take the trouble to exchange them with our neighbors, children, grandchildren, and students.

Medicinal Merits

How did people first learn about the healing properties of herbs? In the beginning, such knowledge was primarily intuitive, similar to the intuitive medicinal knowledge of animals. Pigs know which tubers to root out for food and medicine, and wounded animals know that they should roll in mud. Cats eat grass or catnip when they are not well, and instinctively seek out other herbs.

In the case of humans, however, instinctual knowledge was supplemented at a very early stage with empirical observation and experimentation. The first medicine men and women studied how different animals reacted to herbs. Plants similar to those already in use were tested, and each plant was carefully observed for specific characteristics. Further indications of the healing properties of herbs were given in sacred dreams and visions. Over time, the number of proven herbal remedies increased, and knowledge of the plants' medicinal merits became the treasured property of the shaman or medicine man or woman. This information was passed on to the next generation of healers, in courses of instruction that sometimes lasted up to twenty years. (Knowledge of the healing properties of herbs and plants was considered to be just one of the many healing arts, along with knowledge of the healing properties of stones, animals, charms, poetry, song, drumming, dancing, ritual, hypnotism, exorcism, and the workings of the heavens.)

Western folk medicine still retains some, if not many, reminders of the "primitive" systems of medicine. In the Middle Ages, Western medical folk tradition was strongly influenced by the medicine taught in the monasteries throughout Europe. The herbs widely used in folk medicine were those first grown in the monastery gardens by decree of Charlemagne. Despite this, European folk medicine came to be discredited in later years, for it was associated with the witchcraft practiced by wise women and midwives. Fear of anything "magical," "uncanny," and therefore "unchristian" swept through Europe. Many women were burned at the stake as witches for no other crime than the knowledge of a few basic herbal simples. And much of European herbal knowledge was burned with the witches.

Modern pharmaceutical companies now send herbal prospectors into remote parts of the globe in search of cultures with vital folk medicine traditions. Many modern drugs were first discovered by shamans, and pharmaceutical companies have only recently recognized their medicinal worth. As often as not, the companies then rush to patent the active ingredient of the herb, denying the worth of "primitive" medicine and giving no credit to the original discoverers of the plant.

Many an old wife or country woman doth often more good
with a few known and common garden herbs than our bombast Physicians
with all their prodigious, sumptuous, far-fetched, rare, conjectural medicines.

—ROBERT BURTON, *THE ANATOMY OF MELANCHOLY*

A History of Herbals

Ever since the invention of writing, the history of Western herbal medicine has been closely linked with the history of herbals, those highly treasured treatises on herbal lore that found their way into print. Several ancient Egyptian and Sumerian records have survived until the present day. Through these writings, along with archeological findings, it is possible to piece together a picture of herbal medicinal practice in those times. The Bible often mentions healing plants and herbs, and some references to herbs are also found in the fragmentary works of Greek authors.

But the most important treatises on herbs to survive are the works of the Greek authors Dioscurides (the middle of the first century AD) and Galen (AD 129–199), as well as the great compilatory works of Pliny the Elder (first century AD). These books were the major reference works on herbal matters throughout the entire Middle Ages. Arabian physicians (Avicenna, Averroes, and many others) interpreted these writings, and their writings were in turn widely consulted in the monasteries of the Middle Ages.

The monasteries became important centers for the dissemination and distribution of classical herbal lore, especially in northern Europe. In the ninth century, Charlemagne issued an edict, *Capitulare de Villis,* listing the medicinal herbs suggested for cultivation in monastery gardens. This list became the basis for many modern pharmacopeias. The most important herbals of this monastery period are those of Wahlafridus

Strabo (ninth century), the School of Salernum (also ninth century), Hildegard von Bingen (twelfth century), and the writings of Albertus Magnus (thirteenth century).

A new era in the history of herbals and herbalism began with the invention of the printing press toward the end of the fifteenth century. Peter Schoeffer's *Gart der Gesundheit* was one of the earliest and most important of these printed herbals. His book was followed by the works of Otto Brunfels, Hieronymus Bock, Pieradrea Matthiolus, and Leonhard Fuchs.

In England, the first important herbal was the Anglo-Saxon *Leech-book of Bald and Cild*, which drew heavily on Dioscurides but also included northern beliefs and practices. Many translations or compilations of Latin or German herbals were later printed, ranging from William Turner's *Nieuwe Herball* (1551) to the very important *Herball* of John Gerard (1597), which was the very first to include New World plants. The works of John Parkinson (1629 and 1640) and Nicholas Culpeper followed, and much secondary herbal lore can be gleaned from many books written at the time on the subjects of household skills, cookery, cosmetics, and husbandry.

> *For out of olde feldes, as men seith,*
> *Cometh al this new corn fro yere to yere:*
> *And out of olde bokes, in good feith,*
> *Cometh al this science that men lere.*

—GEOFFREY CHAUCER, *THE PARLAMENT OF FOULES*

Ancient Medicine

In order to understand ancient medicinal practices, and the lore passed down by old herbals, it is important to have some idea of the complexity of early medical doctrines. One of the widespread doctrines of the day was the astrological theory of diseases and herbs. Parts of the body were associated with the various astrological signs (for example, the knees were thought to be in the sphere of Capricorn's influence, the genitals in Scorpio). Herbal cures could be astrologically sympathetic or antipathetic, according to whether the cure was supposed to work with the diseased body part, or against the disease in that part of the body.

The four elements (air, fire, earth, and water), as well as the four vital fluids (blood, phlegm, choler, and melancholy), also helped to identify diseases and herbs. The following shows a simplistic sketch of the relationships between the humors and the four elements.

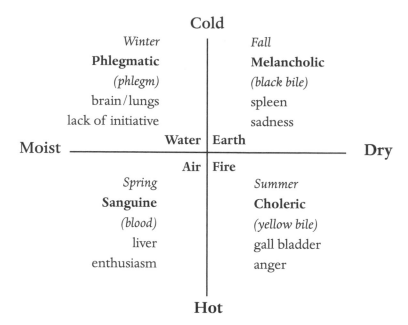

Diseases were classified as sanguine, choleric, melancholic, or phlegmatic, and were cured by herbs that were either hot, dry, cold, or moist in their natures. A medicine considered hot in the first degree could be used to temper cold diseases, but one that was hot in the fourth degree would have to be balanced by a cooler herb in order to make it safe for human use.

The skill with which the best physicians, from ancient to medieval times, cross-referenced and located the herb or herbs suitable for the individual temperament of the patient and the nature of the disease should be the envy of many modern practitioners.

The doctrine of signatures was developed by Paracelsus in the sixteenth century, and later finalized by the German theosopher Jacob Boehme in *De Signatura Rerum*, which revolutionized herbalism. In it, he presented his belief in the theory of signatures, which postulated that the healing properties of herbs can be discovered by studying a plant's "signature." As the determining external characteristic of the plant, the signature was believed to resemble a human organ or body part, signifying which disease it could treat. For example, a kidney-shaped leaf would point to the use of the plant in the treatment of renal disorders, or the bright yellow *curcuma* was used to treat a patient yellowed with jaundice.

Alchemists stressed the importance of isolating active substances through distillation, and of combining metals and chemicals with purely vegetable medicines. In time, "simpling" (the art of curing diseases with one herbal healing substance suited to the individual's needs) was discarded in favor of compound chemical medicines. The sciences of botany and medicine, once united, were irreparably divided. Medicine became more allied with chemistry, and botany with herbalism.

Modern Medicine

In the seventeenth and eighteenth centuries, two developments almost put an end to Western herbal medicine. On the one hand, simple herbal remedies were repudiated in favor of chemical substances and compounds; they were discounted as inexact medicines by the medical profession. A parallel development was the prosecution of folk healers by the Church and temporal authorities. A woman who administered home remedies was considered a witch, and male healers were thought to be conjurors or magicians working in league with the devil. During this era, the scientifically trained doctor became, along with the priest, one of the most important social figures in Western rural life.

Samuel Hahnemann (1755–1843), the founder of modern homeopathy, was one of the first medical men to return to the "simples" of the Middle Ages and to the art of healing with herbal remedies. The most important precept of his system, that "like cures like" (*similis similibus curantur*), was a development of Paracelsus' teachings.

Mainstream interest in herbs did not reawaken in Western society, however, until the twentieth century. Toward the end of the 1800s, herbalism underwent a minor revival in Germany through the efforts of the herbal priests Sebastian Kneipp and Johann Künzle. Their work was not fully appreciated until the time of the world wars, when shortages of materials and trade blockades created an immediate need for inexpensive, readily available, homegrown herbal medicines. Many Western governments then began to support herbalists, and to encourage the cultivation and harvesting of herbs from the wild. It is interesting to note that one of the most important modern English herbals, that of Mrs. Grieve and Hilda Leyel, was published in the years between the wars. Aromatherapy was also developed in the trenches—ethereal oils were used to disinfect and to treat infection.

In the past few years, there has been a tremendous resurgence of interest in herbs and herbal remedies because of their ready availability and their effectiveness as cheap preventive medicine. Herbs are ideal for the regulation of the chronic disorders of modernity, such as stress-related diseases and circulatory and heart troubles. Pharmaceutical companies are now looking more carefully at "primitive" indigenous remedies. Traditional herbal cures are enjoying a renaissance, and more research is being done into the active principles of common herbs.

The current fascination with herbs is a development that should be heartily embraced and appreciated by the experienced herbalist, although with some reservations. Nostalgic over-enthusiasm for all things herbal often results in herbal misuse by the beginner.

Ruthless and systematic harvesting of wild plants by businessmen who want to cash in on a trend is another negative development.

Nothing can be more misleading than the romantic notion that that you "can't do anything wrong" when prescribing herbs. The novice herbalist should concentrate on one or two herbs and try to learn their many uses, instead of harvesting large amounts of many different herbs. It is also important for the more experienced herbalist to learn which applications are practical in terms of the time expended, the availability of the herbs, and the needs of patients. The goal of several years of herbal experimentation should be a small arsenal of time-tried herbal recipes and practices.

True herbalists and herbal specialists are few and far between, especially in industrialized countries. Although we may hope that the renewed interest in alternative forms of medicine will produce a new crop of herbal experts, the novice should keep in mind that much of the information offered by so-called herbalists and herbal remedy producers may be faulty.

The Practical Use of Herbs as Medicine

Modern herbal medicine recognizes three areas of herbal influence on the body:

- Herbs can be employed as tonics, to improve general health and to help prevent diseases. They can be taken in the form of teas, tinctures, juices, herbal wines and spirits, bath additivies, body rubs, and steaming mixtures.

- Herbs can also counteract infirmities, illnesses, pains, and complaints, working specifically to correct and alleviate ailments and to alter harmful tendencies.

- Herbs have the power to strengthen and corroborate weak, damaged, or malfunctioning body parts, restoring them to their normal working order and assisting their functioning.

Before I continue, I must emphasize that the information transmitted in this book is *not* meant to be a substitute for competent medical diagnosis, advice, or treatment, and it is not a do-it-yourself guide for self-treatment. Herbs are by no means harmless or ineffective medicinal substances—many of the strongest drugs, stimulants, and poisons come from plants. Curare, digitalis, and belladonna are all herbal or plant substances; strychnine is of plant origin; tea is made from leaves; penicillin is a mold; coffee is a fruit; tobacco is a leaf; and alcohol is fermented from plant material. Morphine, codeine, and opium are produced from poppies, and cocaine is produced from a shrub. Until the invention of chemical antiseptics, germicides, and antibiotics, herbs were the only known means of killing germs and combating infectious diseases, and were *the* most important therapeutic agents.

The pharmaceutical industry uses many plants and herbs directly as medicines, or else as the blueprints for synthetic drugs. A surprisingly large percentage of the drug products on the market were originally of plant origin. Even the word "drug" originated from the Anglo-Saxon word *dregen*, meaning "to dry." A "drug" was once simply a dried herbal medicine. But chemical drugs based on herbs usually ignore the secondary saponines, glycosides, ethereal oils, and components present in a growing plant in favor of the plant's most effective chemical compound. The healing action of these chemically produced drugs is therefore more specific, but also less universal than that of herbal medicines. This one-sidedness can lead to an imbalance of the natural equilibrium in the body and produce negative side effects. If the correct herb is given in the correct dosage, it will have a balanced effect on the entire body. Its action will be gentle but thorough, specifically counteracting the disease but at the same time strengthening the sickened organ or body area.

Herbs take time to complete their healing action in the human body, just as they took time to grow—one leaf after another, gradually, until the plant was ready to harvest. The plant must be gathered at just the right time to ensure best results, just as the disease should be caught at the right time to ensure healing success. It is better to take small amounts of herbs regularly, over several weeks or months, than to attempt a crash cure in a few days. It is important not to become impatient if the desired healing effect does not occur within a day or two. The consequent use of gentle herbs is often more effective than horse cures, especially for minor or chronic complaints.

Caution and the precise observation of possible individual reactions to herbs are always exercised by careful herbalists. A single herb (for example, stinging nettle) can act as a laxative for one person and have a constipating effect on another. Lady's mantle can act both as a menstrual suppressant and as a menstrual excitant. Others, such as lemon balm or mistletoe, can help to regulate either high or low blood pressure. Some people react to certain herbs only after several weeks of treatment, while others feel the effects immediately. Allergic or highly individual reactions to herbs should never be ignored, be they ever so idiosyncratic. Although tinctures are a practical method of taking herbs, alcoholics may not be able to tolerate the alcoholic content of the preparations.

Patience is essential when dealing with medicinal herbs. A patient who prefers to wait until the last possible minute before beginning a cure, who takes twice the medicine prescribed, or who does not complete the cure and becomes restless if results are delayed more than several days is no stranger to the modern herbal practitioner, and will not have good results with herbs. It should be obvious that gradually effective, long-term herbal medicines do not "work miracles" overnight.

Although I warmly recommend the use of herbal remedies, I would like to point out again that they are not harmless. Opium is not any less dangerous simply because it is herbal. Pregnant women should be especially conservative in their use of herbs that might induce miscarriage. All herbal cures should be interrupted immediately if negative or allergic reactions occur. Expert advice should be followed and herbal medicines used with caution and discretion. It is a real art to learn to mix herbs that complement each other and overlap in their medicinal effectiveness without counteracting each other. I have not listed the chemical constituents of each herb, because this information is available in technical textbooks and journals in a more thorough and up-to-date manner.

Overall, herbal treatments can have excellent results *if* the diagnosis is correct, and *if* the herbs are administered with care and knowledge. Patients should always be treated by a competent medical practitioner or herbalist. Otherwise, important symptoms that can signal the beginnings of a serious disease may be overlooked. If herbs are used wisely, they can be a boon, and save many unnecessary trips to the doctor and even an operation or two. If used irresponsibly, they have been known to kill.

> *Of the simples in these groves that grow,*
> *We'll learn the perfect skill,*
> *The nature of each herb to know,*
> *Which cures and which can kill.*

—MICHAEL DRAYTON, "QUEST OF CYNTHIA"

Tea Preparation

Medicinal herbs are most often taken in the form of teas, especially in Europe. Because of the warming nature of tea and its gradual medicinal action, it is the preferred method of restoring a weakened or indisposed body to health. It is also ideal as a preventive medicine and to strengthen and reattune an impaired physique. A general guide to the preparation of medicinal teas has been given in the Herbal Use Chart at the end of this book.

- A tea can be prepared from leaves, crushed fresh fruits, flowering herbs, and soft stems by pouring boiling water over the herb (in most cases, 1 Tbsp. of the fresh herb to ½ pint of water), covering the container, and then letting the mixture steep for 10–15 minutes before straining and serving. This procedure is generally known as the infusion method.

- Hard seeds, woody roots or stems, bark, dried fruits, and very fleshy leaves and flowers are usually decocted. In other words, they are boiled for 10–15 minutes (1 tsp. of the herb to each 2 pints of water) and left to steep, covered, for another 10–15 minutes.

- Especially woody roots and stems, or herbs that might lose volatile, heat-sensitive substances during the heating process, can be soaked overnight in cold water to draw out the active ingredients. The mixture should be brought to just below a boil in the morning, and allowed to steep for 10–15 minutes.

In this book, when "1 part" of each herb is called for, the part is measured by volume and not by weight. Many herbs are extremely light, while roots are often quite heavy.

Herbal teas are best prepared in glass, ceramic, or enamel containers, and may react if brought into contact with metal, especially aluminum. A tea pot is the best container for steeping tea, and prepared tea can be stored for use throughout the day in a thermos bottle. Warm tea should not be kept for more than 12 hours. Herbal teas lose most of their medicinal properties if reheated.

Herbal teas relished purely for their flavor can be enjoyed lukewarm, chilled, hot, or warm. They should only be consumed in limited amounts to avoid unwanted medical reactions to the herbs. It is best to have several "house teas" and vary them according to mood than to drink gallons of one concoction.

Medicinal herbal teas can be generally divided into two groups: tonic teas and bitter teas. It is best to drink medicinal teas at body temperature or a little warmer. They have a more pronounced medicinal effect if taken in small sips, spread out over the day, than if taken at once in large doses. Their healing effect will be more reliable if they are drunk reliably and regularly. Completing herbal tea cures usually means drinking a tea 2–3 times a day, depending on the herb, for a period of 3–9 weeks. It is advisable to change to another herb with similar properties after this period to avoid jading the body to the particular healing effect of one herb.

Tonic Teas

Tonic teas have a relatively mild taste and are used to tone and strengthen the organs and the entire body. Tonic teas should be enjoyed on an empty stomach in the morning, again in the early afternoon, and once again in the evening about 2 hours before bedtime. Sleep-inducing or nervine teas can be taken in the afternoon, and again as a nightcap at least 1 hour before going to bed. Patients with weak bladders should substitute capsules or tincture for evening tea.

Bitter Teas

Bitter teas have a positive influence on the digestive processes, and strengthen the liver and gallbladder. They should be taken ½ hour to 1 hour before meals, so that the tea can be absorbed before digestion begins. To ensure success, bitter teas should always be drunk before the main meal of the day, and with some regularity before breakfast and the second meal. Bitter teas should *not* be sweetened.

Tinctures

In the United States, herbs are generally taken in the form of tinctures or in gelatin capsules, and tea-drinking is not as widespread. The newest development is to administer herbs in soft gel form, which is a concentrated tincture surrounded by a soft covering. Although this method certainly has its practical advantages, there are several drawbacks. Tinctures and capsules cost quite a bit of money, while fresh herbs can easily be grown in the garden and dried for future use. The cost of alcohol for tincturing is high, and, given the extent of alcoholism in our culture, alcohol is not always advisable. Some herb interactions with alcohol have not been fully researched. For example, valerian tincture is an excitant for some people in tincture form, while for others it can safely be used as a sleep aid. Some active ingredients can only be extracted from a plant with the use of alcohol, other ingredients only with water. Some herbs can easily be given in large doses. Others, like mistletoe, become ineffective if given in too-large doses. Generally, it is easier to learn more about a plant while dealing with the fresh drug, while it is easier to abuse herbs when they are in a concentrated, alcoholic form. People living in the country with a garden should first approach herbs in their natural state, and then experiment with simple preparations such as salves, bath mixtures, syrups, or liqueurs. People living far removed from nature, in big, busy cities with an urban lifestyle, should consult people who have more practical experience with herbs, such as herbalists and organic farmers.

When you begin Physic, persevere and continue in a course: for as one observes, to stir up the humour and not to prosecute, doth more harm than good.

—ROBERT BURTON, *THE ANATOMY OF MELANCHOLY*

Special Herbal Cures

Special herbal cures are cures that are taken at specific times of the year, or to work on specific ailments. The most famous is probably the spring cure, in which blood-cleansing and blood-moving herbs are taken, over a period of a few weeks, to adjust the body to the new season. Similarly, it is possible to strengthen the heart and the circulatory system before summer heat enervates us, to cleanse the lungs before the fall flu season begins, and to strengthen the kidneys and the urinary tract before the cold of winter.

The Spring Cure

For centuries, people have used the spring cure to counteract the lethargy and lack of exercise usually associated with winter, and to cleanse and purify the body in preparation for the activity of the coming summer months. The cure is most effective if combined with a time of fasting, which is usually reserved, in Christian cultures, for the Lenten period.

Taking a spring cure consists of drinking the freshly pressed juice of several spring herbs or drinking herbal tea regularly for 4–6 weeks. Pressed herb juice can be made from the herbs that appear in abundance around the garden in spring: stinging nettles, dandelion, heart's ease, the first strawberry leaves, plantain or yarrow, and small amounts of ground ivy or speedwell. The number of possible herb combinations for tonic teas is almost unlimited.

Spring favorites are yarrow, dandelion, nettle, burdock roots, marigold leaves and flowers, heart's ease, red clover flowers, sorrel, violet leaves, fumitory, lovage and parsley roots, juniper berries, and horsetail. Eating a warm dish of fresh spring greens is an even more pleasant way to greet the spring. Stinging nettles (prepared like spinach) contain many trace minerals and act to purify the system. They also taste surprisingly good. Germans have nicknamed the nettle "nature's broom" because of the plant's thorough cleansing action. Young dandelion leaves, daisy buds and leaves, young dead nettle plants, and strawberry, sorrel, violet, or primrose leaves, as well as watercress and ramsons, have all been used as traditional spring potherbs. Most rural areas celebrate their own culinary traditions by eating spring greens or salads, or Maundy Thursday soups.

> *The season pricketh every gentle heart,*
> *And maketh him out of his sleep to start.*
>
> —Geoffrey Chaucer, *The Knightes Tale*

The Hay-Blossom Cure

Broken blossoms, leaves, and seeds sift down to the floor of the barn as hay settles, forming a feathery powder. It is this sediment that is used in the hay-blossom cure, which has all the healing properties of the scent of freshly cut hay. Hay blossoms are easily gathered in large quantities from a barn, but care should be taken to only use unsprayed hay that was cut that year. Best results are obtained from hay fields with a wide variety of herbs from mountainous areas.

Because of the great number of herbs present in it, a hay-blossom cure is the broadest of all herbal cures in terms of its medicinal action. It helps to invigorate the system and tone body organs, cleanse the body of impurities, support weight loss, relieve minor pains and muscle aches, lessen the symptoms of a cold, and help ward off the flu. A word of warning, however: people with a history of allergies or hay fever should be very careful when using hay blossoms.

Hay blossoms can be applied externally as steaming mixtures, steam baths, baths, poultices, or hot pillows.

- The most common method of using hay blossoms is in steaming mixtures. Add a handful of hay blossoms to every quart of water. Bring the mixture just to a boil, and let it stand, covered, for 15 minutes. Drape towels or sheets over the patient's entire body (or just over the head and chest) to keep the steam from escaping. Place the container with the steaming herbs on a pad on a table or the floor, below the affected area, and take the cover off (taking care to avoid scalding the patient). The steam can be inhaled as long as the mixture remains warm, usually 15–20 minutes. The affected area, which is now very hot, should then be washed with a washcloth and dried carefully before it has a chance to become chilled. Resting in a pre-warmed bed for 1 to 2 hours after steaming will increase the medical value of the steam bath.

- Hay blossoms can also be brewed and strained into a warm tub or hipbath. The remaining hot herb residue can be wrapped in clean cotton cloths and applied as poultices to the hurting body parts after the bath. The patient is wrapped in wool cloths, over the poultices, to maintain body temperature. These poultices may be applied for several hours, although care must be taken to avoid chilling the body or subjecting it to drafts. The area must be dried carefully, and kept evenly warm after the treatment.

- Another method is to place the hay blossoms inside a pillow-like sack and then steam the sack, or to heat it on the closed cover of a water pot. These warm herb pillows, wet or dry, can be applied directly to the body and reused several times. Make sure to keep the area warm during and after the treatment.

The Home Medicine Cabinet

Stocking a home medicine cabinet with herbs and herbal preparations may sound like a major undertaking, but just a few teas, tinctures, and salves are sufficient in most cases. When a home medicine cabinet is stocked with the usual bandages, thermometer, and a few herbal preparations, it is fairly well prepared for minor ailments and emergencies. Listed below are some herbal products that have a wide range of household and medical applications.

- A tea for colds and bronchial, throat, or sinus problems (depending on which is most prevalent in the household) and a cough syrup for children. If these are not available, your spice shelf should always stock fresh sage and thyme for the treatment of these ailments.

- A sleep tea or sedative drops or valerian capsules.

- A tea for digestive troubles, and a light laxative or some fresh linseed kept in the refrigerator.

- A mild diuretic, bladder, or kidney tea mixture or tincture.

- Teas or tinctures for any chronic or recurring illnesses among family members.

- Some powdered oak bark or charcoal tablets, for first aid treatment of mild cases of poisoning and diarrhea.

- A bottle of blended essential oils that can be combined with jojoba, olive, or sesame oil and used as a rub for sore muscles and minor pains, and to relieve headaches. Small stomach upsets, traveling sickness, fainting spells, etc., can be treated directly with the essential oil mixture, a few drops at a time on a piece of bread.

- A sudorific tea, such as linden or elder flower, to induce perspiration and relieve the symptoms of light fevers.

- A chamomile extract for baths, for washing out wounds, for steaming, to gargle, or to use as a disinfectant. Essential thyme oil, suitably diluted, is also a strong antibacterial agent.

- St. John's wort oil or marigold salve. These salves can be used to treat rashes, scars, burns, and wounds, or as massage oils. Aloe plants or house leeks grown in the house or garden can be applied directly to cuts and small wounds.

- An arnica tincture or salve for the first aid treatment of cuts, wounds, sprains, strained muscles, dislocations, and bruises.

- Lavender or rose herbal water, for its deodorant properties and wholesome odor, and for use as a "smelling water" for headaches and fainting spells.

The medicine cabinet can be complemented with fresh herbs when they are in season, and with more potent and specific medicines when they are called for. Once a year, the cabinet should be cleaned out and old herbs thrown away or used for baths. Tinctures can be kept longer, if properly stored in a cool place in dark bottles.

Finding out which herbs are necessary to cure minor complaints and ailments is a skill that takes a certain amount of practice, but it is amazing how little is needed to get by on a day-to-day basis. Many herbal preparations can serve multiple uses; their medicinal action is rarely limited to one area. An experienced and talented herbalist can achieve remarkable results using only a few herbs. Inexperienced herbalists tend to use many herbs and squander large amounts, while knowing little about possible side effects.

If I were asked which herb would be the most important to grow in a garden or have on the home medicine shelf, it would be difficult to decide between sage and chamomile. The School of Salernum exaggerated the simplicity of this decision by asking, *"Cur moriatur homo, cui salvia crescit in horte?"* ("Why does man die, when sage is growing in the garden?")—implying that sage alone has the power to cure all of humanity's ills.

The art of medicine is a question of timeliness: wine timely given helps, untimely, harms.

—Ovid, *Remediorum Amoris*

Miscellaneous Wisdom / Magic and Superstition

In our hectic lives, we leave little room for magic and often consider superstition to be something that was only practiced by Ukrainian peasants in the seventeenth century. We have forgotten that magic is simply a way of approaching something that amazes us and fills us with awe—and that magic rituals are just ways of doing this in a controlled manner. It is precisely because we leave so little room for magic in our modern lives that they are lacking in wonder, amazement, and deeper ties to the natural world.

So, dear reader, bear with me in this book and try to remember that there was a reason for our ancestors to behave in such undignified and superstitious ways. They didn't want to forget that plants are magical creatures, worthy of our admiration and awe. They talked to them, exhorted them, exploited them, and incorporated them into their daily lives. But they also considered plants to be imbued with the divine, and did not believe that humans could lord it over all creatures and get away with it.

Readers may be surprised to see, in the *Miscellaneous Wisdom* sections of this book, so much space devoted to "fanciful" cures. It is true that many "miscellaneous wisdoms" about herbs can be classified as old wives' tales, as mere superstitious practices that should not be taken seriously. These magical herbal remedies have little medicinal worth, but they did satisfy the deep-seated longing of our ancestors to be able to control the natural world by magic, spell, and ritual—and this is as much a part of our herbal tradition as mainstream herbalism and medicine. Some of these herbal superstitions originated in the classical works of Dioscurides and Pliny, and were then assimilated by monks, who transmitted their knowledge to folk healers and midwives—who in turn passed the lore on to "old wives." Other magical remedies are practices left over from pagan rites and religious cults; for example, the great number of beliefs associated with Midsummer's Day or with the Celtic holiday of Beltane (May Day).

However, other "miscellaneous wisdoms" have resulted from empirical observation and experimentation, and are scientifically attestable no matter how unusual they may appear at first glance. The example of the house leek is typical. House leeks have been planted on the roofs of European houses for centuries, and the ability of these plants to prevent lightning from striking the house has been observed again and again. But only recently has scientific experimentation verified this practice by proving that the plant is not harmed by strong electrical currents: the tiny points of each leaf act as miniature lightning rods.

Similarly, such "superstitious" beliefs, arising from centuries of tradition, experience, or just plain fancy, can show us new, unexpected areas for experimentation with herbs, or give us glimpses into areas of the herbal world hitherto overlooked. For example, while the consultation of herbal oracles is usually just a fanciful pastime, it can also point out some of the laws inherent in the natural world and help to reeducate the sensitivities of young people. For example, it is obvious that the way a certain herb grows in spring can hint at the harvest possibilities of another plant, and that the severity of the coming winter can often be foretold by observing the instinctive behavior of certain animals or the growth of certain herbs.

There is a superstition in avoiding superstitions.

—Francis Bacon, *Essays: Of Superstition*

Herb-Gathering Charms and Prayers

Medicine men and women in various cultures have long made a practice of praying to plants before gathering them, or repeating charms and spells during the gathering process. They are very intimate with herbs—their habits of growth, their healing properties, and their idiosyncrasies. Here are a few examples of how people have traditionally asked plants for permission to gather their parts:

When gathering elderberries, flowers, or wood, the plant was once addressed:

> Mother Elder, Mother Elder, give some of your berries
> and I'll give you some of mine when they grow in the woods.[11]

This twelfth-century herb-gathering spell was translated in the Proceedings of the British Academy:

> Earth, divine goddess, Mother Nature who generatest all things … hear, I beseech thee, and be favourable to my prayer. Whatsoever herb thy power dost produce, give, I pray, with goodwill to all nations to save them and grant me this my medicine. Come to me with my powers, and howsoever I may use them may they have good success and to whomsoever I may give them. Whatever thou dost grant it may prosper. To thee all things return. Those who rightly receive these herbs from me, do thou make them whole.[12]

Here are two modern versions of the prayer:

> Earth, you blessed one, Nature, Mother of all things … hear and turn a gentle ear to my prayer. I beg you to give each herb to humans for their health, and beg you to grace me with the knowledge of its healing powers. Come to me, and fill me with that knowledge. I pray that I may use it wisely and give it

---

11. Wilhelm Mannhard, *Der Baumkultus der Germanen und ihrer Nachbarstämme* (Berlin: Bornträger, 1875).

12. Charles Singer, trans. *Early English Magic and Medicine*, vol. 4, proceedings of the British Academy, (London: Humphrey Milford/Oxford Univ. Press, 1924).

wisely when needed. What you give is given wisely. All things return to you. Make the person who receives these herbs whole again.

Please, let me discover the wholeness, the complexity, of existence and of every living being. Let me learn the intertwinings of Nature, like ivy leaves hugging tree bark. Let me comprehend the constant play of opposites, to go beyond duality to an understanding of the whole. Let me see what is not shown, to look with other eyes, beyond sun and moon, to hear inland the roaring of the sea. Let my eyes come to see beyond the surface beyond every leaf, every puddle, every gust of wind. When this has been granted to me, maybe I will come to know the herbs, to know the uses to which they should be put, to know their limits and strengths, as well as my own. Until then, I am infinitely in their debt, a novice, amazed by their complexity.

Literary Flowers

References to herbs in literary works are not always romantically effusive, or dry and tedious. Shakespeare was well acquainted with the many folk names for herbs and flowers, and enjoyed word games and allusions:

> Virtue? A fig! 'tis in ourselves that we are thus, or thus; our bodies are gardens, to which our wills are gardeners, so that if we plant nettles or sow lettuce, set hyssop, and weed up thyme; supply it with one gender of herbs, or distract it with many; either to have it sterile with idleness, or manured with industry, why the power, and corrigible authority of this lies in our wills.[13]

Given the richness and pervasiveness of herbs in literature, I have ended many of the herb chapters in this book with quotations. These quotes are of necessity gleaned from only a few books, and the selection should not be considered exhaustive. My goal was to achieve variety, showcase unusual excerpts, and present various opinions about one herb in varying literary styles. Whenever possible, I made an attempt to return to original sources. (This is especially important in the cases of Dioscurides and Pliny, who were so often quoted and misquoted throughout the Middle Ages that some of the later "quotes" bear little or no resemblance to the original.)

If not otherwise noted, the translations from German and Italian folk texts, as well as from older literary texts in these languages, are my own.

Literature is full of perfumes.

—Walt Whitman, *Uncollected Prose*

---

13.   William Shakespeare, *Othello*, Act 1, scene 3, lines 321-329.

A Concluding Note

It is curious that the majority of healing herbs in nature are lunar, or female, and that the entire science of herbal knowledge has been relegated to women for several centuries. In those decades when scholastic medicine became the jealously guarded territory of men, women continued to practice herbal medicine. But all arts, all practices, are only truly productive, truly fertile, when both the male and the female elements in them are balanced, when each has a voice, and each can influence the other. I would *not* suggest, as William Coles in his missionary zeal did, that we "follow the steps of our Grandsire Adam, who is commonly pictured with a Spade in his hand ... [rectifying] all the disorders" of the garden.[14] I would prefer to suggest that we follow in the steps of both Grandsire Adam and Granddame Eve—that we use our hands as well as the spade, gather from the fields as well as till the garden, get to know the little people of the plant world, that we master the art of simpling as well as compounding, of superstitious remedies as well as established medicine, that we learn to cook with herbs as well as administer them, in order that we may come to have a more complete, unified, and balanced understanding of herbalism and medicine ... and, in the last instance, of life.

In our hectic day and age, it is important to make herbs our friends, because they can help to bring us back into balance. If we want to become healthy again, we need herbs from the garden or the herb store. If we want to eat more balanced meals, then herbs should be part of our diet, tickling our taste buds and harmonizing the properties of foods. If we find pleasure in gardening, then we should take special pleasure in aromatic leaves and flowers. If we like to leaf through old books, then we will also find old acquaintances mentioned with affection by poets and writers with an affinity to nature. Perfume would be unthinkable without the pungent aromas of herbs. Herbs accompany us through the bathroom to the hallway, into the living room and the kitchen, out through open doors into the garden. The one thing we shouldn't do with herbs is ignore them—for they are magical beings that can bring inestimable richness to our lives.

The compilation of this book has taken me several decades and given me many hours of pleasure—as I'm sure it did for the old herbalists, who painstakingly put together herbaria of pressed plants for others to study. I hope that you, my readers, will let this work accompany you on your journey through the fascinating world of herbal lore.

> *Beer with herbs, a patch of strawberries, delicious abundance: haws, yew berries,*
> *kernels of nuts. A cup of mead from the goodly hazel-bush, quickly served:*
> *brown acorns, manes of briars, with fine blackberries. In summer with its*

---

14. Coles, *The Art of Simpling* (London: J. Streater, 1656).

pleasant, abundant mantle, with good-tasting savour, there are pignuts, wild marjoram, the cresses of the stream—green purity!

—"The Hermit's Hut" by an unknown Irish author
of the 10th century, qtd. in Jackson, *A Celtic Miscellany*

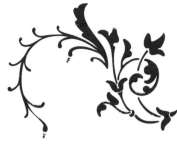

SACRED
HERBS

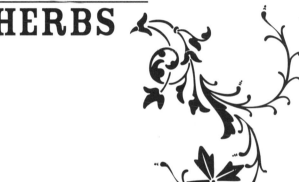

I had No medicine, sir, to go invisible,
No fern-seed in my pocket.

—BEN JONSON, *THE NEW INN*

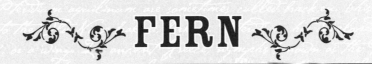

FERN

Name

The name "fern" has evolved from the Old English *fearn*, the Middle High German *varn*, and from the Sanskrit *parna*, which means "feather," "leaf," or "wing."

The most common fern is named *Pteridium aquilinum*. The term *pteridium* developed from the Greek, and (like the Sanskrit *parna*) means a feather, leaf, or wing. In ancient Greece, nymphs known as the Pterides were said to live in clearings where ferns grew. The study of ferns—a science in and of itself—is called pteridology. The use of the term *aquilinum* (in Latin, aquila means "eagle") originated from the resemblance of the fern's fronds to an eagle in flight.

Other ferns are called *Aspidium*, from the Greek word *aspis*, or shield. These plants' spore coverings are similar in form to a shield. The botanical name *Asplenium* is also of Greek origin, and points to the use of these ferns as splenetic medicine. *Dryopteris* is an oak fern. Polypody is, literally, the many-footed fern. The secondary botanical names *femina* and *mas* refer to the ancient division of ferns into male and female orders.

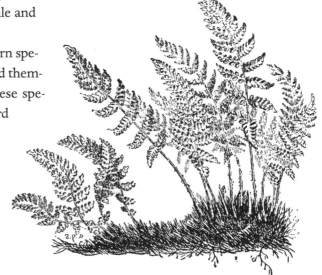

There are thousands of different fern species, and enough botanists have devoted themselves passionately to the study of these species to justify the inclusion of the word "pteridomania" in English dictionaries. Recently, many ferns have been botanically reclassified. Ferns are perennial plants for the most part, and now belong to several plant families. Because of this diversity, it is often hard for beginners to find their way through the forest of ferns. The following are just a few of many noteworthy species:

Folk Names

In folk botany, ferns are rarely differentiated. Most large ferns are called bracken (the word "bracken" is of northern origin, and can be traced back to the Old Norse *brakni, burkni*), and the smaller ferns are usually grouped together indiscriminately. This is not always wise, especially if the plants are being used medicinally.

Pteridium aquilinum is also called bracken, brake, brake fern, female fern, fern of God, or King Charles in the oak ree. German names are *Adlerfarn, Jesus Christwurz, Irrkraut*, and *Federfarn*. French names are *fougère, fougère imperiale, fougère commune*, and *fougère aquiline*. Italians call the plant *felce, filice, felce aquilina, felce da ricotte*, and *erba delle streghe*. The Dutch name for fern is *varen*; the Spanish *helecho comun*; the Irish *raithneach*; the Welsh *rhedyn* or *rhedynen*; the Finnish *sanajalka*; the Japanese *warabi*, and the Rumanian *faletga*. In Hungary, ferns are known as the flowers of the thunder god Perun.

The male shield fern *(Dryopteris filix-mas)* is commonly known as the male fern. German folk names for the plant abound, due to its massive presence in Central Europe. It is called *Wurmfarn, männliches Farnkraut, Farnkrautmännlein, Mausleitern*, and *Hirschzehen*. The French call it *fougère male*; the Italians, *felce maschia*. The lady fern or spleenwort *(Athyrium filix-femina)* is also known as *Waldfrauenfarn* and *Farnweiblein* in Germany.

The regal fern *(Osmunda regalis)* is called royal fern, water fern, and bog onion. The legend goes that a waterman on Lock Tyne once hid his wife and his children from invading Danes among the large ferns growing on the water's edge. From that day, the royal fern has taken on the name of Osmund the waterman. It is sometimes called Heart of Osmund, or Osmund royal fern. The German names are *Königsfarn, Königsrispenfarn*, and *Königsraute*.

Common polypody *(Polypodium vulgare)* is also named rock of polypody, polypody of the oak, rock brake, brake root, wall fern, and oak fern. The common German name is *Engelsüß*, but it is also known as *Baumfarn, Kropfwurz, Marienmilch*, and *grosser Bittersüß*.

Common spleenwort *(Ceterach officinarum)* is occasionally classified as scaly fern, miltwaste, or fingerfern. The German name is *Milzfarn* or *Schriftfarn*.

Hart's tongue (once *Asplenium scolopendrium*, now *Phyllitis scolopendrium*) is called hind's tongue, horse tongue, buttonhole, or God's hair; and *Hirschzunge* in German.

True maidenhair *(Adiantum capillus-veneris)* is spoken of as hair of Venus, and French herbalists call it *capillaire commun* or *capillaire de Montpelier*.

Asplenium trichomanes is the common maidenhair; *Asplenium adiantum nigrum* the black maidenhair or black spleenwort fern.

Asplenium ruta-muraria, once known as *Salvis vitae*, is also called white maidenhair, wall rue, or tentwort. The German name for this herb is *Mauerraute*, and the French classify the three maidenhairs as *Doradilles*.

Botrychium lunaria, moonwort or Grape fern, is sometimes called Unshoe the horse. Its German names are *Mondraute*, *Vexierchrut*, and *Walpurgiskraut*. It is extremely rare in some areas and is therefore protected by law.

Appearance

In times long past, ferns grew as tall as trees, but over the millennia they have slowly developed into smaller species and varieties. Present-day ferns may be a few inches tall, or they may shoot up to a height of 6 ft. or even more. Because they do not produce flowers, but reproduce themselves with the help of spores, they are a botanically unique group of plants. Ferns vary widely according to their location, and a local botanical guide is absolutely essential for the correct identification of all the ferns in the neighborhood.

The odor of all large ferns is astringently unpleasant, as well as unmistakable. The most common large fern has a long, creeping rootstock and wiry stems that may, under some circumstances, even grow to 10 ft. in length. Shoots of young bracken plants, called crosiers, resemble a bishop's staff. Bracken fronds are light green, and spread gracefully outward to cover large areas of ground. Large fronds have a certain similarity to a palm tree. The stems, when cut diagonally at the base, reveal patterns that are said to represent the wingspan of an eagle. Bracken spores are so tiny that they cannot easily be seen with the unaided eye.

The rhizome of the male fern is short and creeping, and lies very close to the surface. It is green on the inside, and is covered on the outside by brown scales. The fronds are 2–4 ft. long and are not arranged in opposite pairs. The spores of the male fern are enclosed in shield-like coverings. The female fern closely resembles the male, but is often smaller. The spores usually form tiny roots while still attached to the fronds of the mother plant, and then "jump" loose, ready to root themselves in nearby soil.

The regal fern has a trunk-like stem and a tuberous rhizome. Its stems are brown and wiry, and the fronds can be as long as 8 or 10 ft. The young fronds are tinged with red; the older are colored a dull green. Some plants of this species are barren, but others have a spiky stem covered with spore cases that ripen in the late spring.

Polypody has a thick yellow rootstock covered with scales. Its fronds may grow 1 ft. long, and occur in opposite pairs.

The rock ferns are much smaller than the wood ferns. Spleenwort grows on walls and in crevices. Its fronds are 4–6 in. long and shaped like the human spleen. Hart's tongue has long, undivided fronds, and is easily differentiated from other ferns because of this. It is evergreen.

True maidenhair grows to a height of 1 ft. and resembles a miniature tree. The stems are black, and the rootstock creeping. White maidenhair only grows 2 or 3 in. high on rocks and walls. It closely resembles garden rue, but is much smaller and more delicate.

Place, Season, and Useful Parts

Ferns can be found in shady, wooded places in all parts of the world except for the extreme south and the extreme north. (As the famed herbalist and physician, Nicholas Culpeper, put it, they grow "but too frequently.") Large ferns are a common sight in woods, copses, recently burnt clearings, damp deciduous forests, stony and shady places, moors, heaths, hedgerows, riverbanks, and gardens. Many of the natural habitats of ferns are being drained, and this is endangering some species. Bracken grows to an altitude of 5,000 ft. and often appears in masses, covering large expanses of the landscape. The male fern can be found growing as high up as 7,000 ft. The regal fern is native to bogs, marshes, moors, and other watery places. Polypody prefers to make its home in old crumbling walls, on tree stumps, or between tree roots and rocks. Spleenwort and the maidenhairs also grow on walls and between rocks, and are found predominately in southern countries.

Bracken generally produces spores in June or July and on into September. The spores of the male fern mature earlier. Fern crosiers are gathered in the spring as they emerge. Maidenhair and spleenwort can be harvested in the summer, and fern roots should be dug in the summer and fall.

Gathering, Drying, and Storage

The young and edible shoots of large ferns are only in season for a few days each spring, just before they begin to unfold. Spleenwort and maidenhair fronds are usually gathered in the early summer, when they are fresh and green.

The roots of the male fern are usually dug in summer or fall. A small section of the rhizome should always be put back into the earth: it will produce a new plant to replace the harvested one. The strongest drug is said to come from plants found in high regions and cold climates, and dug in June or July. The best polypody roots are those gathered from northern plants. Care should be taken when gathering polypody roots, for they can cause skin rashes.

For magical purposes, ferns gathered at midnight on Midsummer's Eve are generally considered to be ideal. Ferns gathered on Easter and Christmas, Whitsun Eve, Trinity Sunday, Groundhog Day, and the Eve of St. Thomas' Day are believed to have great powers. Ferns gathered when a comet is in the sky are also said to have unusual magical powers.

- For those set on gathering fern seed, here is one set of instructions, recorded in Württemberg in 1650: Go to a crossroads on Midsummer's Eve, and in silence draw a circle with a hazel stick around the chosen place. Lay a carefully prepared chicory stalk on a piece of fur within the circle, and only remove it at midnight when ghosts and spirits begin to crowd around the circle. As soon as the chicory is removed, a fern stalk will shoot up in its stead. It will blossom and produce a seed, which will fall onto the fur. The seed should be quickly scooped into a quill-case (or pencil box) and worn next to the skin.[15]

Male fern rhizomes approximately 3–6 in. in length and ½–2 in. in diameter should be washed, scraped lightly to remove the scales, split lengthwise, and then dried in a dark, warm place. Artificial heat can be used to speed the drying process, as long as a temperature of 122° F is not exceeded. The entire root must retain its green color when dried. It should be stored in dark, sealed containers and used within one year. Extremely large fern specimens have been known to produce a root weighing up to 4 lb.

Seed Saving and Germination

Because ferns do not actually produce seeds (despite all the legends), seed saving is not an appropriate term. The plants reproduce with the help of spores, or plant division. The simplest way to reproduce them is to create a situation that closely resembles their wild habitat, and let them reproduce themselves.

Gardening Hints

Ferns are sometimes considered garden pests, but their luxurious growth, majestic size, high value as screening and accent plants, and fertilizing properties should recommend them to gardeners. They actually prefer a shaded, northern position, and will therefore flourish where few other plants will grow. The best soil for ferns is a mixture of peat, humus, sand, and a few pebbles. Ferns can be transplanted in the spring, or the spores are "sown."

Ferns grow well indoors if they are protected from sunlight, excessively damp soil, and dry air. Because of this, they are good choices for the bathroom. The large royal fern, the male fern, and the brake transplant easily. The plants should be dug up in the spring with a large ball of soil, and then set, not too deeply, in the garden. Fern fronds may also be placed, spore-side down, on the earth, and covered with leaves or decomposing wood particles. Young plants should emerge within a few weeks. They must be kept damp until well established, and then need little attention. Wall ferns are a little

---

15. Hanns Bächtold-Stäubli, ed., *Handwörterbuch des deutschen Aberglaubens* (1927–42), vol. II (Berlin: Walter de Gruyter & Co., 1987), 1218.

more difficult to transplant, and should be set under stones. If plants are taken from their natural habitat, care should be taken not to destroy existing stands. Ferns can be fertilized in the fall with leaves and compost as needed. In very warm areas, fern fronds may remain green throughout the winter. Ferns will not grow well under beech trees.

Ferns are an important source of free composting and fertilizing material for the gardener. Fern fronds are rich in potash, and can be used to cover seedlings and frost-sensitive plants, or as a nutrient-rich mulch. They can be chopped and included in liquid fertilizer mixtures. They make excellent mulch material for potatoes and sugar beets. Fuchsia roots can be forced to grow vigorously downward by digging fern fronds deep into the soil before planting. Fern compost is also used to promote tree seeding, and the black wiry rootlets of the Osmund royal fern are used as a potting mixture for orchids.

According to folk belief, existing stands of bracken can only be destroyed on the following days: the four Fridays in May, July 10th, and August 29th.

Culinary Virtues

Although ferns in large amounts can be toxic, fern shoots can be enjoyed in moderate amounts as a blood-purifying meal in the spring. Pregnant women, small children, convalescents, and chronically sick people should avoid ferns, and they do not mix well with alcoholic beverages. The young shoots (also called crosiers or fiddleheads) of such ferns as bracken, the male fern, the lady fern, the esculent brake (or, in North America, *Osmunda cinnamomea*), and the Ostrich fern (*Matteuccia struthiopteris*) can be cut when they are 6–8 in. high in the spring. The fuzzy covering is removed, and the shoots cooked like asparagus in boiling salt water. Fern crosiers are a great delicacy in Japan. There, they are washed in ice-cold water, plunged into boiling water for approximately 2 minutes, removed, and left to soak in very cold water for 2 hours or more. This treatment removes most of the unpleasant medicinal taste and possible toxic qualities of the shoots. They are then heated and served as an asparagus-like vegetable side dish with butter or a cream sauce, or they are puréed as soup. Fiddleheads can also be canned, and are sold in some specialty shops.

The rootstock of the esculent brake was once one of the diet staples of the New Zealand Maoris. The Vancouver Indians also ate bracken roots with great relish. All the ferns have starchy rootstocks that can be ground and used as a flour substitute. Europeans only eat bracken in times of great scarcity, and bracken is generally spoken of there with disdain. The Duke of Orleans once (1745) dramatically presented Louis XV with some fern bread: "Sire, your subjects subsist on *this!*"[16] At the beginning of this century, the

---

16. U. P. Hendrick, ed., *Sturtevant's Edible Plants of the World* (1919) (New York: Dover, 1972), 470.

fern bread made in Normandy was described as "wretched."[17] Young fern fronds are also mixed with bread on occasion, and gruel can be prepared from ground fern roots and barley meal. A beer produced from malt and fern fronds was prepared for centuries in Scandinavia and Siberia.

Household Applications

All the large ferns can be used as bedding material for animals and humans. According to folk belief, the fronds must be dried before use because lying on green ferns will cause blindness. Dried ferns, on the other hand, are believed to have great healing properties. The dried fronds are stuffed into mattress and pillow ticking, or they are placed directly under the sheet. They must be replaced as soon as they begin to crumble. Small pillows filled with fern fronds can be given to infants to ease teething. Fern mattresses also help to reduce minor aches and pains and to soothe rheumatic complaints, cramps, and toothaches. In the days when bedbugs were a cause of sleeplessness, ferns were strewn under the bed to drive away parasites. Roaches flee from burning ferns, as do snakes, flies, gnats, and other insects.

One fascinating aspect of ferns is their ability to photograph themselves in the dark. A fresh fern frond placed on a photographic plate in a darkroom will produce a ghostly shadow print. Ferns are also thought to counteract the unpleasant effects of negative earth and water currents. Mountain climbers swear that a few fern fronds laid in their shoes or worn over their hearts will quickly relieve weariness and cold, making walking easier.

Bracken and all other large ferns can be used to store fruit. The fronds are gathered in quantity during summer, and then dried in an airy attic. In the fall, storage apples can be placed on shelves or in boxes lined with the dried fronds. In Italy, the fronds are used to strain and wrap freshly pressed ricotta (sheep cheese) to keep it from souring. In Galloway the saying goes, "Red bracken brings milk and butter," because the cows begin to produce milk after the ferns turn red on the first frosty nights in October. Bracken can, if desired, be used to produce lye for making soap and cleansing mixtures. The fronds are burned, and the ashes formed with water into tiny balls. The balls are then burned again. The resulting ash is rubbed directly onto linen to scour it, or processed with tallow to produce soap.

Noteworthy Recipes

Fern Ointment: It is a good idea to always keep a jar of herb ointment or tincture in the kitchen for the first-aid treatment of all minor cuts and burns. The wound will heal very quickly if treated immediately. Arnica tincture can be applied to

---

17.   Ibid.

any cut or bruise, or to sprains or dislocations as well as to children's bumps and bruises. If one does not happen to have fern ointment at hand, St. John's wort oil, comfrey ointment, or marigold salve are also excellent for treating burns or scalds. Here is an old recipe for a burn ointment prepared with fern:

> For Scald, or any Burn, an Excellent Ointment. Take of Cream a Quart, Fern-roots a handful: slice and wash the Roots, and thou boil them in the Cream in a Earthen-pot till they Jelly, and at what time there is an occasion to use it: Ferment it with a Spatula, and apply it with a Linnen cloth, often renewing it.[18]

In farmers' households, lard is usually used instead of cream as an ointment base, but it is also possible to prepare a fern ointment with a wax or a lanolin and wax-based salve.

Cosmetic Properties

Aching, tired feet can be refreshed by placing fern fronds in both shoes. Maidenhair fern, which closely resembles human hair, has been praised for centuries for its ability to prevent hair loss, cure dandruff, and make hair grow. The fresh herb is boiled in water or wine, the mixture strengthened with some burdock-root oil or fresh olive oil, and then it is applied liberally, every day, to the scalp.

Medicinal Merits

For centuries, various ferns have helped patients to rid themselves of worms and rheumatic pains. Theophrastus and Dioscurides recommended the male fern for treating colics of the spleen, and Pliny praised spleenwort for its healing effect on the liver, at the same time warning of harmful effects on the reproductive system. Later sources recommended the herb as a contraceptive. Hildegard von Bingen prescribed ferns to cure gout and to restore vision to clouded eyes. Healing ointments were made from ferns to treat hemorrhoids, wounds, and burns, and fern beer was prescribed for patients suffering from disorders of the liver and gall bladder. Ferns gathered from trees were thought effective against a stomachache, and polypody found in oak trees was used to treat melancholy, whooping cough, scurvy, nose polyps, and a hardened spleen. The French believed that a belt of midsummer ferns would protect a person against all internal diseases, and the Swiss hung ferns upside down in the hall to drive rheumatism from the house.

---

18. John Shirley, *The Accomplished Ladies Rich Closet of Rarities* (London: N. Bodington, 1688), 75.

Modern Medicine

Modern herbalists are more cautious than their ancient counterparts when prescribing ferns. They usually prefer the smaller ferns as internal medicine, which are less potent and therefore safer for internal use. Pregnant women, children, convalescents, and those ill with heart, ulcerous, or intestinal disorders should not use fern products. Alcohol should also be strictly avoided when taking fern medicine. If in doubt about the correct botanical classification, avoid taking ferns internally. They are valuable enough as external medicine.

Ferns, especially the male ferns, are still prescribed today as worm remedies. Tapeworms can be paralyzed with the male fern, but hook-and-maw worms *(Ankylostoma and Ascaris)* may resist fern cures. Vermifuges (worm-expelling agents) should always be taken under medical or expert herbalist supervision, and must be administered together with a laxative to avoid absorption by the intestines. Worm cures may only be taken once every eight weeks because of possible cumulative action. The young, diagonal rhizomes of the male fern produce the strongest drug. This is administered in powdered form, or as an ethereal extract.

Of the smaller ferns, the lady fern has the same medicinal properties as the male, but in weakened form. Polypody is often prescribed as a cough herb, as are spleenwort and maidenhair. Polypody and the common maidenhair are mildly laxative herbs. Spleenwort is still used to treat disorders of the spleen. True maidenhair in its fresh state is a glandular drug with a stimulating effect on the female reproductive system. A homeopathic preparation of hart's tongue and golden seal *(Hydrastis canadensis)* is given to diabetics. The royal fern is considered an excellent herb for the treatment of lumbago and jaundice.

All ferns can be applied externally to ease the pains of rheumatism, gout, lumbago, and cramped or stiff limbs. All of the ferns are also said to counteract the negative effects of water and earth currents, and of some forms of radiation. Mountain ferns are generally considered much more potent than lowland plants for these purposes, and the larger ferns more effective than the smaller. The simplest method of using ferns is to lay the fresh fronds on the aching spot. In winter, a tincture can be substituted. Lumbago, sudden rheumatic pains, and cramps in the leg can be alleviated this way. A cushion of fresh ferns, or tiny bags filled with fern spores and placed inside the ears, can help to restore hearing to those afflicted with rheumatic earaches or colds. Cushions of dried fern fronds relieve rheumatic twinges and aches as well as cramps. Writers' cramps and hands strained from computer use can be loosened with an ethereal fern extract.

Warm fern footbaths ease cramps and the pains of gout, and have also been used to treat varicose veins. Fern-root wine is rubbed in to relieve rheumatic stiffness, and fern-root vinegar is an acceptable first-aid treatment for festering wounds before the doctor can be called.

The male fern is used homeopathically as a vermifuge for tapeworms and for inflammation of the lymph glands. In China, thirty-five different ferns are used medicinally, including *Osmunda japonica* and *Matteuccia struthiopteris*, in much the same manner as they are used in the West—to expel parasites and to relieve toxic heat, but also for uterine bleeding due to hot blood. These herbs are toxic enough that they should not be prescribed for weakened patients or children, and should not be taken together with a fatty meal.

Special Cures

The Swiss herbal priest Johann Künzle was of the opinion that the majority of those afflicted with gout could be cured with the help of fern roots, even if they had suffered from the disease for decades. He recommended that a gout-ridden patient take one or two large, fresh, unwashed fern roots, cut them into small pieces, tie them in a linen sack, and place the sack on the aching limb until the pain is gone. If the pains do not lessen, then a warm daily bath prepared with the addition of several crushed (European) juniper berries will help. To make the therapy even more effective, the patient should drink at least a cup of meadowsweet *(Filipendula ulmaria)*, lady's bedstraw, or restharrow *(Ononis spinosa)* tea a day.

> *Fern Tincture:* A tincture of fresh herb fronds can easily be prepared for winter use. Fill a clear, wide-mouthed glass with chopped fresh ferns and cover with clear alcoholic spirits (96 percent wine spirits, or if this is not available, clear grain or fruit spirits). Close the jar securely, and place it in the sun or a warm place for 4–6 days. Strain and filter the mixture, pour it into dark bottles, and stopper well.

Uses in Husbandry

Bracken can be burned, and the potash-rich ashes collected for use in the manufacture of soap and glass. Fern plants gathered in June produce ashes containing up to 20 percent potash, and are therefore an important ingredient in fertilizers. The brake rootstock has also been used by tanners to treat chamois and kid leather. Vintners hung the root in wine casks to keep the wine from spoiling.

In Devon, England, stands of bracken were once set aflame in the hope of causing rain; this practice is still followed to the present day. But ferns provide excellent cover for game and birds, and sportsmen often object to the firing of the hills. Hares love fern plants so much that they are affectionately termed "fern-sitters."

Husbandmen once used to gather bracken to thatch their cottages or to provide bedding material for their animals. For this purpose, the bracken is cut in autumn when it turns yellow, and is dried like hay. Fern is thought to drive away fleas, lice, and other parasites, and is therefore strewn in dog baskets and kennels as well as in chicken coops. Some farmers hang fern fronds in stalls to attract flies. Every evening, they slip a bag over the plants, and then destroy the flies caught in the bag. Some strew the herb in granaries to discourage mice, or even use it as a snake repellent.

Both fresh and dried bracken fronds can be fed to cattle in small amounts, although ferns have been known to cause poisoning in cattle if used as a steady diet. Dried bracken fronds and the fronds and roots of the male fern can be boiled and fed to pigs. Ferns are also believed to be effective against diseases caused by evil influences. Fern plants are hung up in pigsties to keep the animals healthy, and caged birds have their cages strewn with the herb to prevent illness. Sick horses have a piece of fern tied under their tongues, and, in Touraine, France, all the animals are smoked with fern on Midsummer's Eve to discourage disease. In Poland, pigs are given fern tea at midnight as a cure for many complaints. Bracken gathered at midnight on Midsummer's Eve or on Good Friday is fed to the animals at all times of the year to protect them from evil witches. The hand-shaped roots of fern dug on Midsummer's Eve are used to clean animals' troughs. In Germanic countries, cows giving too little milk are fed the roots of a prickly fern.

In countries where bracken is plentiful, it is sometimes used as packing material for breakable goods such as roofing slates.

Veterinary Values

Ferns can be given to animals as well as humans as a vermifugal medicine. Cats and dogs are not as sensitive as humans to the drug, but it is wisest to consult a veterinarian for the proper dosage. Animals with tapeworms are treated with male fern-root oil. The male fern is also administered to horses for the treatment of skin rash.

Miscellaneous Wisdom

According to Johann Künzle, the devil so dislikes ferns that, each and every time he sees the plant, he makes a face like a schoolboy passing by a school building during vacation. Hildegard von Bingen believed that fern fronds could not only drive away witches and lightning, but also the devil. She advised young mothers to place dried ferns in their own beds and in the cradles of their newborn babies. The Wends (a Slavic ethnic group) bathed their children with a fern decoction to wash away the visible and invisible results of a great fright. Northern Italians believed that witches rubbed their hands with the herb in order to direct hailstorms. French fern gathered before sunrise was considered potent against all sorcery and witchcraft.

According to written tradition, fern seeds were considered even more powerful than the legendary mandrake. According to a Swiss report in 1596, the devil himself was forced to set the table for a fern-seed carrier. In 1601, A German was executed as a warlock because he had tucked fern seed in his armpit to make himself invulnerable. In 1611, the Emperor Maximilian legally forbade the use of fern for magical purposes. In

1612, the Synode of Ferrara seconded his prohibition. In 1648, an enterprising Austrian huckster tried to sell fern seeds for 1 Reichstaler apiece. They were advertised as a fail-safe method for protecting travelers from knocks and bruises, and for preventing businessmen from losing profits. Grimmelshausen, Jonson, and Shakespeare also extolled the extraordinary powers of the tiny fern seed.

Ferns found growing on animals' graves in Germany were believed to make a person invisible, as well as rich. Germans also warned against stepping on the herb inadvertently. This would cause even the most experienced woodsman to lose his way until he turned his shoes or clothes backward. In Austria, ferns—or the "quarreling herbs"—were not supposed to be brought into the house.

Magical Powers

Estonians believed that fern fronds gathered on Midsummer's Eve had extraordinary magical powers, if the gatherer could walk unharmed through a ring of snakes without looking back. Such ferns could make him invisible, let him pass through all locked doors, and enable him to steal at will. Midsummer fern was also believed to produce a gold coin every morning if placed under the pillow the preceding evening. Fern plants dug on Midsummer's Eve and then dried in a completely dark room were often hung up in Central European homes to attract good luck and distract lightning. In southeastern Europe, kitchen floors were strewn with fern fronds on Midsummer's Day so that St. John would find a bed of ferns waiting for him under the kitchen table that night.

Fern rootstocks are often gathered on Midsummer's Day for amulet use. The fronds are cut off above the roots so that the remaining piece resembles a hand. This "hand" is then dried over the smoke of the Midsummer fire. The male fern is usually preferred for this purpose, although bracken roots can also be used.

Any person who has fern seed can use it to great advantage. With fern seed in his pocket, a person can go invisible and be able to speak with all animate things, even stones and brooks. He will be blessed with riches tangible and intangible, and with inexhaustible energy and luck. His bullets will never miss their mark if he mixes fern seed with his gunpowder, and he will never be wounded if he wears a fern-seed amulet. The resting places of all treasures will be revealed to him, and he will be able to climb the steepest mountains like a goat. He will always have trumps in his hand, his arrows will always fly true, and his bowling balls will roll so that they knock down all pins.

Some grasping, reckless men covet fern seed so much that they are willing to trade their immortal souls for the tiny seed. They make a covenant with the devil and sign it with their blood. The devil agrees to appear at midnight with the seed in his hand, bringing wealth untold until the day he returns to collect his due.

Magicians place moonwort in a class of its own, apart from other members of the fern family. Because of its lunar nature, it is considered most potent when gathered by moonlight. It is employed in incantations, and alchemists once invoked it to transform quicksilver into the true metal. One popular name for the plant, "Unshoe the horse," comes from its supposed ability to loosen all locks and loosen the shoes from a horse.

Children love to dress up in green-fronded fern skirts and shifts. Adult participants in fertility rituals and processions (including the so-called green men) once also used the fronds as part of their costumes.

The fern's stem is often cut diagonally to reveal patterns that are believed to represent various letters or words. They are also though to represent an eagle, or even the imprint of the devil's foot. In England, witches fear bracken because the letter *C* (Christ) can be found in the stem. The Irish believe that the first letter revealed when a bracken stem is cut will resemble a *G*, the second an *O*, and the third a *D*. In Germany, the letters are believed to be *JC* or *HIC*. In Surrey, England, fortune will smile on anyone who can find the image of an oak tree in a bracken plant. The Finns never use ferns for making mattresses because of the words present in the stems.

Fern Seed and Flower

Although all parts of the fern plant are believed to possess strong magical powers, fern flowers and fern seeds are considered to be supernaturally potent. Botanically speaking, ferns never produce flowers or true seeds, but popular imagination insists that, on certain extraordinary days, the plants suddenly do burst forth into blossom. Fern flowers and fern seeds are believed to be emanations of the sun and are therefore red or golden, or even white. They smell like corruption, or a burning flame, and a fierce storm arises as soon as they are picked or their beauty is spent. The fern flower is the symbol of fiery perfection and golden balance; the fern seed is the quintessence of invisible magical powers. Those people who can manage to win one will have all their wishes fulfilled, and be able to become invisible at will and turn other metals into gold. In Tyrol in southern Europe, they will be able to draw wine from springs on the Eve of St. Jacob's and St. Phillip's days.

A fern plant supposedly only blossoms once a century, on Midsummer's Eve. The fern flower is often associated with fire and snakes. According to the Lithuanians, the snake king slithers out of his lair on this night to catch the "wizard's" seed and places it in his crown. Snakes, and their relatives the dragons, guard the flower all night long. In Sweden, wood trolls protect the plant. Any human smart enough to outwit the fern guardians will be blessed with health, wealth, and good luck, and protected against evil influence. The association of the fern plant with snakes is also widespread in Wales and Germany. In Wales, snakes and adders will follow those who gather fern flowers until they part with them. In Germany, those who use fern seed to make themselves invisible may be betrayed by a snake trailing after them. In Austria, those who meander absent-mindedly and lose their way often are asked if they have fern seed in their pocket. Generally, women are not considered capable of obtaining fern seed—it is considered an area of male expertise.

In Finland, the fern plant is said to have three blossoms, only one of which is white. To gather this flower, a man must spread a white cloth under the plant on Midsummer's Eve and then sit down and wait. Ghosts, spirits, and specters will come and try to distract the gatherer and break eye contact between the gatherer and the plant. The man must then say, "Give me the flower that can be used for forty-four things!" and carefully, very carefully, gather it in a white cloth when it emerges. Then, continuously repeating the Pater Noster, he walks backward until he comes to a field that has been plowed crossways. If he forgets to repeat the prayer, little men will appear and snatch the hard-won blossom from his cradling hands.

According to Silesian tradition in Germany, the man should lay the skin of a yearling black goat under the plant to keep the flower from scorching the earth. He should take off all his clothes to wait for the flower's appearance, and must catch it deftly as it falls.

The Russian belief is that any man who can gather a fern flower at Easter will be able to read the secrets of the earth, and lay its treasures bare. The man should take a knife and a cloth on which the Easter cake has been blessed, and then trace a circle around the plant. He must place himself squarely within the circle, and fix the plant with his eyes. It will blossom just as the words "Christ is arisen!" are sung in church. He must grasp the blossom at the right moment; cover himself with the blessed cloth; and run home without turning to the right or left. In the safety of his own room, he should cut his hand with the knife, and lay the flower in the cut, next to his blood and skin. All secrets will then be revealed, and he will come to know all hidden lore.

The Estonians believe that only an honest man, or an orphan, or three men working together in harmony can gather the fern's devil blossom. The hopeful man (or men) should first try to discover which fern plants will blossom that year, and then chose one growing at a good distance from farmhouses and the sound of cockcrows. He must not say anything to anyone of his hopes and plans and fears, but must go to the plant in respectful silence before midnight on Midsummer's Eve. Then he must enclose the plant in a circle traced with a knife, axe, or sword, or with a twig of juniper or mountain ash, or, if he is a magician, with his bare finger. He then steps inside the circle and prepares a fire from juniper twigs he has brought with him. He lays a holy songbook before him on a blessed cloth, and lights a candle on either side of the book. He must remain within the circle until daylight, reading from the book and using the sword to protect himself from danger. At the stroke of midnight, the plant will produce buds, and then burst forth in a dazzling display of iridescent flowers. Only one of the flowers is the devil blossom: the one that burns constantly with a golden flame. Storms and angry spirits accompany its appearance. The man must, with all his courage and strength, try to keep his eyes fixed on the plant. If he wavers, or if he is foolish enough to step outside of the circle, then the spirits will grab at him and hurl him to his death. If his heart holds true, he will be able to catch the flower in his songbook just before it touches the ground. He presses it close to his skin or places it under his hat, in his left armpit, on his breast, or next to his liver. He must remain in the circle with his flower until daybreak, singing and waking to comfort his heart.

Clever men who do not want to risk their lives hunting fern flowers sometimes enlist the help of a hedgehog. They carefully study the habits of neighborhood hedgehogs until they discover a hedgehog nest. The young ones are separated from their mother with a fence. The mother, anxious for the lives of her babies, will waddle to the woods as fast as she can to find a fern flower. The man must wait patiently and silently until the hedgehog mother returns with the flower in her mouth. As soon as the fence is touched with the flower, it will open and she can go to her young ones. The man can then quickly retrieve the flower from her mouth before she swallows it.

With the flower, it is believed, miracles can be brought to pass and wonders multiplied. If a man moves it in his hand, wishes will come true. If he places it in his purse, his money will have no end. His cellar, pantry, and granary will be filled with the best wines and produce if he lays it on a shelf. If he lays it on the earth, he will be able to find all treasures hidden under the surface. He will be able to heal the wounds, aches, and pains of his fellow human beings, and talk to animals. He can open all locks, loosen all knots, and pass through air and space at will. Any woman who sleeps with the fern blossom next to her skin will be visited by the man who will share her bed.

Harvesting Fern Seed

Fern seed is gathered in much the same manner as fern flowers. It is caught as it falls in nine linen cloths, a handkerchief, a shirt, a blessed chalice cloth, the felty leaves of mullein *(Verbascum thapsus)*, or in a heavy mortar. It is said to burn through an apron or a single piece of paper, and will vanish if touched by a bare hand. In Styria (Austria), the fern plant is said to flower on Christmas Eve. In Swabia and the Palatine (Germany), Christmas ferns can only be gathered by a man who has occupied himself with devilish thoughts during all of Advent. He must then go on Christmas Eve to a crossroads between the church and the cemetery. At midnight, the ghosts of the dead and the living will appear before him, and try to make him talk. If one word escapes his lips, then the devil's claim to his soul will be complete. But if he perseveres, the last ghost will be dressed as a hunter and will present him with several fern seeds tied up in a cloth.

In Lower Austria, fern blossoms at midnight on Midsummer's Eve while thunder growls, storms sweep through the countryside, and all the demons of hell ride the winds.

In Tyrol, the man must stick seven green elder wands in the earth in a circle around the fern and then remove all his clothes, spreading his shirt under the plant and weighing it down with stones. The following morning, he can gather the seed in his shirt, taking care to throw the stones downhill. If he forgets and tosses them uphill, then his work will be undone and the seed will bring more misfortune than good luck.

In Portugal, the traditional way of gathering fern seed is for a man to place his clothes under the plant and weigh them down with silver coins. At midnight, the devil will come to shake the plant and release the seed. The man must then flee to the safety of his house, making crosses behind him with his sword all the way home. He can gather the seed from his shirt the following morning.

Yet another northern German method of harvesting fern seed is to shoot an arrow at the sun on noon of Midsummer's Day. Three drops of blood will then fall from the wounded sun, and the hunter must catch them in a white cloth while they fall. The drops of blood will develop into fern, or blood, seeds.

> *They prepare fern gathered in the summer solstice, pulled up in a tempestuous night,*
> *rue, trifoly, vervain against magical impostures.*
>
> —LEVINUS LEMNIUS, QUOTED IN BRAND'S *POPULAR ANTIQUITIES*

Oracular Worth

In Finland and Estonia, young people anxious to know the names of their future spouses consult fern roots as an oracle. The questioner goes to a crossroads shortly before midnight on Midsummer's Eve, taking care not to say a word. He or she traces a circle around the fern with a rowan stick and steps inside the circle. The entire plant is ripped out just as it begins to blossom, and a letter is revealed in the root. In Cornwall and Sussex, England, lovers simply cut the root to discover the initial of the loved one's name. Austrian and German girls run through a patch of fern plants on Midsummer's Eve. If a fern seed falls into one of the girls' shoes and she cooks it, then the man she will love best in the entire world will appear before her.

In the islands of the Azores, sorcerers make use of the plant to tell the fortunes of their clients, reading the future in the ashes of the burnt flowers. Celtic druids also held the fern in great veneration.

> *When the fern is as high as a spoon,*
> *You may sleep an hour at noon;*
> *When the fern is as high as a ladle,*
> *You may sleep as long as you're able;*
> *When the fern begins to look red,*
> *Then milk is good with brown bread.*
>
> —G. F. NORTHALL, *ENGLISH FOLK-RHYMES*

Legends

In northern German legend, a farmer goes to look for a lost animal in the woods. On his way, he passes through a fern clearing and a fern seed falls into his shoe. After several hours of fruitless search for his lost animal, he returns home. But when he opens the door to his house, his wife lets out a scream of surprise. He tries to reassure her, but she does not seem to hear his words. His children also seem not to see him. In his confusion, the man sits down on a bench and absent-mindedly begins to remove his shoes. The fern seed falls out onto the floor, and the man's wife lets out another scream of surprise at suddenly seeing her husband appear before her.[19]

On one Christmas Eve in Scotland, a man went to a ferny place to harvest fern seed. He soon saw a hare race by with a hound at its heels. A few minutes later, a stranger on horseback came to the ferny place and asked the man if he had seen a dog go by. The man, reticent, shook his head. The uncanny stranger then shrugged his shoulders and replied, "I'll overtake them soon enough." The man waited to see what would happen next. A few minutes later, he saw a stranger come by driving a crippled cow. The stranger asked him if he had seen a dog go by. Again, the man shook his head. The stranger answered, "I'll overtake them soon enough." This was too much for the man. He blurted out, "Ye idiot! Y'ill never get up with them." Because the man had broken his vow of silence, Satan loosened a storm that scattered all the fern seed and blew the man's hopes away.[20]

Literary Flowers

It is a blynde Goose that knoweth not a Foxe from a Ferne-bush.

—John Lyly, *Euphues and His England*

I have news for you; the stag bells, winter snows, summer has gone.
Wind high and cold, the sun low, short its course, the sea running high.
Deep red the bracken, its shade is lost; the wild goose has raised its accustomed cry.
Cold has seized the birds' wings; a season of ice, this is my news.

—An unknown Irish author of the 9th century,
qtd. in Jackson, *A Celtic Miscellany*

---

19. Hanns Bächtold-Stäubli, ed., *Handwörterbuch des deutschen Aberglaubens* (1927–42), vol. II (Berlin: Walter de Gruyter & Co., 1987), 1221.

20. *The Folk-Lore Journal*, vol. 1 (London: The Folk-Lore Society, 1883–89), 26.

The mistletoe hung in the castle hall,
The holly branch shone on the old oak wall.

—Thomas Haynes Bayly, "The Mistletoe Bough"

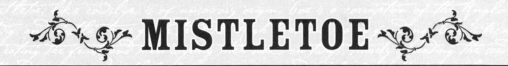

MISTLETOE

Name

The word "mistletoe," like "cowslip," is of unsavory origin. "Toe" is a corruption of the Anglo-Saxon word *tan*, meaning a twig, and "mistle" stems from the Old High German name for dung (this is because birds often propagate the plant by eating the fruits and distributing the seeds in their droppings). Mistletoe berries are viscous and white, hence the botanical names *Viscum* and *album*.

Viscum album is only one of many species and subspecies of mistletoe. It is important to note that American mistletoe *(Phoradendron spp.)* has toxic elements and must not be substituted for European mistletoe in medicinal recipes. The mistletoe found on oak trees is usually *Loranthus europaeus*, a completely different species from normal European mistletoe. Mistletoe is classified as belonging to the family of the **Loranthaceae**, and the order of the **Santalaceae**. According to various definitions, mistletoe is either parasitic or partially parasitic, because it does obtain some nourishment through the formation of chlorophyll in the stem and leaves.

Folk Names

Mistletoe was once known as misseltoe, and now goes by the names of birdlime mistletoe, mislin-bush, misle, devil's fuge, billy goat fodder, all-heal, kiss-and-go, and churchman's greeting. German names are even more numerous: *Mistel, Hexenbesen, Alfranken, Satanskraut, Donnerbesen, Marenstocken, Bocksfutter, Drudenfuß,* and *Donarbesen* (referring to personages of myth and legend). French appellations are *gui, gui commun, gui des druides, gui de chêne,* and *herbe de la croix*.

Italian names are *visco* and *vischia*, and the Spanish call it *muerduago*. In Holland, the plant is known as *düwelnest*; in Denmark as *mistelten*; in Poland as *jemiola*; in Hungary as *fehér byöngy*; in Wales as *uhelwydd*; and in Ireland as *drualus*.

Appearance

Mistletoe is a forked, rounded, evergreen bush that hangs downward from many different types of trees—usually fruit trees, but also birch, hawthorn, poplar, mulberry, hazel, and even evergreens. It is rare on lime trees and maple, and is never found on holly. The stem is thick and short, and the branches are greenish-brown, turning golden-green later on in the year. Each fork of the plant ends in a blossom in spring, and the plants tend to break at the forks.

Mistletoe leaves are leathery, opposite from each other on the stalk, tongue-shaped, greenish-yellow, and look a little like propellers or ears. The leaves fall off after two years, but the stalk remains green. Large balls of mistletoe of 3 ft. in diameter can be up to 30 years old. The flowers are inconspicuous and greenish-yellow, but have a fine smell that attracts flies and bees. Both male and female plants can be found on the same tree. The fruit is pea-sized—green at first, white or yellowish later, and contains one or two seeds enclosed in a sticky substance. Dried mistletoe breaks off into tiny segments at the joints.

Place, Season, and Useful Parts

Mistletoe does not grow in the extreme north, but can be found in southern through central Europe and on into Scandinavia. In North America, poisonous mistletoe species predominate, and their medicinal uses have not been studied extensively.

Mistletoe blossoms in March and April, and the fruit ripens in November or December. Because it is one of the few plants to bear fruit at this time of year, birds (especially the missel thrush) congregate in swarms in the trees and greedily devour the berries, cleaning their beaks on the bark after their feast. Because of the viscous liquid present in the fruits, the seeds stick to the tree and can soon grow into a new mistletoe plant.

In Scandinavia, mistletoe is traditionally gathered on Midsummer's Eve, and in Italy on the first day after the full moon. In other places, it is cut at the new moon. According to the Roman scholar Pliny, the Druids gathered it on the sixth day after the new moon.

Gathering, Drying, and Storage

There are many traditional methods of gathering mistletoe. As the readers of Asterix comics know, the Druids were very partial to oak mistletoe, which was gathered without using iron. Pliny wrote that the Druids ate and sacrificed under the oak tree, then led two white oxen underneath it, ornamented with wreaths on their horns. The priests climbed up into the tree and cut down the mistletoe with golden sickles, catching it in a white cloak before it touched the ground. The oxen were then sacrificed with a prayer for the tree spirit. This magical mistletoe was administered to render all sterile animals fruitful, and placed in water as an antidote against all poisons.

Although mistletoe can be gathered all year, Christmas mistletoe is traditionally believed to be most potent. In Wales, Christmas mistletoe was used to treat epilepsy, and branches that were hit down with a stone were considered more effective. According to one old belief, mistletoe was especially valued for children's diseases if shot from an oak tree with an arrow when the sun was in Sagittarius, on the first, third or fourth day before the new moon. It had to be caught with the left hand as it fell.

Mistletoe branches are usually gathered from November through April, depending on the weather. The leaves and young twigs are harvested for medicinal purposes just before the berries form, and should not be gathered when the temperature is below freezing. The easiest way to gather the herb is while trees are being logged, since this saves using ladders and instruments to cut down bunches of the herb, which are usually high up in the trees.

Mistletoe is largely a parasitic plant, and can stunt fruit and lumber trees if allowed to grow unchecked. When removing mistletoe, remove the branch as well to prevent reinfestation. Anthroposophical herbalists still avoid harvesting the plant with iron, catching it in cloths before it reaches the ground. They also make sure it does not come into contact with electrical or earth currents. This mistletoe is then processed to form the various preparations used in cancer treatment. Mistletoe tea can be kept for one year, and should be re-harvested the following year. It must be dried slowly and thoroughly. Because the plant is so leathery, it is best to cut the drug before drying.

Seed Saving and Germination

If desired, especially good mistletoe plants can be propagated in the same way the birds do it: by squashing the berries on the bark in a tree fork or in a crack where they will not be washed away. There is no information available on storing mistletoe seeds, although theoretically this should be possible.

Gardening Hints

Because mistletoe does not grow in soil, it cannot be properly classed as a garden plant. It can be "planted" by rubbing the ripe fruits onto tree bark, but very few gardeners are willing to have it growing near fruit trees, for it spreads rapidly and can damage the trees. In Switzerland, landowners are required by law to remove mistletoe growing on their property. Nonetheless, the symbiosis between parasite and host tree has not been fully researched. Mistletoe has been known to kill a weakened tree, but in other cases, both host and parasite seem to thrive.

Mistletoe seeds need light in order to germinate, and they also grow best with a little bird dung. The best way to plant mistletoe is to mimic as closely as possible what the missel thrush does when it eats the seeds, and then passes them through its intestinal system. The seeds are pressed into the bark, and then fertilized with some bird droppings or poultry manure. According to the magical law of opposites, mistletoe does not only take nutrients from a tree, but can also be used to make gardens more fruitful. Traditionally, mistletoe leaves were cut up finely, prayed over, and then sown with the desired crop.

Culinary Virtues
Because the berries are poisonous, mistletoe's only use in the kitchen is as a Christmas decoration.

Household Applications
Mistletoe is welcomed into the house during Christmastide as a holiday ornament. The plant was once banned from decorative use in churches because of its pagan associations, and exiled to the kitchen. The servants then kept the pagan traditions alive.[21]

Cosmetic Properties
In the sixteenth century, German botanist Hieronymus Bock wrote down a recipe for a cosmetic product that could strengthen rough and splitting fingernails. The product was composed of equal parts of lime, mistletoe powder, and wine yeast; stirred to a paste-like consistency with a little water; and applied regularly.

Medicinal Merits
According to Sir James George Frazer, British anthropologist and classical scholar, the "golden bough" was a panacea or cure-all for folk communities ranging from the Japanese Aino to the Senegalese Walos and the druids. In many places, mistletoe embodied the mythological healing powers of the bough; Frazer writes that in Holstein, Germany, it was "regarded as a panacea for green wounds," while in Lausanne, Switzerland, and the south of France, "the old Druidical belief in the mistletoe as an antidote to all poisons still survives among the peasantry." As late as the eighteenth century, medical authorities in England and Holland considered it a treatment for the falling sickness. But such enthusiasm among physicians eventually declined: "Whereas

---

21. John Brand and Sir Henry Ellis, *Observations on the Popular Antiquities of Great Britain* (1849). 3 vol. (Detroit, MI: Singing Tree Press, 1969).

the Druids thought that mistletoe cured everything," Frazer notes, "modern doctors appear to think that it cures nothing."[22]

It may be that the modern disdain for mistletoe as a medicinal herb comes from a misunderstanding of its primary medicinal values. It was once used indiscriminately to treat diseases that it could not cure, and employed as a medicine of last resort. Its reputation suffered as a result. St. Vitus' dance, St. Anthony's fire, epilepsy, catalepsy, sudden pains in the chest, muscular atrophy, cancerous growths, sterility, and impotence were all treated with mistletoe. It was believed to have a beneficial effect on the spleen and, in the words of Nicholas Culpeper, to "ripen and discuss" hard knots and abscesses and to heal ruptures. Oak-tree mistletoe was generally considered best for these purposes, followed by pear and hazel mistletoe. There was one ancient oak tree in France, laden with mistletoe, that was a famous pilgrimage site for those troubled with epileptic fits. Willow mistletoe was used in Switzerland to treat St. Anthony's fire, and apple mistletoe was a recognized remedy in England for "the fits." Rings made from mistletoe were thought to be effective against epilepsy, and mistletoe gathered on Midsummer's Day was considered especially effective against all complaints.

Mistletoe has been cultivated for many centuries in the Far East as a medicine used, among other applications, for lowering blood pressure. It has been unearthed in prehistoric archeological sites in Switzerland—evidence that it has been used in medicine and magic for a very long time.

Modern Medicine

It seems strange that there has been little or no research on the different healing properties of mistletoe (*Viscus album*) as opposed to *Loranthus europaeus*. In older medical texts, the mistletoe spoken of was usually *Loranthus europaeus*, but in our time, *Viscum album* is the mistletoe used.

Modern herbalists prescribe mistletoe as a regulatory herb. It can help in the regulation of erratic blood pressure, especially high blood pressure, but can also raise low blood pressure without lessening heart function. It is still administered to those suffering from epilepsy to alleviate that disease. It is used, together with hawthorn and garlic, as one of the most important regulatory herbs for the prevention of heart and circulatory troubles, and is administered, along with valerian, when the patient is especially nervous. Excessive uterine or other unexplainable internal bleeding can be regulated with the help of the herb, and it is also administered to diabetics. After giving birth, women are given mistletoe tea to lessen bleeding and to improve the circulation. It is not generally administered to children.

---

22. Frazer, "Balder and the Mistletoe," *The Golden Bough* (1890–1915) (New York: Macmillan, 1966).

The parts of the mistletoe used medicinally are the leaves and twigs of the European, but not the American, mistletoe—because the berries of the American mistletoe are poisonous. European mistletoe also has toxic properties, especially if the active principle is extracted and injected directly into the bloodstream, or if the berries are eaten in large amounts. But the young twigs and leaves, taken orally in small, regular doses, do not have adverse effects on patients. Even modern doctors recognize the worth of European mistletoe in the treatment of cancer, and recommend it as a treatment when nothing else will work. It is presently one the most widely administered cancer drugs in Germany. It is injected in small doses under the skin or directly into the tumor, and acts to slow the growth of the tumor as well as to relieve pain. European mistletoe found growing on different host trees is used for different types of cancer. But the herb is also effective and valuable as preventive cancer medicine, taken regularly in small doses.

Mistletoe is widely used in Chinese medicine, although there is much confusion between the Chinese and anthroposophical uses of the herb. The preparation Iscador, widely employed in Europe for the supplementary treatment of cancer, is prepared according to the anthroposophical beliefs of Rudolf Steiner and has nothing to do with traditional Chinese methods. It is interesting to note that mistletoe preparations used in the supplementary treatment of cancer are most effective if administered in small doses. Larger doses seem to be ineffective. For other complaints, mistletoe is usually prescribed as an infusion (prepared with cold water overnight), as a fresh juice, or as a powdered drug in capsule form.

Externally, mistletoe is used alone or in combination with horsetail or lady's mantle in baths to treat uterine pains. Cold feet, chilblains, and chapped hands can be warmed with mistletoe foot and hand baths. Mistletoe plasters are applied to facial neuralgia.

A homeopathic remedy of European mistletoe is used to treat epilepsy, chorea, rheumatic deafness, asthma, and Raynaud's syndrome. It is also prescribed for endometriosis and metrorrhagia.

Special Cures

Mistletoe Honey: Mistletoe is usually given in tea or powdered form, or prepared commercially for injection into cancer patients. A simple folk method of taking the herb is to crush the not-yet-fruiting plant with a mortar and pestle and to then add the crushed herb to fresh honey. Mistletoe honey can be enjoyed on its own, a teaspoon at a time, or used to sweeten other herbal teas. Mistletoe can be taken longer than most herbs, but not for longer than a year at a time. Some herbalists recommend using it only during the winter months.

Uses in Husbandry

In ancient Greece and Rome, mistletoe was gathered for its resin, which was fermented and used as glue and birdlime. The sticky yellow glue was spread on tree limbs to catch birds, especially thrushes, which were in great demand as a culinary delicacy. The thrushes, which are primarily responsible for the propagation of mistletoe, were caught in birdlime of their own production. Mistletoe can also be fed to goats, cattle, and sheep, and was once widely used in Europe as fodder. Hares and deer eat mistletoe readily if they can reach it, and martens are rumored to have a weakness for the berries. Bees are often attracted to the plant's tiny flowers

Because it bears fruit at an unusual time of year, mistletoe has played a central role in many rituals to promote the fertility of fruit trees and animals. In Austria, mistletoe was tied to the fruit trees during the twelve days of Christmas (December 25th–January 6th) to ensure a bumper crop the following year. In Pomerania and Bavaria, mistletoe was hung in the house and stall to deter witches and evil spirits. In the British Isles, Christmas mistletoe was given to the first cow to calve in the new year, protecting all the other cattle from barrenness, illness, and witchcraft for the whole year. In the Slavic countries, a cow about to calve was protected by cutting off the tip of a discarded cow horn. Mistletoe, cornelian cherry wood, and gunpowder were wrapped in linen and the bundle placed in the horn, which was then put in a corner of the stall. Central European witches, intent on stealing milk, were said to rub cows with a hazelnut and mistletoe branch before the cows were led out to pasture in the spring.

Transylvanian herders once cut hairs from an unruly stallion's tail and mane to keep him from straying. The hairs were wrapped in a cloth, together with mistletoe collected from a pear tree. Once the horse was safely inside the stable, the herder bored a hole in the threshold, inserted the cloth, and then stoppered the hole carefully with a plug of hazel wood. The horse was then led out until one hoof was across the threshold, squarely placed on the fresh earth. The herder then traced the horse's hoof with a knife and cut out the soil. He poured salt into the hole before replacing the plug of turf. From that day on, the horse would stay close to home and become manageable.

Veterinary Values

Pliny recommended beating barren animals with mistletoe twigs, also known as life rods. Sterile cattle and sheep are still given mistletoe tea in some areas. After birth, a tea prepared from hawthorn or maple mistletoe is also administered to cattle. In ancient times, veterinarians recommended pouring a mistletoe-and-wine concoction up the noses of animals as a preventive measure against infectious diseases. Bewitched animals were beaten with mistletoe switches and given mistletoe beer. In Poland, women added mistletoe to the food of their piglets on April 25th. This was believed to magically free the piglets from disease for one year.

Miscellaneous Wisdom

Mistletoe was once known as the *virga aurea*, because it turns golden at a time when the host trees lose their leaves and the sun is at its lowest ebb—the winter solstice. A golden ball of mistletoe found growing in an old oak is a wondrous sight, and is rightly considered to have magical properties. Like the figure in fairy tales that comes to the King, it neither rides nor walks; it is neither fish nor flesh, naked nor bare, fasting nor full. It does not grow in the earth yet is tied to the soil by its host tree, and is neither herb of the air nor of the earth. It is related to the moon as well as to the sun, fire, lightning, and thunder, and to the colors gold, white, and green. It is sometimes brought to church on Palm Sunday as one of the "palms."

Magical Powers

The many folk names given to this herb point to the plant's association with forces, spirits, and deities that are not quite "canny." Mistletoe is one of the plants we understand the least, and cannot explain and classify by rational means (it is fitting that mistletoe is prescribed for one disease that we also cannot come to terms with: cancer). In the Slavic countries and in Sweden, mistletoe was once hung over the threshold of a house to drive away nightmares. Similarly, it was often hung over beds in Holland and Sweden, to protect sleepers from nightmares. When witches seemed to be causing bad weather in the Tyrolean treetops, a mistletoe wreath was wrapped around a tree to trap them—the weather would then change immediately. In Flanders, mistletoe is believed to grow where a nightmare or a night hag rested on a tree.

The Balder myth of the Edda tells how the young and vibrant spring god, Baldur, is shot and killed by the winter god, Hodur, with a shaft of evergreen mistletoe, all because of the machinations of the troublemaker Loki. Hunters once believed that carrying mistletoe could help to make them "bulletproof" or even invisible. Albertus Magnus, the German philosopher and alchemist, believed that birds would congregate in a tree if mistletoe were hung there alongside a swallow's wing (this is not surprising, seeing how partial birds are to the berries). It is said that if mistletoe grows on a white hazelnut, a treasure can be found as far beneath the tree as the mistletoe is high. In Sweden, this treasure was found with the help of oak mistletoe and Christ's picture, or with a mistletoe divining rod. In other places, magical beings such as alrauns, hazel worms, or snakes are believed to live under hazel mistletoe. In Wales, a snake with a ruby head was thought to protect treasure under ash mistletoe.

The Welsh saying is, "No mistletoe, no luck," and the Welsh believed that mistletoe hung under the roof would bring good fortune. It was carried in Transylvanian weddings to bring luck to the bridal pair. In France, it was believed that a train would not jump the tracks if mistletoe were placed in one of the wagons. Classical writers were convinced that mistletoe, in combination with other herbs such as the martagon lily, could open all locks. In order to be magically effective, mistletoe had to be found growing in a tree, received as a gift, or better yet, stolen. Mistletoe that has been purchased is not considered potent.

The belief was once prevalent that trees with mistletoe growing in them would not be struck by lightning, and that mistletoe could help to put out fires. Houses ornamented with mistletoe would not be hit by lightning, and would not burn down.

In France, children go from house to house at New Year's Eve with a green bouquet of mistletoe to pass on New Year's greetings. They were once protected from bad magic with mistletoe amulets and from witchcraft with mistletoe and angelica amulets. In Wales, it is believed that a sleeper will have prophetic dreams if a sprig of mistletoe gathered at Midsummer is placed under his or her pillow. In Somerset, mistletoe is hung in the hall at Christmas, and each berry means a kiss. In Worcestershire, the bough was hung by the last domestic to join the family. It was decorated with ribbons, apples, and nuts, and could be lowered with a cord so that a lady could remove a berry after being kissed. If there were no berries left on the branch, then it was used to beat fertility into bystanders. Mistletoe was once believed to have fallen from a heavenly tree, and later it came to represent Jesus on the Cross.[23]

Unlike most other Christmas greens, mistletoe was often left in the house after Christmas, and only removed the following year. In other regions, it was believed that all kissers would become enemies if the mistletoe was not burned before Twelfth Night. In Hereford, England, mistletoe was cut from apple trees and poplars on New Year's Eve and hung up just as the clock struck twelve. At the same time, last year's mistletoe was taken down and burned. It was considered bad luck in Wales and the border countries to bring mistletoe into the house *before* Christmas. In Sweden, the golden leaves hanging from a bare tree were taken to be a symbol of life and resurrection.

In the Victorian language of flowers, a gift of mistletoe was taken to mean "I surmount difficulties."

Oracular Worth

In Poland, it is considered a sign of bad times if mistletoe grows on willows or alders. If it grows on a whitethorn in Bretagne, in France, there will be many soldiers

---

23. Wilhelm Mannhardt, *Der Baumkultus der Germanen und ihrer Nachbarstämme* (Berlin: Bornträger, 1875).

for conscription. Generally, a good crop of mistletoe at Christmas is taken as a sign that there will be plenty of corn during the following year.

Literary Flowers

> The doves flew on …
> Alit together on one chosen tree,
> Through whose dark branches shone a glint of gold
> As in the depth of winter—cold in the woods
> The mistletoe is green with sprouting leaf,
> The mistletoe that no tree seeds, that wreathes
> Their trunks with its pale pearl-colored berries - so
> In the evergreen-gloom of the dark ilex-tree
> The leafy gold work—as in the gentle winds
> Jangled its metal foil.
>
> —VIRGIL, THE AENEID

Mistletoe is a child of the sun, generated by lightning, cradled in the top of a tree by the wind and moon. We take it to help the sterile conceive, and to stop cancer from growing hidden in the body. It is balanced between heaven and earth, neither in this world, nor in another, at the branching point between the seasons, a baby oak in the womb. It is known as both golden and silver, yet seems impervious to the flux of the seasons and to the waning and waxing moon. It bears fruit in winter, and fades against the green foliage of its host in summer.

—SISTER CLARISSA'S UNPUBLISHED BOOK OF NATURAL OBSERVATIONS

SOLAR

HERBS

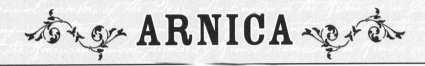

Enclosed in dark bottles, its smell vivifies and restores the sun
to even the darkest sick room in winter.

—SISTER CLARISSA

ARNICA

Name

The name "arnica" is of uncertain etymology, from a Latin base. *Montana* signifies arnica grown in mountainous regions.

The arnicas are perennial members of the **Daisy**, also known as the *Asteraceae* or *Compositae*, family. There is a good deal of confusion between European arnica (*Arnica montana*, which is the one generally referred to in old herbals), and the American arnicas (primarily *Arnica chamissonis* or *Arnica cordifolia*). To confuse matters further, in the American Southwest and Mexico, another member of this family is also known under the name of Arnica: *Arnica mexicana* or *Heterotheca inuloides*, also known as telegraph weed or camphor weed, which is often substituted for European arnica.

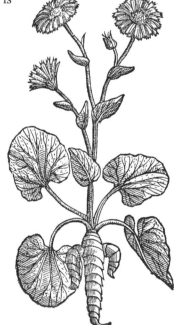

Folk Names

European arnica is also known as mountain tobacco, leopard's bane, or lamb's skin. In German-speaking countries, the herb is called *Arnika, Wohlverleih, Wolfsblume, Gemsblume, Altvatermark, Bergwurz, Berg-wohlverleih, Donnerblume, Kraftrose,* and *Magdalenenkraut*; in French-speaking areas, *arnique, arnica, panacée des chutes, tabac des vosges*; in Italian, *arnica, tabachine,* and *starnudele*. Russian names are *barranik* and *arnika gornaja*. The great German herbalist of the twelfth century, Hildegard von Bingen, called the plant *Wolfsgelena*. (The "wolf" does not refer to the wild animal, but to a skin disease still referred to as *Wolff* in some German dialects.)

Appearance

The most important identifying characteristics of arnica are its unmistakably strong, sunny, spicy smell and the dark egg-yolk color of the flower. The leaves form a rosette, with a few broad leaves placed on the stalk. Arnica is often confused with other yellow-blossoming plants such as dandelion, fleawort, or hawkbit.

The arnica root is dark brown with a whitish marrow, and is surrounded by wiry but brittle rootlets. The leaf rosette lies flat on the ground and the stalk rises to a maximum height of 18 in. with 1–3 pairs of fairly large, medium-green leaves. The herb is aromatic and the taste of the orange-yellow flower is strongly aromatic, even bitter. The flowers are hairy and the flower petals uneven, giving the herb a straggly appearance.

Place, Season, and Useful Parts

Arnica montana is a mountain plant, and grows best from 6,000 ft. on up, although it can also be found at lower elevations (in meadows, moors, heaths, grassy slopes, on humus-rich or sandy soil, or in light coniferous woods). It is often cultivated and can be encouraged to reproduce in its natural habitat. Mountain arnica either grows singly, or appears in great numbers, and is indigenous to Central Europe. It can be found as far north as southern Scotland, as far east as Russia, and as far south as Italy. American arnica grows in the Western part of North America, but has also been cultivated in Russia, East Germany, and Poland in less mountainous areas where *Arnica montana* will not thrive. There are many local variants in North America, and proper identification is necessary before medicinal use.

Arnica blooms from June to August, and it is traditionally gathered on Midsummer's Day. The roots are dug in the fall, or in the spring before the plant blossoms. In many countries, it is illegal to gather wild arnica, and arnica for commercial use must be cultivated.

Gathering, Drying, and Storage

Arnica montana has been over-harvested in many areas, and is sometimes protected by law. It should only be harvested if it grows wild in large numbers. Arnica flowers are gathered on sunny days in summer and packed loosely into baskets, either with or without the calyx (flower receptacle). Arnica leaves are harvested from May to August. The roots of three- or four-year-old plants are collected in the fall after the leaves die, or again in the spring. In order to leave enough plants for reproduction, it is advisable to only harvest one in three roots, taking care to include all the fine side-roots.

Arnica flowers must be dried immediately after picking, before they wilt. It is best to dry them on white paper with the help of artificial heat. Insects are easily visible on the paper and can be discarded. The leaves are dried in the shade, and should be inspected after drying for discolored spots. Discolored leaves must be thrown out. Dried arnica flowers are stored in dark containers for not longer than one year, and arnica tincture must be stored in dark bottles. Then it will keep for several years.

Seed Saving and Germination

Arnica is notoriously difficult to establish from seed, and will often refuse to germinate, driving even the most patient gardener to desperation. The best method of propagation is to find a stand of wild arnica, and then keep the area weeded and tended, encouraging the arnica to reproduce itself in its own time. This way, a whole field of arnica can be obtained for harvesting in a very short time. There are few distinct cultivated arnica varieties, since it is primarily a wild plant.

Gardening Hints

Arnica flowers are usually gathered from wild plants, but the plant has also been introduced into gardens occasionally. It was first grown in Britain in 1759, and has been cultivated since then on rough, high places, in light moors and heaths, and on poor pastures. Arnica grows best in a mixture of loam, peat, and sand, and prefers higher altitudes. It may refuse to grow in rich garden soil or at lower altitudes, and germination is notoriously erratic. In the spring, arnica can be reproduced by plant division; or the seeds can be sown early, in cold frames, and then transplanted in May, or the seeds can be sown in their final position in late spring. To guarantee a relatively even distribution of the seeds, mix them with three parts grass seed (this also avoids the necessity of thinning). The earth must be packed down around the seeds, without covering them completely with soil. If all goes well, the seeds will sprout in two weeks. Arnica flowers can be harvested in two years, and the roots three to four years later.

Arnica is attacked by many insects. Beetles, moths, and the resulting caterpillars are attracted to the leaves. The plant is often a host for molds, and tiny arnica flies lay their eggs in the flower heads. Given all the difficulties involved with the growing of arnica, it is a good idea to study plants growing in the wild and try to duplicate the conditions found there. Growers who have had the best success with arnica have simply naturalized it in a nearby meadow, mown the grass after the plants set seed, and watched the herb reproduce itself.

Household Applications

Arnica was once added to beers and meads as a spice, but this practice has now gone out of fashion.

Cosmetic Properties

Individual reactions to the external use of arnica vary widely. Those with sensitive skin, or who develop a reaction to the herb, should avoid arnica, but everyone else should keep a bottle of the tincture within reach (see the recipe below). It is a gentle disinfectant that can increase the circulation in a wounded area and has a pronounced healing effect on skin infections and blemishes. Arnica tincture, or an infusion of arnica flowers, is often added to strong cleansing mixtures, to soaps, and to acne skin creams. Arnica tincture can be incorporated into bracing facial tonics. Those suffering from hair and scalp troubles can also add arnica to hair tonics to promote scalp circulation.

Medicinal Merits

Mountain arnica was first officially sold in apothecaries in the eighteenth century, and it is still a treasured folk remedy in those countries where it grows wild. Native Americans have used various arnica species as wound remedies for centuries, and the German herbal priest Sebastian Kneipp was enthusiastic in his praise, recommending arnica as the "best first aid for wounds."[24] During the Second World War, the high value of American arnica was rediscovered by mainstream medicine, and it is now considered as potent as the European herb.

Modern Medicine

Most Alpine householders keep a bottle of homemade arnica tincture close at hand for use on cuts, burns, scrapes, bruises, wounds, sprains, blood effusions, and sunburn. Its healing qualities as first aid are truly phenomenal: arnica applied *immediately* to a wound will increase the circulation to the affected area and greatly lessen the possibility of swelling, further bruising, bleeding, or infection. The leaves can also be used as bandages for fresh wounds. Arnica tincture is further employed in the external, and gradual, treatment of rheumatic complaints, arthritis, sprains, and dislocations. It can aid the healing of broken bones, abscesses, and operation wounds, infected veins or fingernails, or, if the skin is still unbroken, it can also be used to paint chilblains. Arnica tincture should be diluted before application, and its use must be discontinued if any signs of skin irritation occur. Singers gargle with diluted arnica tincture to strengthen their voices and counteract hoarseness and exhaustion. A diluted arnica mouthwash can also strengthen bleeding gums. A warm footbath of strongly diluted arnica tea, or very strongly diluted arnica tincture, can warm chilled or tender feet.

There is a great deal of misunderstanding concerning the internal use of arnica. American arnica *(Arnica chamissonis* or *Arnica cordifolia)* should not be taken internally,

---

24.   Qtd. in Richard Willfort, *Gesundheit durch Heilkräuter* (Linz, Austria: Rudolf Trauner, 1973), 53.

but is used in much the same fashion as the European arnica, in tincture or salve form. Mexican arnica *(Heterotheca inuloides)* can, on the other hand, be used internally with caution for menstrual and intestinal cramps. Herbalists are divided on the internal use of the European arnica, *Arnica montana*. Some say that it is poisonous and should never be used internally, while others recommend it as a valuable circulatory herb if used in moderation. The solution to this contradiction lies, as usual, in the middle. The symptoms of a reaction to arnica are a scratching sensation in the throat, difficulty in breathing, nausea, and, in extreme cases, fits of shivering or dizziness. People with weak stomachs should avoid the internal use of arnica altogether. If any allergic reactions to arnica occur, its use should immediately be discontinued. It should only be administered in small amounts in combination with other herbs, and should never be taken for extended periods. Filtering out the tiny flower hairs through filter paper after initial straining can lessen the irritant effect of arnica flower tea. Pregnant women should avoid use of the herb altogether.

Because of its irritant action and its positive effect on the circulation, arnica is employed internally in the treatment of arteriosclerosis, circulatory disorders, water retention, and as a medicine to provoke menstruation. It is further used as a vermifuge and a general stimulant. Arnica plays a role in the treatment of heart muscle weakness, concussions, paralysis, and gout.

Homeopathy makes use of arnica tincture externally and arnica roots internally for the treatment of epilepsy and exhaustion. Arnica is one of the prime remedies for trauma when administered homeopathically. Homeopathic arnica is also given to Alzheimer's patients, and victims of emotional abuse and trauma. Interestingly enough, it is also a good remedy for dogs suffering from abuse or fear of thunderstorms.

Arnica roots are primarily used in folk medicine, taken in tea form to help stop bleeding in the kidney and lungs, and to counteract diarrhea. A dose of 3–6 grains of pulverized roots in 1 qt. of wine is considered useful in the treatment of opium addiction withdrawal, and arnica root tea has been given as first aid for mushroom poisoning.

Special Cures

Arnica Tincture: Arnica is most effective in alcohol, not in salve form, as is the case with several other wound herbs. To make an arnica tincture, loosely fill a clean, clear glass bottle or jar with fresh arnica flowers (they can also be dried, although best results are obtained from fresh flowers). Cover with 90–96 percent spirits, and place the container in the sun for 2–3 weeks. Shake the bottle once every day. After 2–3 weeks, strain the liquid through a strainer, then filter it again through filter paper to remove all flower particles. Dilute the resulting liquid with distilled water, 1 part liquid to 2 parts water. Pour into a dark glass bottle, and store in a cool, dark place. If high-proof spirits are not available, strong clear spirits such as gin, vodka, Slivovitz, or tequila may be used, and diluted with less distilled water.

A Tea for the Regulation of High Blood Pressure: A tea mixture for the regulation and prevention of high blood pressure can be mixed from 3 parts of yarrow, 4 parts melilot *(Melilotus officinalis)*, 2 parts goose grass *(Potentilla anserina)*, 2 parts club moss *(Lycopodium clavatum)*, 2 parts whitethorn leaves and flowers *(Crataegus laevigata)*, 1 part cowslip flowers, 3 parts lemon balm leaves, 3 parts mistletoe (only the European mistletoe, *Viscum album*, should be used here), 1 part vervain *(Veronica officinalis)*, ½ part masterwort *(Peucedanum ostruthium)* roots, 2 parts lavender flowers, 1½ parts angelica roots, and 1½ parts arnica flowers. Mix the herbs together well. Prepare a tea from the mixture once a day and fill it into a thermos bottle to keep it warm. Drink 2–3 times a day over a period of 4–8 weeks. After this cure, switch to another tea with similar effects for at least a month.

Uses in Husbandry

The irritant quality of arnica flowers, with their fine hairs, is so strong that even practiced snuffers can be tickled into a sneeze with arnica snuff. Arnica leaves have also been smoked, especially in France and Sweden, as a tobacco substitute. But the substitute is not always as good as the original, and arnica tobacco can cause yawning and an itching sensation.

Arnica is not a favorite among agriculturalists, because only goats eat it with relish. It robs growing space from other more productive fodder plants. Cows can even be poisoned if they are pastured in an arnica meadow, and their milk will turn red. For treatment of this kind of poisoning, see the eyebright chapter. It is interesting to note that the North American *Arnica chamissonis* was once commercially cultivated as a medicinal plant in Russia, Poland, and East Germany, enjoying more attention and higher praise there that in its native land.

Veterinary Values

Arnica tincture can be applied externally to most of the wounds, sprains, bruises and cuts of household and farmyard animals with good effect. Above and beyond this, it is a good farmhouse disinfectant for minor injuries. The internal use of arnica for animals is not recommended: horses will suffer from exhaustion if injected with arnica, and dogs may react negatively to arnica tea. Nonetheless, a miniscule amount of arnica roots, mixed with other digestive herbs, can be given to animals with colic or those who have lost their appetites.

Miscellaneous Wisdom

Arnica blooms at the time of the summer solstice, and its flowers show a remarkable similarity to the summer sun. This has led to the practice of picking arnica on Midsummer's Day, when the flowers are thought to possess the warm, burning power of the solstice sun.

Hildegard von Bingen thought the plant so strongly imbued with solar influence that she warned of its overwhelming, even poisonous, aphrodisiacal powers. According to her, a wishful wooer only had to rub an arnica leaf against the skin of another person to make him (or her) flame into passion. The passion would then develop into love madness as soon as the arnica leaf withered.

Children in Central and Eastern Europe make a "bed" of arnica flowers, daisies, and bluebells at Midsummer, and then lay a saint's picture on the floral cushion. They expect to find money under the picture in the morning, or to see the image of St. John's head among the flowers. If this happens, then the arnica will have extraordinary healing powers.

Arnica also plays a major role in agricultural and household magic. When it is placed among the rafters or behind a crucifix, or burned in the four corners of a grain field, it is believed to protect the house and crops from hail and lightning (midsummer arnica is considered the best for this). Arnica's solar qualities are called upon during storms, when the herb is burned in an attempt to discourage bad weather. In Austria, the pupae of arnica flies found inside the swollen flower heads were once thought to protect fields against fire, ergot, and insect infestation.

Children with a mind for mischief pulverize arnica flowers and use the fine dust as sneeze or itch powder.

Literary Flowers

The mountain climber last sees in his fall the plant he trampled in his haste to top the mountain. Arnica ... and the miniature sun blazes in his mind, suffusing his fall with its piercing odor. Coming up out of the confusion of hurt, he finds himself bathed in the flower. Arnica ... through its ministrations, his bruised body congeals back to life.

The chamois flower lives in the mountains, not far from wolves and mountain goats, lightning, hail and sun. It comes into bloom on Midsummer's Day, when the sun is strongest. It is gathered on the highest peaks and brought to the valley to protect the inhabitants. A tincture protects animals and humans from hurt, the stalks placed in the corner of the fields or on the roof protect against lightning, thunder and hail as well as crop enemies. The storm is encouraged to move on when arnica is thrown into the fire and its sweet-acrid smoke crawls up the chimney to fight the storm clouds. Enclosed in dark bottles, its smell vivifies and restores the sun to even the darkest sick room in winter.

—Sister Clarissa's Unpublished Book of Natural Observations

A chaplet of herbs I'll make
With Basil then I will begin
Whose scent is wondrous pleasing.

—Michael Drayton, *Poly-Olbion*, Song I

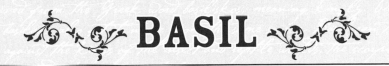

BASIL

Name

The name "basil" is derived from the Greek word *basiliskos*, meaning "kingly." The legendary reptile whose looks can kill, the basilisk, also got its name from this source. According to folk logic, basil can protect humans against the kings of the insect and reptile worlds—the scorpion and the basilisk. Basil is a plant fit for any king, and a king among herbs.

There are countless species and varieties of basil, producing a whole palette of different fragrances, colors, and shapes, but almost all the basils, with a few notable exceptions, are annuals. If taken indoors in the fall, they will usually die back over the winter. Sweet basil *(Ocimum basilicum)* is a member of the **Mint** family (the **Lamiaceae**, earlier known as the **Labiatae)**, and includes both *Ocimum basilicum ssp. basilicum* (large-leaved basil) and *Ocimum basilicum ssp. minimum* (which is often sold as an ornamental). Other basil species include *Ocimum americanum* (American or hoary basil), *Ocimum canum* (camphor or hoary basil), *Ocimum gratissimum* (known as Fever plant or Tea bush and planted as a hedge in Africa and India), and *Ocimum tenuiflorum* (Indian holy basil or Tulsi).

Folk Names

The Anglo-Saxon name for the plant was *nedevyrt*; English names are common basil, sweet basil, garden basil, Josephwort, and St. Joseph's wort. Lesser basil is also known in English as bush basil or monk's basil. Germans call the herb *Basilikum, Basilienkraut, Königskraut, Königsbalsam, Pfefferkraut, Nelkenbasilie, Braunsilge, Josefskräutlein, Hirnkraut,* and *Herrenkraut.* In France, it goes under the names *basile, basilie, basilic, herbe royal, oranger des savatiers, frambasin,* and *pistou*; in Holland, *vol mynte*; in Italy, *basilico, bassilico, basili*; and in Spanish-speaking countries, *albahace menor, albajaca,* or *albahaca.* Sanskrit names are *munjariki, surasa,* and *varvara.*

Appearance

Both sweet and bush basil exude a pleasant, balsamic, spicy fragrance and have a uniquely fiery and peppery taste. Basil is one of the few aromatic herbs that does not have to be crushed to release its oils. When basil is disturbed, a cloud of fragrance is released by the plant. Sweet basil can grow to a height of 3 ft., depending on the variety. The plant has a four-cornered stem and dark green, egg-shaped, shiny green leaves, often wrinkled. According to Nicholas Culpeper in his famous herbal,

> The greater or ordinary bazil riseth up usually with one upright stalk diversely branching forth on all sides, with two leaves at every joint, which are somewhat broad and round, yet pointed, of a pale green colour, but fresh; a little snipped about the edges, and of a strong healthy scent.[25]

The upper leaves are often tinged with purple. Basil flowers are labiate, white, off-white, purple, or pink, and are situated in whorls at the tip of the stem. The plant's fruit is dark brown, containing four tiny black or dark brown seeds that turn slimy when softened in water.

Bush basil only grows to a height of 1 ft. The leaves are much paler, smaller, and more pointed. The seeds do not always ripen in the north. Some basil varieties have miniscule leaves, which form a fragrant "head" of basil. Many green varieties sport a plant or two with dark purple leaves. Other varieties are completely purple or ruffled, or have blistered leaves. Basil fragrances range from spice to camphor, cinnamon, cloves, lemon, or even licorice.

Holy basil has smaller, less shiny leaves and a compact shape.

Place, Season, and Useful Parts

Basil is primarily a garden and a flowerpot herb. It grows wild in most tropical zones and occasionally escapes from cultivated areas, but only rarely survives in the north. Basil is an annual, although the seeds remain fertile for up to five years. The plant blossoms from July to September, according to climactic conditions, and should be gathered before flowering. Basil seeds are gathered as they ripen, in August or September.

Holy or sacred basil, *Ocimum tenuiflorum*, has been cultivated in India for at least 3,000 years, and several other species can be found growing wild in Africa.

Gathering, Drying, and Storage

It is possible, with careful planning and a warm climate, to cut basil twice every season. Cut the plant first on a sunny July day, just before it blossoms, down to the first branches. This first crop is always superior in aroma and quality to subsequent harvests. The second cutting can be made in September, when the plant attempts to blossom a second time.

---

25. Culpeper, *Culpeper's Complete Herbal* (1653) (London: Foulsham, undated), 39.

For kitchen use, the not-quite flowering tops can be nipped off in July, and then cut periodically until September. Do not be afraid of damaging the main stem: bushier plants will form only if the main stem is cut back, allowing the plant to bring forth new leaves.

Basil should be dried quickly in a shady, airy place, or in a dehydrator. The plant can be spread out thinly on trays or on cloths, or tied in bundles and hung upside down. Dried basil must retain a healthy green color on drying, and should be stored in dark containers in a dry place.

Seed Saving and Germination

Basil varieties are easily cross-pollinated by bees, and must be isolated if the varieties are to be kept pure. Many commercial varieties do not come true to type, and some plants from the same seed packet may look completely different from the others. This is because some companies are not taking as much care with the varietal purity of marginally profitable species.

Because bees pollinate the plants, spatial isolation is ideal for maintaining varietal purity. It is also possible to stagger the ripening of different varieties, or to cut back one variety while the other flowers. This way, it is possible to harvest at least two distinct varieties from one plot. Otherwise, the two varieties must be isolated under cages, and bees introduced into the cages to pollinate the flowers.

Basil seeds fall out easily from the seed receptacles, and it is difficult to determine the best time to harvest seeds. If the seed stalks are cut too late, no seeds may be left in them; if cut too early, the seeds will not have ripened. The easiest method is to look at the seed receptacles with a magnifying glass several times to determine when the seeds are fully ripened, and when they begin to fall out. The seed-bearing stalks can be harvested shortly before the majority of the seeds ripen, and allowed to dry on paper in a cool, airy place. Despite the fact that the seeds fall out, others will be difficult to remove. Because of this, it is advisable to rub the seed stalks through a sieve to release the last seeds. The leafy residue can be used for seasoning purposes.

Gardening Hints

Basil was cultivated at an early date, particularly in India. It moved westward, if legend can be believed, with the armies of Alexander the Great. Pyramid findings have proved that the ancient Egyptians cultivated it as early as 3500 BC, and there has been a continuous record of its cultivation in Mediterranean countries since 200 BC. It reached Germany in AD 1100, England in 1548, and the United States before 1806. Basil is now cultivated in most of the world and thrives in warm climates.

Basil is such a temperamental garden plant that the Romans, as Pliny tells us, tried to encourage its growth by contrary magic. It was sown with curses, insults, and prayers to the gods for its destruction; it was plowed under while growing; the young plants were stepped upon, scalded with boiling water, and watered at noon—all in the hopes of getting a good crop.

Despite its difficult nature, basil's fragrance is so pleasant and its taste so enjoyable that a gardening attempt is worth the effort. Fragrance is released each time the leaves are disturbed or touched, imbuing the garden with a pungent aroma. There is a bewildering array of basil varieties available in the most exciting fragrances: cinnamon, cloves, lemon, and spice. Many gardeners suffer from something akin to basil addiction, hunting for ever-new fragrances and leaf forms. Small bush basil is best suited for planting in flowerpots, and broad-leaved basil is ideal for large-scale cultivation and drying. Basil does not always do well in the north: it is extremely frost sensitive, "freezing" at temperatures above the freezing point, and it matures so slowly in colder climates that it is easy prey for snails, who adore it.

Basil requires rich, well-fertilized, loose soil and cannot compete with aggressive weeds. Because almost all basils are annuals, they must be re-sown each year. The best results can be obtained by sowing the seeds at the end of March under glass or in peat pots, and then transplanting them into bigger pots without disturbing the roots. The plants are only placed in their final position when all danger of frost is passed. Outdoor sowings are only advisable in warmer, humid climates. The young plants should be shaded for a few days after transplanting and protected from wind during the entire growing season. They are thankful for a sheltered southern position and do well in pots. Basil has few insect enemies, but snails make up for that and can mow down basil plantings overnight.

It is possible to prolong the season by transplanting basil into pots and bringing them into the house before the first frost, but the plants will eventually die back. Many windowsill gardeners are too timid to cut the plant's main stem back in summer, with the result that the plant soon sets seed and dies. If you want to keep basil producing leaves in a pot, nip out the main stem and keep cutting back any flowers. New leaves will soon form at the nodes, producing bushier, healthier-looking plants.

One old scrap of gardener's wisdom: if rue and basil are planted together, the basil will be overpowered by the stronger herb, and eventually curl up and die.

Culinary Virtues

Basil is one of the most valuable aromatic kitchen herbs. A cook who has made the acquaintance of the fresh plant will never want to be without it, and may overuse it. Basil stimulates the digestive glands and should be added to heavy foods. It has pronounced antiseptic properties, and helped to preserve meat and fish before the era of refrigeration. It has been used as a pepper substitute and curry ingredient, and is often combined with savory and rosemary as a basic seasoning mixture. Unlike most herbs, dried basil's flavor increases with cooking, and it should be used sparingly or it will overpower more subtle flavors.

Uncooked fresh basil is often added to cold tomato dishes, to cucumber and tomato salads, and to dips and cold sauces. According to country Italian cooks, the herb should never be chopped, only torn or pounded in a mortar in order to fully retain the aromatic properties of the leaves. They are a spicy addition to vegetable juices, to seafood cocktails, and to cottage cheese or cream cheese mixtures. Some cooks like to aromatize olive oil with a sprig of basil. Basil is an indispensable ingredient of famous Italian *pesto* and *salsa verde* sauces. Unusual kitchen presents can be prepared from sprigs of scented basil placed in decorative bottles and preserved with high-quality wine or cider vinegar.

Many cooked dishes are flavored with the dried herb. It is an important ingredient in spaghetti sauces, tomato soups, ketchup, mushroom dishes, omelets, stuffed tomatoes, and casseroles or soufflés using tomatoes. It is often added to mixed soup seasonings, and is a traditional French flavoring for turtle soup, bouillabaisse, pistou and eel dishes. The famous Fetter Lane sausages contained basil, and it is still added to patés and liver wurst. Duck stuffed with a few sprigs of fresh basil leaves loses some of its heaviness, as do pork, mutton, legumes, pulses, cabbage, and grain dishes. It can be used as a seasoning for eggplant and eggs.

Basil leaves can be preserved by washing them, drying them on kitchen towels, and freezing them whole. The leaves can be easily crumbled while still frozen, and retain most of their aroma. They can also be stored in sterile jars under a layer of olive oil, or dried for winter use. Pesto is a very agreeable way of making the aromatic herb available all year round. Basil's fragrant stalks can also be dried and added to pickling spices.

The mucilaginous seeds of some basil species, such as camphor basil, are used to prepare drinks. The leaves are used sparingly in the kitchen, as is holy basil.

Noteworthy Recipes

Basil Vinegar or Wine: In the nineteenth century, food writer and cook William Kitchiner offered a recipe for basil vinegar in his bestselling book, *The Cook's Oracle*:

> Sweet Basil is in full perfection about the middle of August. Fill a wide-mouthed bottle with the fresh green leaves of basil (these give a much finer [flavor] and more flavor than the dried), and cover them with Vinegar or Wine, and let them steep for ten days; if you wish a very strong Essence, strain the liquor, put it on some fresh leaves, and let them steep fourteen days more.
>
> Observation. This is a very agreeable addition to Sauces, Soups, and to the mixture usually made for Salads. It is a secret the makers of Mock Turtle may thank us for telling; a table-spoonful put in when the Soup is finished

will impregnate a tureen of Soup with the Basil and Acid flavours, at very small cost, when fresh Basil and Lemons are extravagantly dear.[26]

Flavoring Powder: Here is another old recipe, which I've adapted from one first published in 1861: A seasoning powder for everyday use can be prepared from 1 oz. dried lemon thyme, 1 oz. dried savory, ½ oz. dried sweet marjoram, ½ oz. sweet and dried basil, 2 oz. dried parsley, and 1 oz. dried lemon peel. Remove the dried leaves from the stems, pound them in a mortar together with the lemon peel, and then pass them through a fine sieve. The resulting mixture can be stored in airtight jars or bottles in a cool place within easy reach of the stove.[27]

Soup Greens: A similar mixture is used to season soups during the winter months. One part each of finely-diced dried parsley leaves and carrots, ½ part dried leeks, ⅙ part dried parsnip or celeriac roots, ⅙ part dried lovage leaves, and ⅛ part each of dried sweet marjoram and sweet basil are placed on paper in a dehydrator at the lowest temperature to remove the last vestiges of moisture, mixed well together, and stored in airtight containers in a dark, cool place. The mixture can be stored until it begins to lose its aroma, up to 12 months. Dried soup greens should be soaked for an hour in a little cold water, and then cooked until completely soft.

Basil Jelly: A novel way to use and preserve herbs is in jelly form. These tart jellies are served with beef, pork, mutton, game, or chicken in much the same way as mint jelly. Basil jelly is made from crabapple or green apple juice sweetened with as little sugar as possible. Add 1 Tbsp. of cider vinegar and a large sprig of finely pounded basil (the scented basils are particularly good prepared this way) to each pint of sweetened apple juice. Let the mixture cook gently over a low flame until the jellying point is reached (that is, until the mixture sheets off a spoon, and the last drop seems to contract into a ball before falling). Strain out the basil while pouring the jelly into sterile jars. Seal with any of the traditional methods. A sprig of fresh basil can be placed in the middle of the glass after it has been filled as a decoration. Adventurous cooks can also make basil-chili jelly in the same manner.

Basil Sandwiches: Basil can be used with amazing results even in the simplest recipes. Basil sandwiches are ideal tea accompaniments, and can be served as a light but cheery meal. First, hard-boil several eggs, and let them cool. Then mince or pound several sprigs of fresh basil. Combine the basil with some softened, unsalted but-

26.   Kitchiner, *The Cook's Oracle* (1817) (London: Samuel Bagster, 1860), 262.

27.   Adapted from Mrs. Isabella Beeton, *The Book of Household Management* (1861) (New York: Farrar, Straus & Giroux, 1977), 214.

ter. Toast several slices of rye or whole wheat bread, and spread generously with basil butter. Fill the sandwiches with the finely chopped hard-boiled eggs, season with a little salt and lemon juice, cut into shapes, and serve.

Potatoes with Basil: This is one of the simplest methods of turning ordinary and cheap potato meals into special occasions. Peel, slice, and quarter 4 medium-sized potatoes for every person, and then cook slowly, without browning, in butter and a little water in a covered pan, adding a little more water if necessary. When soft, season with salt, and turn into a pre-warmed serving dish. Sprinkle the top of the bowl with finely chopped fresh basil.

Freshly gathered parsley, chervil, chives, or even mint can be substituted when basil is hard to come by. Fresh sage leaves also complement potatoes, but they should be added while the potatoes are still boiling and removed before serving.

Basil Butter: Another simple method of exploiting basil's aromatic properties is to combine the herb with sweet butter. Soften 8 oz. of butter and add the juice of 1 lemon. Finely chop 4 heaping Tbsp. of fresh basil, or pound in a mortar. Combine the softened butter with the basil, mix well in a food processor, form into a roll, wrap in aluminum foil, and place in the refrigerator until hardened. Large amounts can be frozen for later use. This butter is served on bread, with grilled meat, fish, or boiled potatoes, or it can be added as a flavoring to vegetable dishes, sauces, and soups.

A spicier, less delicate basil butter is obtained by adding several cloves of pressed garlic, half as much finely chopped parsley, several minced olives, a touch of anchovy paste, and some freshly chopped rosemary, savory, and thyme leaves.

Pistou: This traditional French soup of Italian origin reminds us of the pleasant fragrance and tastiness of a simple dish prepared with the freshest ingredients. The vegetables are prepared as follows: chop 1 onion and 1 leek, peel 3 or 4 large tomatoes (preferably ripe plum tomatoes), string and cut 2 lb. of string beans, and peel and dice 3 medium-sized potatoes into medium-size cubes. Then heat the onion and leek gently in 1 Tbsp. butter or olive oil until the onion turns glassy, add the tomatoes and simmer until soft. Add 1½ qt. of vegetable stock or water, and let the mixture come to a boil on high heat. Add the beans and the diced potatoes as soon as the soup begins to boil. Season to taste with salt and a little freshly ground pepper, and let simmer until the vegetables are soft, but not overcooked.

While the soup is cooking, peel and pound 2 cloves of garlic and 2 small sprigs of fresh bush basil in a mortar. Add 2 Tbsp. of olive oil, and continue to pound. Mix this finely crushed basil mixture into the cooked soup, sprinkle with freshly grated Parmesan cheese, and serve. If fresh Parmesan is not available, substitute a tasty local cheese instead of using packaged and pre-grated Parmesan, which often has an unpleasantly biting taste. If a mortar is not available, use a food processor.

Pesto: There are many, many variations on the pesto theme. Basically, pesto is a garlic and basil sauce that preserves the herb's fragrant and very volatile aroma for winter use. The simplest pesto is made with a generous amount of fresh basil leaves, half again as much garlic, and a little parsley ground fine in a mortar. If desired, a salted anchovy can be added and crushed with the other ingredients. The mixture is then stirred into a paste with a little olive oil and lemon juice.

The refined, traditional pesto recipe calls for 1 cup of basil leaves pounded with 4 large cloves of fresh garlic and ½ cup of piñon nuts in a mortar. Then add 1 tsp. of salt and ½ cup of freshly grated Parmesan cheese, pounding all the while. Pour a thin stream of olive oil into the mortar, still continuing to pound, until the mixture attains the consistency of creamed butter. Pesto can be served fresh, sealed in small jars, or frozen.

Many modern cooks prefer to mince pesto ingredients in an electric blender. This saves times, but does not always improve the taste of the sauce. If fresh Parmesan is not available, it is best to simply omit it. The piñon nuts can, if necessary, be substituted with fresh, unsalted cashew nuts or pecans, unhulled and unsalted sunflower seeds, or even walnuts.

Pesto is used as a concentrated seasoning, and added a teaspoon at a time to sauces, soups and cooked dishes, or it is served on hard-boiled eggs, baked potatoes, bland fish, stuffed tomatoes, pasta, or gnocchi. If used sparingly, it can also be mixed with fresh ricotta or cream cheese as a spread for crackers or toast.

Household Applications

Freshly growing green basil is a cheerful ornament for any house. It exudes a pleasantly powerful aroma that can brighten and freshen a room, helping to drive away flies and mosquitoes. Holy basil has been grown for millennia in India to help purify the air. In winter, small sacks of dried basil hung in a room discourage insects and freshen the air. Pots of basil are set on the tables of French restaurants to drive away flies; in India, fresh basil is used as living incense to honor the Krishna, Vishnu, or his mate, Lakshmi. In Tudor England, farmers' wives presented their departing guests with small pots of basil. The plant is also a delightful addition to potpourri, sachets and nosegays. In John Parkison's words,

> The ordinary Basill is in a manner wholly spent to make sweete or washing waters among other sweet herbs, yet sometimes it is put into nosegays. The

Physicall properties are to procure a cheerfull and merry hearte whereunto the seeds is chiefly used in powder.[28]

Cosmetic Properties

Basil is treasured as much by cosmeticians as cooks for its fresh, aromatic fragrance and its antiseptic, invigorating qualities. Fresh basil leaves can be added to facial steaming mixtures, or used as bath herbs. Steaming with a small amount of basil mixed with a larger amount of a neutral herb such as mallow or chamomile is said to clear the head as well as the face. Maurice Messengué recommends poultices of basil leaves to firm the breasts, and for cleansing and softening the skin. The plant has also been added to mouthwashes and gargles. Essential basil oil (the best oil comes from France) is widely employed by the perfume industry, and is often added to sauna oils. In the Middle Ages, basil was known as the "Italian eye herb" and was used in inordinate quantities as a brightening eyewash.

Medicinal Merits

Basil seems to be a plant that is either liked inordinately or disliked intensely. Early supporters of the herb praised it as pectoral, cordial, cleansing, comforting, and pleasing. It was used to strengthen a "damp brain," to warm chilled veins, to aid the digestion and to expel wind, to excite the kidneys, to break a fever, and to help clear up head and lung colds. Basil was considered to be an excellent aphrodisiac. In Culpeper's words, "it expelleth both birth and after-birth; and as it helps the deficiency of Venus in one kind, so it spoils all her actions in another. I dare write no more of it."[29]

Other authors believed basil to be an "enemy to sight, and a robber of wits." Despite these differences of opinion, all authors agreed that basil was a sovereign remedy, taken internally or applied externally, to treat wasp and scorpion stings and snake bites. Basil's association with scorpions, with the zodiacal sign Scorpio, with the planet Mars, and with sexuality has prompted many negative evaluations of this pungently aromatic herb, and many disagreements about its medicinal merits.

Camphor basil has been cultivated at various times as a source of camphor for medicinal purposes.

Modern Medicine

Modern healers make restricted use of sweet basil, preferring holy basil as a medicinal herb, and little research has been done on the herb's chemical constituents. It exerts a mildly stimulating influence on all the glands, and has antiseptic and cleansing properties.

---

28. Qtd. in Mrs. Maude Grieve, *A Modern Herbal* (1931) (London: Penguin, 1976), 86.

29. Culpeper, *Culpeper's Complete Herbal* (1653) (London: Foulsham, undated), 39–40.

A tea of the leaves, flowers, or flowering tops has a refreshing effect on the entire organism. This tea can be taken by nursing mothers to help increase the milk flow, by the feverish to provoke perspiration, and by those suffering from colds to clear the chest, throat, and lungs of mucus. Basil has a strengthening, stimulating effect on a sluggish stomach. It can help to relieve nausea, prevent travel sickness, lessen the pressures of flatulence, increase the appetite, discourage worms, and generally cleanse and tone the digestive system. Basil leaves infused in white wine can be administered as a mildly laxative digestive tonic.

To complete the list of basil's medicinal uses: snuff prepared from basil leaves is used to treat nervous headaches and nasal colds, and a wound salve is made from the leaves. Basil tea also serves as a gargle, and cooked basil seeds are administered to expel mucus and catarrh. Aromatherapy makes extensive internal use of the essential oil to treat migraines and weak nerves due to overwork, as well as stomach cramps and sleeplessness.

Holy basil has been used for centuries in Ayurvedic medicine, but has recently been rediscovered as an effective herbal medicine for stress-related complaints such as gastro-intestinal disorders, diseases of the immune system, and elevated cholesterol readings.

Camphor basil *(Ocinum canum)* is the homeopathic remedy, prescribed for kidney pain with violent vomiting, kidney colic, red sand in the urine, and kidney stones, especially on the right side.

Basil helps to dispel cold, according to Chinese medicine, and to resolve dampness and toxins. It can be of help when the stomach erupts upward with belching, and in treating headaches due to colds and cold invasions.

Uses in Husbandry

Basil is a cash crop in the Mediterranean countries, and the extraction of its oil a commercial venture since 1582. It was once used as a trade sign for cobblers in France, and was hung in front of the shops to attract customers (as well as luck) to the business.

Bees appreciate basil tea sweetened with sugar or honey from another hive. They avidly visit the plants. Basil leaves are included in herbal snuff mixtures, and they are also valued as a pleasant, spicy pipe tobacco substitute. Those who want to stop smoking may try smoking pipes or cigarette papers filled with basil when the craving overcomes them.

Camphor was once obtained from the camphor basils, and used both medicinally and for the production of fireworks. Holy basil is often used as a mosquito repellent.

Veterinary Values
Horses suffering from cramps are rubbed down with basil-leaf spirits.

Miscellaneous Wisdom

Basil has been associated with scorpions and snakes since the beginning of recorded herbalism. This may be because the herb's roots resemble these animals, or it may also be because both the plant and the animals prefer warm, sunny places. Snakes and scorpions can often be seen sunning themselves next to basil plants. Simply smelling the herb, or crushing it, was once thought to breed scorpions in the brain. Antonius Mizaldus (a sixteenth century physician and astrologer) wrote that basil would breed venomous beasts if laid in horse manure. In the Middle Ages, scorpions were supposedly generated by rubbing basil between two stones and then covering the herb with a glass container. By the logic of sympathetic magic, basil was thought to protect humans against scorpions, serpents, and the basilisk. According to the ancient Greek physician Dioscurides,

> Being applyed with the flour of Polenta, & Rosaceum, & vinegar, it doth help inflammations, & ye stroke of ye sea dragon, and of ye scorpion ... It [the seed] causeth also many sneesings, being drawn up by the smell, & the herb doth the like. But the eyes must be shut whilst ye sneesing holds. Somme also doe avoyd it and doe not eate it, because that being chewed, and set in the Sunne, it breeds little wormes. But the Africans haue entertained it, because they which eate it and are smitten of a scorpion, ye remaine without paine.[30]

In ancient times, some herbalists believed that it could engender lice (Dioscurides) and that it was too fiery for normal use (Galen). In fact, poverty was even represented in Greece as a woman looking at a basil plant. A modern French idiom for slander is to *"semer le basilic."* In the nineteenth century, basil's association with the zodiacal sign Scorpio and the planet Mars caused it to be associated with fiery anger. The herb has also attained all the evil connotations of a grave plant from being scattered on graves in Egypt, planted on graves in Persia and Malaysia, and placed on the breast of Hindus at death.

Basil is a plant of magical extremes: many are ready to sing its praises; others malign the plant with invective. Basil, especially Holy basil, is honored as a sacred plant by the Hindus, and placed before the door to keep away evil spirits. It was once considered such a "kingly" herb that only a king had the right to cut it, and then only with a golden sickle. The dual nature of the herb is characterized in this verse:

> I pray your Highness mark this curious herb:
> Touch it but lightly, stroke it softly, Sir,
> And it gives forth an odor sweet and rare;
> But crush it harshly and you'll make a scent
> Most disagreeable.[31]

---

30. Robert T. Gunther, ed., *The Greek Herbal of Dioscurides* (New York: Hafner, 1959), 182.

31. Charles Godfrey Leland, "Sweet Basil." Qtd. in J. K. Hyott, *The Cyclopedia of Practical Quotations* (New York: Funk and Wagnalls, 1896; original from U of Wisconsin; digitized 2007), 246.

Even the aphrodisiacal qualities of the plant are considered to be contradictory, visualized by the symbolical representation of the herb as "love washed with tears." The plant symbolizes both the feverish qualities of passionate love and the binding qualities of gentle friendship. It is thought to awaken sympathy between humans. It was added to love philters in the Middle Ages, and is still presented as a love token, or included in charms and spells. In Moldavia, a man who takes basil from a woman is considered bound to her in love. In northern Italy, a man who accepts basil from his sweetheart is believed to remain constant. The aphrodisiacal qualities of the herb give support to the time-honored adage that "the way to a man's heart is through his stomach."

Oracular Worth

In keeping with its aphrodisiacal powers, basil was used in the Middle Ages to prove a woman's chastity. A sprig was placed under the bowl of a woman to be "tested." If she ate her meal, then she was undoubtedly chaste, but if she turned down her food, she had to face the verdict of wantonness.

Legends

According to Bulgarian belief, it was Satan who told God how to make a virgin conceive. During one of their talks, Satan told God to pick a bunch of basil flowers, lay them under his pillow, and sleep on them overnight. In the morning, God should take them to a virgin, have her smell them, and she would conceive.

> This one time, God followed Satan's advice, and slept with the basil flowers under His pillow. In the morning, He sent the Archangel Gabriel to Mary. Gabriel presented her with the basil flowers. The Virgin Mary took pleasure at the odor of the herb. As a result, she conceived, and gave birth to Jesus.[32]

A Catalan legend also depicts the relationship between Mary and the basil plant:

> The Virgin Mary was looking for a hiding place for herself and her baby when she saw a farmer sowing grain.
> "Farmer! Farmer!," she cried, "go and call your family, for it's time to harvest!"
> At first the farmer didn't want to listen to her, but then he decided to humor her. He went home and gathered his family together. When they got back to the field, the grain was already ripe. He and his family set to work to harvest the field. Mary hid herself and the baby Jesus inside the last sheaf. The grain plants covered her completely, except for a piece of her cloak that peeped out from the bottom. Some basil plants growing nearby saw what had happened, and bent over to cover the scrap of cloth.

---

32. Oskar Dähnhardt, *Natursagen*, vol. 1 (Leipzig, Germany: Teubner, 1909), 3.

A moment later, Herod rode up. He asked the farmer if he had seen a woman go by with a child in her arms.

The farmer answered, "Yes, I saw them, when I began to sow this field."

Herod knew that must have been several months ago, and hurried on. In his haste, he didn't hear the mint plant rustling, "Under the sheaf! Under the sheaf!" and ignored the jay cawing overhead: "Under the sheaf! Under the sheaf!"

Jesus and Mary were safe from Herod, despite the mint and the jay. As punishment for their betrayal, Mary told the mint that it would never blossom, and decreed that the jay would never have a full stomach. But she blessed the basil plant, and said that it would flourish. Since then, basil has always grown fragrant and aromatic. It is known as Mary's plant, and is worn by girls and women under their blouses.[33]

Literary Flowers

For as by basil the scorpion is engendered, and by means of the same herb destroyed: so love which by time and fancy is bred in an idle head, is by time and fancy banished from the heart.

—JOHN LYLY, *EUPHUES AND HIS ENGLAND*

Scorpions like to sun themselves in the shade of a green and fertile plant, in basil's aura. There they die, and are reborn, and metamorphose like basilisks: to be engendered in the brain by basil's pungent odor and there to scuttle in melancholy corners as incubi of the night, there to sting, and to prick and to irritate their uneasy host throughout the winter's dark months. But when spring comes, the scorpion flees back to the shading roots of the kingly basil plant. It is then that basil has the power to heal and to gently soothe, and to cleanse and remove all winter's superfluities.

—*SISTER CLARISSA'S UNPUBLISHED BOOK OF NATURAL OBSERVATIONS*

---

33. Oskar Dähnhardt, *Natursagen*, vol. 2 (Leipzig, Germany: Teubner, 1909), 62.

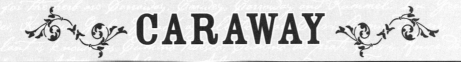

CARAWAY

Name

The word "caraway" has evolved from the Latin *carum*, and that in turn from Greek and Arabic. The plant is sometimes confused with the much stronger-tasting cumin (*Cuminum cyminum*) or black cumin (*Nigella sativa*).

Carum carvi (or, as it is sometimes called, *Carum officinalis*) is a biennial member of the *Apiaceae*, earlier known as the **Umbelliferae** (**Carrot**) family.

Folk Names

English names for the herb are carraway, carwey, carroway, and kummel. In German, it is known as *Kümmel*, *Karwei*, *Kümmi*, and *Garbe*. French appellations are *carvi*, *cumin des prés*, and *anis des vosges*. In Italian, the plant is known as *cumino tedesco*, *cumino dei prati*, *carvi*, *anice dei vosgi*; in Spanish, it's *carvi*; in Portuguese, *alcaravia*, *alcorovia*, *alcaravea*; in Russian, *tmin obyknovennyj*; in Scottish, *carvy* and *kervie*; and in Irish, *cearbhas*.

Appearance

Because caraway belongs to the family of umbels (also called the **Carrot** family), it can easily be confused with poisonous plants. Caraway's most important identifying characteristic is the pungent odor and flavor of the seeds. The plant has a long, spindly white root resembling a parsnip or a carrot, a wrinkled outer skin, and tiny fibrous rootlets. The taste of the root is spicy, but less pronounced than that of the fruits. In its first year, caraway pro-

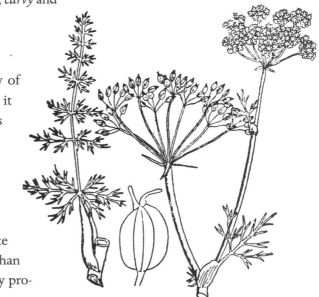

duces a leaf rosette, and in the second, a flower stalk that rises up to 2–3 ft. above the ground (the plants are often quite small). The stalk is slightly furrowed and branched, and supports grass-green leaves similar to those of the carrot and umbels of tiny white or reddish-white flowers. These flowers produce fruits containing two seeds, seeds that are, according to Culpeper, "smaller than the aniseed, and of a quicker and better taste."

Place, Season, and Useful Parts

Caraway is cultivated in Holland, England, Germany, Iceland, Syria, European Russia, and Morocco, as well as in gardens the world over. It is found growing wild in Europe, Asia, New Zealand, and North and South America to an altitude of 6,000 ft. on mountain pastures, meadows, flooded areas, rubble, roadsides, banks, and in stony riverbeds. Caraway fruits grown in northern regions usually contain more essential oils than those grown in the South. The plant flowers from May to July, and sometimes again in the fall.

Gathering, Drying, and Storage

Caraway can be harvested in the summer of the plant's second year, just as the fruits begin to turn brown. The upper part of the plant is harvested with a sickle or garden shears, and then placed on a cloth and carried to a dry, shady place to ripen. The plants are threshed when dry to release the seeds. The umbels can also be cut singly, and dried quickly on trays in the sun or in heated rooms. Properly dried caraway seeds keep well, preferably in a cool, dry place. Caraway roots should be dug in April.

According to German folk belief, the best caraway is gathered on Midsummer's Day before sunrise or while the noon bells are ringing, or on St. Vitus's Day (June 15th). Caraway is supposedly more effective against a stomachache if bitten off during the Ave (evening) bells.

Seed Saving and Germination

Many gardeners believe that there is little variability in herbs. This is a general misconception, for even the wild-growing caraways vary widely in different growth habits, seed size and oil content. Generally, only one or two varieties are available commercially. The caraway enthusiast would do well to experiment with various varieties available from specialist nurseries, seed-saving organizations, and gene banks. Some have been selected for their thick roots, others for their oil content, and still others for the quantity of fruits they produce. They will cross with each other, and should be isolated to keep the varieties pure.

It is important to remember that the plant only sets seed in its second year, and garden space should be apportioned accordingly. The best seeds for propagation are formed in the plant's central umbel, which ripens first. The seeds dry well, and are easily removed from the stalk. They remain viable (fertile) for 2–3 years, if dried and stored well.

Gardening Hints

Although the seeds of the wild caraway plant generally contain more ethereal oils than those of cultivated plants, it is easier to harvest cultivated caraway seeds. This consideration has led to the widespread cultivation of the herb. Some adventurous gardeners grow the plant for the sake of its parsnip-like root.

Caraway is an unusual garden plant because it actually prefers heavy clay soil, a shady position, and wet weather. Granted, the soil should be aerated with a little sand or gravel so that the plant's tap root can work its way downward, and the herb appreciates a little organic fertilizer and some limestone, but it can be grown where few other plants will survive. Gardeners often sow caraway next to peas, poppies, beans, or grains, and avoid planting caraway next to fennel. Commercial growers sometimes sow mustard, pea, bean, flax, grain, clover, or poppy seeds together with caraway, and harvest the companion crop the first year, and the caraway one year later.

Caraway seeds should be sown outdoors in the fall as soon as the fruits ripen for best germination, or again the following spring. They will usually germinate in 2–4 weeks. Some gardeners are convinced that they sprout better if left uncovered in very damp soil; others recommend a sowing depth of ¼ in. (According to the ancient Greek scientist Theophrastus, caraway grows best if it is cursed while being sown.) Caraway seedlings should be thinned to allow 1 ft. between plants. They do not transplant well. It is important to weed and cultivate the plants regularly. In the fall, caraway plants form a winter-hardy rosette that brings forth flower stalks the next spring, and fruits in the late summer or fall.

Culinary Virtues

Caraway has been widely used by cooks since ancient times. It was one of the few herbs found in the prehistoric kitchens of Switzerland, and is indispensable for German, Swiss, and Austrian cooking to this day. Caraway seeds have a warming effect on the digestive organs, and are a perfect seasoning for "windy" foods. They also improve the appetite and freshen the breath. Fresh caraway seeds are much more aromatic than dried seeds, and freshly powdered caraway seeds are more potent than whole caraway seeds.

Young caraway leaves have a sharp, pungent taste, and can be included in spring salads and soups. Larger caraway leaves are cooked in soups, or added to spinach dishes, or used to flavor marinades. Caraway roots are edible, and are occasionally cultivated. Caesar mentioned a bread prepared with milk and caraway roots. Caraway roots can also be boiled like parsnips and served with melted butter, or grated raw into salads.

German cooks use caraway seeds extensively as a seasoning. The seeds help to make fatty foods more attractive and digestible, as well as giving them an unusual flavor. Caraway seeds are often added to pork roasts, sausages, sauerkraut, black bread, pickled beets, cooked cabbage, potato dishes, cheeses, cottage or cream cheeses, soups, cooked vegetable salads, mushrooms, and to various boiled vegetables. Boiled potatoes and steamed cabbage are often seasoned with caraway seeds. Caraway seeds are also, like coriander seeds, used to cover up the taste of musty flour, and are also, like coriander, made into comfits. Caraway seeds, laurel leaves and juniper berries are considered the appropriate seasoning for boiled rye, and rye bread is traditionally flavored with whole caraway seeds. Thyme and caraway seeds are added to oats. A traditional English dish, mentioned by Shakespeare and served at Trinity College, is roast apples with a side dish of caraway seeds. In Scotland, "carvi cakes" were once a familiar sweet, almost as familiar as "salt-water-jelly." This "jelly" consisted of a dish of caraway seeds into which the family members dipped their buttered bread at tea time.

Caraway seeds are also extensively employed by distillers. Caraway liqueur should not be taken regularly for an extended amount of time, but an occasional glass of caraway liqueur taken after a heavy meal is an excellent cordial and digestive medicine, warming and comforting. Unfortunately, the liqueur commercially sold as Kümmel often contains no caraway whatsoever. In the Middle Ages, caraway roots and caraway seeds were used to flavor and to preserve beer.

Noteworthy Recipes

Austrian Pork Roast: Choose a not-too-lean but solid, medium-sized piece of pork with a piece of fat on top. Season the roast with salt and freshly-ground pepper, a little Hungarian paprika (optional), and rub it with a clove or two of garlic, tucking the remaining garlic under the meat when done. Decorate the fatty top of the roast with a crosshatch pattern by cutting deeply into the fat with a sharp knife. Sprinkle the entire roast with whole caraway seeds. Put in a heavy casserole or baking dish for 10–15 minutes in a very hot oven, or until the fat begins to brown on top, and then turn down to complete the roasting process at moderate heat until very well done. Add a little water during the roasting process if necessary. Use the drippings in the pan to make a sauce, and serve with dumplings or boiled potatoes. Cabbage complements the taste of this pork roast, especially if the cooked cabbage or coleslaw has also been seasoned with caraway seeds.

Caraway Potatoes: This is an excellent way to reheat boiled potatoes, or make a quick, nourishing meal. Cut cooked, half-cooked or raw potatoes in half lengthwise. Sprinkle the cut side with coarse salt and caraway seeds and place face up on a baking sheet. Bake in a moderately hot oven until warm (approximately 10 minutes), or cooked through (30 minutes), and brush with a little oil if necessary. Serve piping hot with cottage cheese, sour cream or guacamole. It is also possible to grill the potatoes on an electric grill, adding the seasoning later.

Household Applications

Pungent caraway seeds are occasionally added, in small amounts, to sachets. This practice probably dates back to the time when fleas were a serious household problem. Then, it was also customary to strew caraway in the house and to sprinkle the floor with caraway seed tea. The Wends, a Slavic ethnic group, prepared and ate caraway-seed biscuits every Maundy Thursday in the hopes of freeing themselves from the bothersome parasites for an entire year.

Cosmetic Properties

In the days when lice were a cosmetic problem, women rubbed their bodies liberally with caraway and anise oil to drive the insects away. Caraway oil is now primarily used by perfumers to create exotic scent mixtures. Soap is sometimes aromatized with a by-product of caraway distillation.

Medicinal Merits

Caraway was once classified as one of the *Semina quatuor calida maiora*, the four herbs with the most pronounced warming properties. These helped to ease colics and flatulence and to dispel mucus from the digestive organs. A caraway salve and sacks of crushed and roasted caraway seeds were rubbed or laid on children's stomachs to relieve colics, and placed on other parts of the body to ease aches and pains and to loosen mucus and phlegm. Caraway seeds in wine were considered an effective remedy for a cough, and birthing mothers in Bavaria were fumigated with caraway seeds or laid on a bed of caraway to ease their delivery.

Modern Medicine

Caraway roots and caraway seeds are still thought to have excellent carminative, or wind-dispelling properties, and are considered comforting and strengthening for all the digestive organs as well as the lungs. Caraway fruit tea can help relieve gall bladder spasms; it can whet the appetite, and can even be given to an appendicitis patient before arrival at the hospital. Caraway stimulates the bladder and the kidneys, and can help to bring on a period, or to increase the milk of a nursing mother. Through the mother's milk, the baby's colicky pains can also be eased.

Ethereal caraway oil is a strong antiseptic, and is used externally to treat rheumatic pains. Caraway leaf poultices are applied to wounds, boils, pustules, and infected fingernails. Warm caraway seed sacks are used to ease rheumatic headaches and toothaches. Children with rickets will begin to mend if exposed to enough sunlight, fed with calcium-rich foods, and rubbed with caraway oil, or bathed in caraway seed baths.

Caraway seed is used in Chinese medicine, as in Western, to treat indigestion, nausea, no appetite, and hiccups. It is also thought to move the liver and warm the kidneys.

Special Cures

Kümmel Liqueur: A medicinal Kümmel liqueur is prepared by placing 2 oz. of caraway seeds and 8 oz. of brown sugar in a bottle together with 1 qt. of wine spirits. Let the mixture stand, stoppered with a valve cork (otherwise, the bottle may "blow its top"), in a warm place for 14 days, and then strain, filter, and bottle. This liqueur is a fortifying stomachic medicine and can be taken in small doses, after an especially large meal.

Uses in Husbandry

Caraway is a good fodder plant, and its presence in a pasture is generally appreciated. Press-cakes left over from the distillation or oil-pressing process can be fed to cattle with good results. Bees visit caraway flowers, and pigeons can be encouraged to remain in a new home if given a piece of caraway bread on arrival. However, large amounts of fresh caraway seeds have been known to poison birds.

Miscellaneous Wisdom

Caraway has been associated with both marriage and death for centuries. In Great Britain, it was included in love potions and philters destined to bind two lovers to constancy. In Germany, it was laid in coffins, together with salt, to protect the deceased on their passage to the other world.

Caraway was also believed to have important antidemonic properties. Witches, spirits, and elves supposedly feel uncomfortable around any part of the caraway plant. In Eastern Europe, a pot containing boiled caraway seeds was placed under the bed of an uneasy, demon-ridden child and a few seeds were sewn into a baby's diapers to keep him from suffering the pains of colic. Diapers left out overnight and exposed to the dangers of the Romanian night had to be smoked with caraway seeds before they could be used.

Legends

According to legends and folk tradition, elves, dwarves, and wood women flee from caraway and are incensed when they see humans kneading the seeds into bread dough. The following are some of the exclamations recorded at the sight of this "disgusting" spectacle. "Caraway bread brings dearth and dread"; "Caraway bread will hasten our end"; "Now this house will suffer need, because in my bread they baked caraway seed"; and "May God help you in your need, if in your bread you bake caraway seed."[34]

---

34. Hanns Bächtold-Stäubli, ed., *Handwörterbuch des deutschen Aberglaubens* (1927–42), vol. 5 (Berlin: Walter de Gruyter & Co., 1987), 806.

The dried leaves of coltsfoot and of other plants, as milfoil or yarrow,
are still frequently smoked in the country and generally mixed with tobacco.

—NOTES AND QUERIES

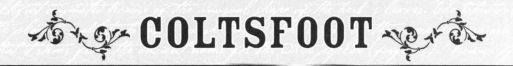

COLTSFOOT

Name

The name "coltsfoot" originated because of the unusual shape of the herb's leaves. It is a
perennial member of the **Daisy** family (***Asteraceae***, once ***Compositae***), and is known under
the botanical name *Tussilago farfara*. The word *tussilago* alludes to the plant's ability to
ease a cough *(tussis)*. The origins of *farfara* are uncertain. Some experts say that it stems
from the ancient name for the white poplar *(farfarus)*. Others associate the herb with the
Latin word for flour, pointing to the floury color of coltsfoot leaves, and also to the plant's
adverse effect on grain grown in its vicinity (from *far,* meaning grain, and *fugere,* to flee).

Folk Names

Obsolete names for coltsfoot are coltefoote, horse hove, pole foote, bull foote, field-
hove, personatia, pes pulli, bethicon, and tussyllage. Modern English names are colt's
foot, horse-foot, horse-hoof, foal-foot, colt herb, hall foot, ass's foot, sow-foot, bull-foot,
calves' foot, cow heave, hogweed, son afore the father, tushalan,
tushy-lucky, gowan, yellow stars, dummy weed, dove-dock, poor
man's baccy, yellow trumpets, wild rhubarb, hoofs, cleats, clat-
terclogs, coughwort, clayweed, ginger, and ginger root. German
names are *Huflattich, Eselshuf, Butterblätter, Sohn vor dem Vater,*
Sommerthürlein, Hustenkraut, and *Hasentatze.* The French call it
tussilage, pied de cheval, pas d'âne, pied de poulain, quirin, taconnet,
and *filius antre patrem.* Ancient Italian names are *erba ungula*
cavalina, striginon, manicum, dorigion, cechalion, herba bactina,
and *betico farfarum.* Modern Italian names are *tussilagine, ung-*
hia cavallina, farfaraccio, farfaro, farfarello, and *falsa vaniglia.* The
Dutch call the herb *zoon-voor-de-vater;* the Irish call it *sponc.*

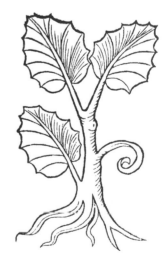

Appearance

Coltsfoot has long, creeping white roots that may grow to a length of 6 ft. The tiniest root segment can produce a new plant, which is why coltsfoot is such a persistent weed. The flower stalks are approximately 1 ft. in height, and are covered with small scales like those of the asparagus plant or the flower stalk of the house leek. These scales or bracts are of a reddish color, as is the flower calyx. Small, bright yellow flowers that resemble small dandelion blossoms can be found at the end of the stalks. Young coltsfoot flowers let their heads droop, but full-grown blossoms show their faces to the sun. When rain or darkness threatens, coltsfoot flowers close their petals tightly. Coltsfoot seeds are found at the bottom of tiny seed parachutes.

Coltsfoot leaves develop after the flowers and flower stalks have died back. They are shaped like hooves (hence the many folk names) and can be as large as rhubarb leaves when fully grown. They contain nine nerves. Young leaves are downy underneath, and covered with tiny felty hairs above. Older leaves lose their felty upper covering and turn an even dark green. In general, coltsfoot leaves are greener, thicker, and smaller than the leaves of the butterbur. The coltsfoot plant has little or no odor after the flowers have spent their perfume, and the leaves taste bitter, salty, and a little slimy.

Place, Season, and Useful Parts

Coltsfoot is a very common plant in Europe, Asia, North America, and northern Africa to an altitude of 7,500 ft. It is one of the first plants to produce flowers in the spring, as soon as the snows melt. It blossoms from March to April and, on some occasions, once again in the fall. The leaves appear from May on. The plant can be encountered in fields, vineyards, and furrows, and in gravel pits, rubble heaps, and disturbed soil (especially around new house foundations). It also thrives in quarries and clay pits, on railway embankments, and along roadsides, rivers, and sea shores.

Gathering, Drying, and Storage

One of coltsfoot's names, *Filius ante patrem*, refers to a botanical peculiarity of the plant. Coltsfoot blossoms long before the first leaves appear; hence, in folk logic, the son of the plant comes into the world before the father. Coltsfoot flowers should be gathered before they fully open and begin to develop seeds, in March and April. Coltsfoot leaves are gathered from May through July. Old, tough leaves should be discarded and the stems removed. Care should always be taken to avoid bruising the leaves, and plants found growing in very dark and gloomy places should also be avoided. It is wise to make note of good gathering spots in the spring when the plants flower, to avoid confusion with the very similar butterbur.

The flowers are dried in shady, airy places on paper. Carefully remove any insects that fall out of the flower heads on drying. The fleshy leaves must retain their green color on drying, which is usually brought about with the help of artificial heat or by drying them quickly in a warm, airy place.

Seed Saving and Germination

There is little variation between coltsfoot plants, so seed saving is not often practiced, although some selection can be done in order to obtain the largest and most tender leaves. Wild plants are reproduced by root and plant division.

Gardening Hints

Coltsfoot is rarely welcomed in any garden, although some smokers like to sow wasteland with the fast-spreading plants. Coltsfoot seeds germinate easily if they are broadcast, and not covered with earth in early spring. Mature plants can be divided in the fall. Coltsfoot will pop up spontaneously on clayey soil, or on earth disturbed by bulldozers, for example when digging out foundations. Coltsfoot prefers a sunny, yet damp position. It grows well in poor soil or on waste ground. In fact, the presence of large numbers of coltsfoot plants can give the trained specialist an indication that marl (soil containing clay and carbonate of lime), zinc, or coal deposits are present. The plant usually refuses to grow on limestone.

Eradicating existing coltsfoot patches is a much more difficult undertaking. Sheep or goats can be allowed to graze on the land to keep the plants from going to seed, or the ground can be tilled or hoed, and sown thickly with green manure crops. Since coltsfoot grows best on clayey soil, repeated tilling with organic matter or compost, and the addition of limestone will also help solve the problem. Some gardeners who have reached the end of their rope go to the extreme of draining the area, and then salting the plants liberally. This will kill them, but will also negatively affect the soil for future plantings. Others believe that the weeds can only be killed by digging them up on Whitsun Day, July 30th, or the evening of August 14th.

Culinary Virtues

Young and tender coltsfoot leaves can be used in many different kitchen recipes. For example, they can be substituted for cabbage leaves to wrap stuffing and forcemeat. They can also be cut into strips, cooked and flavored with savory or dill and few drops of wine vinegar, and served as a side dish, or puréed into thick soup. Other cooks mix young coltsfoot leaves with nettles and a little ground ivy (Glechoma hederacea) as cooked spring greens. Still others prepare a simple dish prepared from cooked potatoes seasoned with coltsfoot, young lungwort (Pulmonaria officinalis), comfrey, and salad leaves. Shredded coltsfoot leaves can be added to pancake batter and to egg and cheese dishes as well as to vegetable juices, salads, and soups. Coltsfoot wine, prepared from the flowers, does not have as pleasant an aroma as dandelion wine, but it is useful medicine. Coltsfoot cough drops, coltsfoot rock candy, and coltsfoot sticks are used, like horehound candy, for easing a cough. They are more pleasant, and less bitter in taste.

Noteworthy Recipes

Coltsfoot Wine: Coltsfoot wine is prepared like dandelion wine. Mix 2 qt. of dried coltsfoot flowers and 1 lb. of raisins in a large container. Stir 2 lb. of sugar into 1 gal. of water in a large pot, and bring the mixture to a boil. Skim off all impurities, and then pour this liquid over the coltsfoot leaves and raisins in the large container, and let cool until lukewarm. Stir a cake of yeast into a little of the lukewarm liquid, and then spread it onto a thick slice of toast. Float the toast carefully on the surface of the liquid, and cover the container. Remove the toast the following day, and cask the liquid, stoppering it with a thistle tube to let fermenting gases escape. Only close the cask when the liquid has stopped fermenting violently, after 2 or 3 days, depending on the temperature. Open the cask 3 months later, and add the juice of 2 lemons and 2 oranges, along with a small glass of brandy. Siphon the clear wine into sterilized bottles, cork the bottles securely, and then store in a horizontal position for at least 3 months before tasting.

Household Applications

In the absence of paper or other wrapping material, large coltsfoot leaves can be used to wrap food and butter. The plant's silky seeds were once gathered by Highlanders to stuff pillows and mattresses. The felt on the underside of the coltsfoot leaves was also rubbed off and wrapped in pieces of cloth dipped in saltpeter. These packages were carefully stored in a tin for use as tinder for starting fires. A green dye can also be produced from the herb.

Cosmetic Properties

Coltsfoot is a cooling herb, and its large leaves are bruised with a rolling pin and applied, green side down, to inflammations and sores. Compresses of bruised coltsfoot leaves are used to reduce swellings. Sore feet can be treated with poultices of fresh coltsfoot leaves, or with footbaths prepared from the dried herb. Infected eyes are bathed in filtered coltsfoot infusions. A paste of coltsfoot tea and Bentonite or French green clay is applied to pimples and acne with good results, and coltsfoot compresses are used to soothe skin disfigured by thread veins. Facial waters prepared with coltsfoot leaves have mildly astringent and cleansing qualities, but also cause the skin to freckle more easily.

Noteworthy Recipes

Facial Water: Place ½ handful each of coltsfoot, rosemary and sage leaves, as well as lavender and chamomile flowers, in a bowl, jar or enameled pot with a closely fitting lid. Pour 2 oz. of 96 percent alcohol (or proportionately more high-proof spirits) and distilled water over the herbs until they are completely covered with the liquid. Cover the container, and place it in a warm place, or in direct sunlight. Stir the mixture, and replace any moisture that has evaporated daily with distilled water. On the 7th day, strain the mixture and filter it. Add a few drops of rose or lavender water as desired. Bottle the liquid and cork the bottles securely. Store in a cool place. This facial water has mild astringent properties, and can also be used as an after-bath tonic. It will not keep indefinitely, and can be frozen with good results.

Medicinal Merits

In Italy, the belief was once prevalent that fumigating a patient with coltsfoot was the best general guarantee of recovery. To this day, French apothecaries proclaim their trade by painting coltsfoot leaves on their doors. Apuleius recommended a coltsfoot-leaf belt worn on the body against fever and pain. Roman gladiators bound the large leaves on their heads as protection against wounds, and used them as emergency bandages. The roots of alpine coltsfoot and of the butterbur *(Petasites hybridus)* were given in powdered form as preventive medicine against the plague. The recovery of the plague patient was guaranteed if the herb could make him or her perspire enough to "break" the fever. Coltsfoot leaves were applied to wounds, inflammations, sores, pustules, cancerous growths, and used to cool heated conditions in the "privy parts." Similarly, St. Anthony's fire, wheals, piles, "hot" livers, and the fire of rheumatic and arthritic pain were all treated with the herb. Coltsfoot leaf and flower tea was given to patients with colds, coughs, and all other disorders of the respiratory system.

Modern Medicine

Modern physicians view coltsfoot primarily as an expectorant herb. Like the mallows, coltsfoot soothes and gently cleanses the mucous membranes and helps to heal inflammations and infections, dispelling mucus from the lungs. It is therefore one of the most famous cough and cold medicines, in tea, syrup, candy, or cough drop form. People troubled with asthma, bronchitis, or hoarseness also benefit from repeated use of the herb.

The juice extracted from fresh coltsfoot flowers and young leaves, as well as coltsfoot soup, dried and powdered coltsfoot leaves, or coltsfoot tea can be taken in spring to cleanse the blood, kidneys, and the entire lymphatic system. A tea for the treatment of scrofula is prepared from equal parts of coltsfoot and walnut leaves, and flavored with a few drops of red wine. Scrofulous skin diseases, swellings, allergic rashes, and even benevolent growths are treated with renewed applications of coltsfoot-leaf compresses and a coltsfoot-tea cure. Coltsfoot roots are more radically cleansing than the leaves, and are therefore occasionally given, a pinch of the powdered drug at a time, to patients with rheumatism, rashes or scrofula, or as a sudorific to break a fever.

Because of their large size, coltsfoot leaves can be very helpful in the external treatment of wounds, inflammations, swellings, sprains, sore feet, and can also be used to cool the brow of a feverish patient. They are used as emergency bandages until medical treatment can be obtained. The green side of the leaf is applied directly to the skin after being bruised with a bottle or rolling pin, or the leaves are shredded, and applied on a large leaf. They can also be mixed with honey spread on a gauze bandage. Homeopaths prescribe coltsfoot for tubercular diseases and coughs.

Chinese doctors call the herb *Kuan dong hua* and use it, just as in the West, for coughs and to strengthen the lungs. It is especially warming for the lungs when it has been prepared by roasting it in honey.

Special Cures

Coltsfoot is a major ingredient in most bronchial tea mixtures, along with other herbs such as sage, plantain, comfrey, marshmallow roots, fennel seeds, thyme, burnet saxifrage roots *(Pimpinella saxifraga)*, speedwell *(Veronica officinalis)*, lungwort *(Pulmonaria officinalis)*, betony *(Betonica officinalis)*, mullein flowers *(Verbascum thapsus)*, elecampane *(Inula helenium)* and licorice roots *(Glycyrrhiza glabra)*, elder flowers *(Sambucus nigra),* and linden *(Tilia europea)* flowers.

Coltsfoot Tea: This is usually composed of 1 part of the flowers and 1 part of the leaves. The Swiss herbal priest Johann Künzle recommends a pleasant-tasting and mild cough tea prepared from 1 part coltsfoot flowers and 1 part cowslip flowers. Sir Thomas Browne, a seventeenth-century English author, offers an antiquated recipe for whooping cough that is still applicable for children with persistent coughs (omitting the rhubarb roots, which may be too strongly laxative):

> Sʳ Tho. Brown's drink for a hooping cough Take of Raysons of the Sunne ston'd an ounce, Currance a Spoonfull, 5 or 6 figgs, 8 or 9 Coltsfoot leaves, marrygold & cowslip flowers of each a few, Liquorice half a quarter of an ounce, Anniseeds a thimble full, China (rhubarb) roots a quarter of an ounce: boyle all these in a Pint & a half of Barly water to a Pint, then strein it & give it 2 or 3 Spoonfulls at a time warme when you see occasion, adding to it a little Syrup of Violets or Sugar Candy: it's good without either.[35]

Coltsfoot Syrup: This is often given to children with colds and coughs who refuse other less pleasant-tasting medicines, and to adults with chest congestions and coughs.

---

35. Browne, *The Works of Sir Thomas Browne*, vol. 3 (London: Faber & Faber, 1965), 463.

A historical recipe for this popular remedy was recorded by John Shirley, a seventeenth-century writer on the cosmetic arts for fine ladies. It has great similarity to Sir Thomas Browne's recipe:

> An Excellent Syrup to preserve the Lungs, and for the Asthma.
>
> Take of Nettle-water & Coltsfoot-water each a pint, Anniseed and Liquorish powder, of each two Spoonfuls, Raisins of the Sun one handful, sliced Figs, number four: boil them together until a fourth part be consumed, strain the liquid part, and make it up into a Syrup, with a pound of white Sugar-candy bruised into Powder, and take two Spoonfuls of it each morning fasting.[36]

Alpine Syrup: A more modern recipe calls for a different approach. Cover the bottom of a stoneware jar with a layer of freshly-gathered, washed and dried coltsfoot leaves, and sprinkle it with brown sugar. Continue alternating layers with sugar until the pot is full, and then add a sprig of rosemary. Cover, and let the mixture stand for 24 hours. Add several more alternating layers of coltsfoot leaves and sugar until the jar is filled again. Seal the jar closely and carefully with parchment or thick waxed paper and a tightly fitting lid. Dig a hole in the garden, and set the jar in it so that the top is below ground level. Weigh it down with a board, and place a large stone on the board to mark the spot. Cover the hole with earth, and let the syrup ferment in the earth for at least 8 weeks. Then dig it out and strain the resulting mass through cheesecloth. Bring the liquid to a boil, pour it into sterilized bottles and seal for future use (freezing is also an alternative). The slow fermentation of the coltsfoot leaves makes this syrup preferable to syrup made the easy way. To do this, add bruised and freshly washed coltsfoot leaves to white sugar, and heat slowly until liquid. Strain the resulting mixture, pour into bottles, and use quickly.

Coltsfoot Candy: The following coltsfoot candy recipe is of medicinal as well as culinary interest. Coltsfoot candies, like horehound drops, were once found in most households as a pleasant treatment for coughs. It can be prepared from approximately 2 oz. of coltsfoot leaves brewed with 1 qt. of boiling water. Boil until half of the liquid evaporates, and add 4 cups of sugar. Stir until dissolved, and then boil, stirring constantly, until the hard-ball stage is reached. Pour the boiling candy carefully into a buttered cake tin, or onto a buttered marble slab, and cut into shapes quickly with a buttered knife before the mixture cools. Roll the individual candies in granulated sugar (or in slippery elm powder) to prevent them from sticking together during storage. Store in a candy jar or tin.

---

36.   Shirley, *The Accomplished Ladies Rich Closet of Rarities* (London: N. Bodington, 1688), 23.

Uses in Husbandry

Animals are more partial to fermented coltsfoot leaves than to the fresh plant. Swiss farmers sometimes pick coltsfoot leaves in the summer, press them down into barrels, and then bury the barrel in the earth. The barrel is dug up in winter when fresh fodder is not available, and the fermented coltsfoot fed to the pigs. Bohemian farmers used to feed their horses a little coltsfoot to give them a "fiery" look on market days. Another animal, the goldfinch, makes extensive use of the plant: the silky seeds are gathered to line its nest.

Humans, on the other hand, use coltsfoot leaves to prepare herbal smoking mixtures and snuffs. British herbal tobacco contains a large amount of coltsfoot leaves. Coltsfoot tobacco is said to heighten one's powers of perception, and it has been used for centuries to treat colds, sinus problems, bronchitis, asthma, and tuberculosis. To make coltsfoot tobacco, the leaves are dried, heaped, fermented, and then dried again in much the same manner as Virginia tobacco. They are hung in a warm, dry place until they attain the yellow-brown color of chamois-leather. The midribs are then ripped out, and the leaves packed into stone jars with the addition of a little brandy. After a month, they are removed in layers, rolled out, and pressed under weights before being shredded into tobacco. During World War II, herbal tobacco consisting for the most part of coltsfoot leaves was sold in Flemish cities with the mysterious words printed on the label: "Not tobacco, but also not chestnut tree." Smoked coltsfoot leaves are still sold and smoked in China as a substitute for tobacco.

Veterinary Values

Large coltsfoot leaves can be used as emergency bandages for all animals, and as poultices to cool infected or inflamed areas.

Miscellaneous Wisdom

In Switzerland, witches were once thought to steal milk with the aid of coltsfoot roots. According to the written report of one witch trial, the roots were dug in the secrecy of night in complete silence. They were wrapped in white linen, and the linen bundle was buried underneath the stall door before the break of day. The witch then waited for the cow to step on the roots. From that day on, the milk of that cow would flow into her pail, and the rightful owners could only draw bloody liquid from the beast.

Children use coltsfoot leaves interchangeably with dock leaves to "rub out" nettle stings (see nettle chapter), often with the same rhymes. The plant's large leaves are used as umbrellas during unexpected downpours, as plates on picnics, and as roofing material for children's thatched houses.

Though you like the fat and meat which are eaten in the drinking-halls,
I like better to eat a head of clean water-cress in a place without sorrow ...

—"The Wild Man comes to the Monastery," *A Celtic Miscellany*

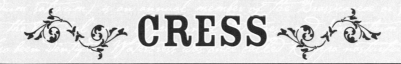

CRESS

Name

Because the smell of this herb is so pungent, the botanical name for cress (*Nasturtium*) evolved from the Latin words for "a twisted nose"—*nasus tortus*.

Garden cress (*Lepidium sativum*) is an annual member of the **Brassicaceae** or **Cruciferae** family. *Nasturtium officinale* is the botanical name of perennial watercress, and *Nasturtium microphyllum (Rorippa microphylla)* has also been identified. Watercress was once called *Rorippa nasturtium-aquaticum*. An interesting local garden cress, *Lepidium virginicum*, or Virginian peppercress, can be found in North and Central America. *Lepidium meyenii*, or maca, has been grown for centuries in Peru for its tuberous roots.

Folk Names

Garden cress is also called garden pepperwort, peppergrass, and pepperwort; *Gartenkresse* in German; *mastuerzo, berro alenois*, and *nastuerzo hortense* in Spanish; *passérage, cresson alénois*, and *cressonette* in French; *crescione inglese* and *masturzio ortense* in Italian; and *teretura* in Turkish. The Sanskrit name is *chandrasura*.

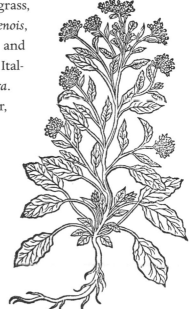

Virginian peppercress is known as poor man's pepper, and in Mexico it is called *rochiwari*.

Watercress is also called brooklime, tang-tongues, tongue-grass, water-grass, carpenter's chips, wild water cress, common water cress, and cuckoo flower. It is named *Brunnenkresse, Kirchen*, and *Wassersenf* in German; *cresson, cresson des fontaines, cresson d'eau*, and *crinson* in French; *crescione, crescione, crescione aquatico, crescione dei sorgenti, nasturzio aquatico*, and *sisimbro aquatico* in Italian; *berwr dŵr* in Welsh; and *bidar* in Irish.

Appearance

Garden cress is such a familiar plant that it needs little description. Fresh cress plants are often sold in packages in grocery stores. If cress is allowed to grow outdoors, the leaves will be larger, but the fresh green color will remain the same. The fruits of the plant are unusual: the seed capsules are placed very close to the main stem, and are shaped like coins that open up to reveal the seeds.

Watercress usually only grows to 3 ft. in length, and can be found in running or in very clean water. Its true roots disappear early in the year and are replaced with silvery fibers growing on one side of its creeping, hollow stems. The stems are weak, thin, and full of sap, and produce unpaired dark green, fleshy leaves. The end leaf is always rounded, although the number of leaves on a stalk varies. Watercress is evergreen, and continues to grow under ice. It has no particular smell, but a sharp and spicy taste that is most pronounced while the plant is flowering. Watercress flowers are small and white, with four cross-shaped petals. The seeds grow in pods.

Place, Season, and Useful Parts

Garden cress flourishes in moist soil, and occasionally escapes from cultivated areas. If the situation is too dry, stunted plants will be the result.

Watercress grows in clear, slowly running brooks, in springs, or their runoffs. It can occasionally be found in standing or even salt water to an altitude of 6,000 ft. Watercress grows in most of the northern temperate zone. It can be gathered at all times except when blossoming, or covered with ice. The herb usually blossoms from May on intermittently until October.

Gathering, Drying, and Storage

Garden cress can be cut as needed and re-sown periodically. It should only be eaten fresh, since it neither freezes nor dries well. Juice can be extracted from both the cresses, and frozen or canned for later use.

Watercress that has not yet flowered can be harvested from February on into the fall. It should only be gathered from clean, freshly running brooks, and never from standing or polluted waters. The herb can be confused in Europe with other aquatic plants such as the fool's watercress *(Apium nodiflorum)*, generally considered to be poisonous. Small watercress leaves or the entire young plant are gathered and packed loosely into baskets to prevent bruising. Snails and small aquatic insects often adhere to the plant, and the leaves should therefore be washed carefully in salt or vinegar water. Watercress is at its best when fresh, but can also be dried quickly in a shady, airy place, without turning, or with the help of artificial heat. It does not keep long.

Seed Saving and Germination

A number of garden cress varieties exist, and there is also local variation among wild species. Single varieties should be isolated to maintain varietal purity. The easiest method of doing this is temporal isolation. The flowering of different varieties is staggered by sowing them several weeks apart. This way, they can pollinate without interference, and more seed can be obtained. It is easy to harvest garden cress seeds by cutting the entire plants when the first pods ripen and letting them dry on cloths or head down in paper bags. The ripe seeds are stripped from the plants by hand.

Watercress is usually propagated by letting it seed itself, or by distributing the seeds in lightly running water (they will not do well in stagnant water). Plants can also be transplanted to suitable habitats with good success.

Gardening Hints

Garden cress is so easy to grow that the crop can be entrusted to a child. Cress prefers damp and sandy soil, but will germinate under most conditions. Seeds should be sown every two weeks from spring to autumn to ensure a continuous crop. They sprout quickly, and produce greens that can be harvested as soon as the first true leaves begin to appear. The tips of the plants are nipped out, or the entire plant cut fairly close to the ground. It should quickly recover from the cut to produce a second crop of leaves. A few plants should always be allowed to go to seed, so that there will be seed for the next sowing. Before winter, more plants can be allowed to set seed, and the excess used for sprouting in winter. Cress plants grow well in the vicinity of lettuce.

Children who are fascinated by growing plants but are still too impatient to have their own gardens can be given cress seeds to grow indoors on damp cotton or paper towels. Even under adverse conditions, the seeds will sprout within a couple of days. Mustard seeds can also be sown along with the cress in different patterns. This way, it is possible to spell the child's initials with the growing plants.

Watercress is more difficult to raise, and is usually gathered from the wild. But it does propagate itself once established, and is worth a try in the garden. The seeds remain fertile for as long as 5 years, and are spread by running water or birds. Although its rootlets die off each year, watercress is a perennial plant, and its stem quickly produces new roots. Watercress seeds can be sown by scattering them in 1–6 in. deep, very slowly running water, or started indoors and then transplanted to a nearby brook or a large outdoor container with some water movement.

The Tarahumara Indians grow Virginian cress, also known as poor man's pepper or rochiwari, as a companion plant in cornfields. It is harvested before the corn grows tall, allowing two crops to be gathered in the same season.

Culinary Virtues

Garden cress sprouts in two or three days, and should be sown repeatedly outdoors to ensure a continuous supply of fresh greens. In winter, the seeds can be sprouted on dampened cotton placed on a plate on a warm windowsill, and harvested with scissors a few days later. Some windowsill-gardeners like to combine a few pungent mustard seeds with the cress. Others sprout cress and other sprouts such as alfalfa or fenugreek in special sprouting pots.

Garden cress greens are cut before the plant develops true leaves. The cuttings are then chopped finely and served in green or potato salads, on buttered bread, baked potatoes, in herbal butters, as a garnish for potato or egg salads, or as a seasoning for scrambled eggs, meatloaf, hamburgers, steaks, or cutlets. Spring salads can be prepared from spinach, head lettuce, dandelion and nettle greens, and seasoned with some freshly chopped garden cress.

Watercress is gathered before it blossoms from clear, unpolluted springs or brooks. It should be carefully washed in vinegar or salt water to destroy insect eggs or larvae still adhering to the plants (there is danger of liver fluke infestation). Watercress remains green through the cold months of February and March. It contains surprising amounts of iodine, as well as other mineral salts and vitamin C, and is somewhat more "peppery" than garden cress. It is included in spring salads, or served alone, seasoned with lemon juice, before a main course. Creamy soups thickened with cream or eggs, béchamel sauce, or semolina can be seasoned with watercress. It is stir-fried with a little ginger, and served with meat or fish, or used as a fresh garnish. Cooks sometimes employ the expressed juice of watercress as a seasoning for spicy sauces, and the pounded seeds are occasionally used as a seasoning or in the manufacture of mustard.

Watercress soup can be prepared in much as the same manner as sorrel and potato soup (see sorrel chapter). Milk can be substituted for the broth, and the mixture puréed carefully to mince the tougher stems. Watercress sauce is served hot with chicken or salmon. Meat can also be seasoned with the tender young herb. The meat is browned over a high flame to seal in the juices. Turn down the heat, add some chopped ginger, followed by chopped garden cress or watercress, soy sauce or salt, and, if necessary, a few drops of white wine to keep the herbs from burning. The heat is lowered even more, the pan covered, and the meat allowed to cook gently until tender. A dab of cress butter can also be served with meat dishes, or they can be seasoned with cress vinegar.

Noteworthy Recipes

Watercress Purée: Watercress purée is made by wilting the cleaned leaves in melted butter, passing the mixture through a sieve or putting it through the blender, and then stirring in fresh mashed potatoes, a little butter and cream, and salt and pepper. Watercress purée is a meal in itself, or it can be served as an accompaniment to meat.

Cress Butter: Cream ¼ lb. of fresh, unsalted cream butter, then add 1 Tbsp. of minced chives, watercress and chervil or parsley, and a pinch of salt if desired. Roll the butter, wrap it in aluminum foil and place in the refrigerator or a cool place to harden. Serve with bread, vegetables, or meat.

Cress Vinegar: William Kitchiner offered this recipe in the nineteenth century:

> Dry and pound half an ounce of Cress-Seed (such as is sown in the garden with Mustard), pour upon it a quart of the best Vinegar, let it steep ten days, shaking it up every day.
>
> Obs –This is very strongly flavoured with Cress, and for Salads, and Cold Meats, &c. it is a great favourite with many;–the Quart of Sauce costs only a Half-penny more than the Vinegar.[37]

Cosmetic Properties

Fresh watercress compresses cleanse and bleach blemished or freckled skin, and can help to arrest hair loss caused by fungal infections.

Medicinal Merits

Garden cress was once thought to inflame the passions and warm the heart, as well as renew one's lust for life. It was included in many spring tonics and men were warned against excessive use of the plant. Cress was though to sharpen the senses and clear the brain, and to cleanse the spleen and lungs. Powdered cress seeds were inhaled to induce sneezing. Culpeper wrote that cress helps with headaches and "consumes the gross humours winter hath left behind," also noting that "those that would live in health may use it if they please; if they will not, I cannot help it. If any fancy not pottage, they may eat the herb as a salad."[38]

Watercress was not, according to ancient authorities, quite as violently effective as garden cress, which was administered to treat lethargy, scurvy, and drowsiness, to expel worms, and to treat tuberculosis and hepatitis. It was applied to fungal diseases such as ringworm, and to feverish growths. Watercress was considered a good diuretic, capable of expelling poison from the body and the kidneys. In the words of the Anglo-Saxon Nine Herb Charm,

> This herb is called Stime; it grew on a stone,
> It resists poison, it fights pain.
> It is called harsh, it fights against poison.
> This is the herb that strove with the snake;

---

37. Kitchiner, *The Cook's Oracle* (1817) (London: Samuel Bagster, 1860), 263.

38. Culpeper, *Culpeper's Complete Herbal* (1653) (London: Foulsham, undated), 104.

This has strength against poison, this has strength against infection,
This has strength against the foe who fares through the land![39]

In this case, the "foe" was understood to be the contagious diseases that swept as epidemics through the land, often decimating the population.

Modern Medicine

Watercress is invaluable as a spring tonic because of its high vitamin C and mineral salt content, and because it is one of the very first green spring plants. Due to its high iodine content, it helps to activate the thyroid gland in particular, and is an important aid against the current epidemic of hypothyroidism. Watercress can help to rid the body of excess fluids, counteract anemia, cleanse the lungs, stimulate the digestive organs, reduce swellings of the spleen, and lower fevers. Recent experiments have discovered an antibiotic agent effective against *Candida* and other fungal diseases, and suspected of having a deterrent effect on some influenza viruses. Given the increasing stubbornness and epidemic nature of these diseases, this discovery should be of great interest to the modern herbalist. A homeopathic essence of the freshly blossoming plant is administered to patients suffering from fever and nerve pains. A watercress salve, prepared like a marigold salve (see that chapter), is also said to have a curative effect on burns.

A daily watercress salad is recommended for patients with pulmonary complaints. Children troubled with worms are encouraged to eat watercress salads seasoned with oil and vinegar. Pregnant women should shun the spicy herb because of its unpredictable effect on the glandular system. Patients with an overactive thyroid should also avoid the plant, but it can be of great help to those with thyroid insufficiency or imbalance.

Although most herbalists now consider watercress to be the more potent of the two cresses, garden cress has recently been recognized as having medicinal properties beyond its obvious nutritional qualities.

Watercress is considered a cooling and bitter food in Chinese medicine, used to clear heat, to lubricate the lungs, and act as a diuretic while alleviating thirst and dry cough.

Special Cures

Watercress Juice Cure: Watercress juice can be taken for up to 4 weeks in the spring as a tonic cure. The juice of the fresh plant is combined with the juices of other cleansing herbs such as brooklime *(Veronica beccabunga)* and borage, or it is taken alone. On the first days of the cure, take 2 tsp. of the juice, thinned with water or fruit juice, and slowly work up to 6 tsp., and then back down to 2 tsp.

---

39. Qtd. in Paul Huson, *Mastering Herbalism* (New York: Stein and Day: 1974), 231.

Veterinary Values

Fresh green garden cress can be added to the diets of dogs and cats with good results. Crushed cress seed is given to dogs suffering from lack of appetite. In the Far East, sick water buffaloes and cows are fed with cress.

Miscellaneous Wisdom

In ancient Rome, lazy sluggards were told to *"Edc nasturtium!"* (eat cress). In Greece, the saying went, "Eat cress and learn more wit." The plant was believed to cure lethargy and anemia, and to clear the brain.

Legends

In a Swiss village, a special mass was once called to invoke God's intervention against the ravages of the plague. The people praying in the church were astonished to hear a voice coming from above the altar: "Eat pimpernel and watercress, the Death will want you less!"[40]

Literary Flowers

Good its clear blue water, good its clean stern wind,
Good its cress-green watercress, better its green brooklime.
Good its pure ivy, good its bright merry willow,
Good its yewy yew, better its melodious birch …

—AN UNKNOWN IRISH AUTHOR OF THE 12TH CENTURY,
QTD. IN JACKSON, *A CELTIC MISCELLANY*

And in his left hand he held a basket full
Of all sweet herbs that searching eye could cull:
Wild thyme, and valley-lilies whiter still
Than Leda's love, and cresses from the rill.

—KEATS, *ENDYMION*

And sprouting from the bottom purply green
The watercress neath the wave is seen
Which the old woman gladly drags to land
Wi reaching long rake in her tottering hand …

—JOHN CLARE, *THE SHEPHERD'S CALENDAR*, "MARCH"

---

40. *Schweizerisches Archiv für Volkskunde*, vol. 3 (Zurich: Société Suisse des Traditions Populaires, 1897–present), 135.

CRESS

The brook resumes its summer dresses
Purling neath grass and water cresses
And mint and flag leaf swording high ...

—JOHN CLARE, *THE SHEPHERD'S CALENDAR*, "MAY"

Star-disked dandelions, just as we see them lying in the grass,
like sparks that have leaped from the kindling sun of summer.

—O. W. Holmes, *The Professor at the Breakfast Table*

❧ DANDELION ❧

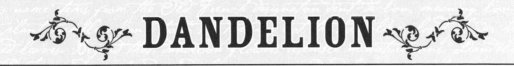

Name

Dandelion's name stems from the Old French designation *dent-de-lion*, meaning "lion's tooth." Several parts of the plant resemble a lion's tooth: the tapering root, the tooth-like, closed flower head, and the ferociously jagged leaves. Beyond that, dandelion flowers resemble miniature suns, and these are associated with the zodiacal sign Leo, or lion. One or all of these facts may have led to the herb's name.

The origin of dandelion's botanical name, *Taraxacum*, is uncertain, but folk names for the plant are numerous and graphical.

Dandelion is a perennial member of the **Daisy** family (**Asteraceae** or **Compositae**), and is commonly termed *Taraxacum officinale*, although some other synonyms are occasionally used: *Leodonton taraxacum, Leodonton vulgare,* and *Taraxacum vulgare.*

Folk Names

Here are just a few of the plant's innumerable titles: piss-a-bed, piss pot, pissimire, pishamoolog, pittle bed, pee-a-bed, wet-a-bed, wet-weed, mess-a-bed, shit-a-bed, lay-a-bed, bum-pipe, stink Davie, bitter aks, devil's milk-plant, devil's milk-pail, milk gowan, puffball, heart-fever grass, swine's snout, lion's tooth, golden suns, male, burning fire, monk's head, priest's crown, dindle, canker, cankerwort, dog-posy, blowball, puffball, wishes, combs and hair-pins, clocks and watches, tell-time, time flower, time teller, what o'clock, clock flower, clock, fairy clocks, old man's clock, farmer's clocks, schoolboy's clock, shepherd's clock, one o'clock, one two three four o'clock, twelve o'clock, and doon-head clock. German names are *Löwenzahn, Butterblume, Teufelslichter,*

Hexenlichter, *Sonnenwirbel*, *Lämmchen*, and *Kuhblume*. The French call it *dent de lion*, *pissenlit*, *laiteron*, *groin de porc*, and *coq*; Italians, *tarassaco*, *piscialetto*, *capo di fratre*, *radichiella*, *pisciacane*, *stella gialla*, and *dente di leone*. A Dutch name is *beddepissers*. Spanish terms are *diente de léon* and *anagrón*; Welsh, *dant y llew*; and Russian, *oduvančik lekarstvennyj*.

Appearance

Although the dandelion is the one herb that supposedly every child can identify, there are many botanical variations and malformations to confuse amateur botanists and herbalists. The most imposing feature of the dandelion is the yellow sun-shaped flower that moves its head with the sun and closes its petals when rain or darkness threatens. Dandelion stems are milky, hollow, and hairless, the leaves toothed and deeply gashed, gathered at the root in a rosette. They have a bitter taste. The spent flowers resemble a swine's snout. Dandelion seed globes are composed of tiny white parachute seeds that blow away to reveal a flat disc that looks like a priest's tonsure. The tapering roots are brown on the outside, white or whitish on the inside, and filled with a milky sap. Their smell is intensively earthy.

Place, Season, and Useful Parts

The dandelion is such a common cosmopolitan that it is more appropriate to list the places it does not grow than the places it does appear. It does not grow in most of the Southern Hemisphere, on moors and dunes, at extremely high altitudes or in extremely cold or arid climates. It flourishes in meadows and well-fertilized fields, and has even been known to settle in trees and on top of thatched houses. Meadows colored a rich yellow by dandelion flowers or a soft white by dandelion seed heads are a common sight. Dandelions flower in April and May, and some bloom off and on until the first snowfall. Dandelion roots are perennial and the plants will continue to grow until mowed down by frost. New plants spring up as soon as the snow melts in spring.

The entire dandelion plant can be put to good use, from its downy seed heads to its roots. Flowers should be gathered when fully blooming late in the morning on a sunny day. Leaves and young plants should only be gathered from second-year plants in the spring or fall. The spring roots are bitter, the fall roots sweeter and firmer.

Gathering, Drying, and Storage

Dandelion flowers should be picked together with the calyxes, or flower receptacles, but without stems. The leaves can be picked singly, or the leaf rosette cut above the root and rinsed quickly under running water to remove dirt. Do not pack too tightly into baskets or gather the leaves in plastic or metal containers. Dandelion leaves should be processed immediately, or spread out to dry as soon as possible. Shake the roots to free loose dirt, then scrub them with a dry brush and, if necessary, wash them quickly under running water. Commercial growers plow the soil to unearth the roots and then sort, wash, and dry them.

Dandelion leaves, flowers and roots need to be dried quickly in dark, airy rooms. The cleaned roots can be split and hung up to dry on strings for 7–10 days and then transferred to heated rooms. In damp climates, it is best to split and cut the roots into small pieces, and dry over a very slow oven or in the vicinity of another source of low heat.

Dandelion greens and flowers must be completely dry before they are stored. The roots should be crisp to the touch, and retain a white core. Dried roots are sometimes subject to maggot infestation. They must be stored in closed containers and checked regularly.

Seed Saving and Germination

Some gardeners attempt to save seed of their favorite dandelion plants without isolating them, forgetting that dandelions are pollinated with windblown pollen. Every wild plant within half a mile radius is going to be contributing pollen to the seed plants, and they will not come true to type. In order to save seed from cultivated varieties, the plants need to be isolated in isolation greenhouses, or placed under a floating row cover with introduced pollinators, or grown so that they will flower at a different time from wild varieties. This will take some doing, but can be accomplished by sowing the plants indoors or in a cold frame so that they flower in late summer or early fall. If the timing is not right, then "off with their heads!" In other words, mow the plants down so that they stop blossoming, and then let them bloom when wild varieties have stopped flowering. Seed obtained this way should come true. The ripe seed heads are gathered, and then rubbed against a sieve to remove the down.

A surprising number of cultivated dandelion varieties exist, and the wild plants often vary dramatically. Mutations and malformations are quite common, making the task of identifying different subspecies quite difficult. As a rule, cultivated varieties have been selected to produce larger, softer, less bitter leaves that respond well to blanching. Wild plants are usually more medicinally potent.

Gardening Hints

Dandelions can be classified as hated weeds or appreciated as a marketable delicacy. When the plants invade hay, alfalfa, or clover fields, or force their way into gardens, inhibiting the growth of other plants, and rooting deep into the soil, they are justly despised as persistent pests. On the other hand, cultivated varieties are healthful delicacies that can be grown successfully by the commercial as well as the home gardener. This is the case in Europe, India, and Japan. Another method of putting dandelions to good use is to root out the not-yet blossoming plants, and then ferment them in rainwater as a valuable liquid fertilizer. Be careful not to include flower heads, or you may end up sowing the seeds all over the garden! This dandelion brew can be used to water the compost heap, and to add valuable nutrients to the soil.

Dandelion seeds germinate best if sown loosely on porous soil without covering the seeds. The plants should be thinned rigorously, and kept neatly in a line to avoid confusion with wild volunteer plants. They can be forced under sawdust or blanched under an inverted flowerpot or weighted board to make the leaves more tender and also less bitter. The flower heads should be removed as soon as they appear in order to lengthen the leaf harvest. As the year progresses, and the soil warms, the leaves will become tougher and less palatable. If you are saving seed, it is a good time to let the plants blossom, after all of their wild neighbors have gone to seed.

Gardeners often look at the way dandelions blossom in the spring to determine how the gardening year is going to turn out. A few scraggly dandelion blossoms presage a bad year for the garden, but if the fields seem to explode with large dandelion heads, it is taken as an especially good sign.

Culinary Virtues

Long before its generally accepted use in Europe, the dandelion was a food staple of Native Americans. Although it was eaten in Italy as early as 1650, it remained a primarily lower class or emergency food until recent years. It has now gained the reputation of an exotic delicacy bought at high prices in specialty stores. In order to meet demand, gardeners have developed new varieties with large leaves and mild taste. Both wild and cultivated dandelion greens can be canned or frozen for winter use.

The dandelion is one of the most versatile and common wild food plants available to humankind. It would be theoretically possible to serve an entire meal based solely on dandelions. The sweet fall roots can be boiled, baked, or grated and eaten raw. Dandelion roots, crowns, and leaves are added to vegetable soups. The crowns are steamed and served with butter; and the cooked leaves mixed with spinach, potato salads, egg dishes, savories, and soufflés. Small dandelion buds are sometimes pickled as caper substitutes, and tender young dandelion leaves added to sandwiches. Dandelion salads can be flavored with some crumbled crisp bacon or croutons. A little hot bacon fat poured over the crisp leaves will also improve the salad's texture and taste. Another method of preparation is to dress cooked dandelion greens with olive (or flax) oil and vinegar, and garnish them with chopped boiled egg. A simple green lettuce salad can be "refined" with the addition of a few fresh dandelion leaves. Dandelion wine and dandelion beer round out a meal prepared with dandelions.

One of the best-known ways to use dandelion flowers is in dandelion syrup. This springtime delicacy is used as a honey substitute at a time of year when fresh honey is not yet available.

Before coffee became a universally accepted morning drink, coffee prepared from roasted dandelion roots was very popular. It is now enjoyed by those who have learned to savor its bitter medicinal properties.

Noteworthy Recipes

Dandelion Syrup: Pick 5–6 handfuls of dandelion flowers and remove the stems. Carefully rinse and strain the flowers to remove insects and dust, and then place them in a large saucepan. Barely cover with water. Let the mixture boil for 10–15 minutes, and strain. Return the strained liquid to the saucepan, and stir in 3 lb. of sugar and the juice of 2 lemons. Bring to a boil, stirring all the while. Strain, and pour into clean jars. If a thicker consistency is desired, the syrup can be boiled longer until the thread or softball stage is reached. Dandelion syrup should be sealed in canning jars for extended storage, or it can be frozen.

Dandelion Rhubarb: This is a novel way to prepare dandelion flowers. Dandelion rhubarb is a cleansing spring medicine as well as a refreshing dessert. Pick several handfuls of dandelion flowers, rinse them carefully, and barely cover them with water in a saucepan. Boil for 10–15 minutes. The strained juice, sweetened with sugar, is used as cooking water for fresh rhubarb stalks.

Dandelion Beer: Dandelion beer is made in the same fashion as nettle beer (see the stinging nettle chapter). Mixed herbal beers can be prepared from mixtures such as dandelion flowers, nettle leaves, cleavers *(Galium aparine)*, white dead nettles, curled dock, lemon or orange juice, and ginger.

Dandelion Wine: Because winemaking is such a delicate art, it is advisable to seek help from an expert, or to study a detailed and accurate account of the winemaking procedure. Some brewers insist that the quality of their wines is due to jealously guarded secrets, such as only preparing wine from flowers gathered early in the morning on May Day in utter silence.

To make the wine, pour 1 gal. of boiling water over 1 gal. of loosely packed, stemless dandelion flowers, and let stand, covered, in a crock for 3 days. Strain through muslin and then squeeze the juice out into a large saucepan. Add 1 lb. of sugar for a dry wine, or up to 3 lb. of sugar for a sweet, heavy wine. Raisins can be substituted for some of the sugar in the recipe if desired, and the juice of 2 lemons and 2 oranges added for flavor. Boil the mixture for 30 minutes, skim, and then let it cool until lukewarm. Stir ½ cake of yeast (or ½ oz. of dried yeast) with a little water until soft, and spread onto a slice of toasted bread. Float the toast on the surface of the brew and let stand, covered with a clean cloth, for 3 days. Then strain once again through muslin into a sterile fermentation flask, equipped with a thistle funnel or valve cork. Let the wine "work" until fermentation stops completely, feeding the mixture every couple of days with a few raisins to increase its potency. Decant, bottle in sterilized bottles, and cork carefully. Dandelion wine improves with age, and should be stored for at least 6 months before drinking.

A much more delicate wine can be produced by using a Mosel wine yeast, bought at a specialty store, and a very small amount of sugar, 1 lb., for every gallon of water.

Household Applications

Ethereal dandelion oils have been occasionally used to flavor liqueurs. For centuries, thirst-quenching dandelion beer has been traditionally served to farm workers. The task of making dandelion wine, beer, and stout has in the meantime been elevated to a high art, and dandelion wine is often considered the best herbal wine of all. The joke about the little drunk old ladies and their secret supply of dandelion wine in the parlor is not as far-fetched as it may seem: a carefully prepared and well-aged dandelion wine has all the potency and good flavor of superb mead.

One of the most exasperating things about dandelions is their ability to stain hands and clothing dark brown. The pithy sap found in leaves and roots is very difficult to remove. But this drawback also has its positive side: a yellow-brown, fairly stable dye can be produced from the roots, and a purplish hue prepared from the leaves. The whole plant, roots and all, can also be used with alum, iron, or tin as mordants to produce tones from beige to gray to yellow-brown.

Cosmetic Properties

Dandelion leaves are used as a cleansing tea cure to clear the skin of impurities and remove blemishes. Because of its milky sap, the plant is rarely used externally.

Medicinal Merits

According to the doctrine of signatures popular in the late Middle Ages, a plant reveals its medicinal merits though its most striking external characteristics. In the case of the dandelion, these were the milk sap and the bright yellow color of the blossoms. The milky sap was thought to increase the milk flow of humans and animals, and to remove milky films over eyes (cataracts). The yellow color of the herb's flowers pointed to dandelion's major modern medicinal merits: a gall bladder and liver drug as well as an excellent diuretic medicine.

Modern Medicine

Dandelion, both root and leaf, has a beneficial effect on the liver, a stimulating effect on the gall bladder and its secretions, and a positive strengthening effect on the stomach and intestines. It has been used with success to treat hemorrhoids, the early stages of jaundice and hepatitis, and some forms of diabetes and anemia. It is a blood-cleansing medicine effective against certain types of rashes and eczema, and can also be taken as a bitter tonic for the stomach, and a light tonic stimulant for the entire system.

The diuretic, or, to use the language of the old herbals, water-provoking action of the dandelion plant is so notorious that it has been nicknamed Piss-a-bed. It is useful in the treatment of kidney insufficiencies, water retention, and mild forms of rheumatism and gout, as well as all conditions that arise from a malfunctioning liver or kidney.

Dandelion roots and dandelion leaves are often used in combination in tea form, or as an alcoholic tincture or extract. They are quite potent, and should only be taken for a short time. Cooked dandelion greens are also medicinally valuable. The expressed juice of the fresh plant as well as the dried milky sap of the fresh plant were once commonly sold as medicine, but have now gone out of favor in most countries. *Taraxacum* is an important homeopathic remedy prepared from plants harvested before they blossom, and used like the fresh herb for liver and spleen. It is prescribed for those with a patchy white-coated tongue, who are impatient and irritable, and have cold fingertips. It can also be used to treat patients with night sweats, who have an urge to urinate frequently.

Dandelion is used in Chinese medicine to counteract food poisoning and to treat breast disorders, as well as being employed as a liver and gallbladder drug, especially for hot conditions. It can effectively detoxify the blood, liver, and kidneys, and promote lactation in nursing women as well as urination. The main species is *Taraxacum mongolicum*.

Special Cures

A Tonic Tea for the Immune System: In order to strengthen the immune system and constitution and restore the entire body to its former health, German herbalists suggest abstinence from all beverages except water and a tea prepared from 1 part of angelica seeds, 1 part of dandelion roots and leaves, and 2 parts of stinging nettle leaves. The herbs should be brewed 1½ tsp. to ½ pint of cold water, and left to stand overnight. In the morning, heat the mixture, but do not let it come to a boil. The tea should be taken for 4 weeks and 4 weeks only for best results. After a pause of 2–4 weeks, it can be taken again if no negative results have been observed.

Uses in Husbandry

Dandelion is a very important bee plant because it blossoms profusely in spring, and then continues to bloom off and on again until fall. It has been computed that a bee has to visit 125,000 dandelion flowers in order to produce 2 lb. of honey.

A rubber substitute has been produced at various times from Russian dandelion, *Taraxacum kok-saghz*, and the plant cultivated for this purpose.

Dandelions serve as fodder for both wild and domesticated animals. The seeds are eaten by pheasants and grouse; the leaves by deer and hares. Sheep will eat dandelion with reluctance, and horses will not touch it. Puppies profit if very finely chopped dandelion greens are added to their diet, as will mature dogs troubled with jaundice, baldness, loss of hair, or heart troubles. The leaves and powdered roots are included in some commercial rabbit pellets, and dandelion is often added to silage. Farmers do not appreciate the presence of dandelions in hay fields because they rob growing space from more profitable feed plants. Dried dandelion leaves also tend to crumble and turn to powder, sifting down to the bottom of the hayloft.

Because dandelions contain white "milk," some farmers believe that dandelions can restore milk to bewitched cows. In Germany, hexed animals are fed a mixture of dandelion, salt, and clay. Danish sorcerers are said to make use of the milky plant to steal milk from the cows of their enemies.

Miscellaneous Wisdom

Dandelions are universally believed to cause bed-wetting. In northern Italy, even touching a dandelion can have disastrous results. In France, blowing away the seed will result in a wet bed, and in other places, children are warned never to take dandelions to bed. One isolated English belief turns the whole thing around by saying that children will *not* wet the bed for twelve full months if they are given dandelion flowers.

Another widespread folk belief is that anyone who finds the first three spring dandelions will remain in good health for the rest of the year. Such an undertaking may sound simple enough, but dandelions have a way of springing out of the ground all at once, and finding the very first three flowers is often a difficult task.

In Lincolnshire, the memory of a woman who could once miraculously cure anemia is still alive. She would hollow out a dandelion root, fill it with a mixture of ground iron filings, honey, and butter, and give her patients these "pills" to swallow. Another drastic Lincolnshire remedy was to give birthing women cakes to eat before delivery. These pain-killing biscuits were made of a combination of whole wheat flour, crushed hemp seed, grated rhubarb root (medicinal rhubarb, and not kitchen rhubarb), dandelion roots, egg yolks, milk, and gin. They may have been pain killing for the mother, but rhubarb is a strong laxative, and the other ingredients may have negatively affected the unborn child.

Legends

The dandelion plant often brings forth one blood-red leaf among the green. The inhabitants of Lechrain believed that several drops of Mary's menstrual blood fell on the plant after she conceived Jesus. The blood was taken as proof of her immaculate state, and the red dandelion leaves thought to bear living witness to her virginity.

Oracular Worth

The dandelion is indisputably the most famous oracular plant. Children love to blow on the full seed "lanterns" and count the remaining seed parachutes. The resulting number tells the time of day, or how many years they will live, how many years will pass before they marry, how many children they will have, how many sins they have committed, or how many lies they have told in one day. If all the seeds fly away, it means that something nice will happen: a good dinner at home, a gift of new clothes or toys. If the disk of the seed head is white, it is taken as a promise of heaven, but a black one is a sure warning of hell. Czech children blow dandelions in the direction of an adult to find out how many sins he or she has committed. Each seed head that sticks to the adult's clothes represents one sin. In Holland, girls ask the full seed heads, "Does he love me?" If all the seeds blow away when the girl blows "Yes," then he loves her. If they blow away when she blows "A little," then he loves her a little. If they all blow away at "Much!" then he loves her dearly. If it happens when she blows "No," then she will become an old maid, or have to wait for a new sweetheart.

If dandelions grow high in spring, Austrian and Slovakian farmers take it as a sign that the flax will also grow to a good height. When fields are yellow with dandelion flowers, then the year will be fruitful. Rain is thought to be imminent if the down flies off dandelions on a windless day.

Herbal Pastimes

Because they are so common, dandelions are often used by children as playthings. Adults rarely employ the quickly-wilting flowers for ornamental purposes, but children take hedonistic delight in forming dandelion rings, chains, wreaths, and crowns, and their quick-witted imagination can turn two joined flowers into a pair of glasses, and dandelion stems into trumpets. Stems that have been split and soaked in water make good doll's curls. Some budding architects even use the stems as plumbing for miniature cities. No warnings, or scoldings by adults that they will stain their clothes, can keep children away from dandelions. There have even been cases of poisoning when small children insisted on stuffing themselves with dandelion flowers.

Literary Flowers

Dandelion suns rise eager with the morning. Leonine heads soak in the sun's warmth, transmit its heat along hollow shafts, past leaves to the receptive rosette, where it meets water trickling down to the root. Dark bark hides the process of transformation of warmth and dew into milky juice. The sap then travels up the stalk with fresh energy to nurture new leaves and the developing seeds. The seed heads turn full like a field of downy stars suspended in whiteness on hollow stalks. A coming rain draws circles around the moon and the single plumes from their clusters. A gentle wind or a child's breath sends the parachute stars into orbit.

—SISTER CLARISSA'S UNPUBLISHED BOOK OF NATURAL OBSERVATIONS

You see here what virtues this common herb hath, and that is the reason the French and Dutch so often eat them in spring; and now if you look a little farther, you may see plainly without a pair of spectacles, that foreign physicians are not as selfish as ours are, but more communicative of the virtues of plants to people.

—NICHOLAS CULPEPER, CULPEPER'S COMPLETE HERBAL

Vervain and Dill
Hinders witches from their will

—English Folk Saying

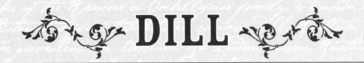

DILL

Name

The final etymology of the word "dill" is uncertain. The Danish form was *dild*, the Anglo-Saxon *dile*, and the Old High German *Tillj*. Some scholars suggest that the word originated from the Norse *dilla*, meaning "to lull."

The ancient Greeks and Romans also called dill *anethon*, or *anethum*. Aristophanes mentioned a plant called *anethon*, which was derived from the Greek word for wind (flatulence).

Dill, an annual member of the **Apiaceae** or **Umbelliferae** family, is known under the botanical name of *Anethum graveolens*. Botanists differentiate between common dill, *Anethum graveolens var. graveolens*, and garden dill, *Anethum graveolens var. hortorum*. An Indian version, *Anethum graveolens var. sowa*, has been described and is widely grown in the East as a medicinal herb.

Folk Names

Dill is generally called by its proper name, and has few nicknames. The seeds are called meeting house seeds in English. *Dill*, *Hexenchrut*, and *Gurkenkraut* are German names. It is called *aneth*, *aneth odorant*, *fenouil puant*, and *fenouil bâtard* in French; *aneto*, *aneto puzzolente*, and *finocchio fetido* in Italian; *anethon* in modern Greek; *eneldo*, *hinojo*, and *inoldo* in Spanish; *endro* in Portuguese, and *ukrop* in Russian.

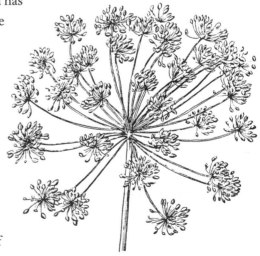

Appearance

All members of the **Carrot** family can easily be confused with each other. Since many members of this family are poisonous, caution is the major rule to be observed when dealing with them. Dill can best be identified by its earthy, penetrating smell, which is unique, and by the feathery appearance of its leaves, similar to fennel. Dill leaves and fruits have a pleasant and warming taste, and are similar in growth to fennel, until the umbels form.

Dill has a small and spindly, woody root. Its round and hollow stem can grow to a height of 3 ft. and is scored lengthwise with miniscule green and white stripes. Dill leaves are feathery and threadlike, and of a rich green color with a blue tinge. The entire plant is hairless, and the upper leaves hug the stalk closely. Dill, unlike fennel, usually has only one stalk. Dill flowers are yellow and are formed into umbels up to 6 in. in width. Dill fruits have a spicy taste, are typically flattened, and look a little like lentils. They are greenish-brown in color.

Place, Season, and Useful Parts

Dill grows wild in grain fields in southern Europe, northern Africa, the Americas, and the Orient, and is cultivated in most areas. It either originated in the Caucasus or in the Mediterranean region, and was widely used by ancient Egyptians, Greeks, Romans, and Jews. It often escapes from gardens, and can be found on rubble, sandy banks, and riverbanks, as well as in fields, near fences, paths, and houses. Under favorable conditions, it can be grown to an altitude of 3,800 ft. Dill blooms from June to August. The fruits usually ripen in July, August, or September, and sometimes into October.

Gathering, Drying, and Storage

It is a good idea to plant two plots of dill in the garden for kitchen use. The first can be cut repeatedly, and re-sown as needed, and the other allowed to go to seed for pickling time. Dill leaves should be cut repeatedly for kitchen use before the plant begins to blossom. The ripe seed heads are gathered in the morning as soon as the dew has dried. Each umbel can be cut separately, or the entire plant harvested in August or September, as soon as the lower seed heads ripen. The harvested plants should be handled as little as possible to prevent loss of seeds. Dry on cloths in an airy, dark place. Another possibility is to bind them in bundles and then thresh them outdoors on dry, sunny days onto sheets. The threshed fruits must be dried quickly, if necessary with artificial heat. The thoroughly dried fruits are stored in airtight containers.

Dill leaves taste best fresh, but they can also be chopped and frozen, either dry and loose in plastic bags, or damp in ice cube trays. The single dill cubes are then transferred to a plastic bag and stored in the freezer for use throughout the winter. The seeds keep well if they have been dried properly, and maintain their aroma longer than most herbs. Ethereal dill oil is clear and yellow when fresh. Dark or murky oil should be discarded.

Seed Saving and Germination

Different dill varieties will cross with each other. Valuable dill varieties should therefore be grown out singly and in isolation to keep the variety pure. Some modern dill varieties have been developed so that they form a mass of leaves, and do not seed as easily.

As is the case with most members of this family, the best fruits are formed in the first, central umbel, and this should be put aside as seed for the following year. The seed of the secondary umbels are inferior in quality and can be used in the kitchen, especially for pickling. The seeds remain fertile under cool conditions for 2–3 years, and are not as short-lived as some other members of the carrot family.

Gardening Hints

Dill will propagate itself quite happily if allowed to go to seed. It grows well in most soils, but does best on rich, well-drained humus. It dislikes the extreme heat of the south, but prefers a fairly dry climate and a somewhat sunny position, for it is susceptible to mold.

Because dill has very short roots and rarely survives transplantation, it should be sown directly outdoors in the spring. Dill seeds usually sprout in less than 2 weeks, and should be thinned to allow 4–5 in. between plants. Succession plantings are recommended every few weeks. Dill patches should always be kept well weeded. The plants will thrive if protected from wind and extreme heat.

Dill can be sown alone, or it may be sown between other plants to aid their growth. Onions, parsley, asparagus, salad, and spinach are all said to prosper in the vicinity of dill, and it can help to improve the flavor of cabbage. Tomato plants will mature faster if dill is nearby, but the dill should be removed before the tomatoes attain full growth. The same thing is true for carrots. Dill and fennel should never be grown next to each other.

According to German gardening superstition, dill, salt and linseed (flax) sown along the whole length of the house on New Year's Day will supposedly secure the house from harm for the whole year.

Culinary Virtues

As a general rule, dill leaves are not as strongly flavored as dill seeds, and are generally preferred for kitchen use. Both can help to make foods more easily digestible, and "windy" foods more agreeable. Although rarely eaten, the roots of the dill plant are edible, and were once included in the diet of the North American Snake or Shoshone nations.

Finely chopped dill leaves serve as an excellent salad seasoning, and are superb in fresh cucumber and tomato salads. Dill is a good seasoning for bland vegetables such as young potatoes, cabbage, Brussel sprouts, broccoli, beets, turnips, green beans, and tomatoes. Herbal dill butter adds flavor to fish or vegetable dishes. Fresh dill leaves can be used to season mayonnaise, dips, cold sauces, soups, Bloody Marys, deviled eggs, cream cheese spreads, avocado salads, and fish cocktails, as well as millet. Fish is traditionally served with a dill sauce, or cooked on a bed of dill or fennel leaves to make it less "fishy." Crab and dill also complement each other.

The flowering dill plant, without roots, or just the seed umbels are added to pickling mixtures and vinegar. Ornamental dill vinegar can also be prepared by infusing several flowering or seed-bearing stalks in fresh cider vinegar.

Dill seeds, or, to be more precise, dill fruits, are widely used in baking, distillation and pickling. They are also added as a seasoning to lamb stews, fish soups, and rice dishes. Ripe dill fruits can be added to pickling spice mixtures, chutneys, and Indian curries, and they are occasionally substituted for caraway in sauerkraut. Ground dill seeds are a passable salt substitute for those on salt-free diets. Commercial dill salt is often not worth its price: it is usually made from normal table salt flavored with dill extract. The fruits of the various members of the carrot family such as anise, caraway, coriander, fennel, and dill are often used to flavor bread, because they counteract its windy nature and make it more easily digestible.

In Saxony, women used to carry dill fruits with them while baking to prevent the dough from being hexed. They are still added to many traditional types of bread, and French cooks use them to flavor some cakes and pastries. The oil obtained from ripe dill fruits is a good flavoring for liqueurs. The leftover fruit pulp can be roasted at a low temperature (375° F) as a coffee substitute.

Noteworthy Recipes

Dill Pickles: There are as many ways of making pickles as there are of eating them. The following is only one of many traditional recipes.

Peel and halve 8 lb. large cucumbers, taking care the cut off the bitter ends. Scoop out the seeds with a spoon, and taste for bitterness. Discard any bitter cucumbers, or they may ruin the whole batch. Then cut the remaining cucumbers into 2-in. cubes. Boil 1 qt. of watered vinegar with at least ½ lb. (according to taste) sugar, 2 chilies, 4 Tbsp. of mustard seeds, 4 bay leaves, and several unripe dill fruit umbels, or dill flowers. Stir in the cucumber squares, let boil for 5 minutes, and let cool. Pack the cucumbers into sterilized jars, pour the vinegar mixture over them, cover with cellophane or canning lids, and let stand in a cool place for one week. Then pour off the juice, bring it to a boil, let it cool, and pour it back over the cucumbers. Seal and place the jars in a cool, dry and dark place. Those who like a sweet pickle may want to omit the chilies, and increase the amount of sugar.

Household Applications

Dill seeds can be added in minute amounts to herbal sleeping pillows.

Cosmetic Properties

Dill fruits are chewed to sweeten the breath and to prevent hunger pains, hence the name "meeting house seeds" (churchgoers got hungry during the long service, waiting for their Sunday dinner). The oil extracted from dill fruits is used in perfume for its fresh, herbal odor, and in soaps.

Medicinal Merits

An ancient Egyptian papyrus mentions the use of dill to treat headaches. Pythagoras reported that dill held in the left hand could cure epilepsy. Dioscurides believed it would weaken the sight if used for a long time, but on the other hand recommended it to provoke urine, to counteract nausea, and to increase milk flow:

> It stayeth ye hickets, & being drank too long together it both dulls the sight & exstinguisheth geniture, but ye decoction thereof is good by way of Insession for women troubled with womb-griefs, but the seed being burnt & sprinkled on takes away ye Condylomata.[41]

The leaves and flowering tops of the dill plant have been applied for many years as warm poultices to hernias and damaged navels.

Modern Medicine

Modern herbalists usually only prescribe dill fruits for medicinal use. Dill is similar in its action to fennel, anise, coriander, and caraway, and the fruits are so mild that they can be given to infants to lessen colicky pains. People with diseased kidneys should, however, avoid taking dill for extended periods or in large amounts. The fruits are warming and have a stimulating effect on the digestive organs, on the kidneys, and on the milk glands. Dill can help to expel mucus from the body, and can also be taken to relieve the sleeplessness resulting from digestive disorders.

Nursing mothers drink warm milk in which dill leaves have been steeped, or drink dill fruit tea to increase their supply of milk. Babies with digestive disorders can also be given a little of the tea. The expressed juice of the fresh plant has sometimes been applied to piles. A medicinal oil is prepared from the ripe fruits and used as an antiseptic painkiller.

Dill helps to disperse cold and warm the yang in Chinese medicine, and combines well with fish and meat to make them more readily digestible. It also counteracts indigestion and lack of appetite.

---

41. Robert T. Gunther, ed., *The Greek Herbal of Dioscurides* (New York: Hafner, 1959), 301.

Uses in Husbandry

Dill is a plant favored by bees, but usually avoided by birds. Since birds rarely disturb newly sown dill seeds, some farmers place dill, caraway, and salt in a corner of the field before sowing. They are convinced that this will magically prevent animal interference with their crop.

Dill fruit pulp left over from the distilling process can be roasted and fed to cattle, as can the fresh fruits. Both are believed to protect the animals against evil influences. Whole dill plants are hung in stalls or around the animals' necks to keep them healthy. In the late Middle Ages, cows were given dill fruits, and dill and salt were strewn in the stalls on the Eve of the first of May (Walpurgis Night) to secure them from witches. Cows are still given dill after calving to discourage disease and encourage the flow of milk. It is also considered wise to carry dill and salt in a vest pocket when buying animals. Each newly born or newly bought calf should be sprinkled with dill and salt, and all the animals treated the same way in spring, before they are led to pasture the first time.

Dogs also profit from a little finely chopped dill added to their diet. A tea of dill fruits or the addition of crushed dill seed to the food of a nursing bitch can help to increase her flow of milk.

Miscellaneous Wisdom

Dill, fennel, and celery were once associated with the Dionysian cult in ancient Greece. Dill was also grown in Adonis' garden, and placed as an offering on his grave every year. The ancient Romans classified dill as a plant of Bacchus, and fashioned it into wreaths and balls as a symbol of joy.

In modern folk belief, dill is associated with marriage, birth, and young children. It was once customary in Germany for the bride and groom to strew dill in their shoes before going to church. Some brides secretly tucked bread, dill, and caraway seeds into their pockets before the ceremony to protect themselves and their new houses. In northern Germany, a bride who carries mustard and dill seeds during the sermon and says, "I have mustard and dill; When I talk, husband, be still!"[42] will be able to command her husband.

Dill is said to lessen the pains of childbirth when placed in the mother's bed. If she has a silver coin in her bed as well, and says,

> I say, on my bed of silver and of dill,
> Do, child, what I want you to do,
> Be, child, what I want you to be![43]

---

42.   Gustav Hegi, *Illustrierte Flora von Mittel-Europa*, vol. V/2 (Munich: Lehmanns, 1913–1918), 1294.

43.   Hanns Bächtold-Stäubli, ed., *Handwörterbuch des deutschen Aberglaubens* (1927–42), vol. II (Berlin: Walter de Gruyter & Co., 1987), 296.

then she will have complete control over her newborn baby. Dill fruits were also hung around babies' necks to protect them from harm until they could be baptized.

Dill is generally believed to counteract magic and evil influences, especially if worn next to bare skin. Czechs troubled by witches and nightmares can be cured if someone secretly places dill under their pillows. According to an English saying, "Whosoever weareth Vervin or Dill, may be bold to sleep on every hill." (In other words, the protective power is so great that they can even sleep on a faery hill.) Northern Italians who wish to gain more physical strength can eat bread made with flour, beer, and dill seeds. Serbians note that a person who keeps popping up is "like dill in every broth."

Last, but not least, dill is supposed to give its wearer power over the outcome of court cases, and directly influence lawyers and judges, those stubborn and inscrutable members of the human race. All that has to be done is to place dill and oat straw in one shoe before going to court, and then to say, "Oat straw and dill, Gentlemen, be still!"[44]

Legends

An Eastern European wood woman was once on the verge of divulging the secret of the four-leaved clover and dill seeds to a human listener. But before the words could pass her lips, her sister called out to her, "Whatever you do, don't tell the secret of the four-leaved clover and the dill plant!" The wood woman obeyed her sister, and human beings have not yet been able to discover the secret powers of these plants.

Literary Flowers

This man, that is alone a king in his desire,
…but absolutely free,
His happy time he spends the works of God to see,
In those so sundry hearbs which there in plenty growe:
Whose sundry strange effects he onely seeks to knowe.
…The wonder-working Dill he gets not farre from these,
Which curious women use in many a nice disease.

—MICHAEL DRAYTON, *POLY-OLBION*, SONG XIII

---

44. Hanns Bächtold Stäubli, ed., *Handwörterbuch des deutschen Aberglaubens* (1927–42), vol. II (Berlin: Walter de Gruyter & Co., 1987), 297.

Above the lower plants it towers, / the Fennel with its yellow flowers,
And in an earlier age than ours / was gifted with the wondrous powers
Lost vision to restore.

—Henry Wadsworth Longfellow, "The Goblet of Life"

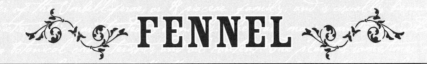

FENNEL

Name

The English name "fennel" and the botanical term *Foeniculum* are both derived from the Latin *faeniculum*, which means "little hay." *Foeniculum vulgare* is the most common fennel.

Fennel is a member of the **Umbelliferae** or **Apiaceae** family, and is usually biennial to perennial except for some garden varieties, which are treated as annuals. There are many varieties of wild and cultivated fennel with widely varying botanical characteristics and oil content. The plant is sometimes confused with Hog fennel (*Peucedanum officinale*) or even with other poisonous members of this family, and care must be taken when gathering it.

Foeniculum vulgare var. vulgare is the botanical name for wild fennel. Two varieties are generally known to gardeners: *Foeniculum vulgare var. dulce* (sweet fennel or seed fennel, which is cultivated for its fruits and seeds), and *Foeniculum vulgare var. azoricum* (which is grown for its bulbs and stalks). There are also various distinct varieties of wild fennel.

Folk Names

Fennel was called *marathron* by the ancient Greeks, and *flonel final* by the Anglo-Saxons. The Old English name for it was *finugl*, which later became *finkel*, *fenkel*, and *spingel*. Wild fennel is now called common fennel; the cultivated forms are known as sweet fennel, florentine fennel, florence fennel, mild fennel, devil-in-a-bush, and love-in-a-mist. German names are *Fenchel*, *Finkel*, *Fenigl*, *Enis*, *Brotsamen*, *Knollenfenchel*, and *Kammfenchel*; the French call it *fenouil*, *aneth doux*, *aneth fenouil*, and *anis vert*. Italians speak of *finocchio*, *finocchio di Bologna*, *finocchio di Chioggia*, *carosella*, *finocchione*, and *finocchini*; the Spanish speak of *hinojo*, *comino*, and *anis*; the Russians of *krop*; and the Chinese of *hui-hsiang*.

Appearance

The best way to recognize fennel is by the smell of the crushed plant or seeds. They taste like licorice, and are very sweet, with little bitterness. Wild fennel is somewhat acrid, but cultivated fennel is very pleasing to the palate. The plant is similar in appearance to dill when young, but then develops marked characteristics. Its root is white, thick, long, and tapering, and the erect main stalk is scored lengthwise, and is of a blue-green color. It is filled with a white pithy marrow, and grows to a maximum height of 6 ft. The base of the thick leafstalks is as large as a fist, and forms the "bulb" of cultivated varieties. Fennel leaves are feathery, but coarser than those of dill, and of a darkish green or even reddish color that sets off the plant's small bright yellow flowers. Fennel flowers are gathered in umbels that may reach a diameter of 6 in. The fruits are half-moon shaped, and are composed of 2 seeds, each marked by 5 vertical gray stripes.

Place, Season, and Useful Parts

Fennel was originally a Mediterranean plant, and therefore prefers dry and sunny southern slopes, terraces and vineyards, railroad embankments, riversides, and meadows. It often escapes from cultivated areas, and has established itself as a wild plant in temperate areas the world over, especially near the sea. Although the plant may not form fruits in the extreme north, it can still be cultivated there for its leaves and fleshy stalks. Fennel "bulbs" should be gathered from July to October and occasionally on through the winter. The seeds are harvested from August to October. The roots are dug in September to November or in the early spring.

Gathering, Drying, and Storage

Fennel roots can be dug, and then cut into small pieces for drying in September. The leaves, or fronds, are cut from spring on into the summer, and the plants cut back to encourage new shoots, which are more delicate in taste and texture. The so-called bulbs are harvested in the late summer and fall on into spring, depending on the microclimate. The seeds, or, to be botanically correct, the fruits, are gathered in the fall as soon as they turn yellow or brown and are marked with gray stripes. The first harvest is usually the best, since late-ripening fruits usually do not have a high oil content. Fennel seeds can be gathered singly, or with combs. The umbels may also be cut with scissors, or the entire plant, without the roots, cut and spread out to dry on tarps or sheets. As soon as they are dry, the plants should be threshed to remove the seeds. If the season is unusually damp, the drying process can be completed with the help of artificial heat. Fennel roots should be dried slowly with artificial heat. Fennel leaves and stalks do not dry well, but may be frozen with good result, especially in purée form.

Seed Saving and Germination

Sweet fennel seeds remain fertile under cool, dark, and dry conditions for about three years, and germinate in approximately two weeks. The best seeds are formed in the first central umbel. Many different fennel varieties have been developed over the centuries, above and beyond the wild forms. So-called bronze fennel has become popular in the last few years, and is often sold as a bulb fennel, although it is actually a seed variety. Care should be taken when choosing vegetable fennel varieties, for they differ widely, and may not do well in your area. A fair amount of experimentation is necessary until you find a variety that will do well with your local climate. When you do, stick with the variety or a similar one, and try to save seed from this variety, so it will further acclimatize itself to your needs. Seeds can only be saved from two-year plants, so the seeds should be sown in late summer and allowed to overwinter outdoors, or sown in spring, and the roots dug out, lifted, and stored indoors over the winter. They should be replanted in spring as soon as possible, and isolated from other varieties to maintain the desired characteristics.

Gardening Hints

Sweet fennel is grown for its seeds in Europe, Asia, and the Americas. It is not a difficult plant to raise, and may even volunteer, coming up year after year. It generally does well even under adverse conditions. Fennel prefers light, well-drained, rich yet not freshly fertilized soil with a fairly high lime content, and likes to be watered frequently. It grows best on southern slopes in areas where the late summer and the fall are warm and dry. Fennel should be moved to a new position each couple of years so as not to deplete the soil. According to one superstitious belief, fennel should always be sown together with a few silver coins, bread, and salt to ensure a good harvest.

Bulb fennel was at one time only available in France and Italy, but has become much more popular in recent years. It is an ideal diet food, helping to rid the body of excess liquids, and supplying minerals and nutrients without many calories. It is sensitive to frost, and should only be sown after the last freezing spring days, or even a little later. If the summers are not cool and moist enough, the plants may begin to bolt and go to seed. In Italy, it is sown in the fall, and the stalks thicken into "bulbs" in the early spring. An intimate knowledge of local weather is necessary to grow large fennel bulbs, which are actually thickened stalks. Fennel requires rich, but not freshly fertilized, soil. If fertilized with fresh manure, the plants may be subject to attack by snails and aphids. After the plants are well established, they must be kept moist, and mounded over with soil or mulch to whiten and sweeten the bulbous stalks.

Fennel fruits will mature during the first year in most climates, but may take two years in very cool areas. Depending on the length of the growing season, fennel may be sown in the spring after all danger of frost is past, or in the fall. The seeds are direct-sown and well-covered with earth. The plants are then thinned until they stand 1 ft. apart. It is advisable to harvest the seeds before cold weather, or they will fall off. After harvesting, the perennial plants should be cut back, covered with composted manure or a thick mulch layer of straw, leaves, or other organic matter as protection against the cold. The roots can also be lifted with at least 4 in. of stalk, and placed in a deep ditch covered with earth, or stored in sand in a container in the cellar. Carefully check the plants during the winter and remove any moldy material. The roots can be replanted in the spring with good results, or even raised in window boxes as soon as the weather warms up.

Culinary Virtues

Fennel was already used in the Pharaohs' kitchens, and it was cultivated by ancient Romans. According to John Parkinson, fennel's

> leaves, seeds and rootes are both for meate and medicine; the Italians especially doe much delight in the use thereof, and therefore transplant and whiten it, to make it more tender to please the taste, which being sweete and somewhat hot helpeth to digest the crude qualities of fish and other viscous meats. We use it to lay upon fish or to boyle it therewith and with divers other things, as also the seeds in bread and other things.[45]

In modern culinary practice, fennel leaves are used fresh as a seasoning herb and substitute for dill. The thick stalks of cultivated varieties are eaten as a vegetable or salad, and the ripe seeds are valued for their aromatic oil, adding flavor to pickles and baked goods, as well as distilled spirits.

Fennel leaves are primarily used to season oily fish, in much the same manner as caraway is used to season heavy meats such as pork. Culinary historians conjecture that this custom might have originated in coastal areas, where fennel can usually be found growing wild. An English saying ridicules the association of fennel with fish dishes: "Crabs, Salmon, Lobsters are with Fennel spread/Who never touched that Herb until they were dead.[46]

---

45.   John Parkinson, *A Fragment from Theatrum Bontanicum* [1640], *"or An Herball of a Large Extent"* (Falls Village, CT: Herb Grower Press, 1967).

46.   Marcel Boulestin, *Boulestin's Round-the-Year Cookbook* (New York: Dover, 1975), 40.

Fish are often boiled on a bed of fennel leaves. Italian cooks sometimes wrap fish in fennel leaves before baking or grilling them on an open fire. Salmon is traditionally served with fennel sauce, bass and mackerel are stuffed with the herb, and eel soup is seasoned with finely-chopped fennel. In the Middle Ages, fennel was a recommended seasoning for fish eaten during Lent. Fish caught under the influence of Pisces was considered unfit to eat until tempered with fennel.

Fennel leaves are also added to salads or vegetable soups (borscht), and they may be used to flavor herbal butters and vinegar. Sometimes, a fennel frond is included in mixed green herbs. Finely chopped young fennel leaves can be used to season poultry or added just before serving to various vegetables such as potatoes, carrots, and peas. Some bakers place their bread dough on a bed of fennel fronds before baking. The leaves of wild fennel plants can occasionally be used as a substitute for garden fennel, although their flavor is not as delicate.

Unripe fennel flower heads are often added to pickling spices, or used together with black currant leaves and horseradish roots to flavor pickled cucumbers. Ripe fennel flower heads make a pretty garnish, especially when complemented with blue borage flowers.

Some cultivated varieties of fennel have sweet-tasting, large, white, bulb-like leaf stalks. They can be eaten raw, thinly sliced into salads, or they are steamed as a vegetable, baked in the oven, puréed, or even juiced. Broth made from the fresh plant has few calories and is recommended for those on a diet. Infants also thrive on fennel purée, for it is soothing and easy to digest. Fennel is a favorite dish in Italy, where it is often served as an appetizer or salad, or braised in butter, and seasoned with grated Parmesan, salt, and pepper.

Fennel seeds are widely used as a seasoning. The fruits of first-year plants are sweet in flavor, but become progressively bitter in subsequent years. Several garden varieties of fennel have been selected to produce the sweetest, most aromatic fruits. Apple dishes are sometimes flavored with fennel and dill seeds. Fennel seeds were used in ancient times to preserve foods, and a memory of this custom has survived to the present day. Fennel, anise, caraway, and coriander seeds are sometimes added to bread to cover the taste of old or musty flour. Fennel seeds are employed to season olives, pickles, cheese, and sauerkraut. They are also widely used by distillers: absinthe and sambuco usually contain distilled fennel and anise seeds, Saragossa wine or English sack is prepared from fennel roots, and a fennel liqueur can be distilled from fennel stalks. Chewing fennel seeds is supposed to ease hunger pains, and the dried seeds are usually included in the herbal digestive mixtures served after meals in India.

Noteworthy Recipes

Fennel Sauce for Mackerel: Here is a "Fennel Sauce for Mackerel" from Mrs. Isabella
Beeton in 1861:

> Ingredients. ½ pint of melted butter, rather more than a tablespoonfull of
> chopped fennel.
>
> Mode. Make the melted butter very smoothly; chop the fennel rather small,
> carefully cleansing it from any grit or dirt, and put it to the butter when
> this is on the point of boiling. Simmer for a minute or two, and serve in a
> tureen.
>
> Time. 2 minutes.
>
> Sufficient to serve with 5 or 6 mackerel.[47]

Cazzo del Imperatore: This farmers' dish received its rather vulgar name because of
its supposed aphrodisiacal properties. It is a very simple appetizer traditionally
served in Italy when fennel is in season.

> Very fresh and sweet fennel bulbs are washed and any unsightly bruises care-
> fully cut out. Then they are quartered and cut into eighths or sixteenths, depend-
> ing on the size of the fennel. Arrange tastefully on a plate, garnishing with other
> aphrodisiacal flowers such as nasturtium. Flavor with just a pinch of fine sea salt,
> plenty of the best extra virgin olive oil, and season lavishly with freshly ground
> black pepper.

Household Applications

Fennel is included in many household potpourri and sachet mixtures.

Cosmetic Properties

Fennel's major merit as a cosmetic herb is as a breath-freshener. Fennel seeds are chewed
after a meal to sweeten the breath, fennel oil is added to commercial toothpastes and
mouthwashes, and fennel breath lozenges are available at drugstores and pharmacies.
Fennel oil is further used in the manufacture of perfumes.

Infusions of fennel seeds are added to facial lotions, beauty packs, eye rinses, and
moisturizing creams. Fennel facial lotion is mildly astringent and cleansing. A beauty
pack of fennel tea and honey can be of help in the treatment of wrinkles, a facial pack
of fresh mayonnaise and fennel tea is recommended for dry skin, and creams prepared
with fennel are said to prevent wrinkles and heal dry skin. Fennel steam baths help to
soften rough, dry skin, and fennel baths have a stimulating and invigorating effect on the

---

47. Beeton, *The Book of Household Management* (1861) (New York: Farrar, Straus & Giroux, 1977), 198.

entire body. Fennel tea may, in the absence of anything better, be used as a hair rinse. Compresses of crushed fennel seeds or boiled fennel roots are applied to the breasts to help tone and firm the skin.

Medicinal Merits

Fennel is one of the oldest medicinal herbs. It has been employed in China for thousands of years, and Indians, Egyptians, and Arabs have sung its praises for centuries. Dioscurides and Pliny wrote about it, and it was widely used in Spain around the turn of the first millennium. Charlemagne ordered its cultivation, Hildegard von Bingen recommended it, John Gerard wrote of its eye-strengthening properties, and Nicholas Culpeper listed a variety of possible applications. Its hot and dry nature suggested it be used to draw out fevers, to aid digestion, and to counteract sleeplessness, melancholy, psychic illnesses, and colds. It was taken to expel excess water from the body and given to women after childbirth. It was also thought to ease inflamed or engorged breasts and to make them produce more milk. Fennel was administered to dry out the poison of snakes, scorpions, mad dogs, and harmful herbs, as well as ear worms, and to cure a great variety of eye diseases.

> *In Fennel-seed, this vertue you shall finde,*
> *Foorth of your lower parts to drive the winde.*
> *Of Fennel vertues foure they doe recite,*
> *First, it hath power some poysons to expell,*
> *Next, burning Agues it will put to flight,*
> *The stomack it doth cleanse, and comfort well:*
> *And fourthly, it doth keep and cleanse the sight.*
> *And thus the seed and hearbe doth both excell.*
>
> —*THE SCHOOL OF SALERNUM*

Modern Medicine

Fennel's reputation as an effective healing herb has not been impaired in modern times. Both herbalists and homeopaths recommend it as an excellent herb for nursing mothers and their babies, especially because of its mild laxative qualities and its positive action on the digestive organs. Fennel juice and fennel tea are still used to wash out weakened or infected eyes, and the seeds added to cough mixtures and used to flavor cough drops. The use of fennel as a folk remedy for epilepsy has recently been corroborated by scientific research: large doses of fennel oil will produce epileptic symptoms in humans. According to the doctrine that "like cures like," minute doses of fennel taken over a long time are believed to have a curative effect on the malady. The roots are also cooked and administered as a mild laxative.

Fennel is employed in Chinese medicine, as in Western, to disperse flatulence, indigestion, and abdominal fullness, as well as increase the appetite, warm the stomach, and disperse cold in the liver meridian (leading to hernias). The seeds are known as *Xiao hui xiang* and are roasted in a dry skillet, and then ground to a powder. The powder is used as a kitchen seasoning herb. Other sources combine the powder with other herbs in rice wine and take it for complaints such as hernias and intestinal pain due to cold. Excessive use of fennel is believed to harm the eyes, and it is not recommended for hot diseases, or for men suffering from premature ejaculation.

Special Cures

Fennel roots and fennel fruits are either taken alone, or processed as fennel water, fennel syrup, fennel tincture, fennel honey, fennel electuary, and fennel oil. Fennel seeds prepared as tea or steeped in warm milk can help to increase the milk supply of nursing mothers. A diluted fennel seed tea can also be given to infants as a calming drink to alleviate digestive disorders. A tea with a more pronounced effect on lactation can be made by combining equal parts of dried fennel, anise and dill seeds, and lady's mantle leaves, or, if available, the leaves of the alpine lady's mantle.

Uses in Husbandry

According to an old adage, one should plant "fennel near the kennel" to keep away fleas. Incidentally, fennel also acts as an aphrodisiac for dogs, and can be added, finely chopped, to a raw meat diet to increase fertility, and, later, to increase the milk flow of nursing bitches.

Dried fennel stalks and leaves, and the residue left over after distilling can be fed to cattle, horses, and sheep, resulting in improved appetite and increased milk production. Fennel may be rubbed onto beehives to keep the bees from swarming, and the insects can be fed with sweetened fennel tea.

Veterinary Values

Animals given powdered fennel seed in addition to their regular diet usually have a good appetite and few digestive problems. Fennel seeds are heated in sacks and applied as warming poultices for various complaints.

Miscellaneous Wisdom

Fennel was one of the garlanding herbs used by participants in the Attic mysteries, and was considered sacred to Aphrodite and Artemis. According to ancient accounts, snakes used fennel as a healing herb when their eyesight was clouded, and rubbed themselves against it when shedding their skins. Anglo-Saxons considered fennel an important magical and anti-demonic herb, and it was included in the famous Nine Herb Charm:

> Thyme and Fennel, a pair great in power
> The wise Lord, holy in heaven,
> Wrought these herbs while He hung on the cross;
> He placed them and put them in the seven worlds to aid all, poor and rich.[48]

In the Middle Ages, fennel was used together with St. John's wort to protect humans against witchcraft, demons and dwarves. It was hung over the house and stable doors on Midsummer's Eve to avert evil, and the udders and horns of cows were rubbed down with the herb to keep them free from disease. It is still used as an antidemonic plant in most European countries, and as an aphrodisiac in some. Italians wear the plant as an amulet against evil spirits, and use its name in endless sexual puns and innuendoes. Witches in the province of Friaul fight against each other with fennel branches. The inhabitants of Somerset consider fennel to be a "good" herb, and hang it over the doors of houses to protect the house and its inhabitants from fire. In some versions of the Prometheus myth, a hollow fennel stalk served as the hiding place for the coal used to bring fire to humans.

Oracular Worth

According to popular myth, pregnant women with cravings for fennel will certainly give birth to a son. Good fennel years are also believed to presage good vintages.

Literary Flowers

> Let us not forget to honor fennel. It grows
> On a strong stem and spreads its branches wide.
> Its taste is sweet enough, sweet too its smell;
> They say it is good for eyes whose sight is clouded,
> That its seed, taken with milk from a pregnant goat,
> Eases a swollen stomach and quickly loosens
> Sluggish bowels. What is more, your rasping cough
> Will go if you take fennel-root mixed with wine.
>
> —WAHLAFRIDUS STRABO, HORTULUS

---

48.   Qtd. in Paul Huson, *Mastering Herbalism* (New York: Stein and Day: 1974), 231.

A damned death!
Let gallows gape for the dog; let man go free,
And let not hemp his windpipe suffocate.

—William Shakespeare, *Henry V*

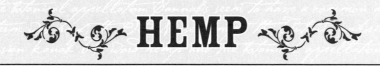

HEMP

Name

The word "hemp" and the botanical appellation *Cannabis* seem to have a common and very ancient origin. The Old High German term was *Haaf*, the Old Norse *hampr*, the Teutonic *nahpi-z* or *hanapi-z*, the Latin *cannabis*, and the Persian *kanab*.

It is interesting to note the importance of the word "hemp" for gallows humor. Hemp fibers were at one time used to manufacture the ropes used for hanging criminals, and these malefactors came to be known as hempseeds or hempstretches. Their widows were called hempen-widows, and they were said to wag hemp, to taste hemp, or to die of hempen fever. In Scottish dialect, a young person in the process of sowing wild oats (purists will shudder at the botanical confusion) is called a "hempie." In Germany, a criminal was said "to avoid passing by a hemp field" or to "be growing to hemp size."

Hemp is closely related to hops, and is an annual member of the **Cannabaceae** family. The botanical name for hemp is *Cannabis sativa ssp. sativa*. The medicinally more potent herb, also called Indian hemp, is known as *Cannabis sativa ssp. indica*. A wild species can be found in Siberia and Central Asia, *Cannabis sativa ssp. spontanea*, and there are many local variants.

Folk Names

Hemp is nicknamed neckweed, devil's flower, and gallows grass. Indian hemp is known as bhang, ganja, dagga, marihuana, pot, grass, and a host of other endearing names that have sprung up in the last decades. The female plant was once, because of its stately size and flowers, thought to be the male of the species. Botanists have since corrected this misconception, but the old folk

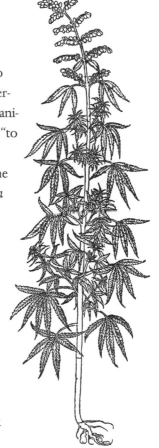

names persist. The female plant is therefore called winter hemp, Carl, Carl hemp, churle hemp, and Charle hemp. The male plant is known as summer hemp, fimble, femble, flembe, fyrble, and barren. This division is also prevalent in Germany. Female plants are called *Samenhanf, Mastel,* and *Sämer;* the males are known as *Femmel, Fimmel,* or *Geilhanf.* Other German names are *Hanf, Honif, Semmelhanf,* and *Bästling.* The French call the herb *chanvre;* the Spaniards call it *canabo, cañamo, mariguana,* and *marijuana;* the Italians, *canapa;* the Dutch, *hennep;* the Swedes, *hampa;* the Danes, *hamp;* the Welsh, *cywarch;* and the Irish, *cnáib.* Russians name it *konopija posevnaja* and *konopija indijskaja,* and the Hindi name is *kimab.*

Appearance

Hemp is a handsome, tall plant, probably the largest in the garden, despite the fact that it is an annual. It will easily grow to a height of 10 ft. and has a white spindly tap root, as well as an angular, tough, upright stem. The entire plant exudes an unmistakably powerful and resiny odor that can become literally overpowering when a hemp field begins to blossom. Even the relatively insensitive human nose can smell a hemp field hundreds of feet away. As Culpeper explains, the plant has many

> fingered leaves, each leaf composed of five, six or seven (9) parts, long and narrow, sharp-pointed, and serrated about the edges, the middlemost being longest, set together upon one long footstalk; they are green above, hoary underneath, and rough in handling.[49]

Anyone who has handled hemp knows the difference between male and female plants. The males are small, and quickly die. They have yellowish-green or whitish-green flowers clustered in bunches at the top of the stalks. These flowers do not produce seeds, but pollen. The female plants are much bushier and grow to a great height. The flowers and seeds of the female plants are not always easily visible, since they are greenish in color.

Place, Season, and Useful Parts

Hemp can be found growing wild in India, Siberia, China, and Persia. Indian hemp originated in northwest India, Iran, and Afghanistan. It often escapes from cultivated areas and is spread by birds, or from birdseed discarded on dumps and rubbish heaps. It has now naturalized itself in most warm climates. Hemp grows on rubble, barren fields, on walls and in hedges, or on forested slopes to an altitude of at least 4,500 ft. Hemp has been cultivated for at least several millennia before the birth of Christ. At the beginning of the century, it was grown in the Blue Grass region of Kentucky as a

---

49. Culpeper, *Culpeper's Complete Herbal* (1653) (London: Foulsham, undated), 183.

fiber crop, but later fell into disfavor as a narcotic and was systematically eradicated in North America. Hemp flowers in the months of July and August.

Gathering, Drying, and Storage

Hemp was once called the Devil's flower by workers in hemp fields because it gave them headaches and was reputed to make young women barren, and caused old women to break out in rashes.

The flowering tops of the female plants should be cut in full bloom in August or September for medicinal purposes.

Mechanical harvesters have been developed to harvest hemp fibers, and easier methods developed to separate the fibers from the woody parts of the stems. A few decades ago, the stalks had to be cut by hand, bundled, stacked, and "retted", i.e., subjected to the elements to isolate the fibers. Small male hemp plants were harvested in summer. The larger female plants, known as Carl hemp, were cut in September when fully mature. Carl hemp was cut with a sickle or machete as close to the ground as possible, and then allowed to dry in the field. The stalks were sorted according to length, and left out in the rain or soaked in water for 2–4 weeks until they began to soften. They were dried again, and pressed or beaten to separate the fibers. Careful observation has shown that plants harvested during the waning moon are drier, and contain sturdier fibers than those harvested during the waxing moon. These plants are, on the other hand, much more aromatic and full of resin, and are better suited for medicinal purposes.

If you want to harvest hemp seeds, you will have to do something about the birds that have been known to strip a plant within a few days. Nets are not very practical, for the gluttonous birds will creep up under the nets and get caught in the mesh. One method is to allow the birds to begin feeding, and then to cut down the entire plant without roots. Place the harvested plants on cloths in an airy, dry place indoors, and most of the seeds will ripen, but will have to be threshed out. Another disadvantage is that the leaves may begin to mildew in damp climates, and the plants will have to be turned regularly and checked for spoilage. Yet another trick is to offer the birds a somewhat earlier variety as a decoy plant, which will keep them busy until the seeds of the main variety ripen.

In an ideal world without birds, the best method of gathering hemp seeds is to shake the plants daily into a paper or cloth bag, and then to dry them in a dry, dark place. One female plant will produce an amazing number of seeds, but it is necessary to gather seeds from several plants in order to maintain the genetic diversity of the variety.

Hemp leaves are usually collected from the female plants as soon as the plant begins to flower or when the seeds are being set by cutting branches off the plant, and immediately stripping the leaves, flowers, and seeds from the pithy stems and drying them quickly in a cool, dry and airy place. Some plants are so high in resin that it will take the leaves quite a while to dry completely. They deteriorate rapidly, especially if they are damp, and must be stored in a dry place.

Seed Saving and Germination

There are innumerable hemp varieties, especially in the more temperate zones. The plant self-seeds and is distributed by birds descending in swarms on seed-bearing plants. In recent years, several collecting expeditions have taken place in the former Soviet Union and Asia to search for neglected hemp varieties. Generally, hemp varieties can be divided into fiber plants and medicinal herbs, although the differences are not clearly defined, but the alkaloid content can vary dramatically from one variety to another. In the European Union, most commercial varieties have fewer alkaloids, and higher fiber content.

The most important thing to remember when trying to save hemp seed is that both male and female plants are necessary for reproduction. The male plants are smaller and dry up quickly, the female larger and bushier, and sport light green to yellow tiny flowers. These are more aromatic. Hemp varieties will cross with each other if grown in the immediate vicinity. In order to maintain pure strains, hemp varieties must be isolated or grown at least half a mile apart.

Hemp seeds keep well in a cool, dry, and dark place. They have been known to germinate even after being forgotten for years in some attic.

Gardening Hints

Hemp has been cultivated for a very long time. It was a recognized medicinal herb in China in AD 220, and was cultivated by the ancient Egyptians, Greeks, Romans, and Celts. It matures in 90–150 days, and can therefore be grown in northern areas as well as in the south. Southern hemp is medicinally more potent than hemp grown in the north. As a result, fiber varieties usually predominate in northern countries. Local legislation varies, but it is often illegal to grow the plant for sale as an intoxicant, and legal to raise it for bird food, oil, or fibers. In some cases, it is illegal to buy hemp seeds in a herb store, but possible to go to the next seed shop and buy them in sacks as bird food. Restrictive legislation has been eased in the European Union, and subsidies are now being paid for the production of alkaloid-poor varieties for fiber production. In the United States, exceptions for the medicinal use of marihuana are only just being allowed, and it is illegal to grow the plant.

Hemp will grow on any soil except especially cold, wet, totally barren, or ecologically damaged land. It will grow, but does not thrive, on thick clay, and is perfectly happy on poor, sandy soils. Hemp prefers soil with a slightly basic pH, and responds well to direct sunlight and some shade. It should be sown in the spring. It requires little attention until harvest, for it is an extremely hardy plant, and will poison most of the weeds growing next to it, or take so many nutrients from the soil that weeds pine and die. Despite its extremely rapid growth and greedy habit, it does not need fertilizer input to grow well, and is a good crop for clearing the soil in a rotation system. Pests generally avoid the plant. Hemp may be dwarfed in very hot summers because of lack of moisture. Organic gardeners like to keep a hemp plant in the garden as a decoy or a special attraction for birds. Rust on members of the mallow family such as marshmallow and hollyhocks can be prevented with a companion planting of hemp.

Gardening Superstitions

As a general rule, hemp should be sown according to the uses to which the plant will be put. Seed crops are usually sown early, so the seeds have enough time to ripen. Fiber or drug plants should be started a week or three days before the full moon. Plants sown during the waning moon will be shorter than other plants. Auspicious traditional sowing days are April 11th, or the 100th day of the year; May 1st and 3rd; and the days allotted to the Saints Urban, George, Christian, and Job. In Baden (Germany), peasants believe that the herb should be sown on the 11th, 12th, or 13th of May, the days devoted to Saint Bonifatius, Saint Pankratius, and Saint Servatius. These three saints are irreverently known in Central Europe as the "ice men" because of the cold spell that usually accompanies them. Fiber hemp should be started during the "ice days" because these three saints were the tallest men, and the hemp will, by association, grow straight and tall. Swabians believe that hemp sown under the astrological sign of Leo will have long fibers, and that hemp sown under the influence of Pisces will make smooth strings.

According to popular belief, it is easy to foretell how good a hemp harvest will be, and to influence the height of the crop. If the weather is bad on Shrove Tuesday (the last day of Carnival, before Ash Wednesday), then the hemp will grow well that year. If the weather is bad when the first stork arrives in northern Europe, then the hemp will be short. If the cowslips and primroses have long stalks in the spring, then the hemp stalks will also be long. In France and Germany, a willow wand is stuck into the ground when the hemp is sown in order to show the plants how tall they should grow. The hemp will be tall if sown by a tall person, or the person sowing it can jump high, or if the last person in church on Ash Wednesday is tall. Similarly, the hemp will grow tall if couples jump high while dancing on Shrove Tuesday, or if they jump high over the Midsummer's fire. In Swabia, the dancers cry out, "Three ell-long hemp! Three ell-long hemp! Let the hemp grow three ells long!"[50]

---

50.   Hanns Bächtold-Stäubli, ed., *Handwörterbuch des deutschen Aberglaubens* (1927–42), vol. 3 (Berlin: Walter de Gruyter & Co., 1987), 1436.

In Bavaria, straw wheels are rolled down mountainsides at Midsummer to make the hemp grow better. In northern Italy, women prepare a special pasta dish on the last Thursday in January. The longer they stir, the higher the hemp will grow. In Poland, girls who oversleep Mass on Easter Sunday are "watered" by churchgoers to make the hemp grow taller.

Culinary Virtues

Hemp seeds have a very high oil content, and are often pressed to produce an oil of excellent nutritional value (including omega-3 essential fatty acids), but only fair keeping quality. It is now being produced and marketed in the European Union and Canada as a salad oil. Roasted hemp seeds have been enjoyed since antiquity, and are still traditional fare in Russia, Poland, and other parts of Central Europe. A traditional Silesian (German) Christmas menu consists of hemp soup, fish, poppy dumplings, and stewed fruit. Russians once made hemp butter from the seeds. Austrians are now using hemp seeds in traditional bakery products in place of poppy seeds. Both hemp and poppy seeds have a high oil content, and can be added to bread, cookies, and heavy cakes such as fruitcakes to make them more nutritious and appetizing. Only Indian hemp is so potent that it has a narcotic effect when used in bakery—normal everyday hempseed is ineffective, even if eaten in large amounts. The seeds can also be ground and used as a filling for cookies. Fresh hemp is occasionally used to flavor and to strengthen beer, or is processed as a milk substitute or nutritional powder.

Household Applications

Green hemp plants are said to drive away bed bugs, and dried hemp stalks can be employed as primitive "matches." The dried stalks can be used in the garden to unobtrusively stake smaller plants.

Hemp, just like jute *(Corchorus capsularis)* and sisal *(Agave sisalana)*, is used to manufacture rope and twine, and its fibers can also, like those of flax and nettles, be woven into very sturdy cloth. The Chinese used it for this purpose at least 4,500 years ago. At one time, barren plots of land were designated in land deeds as "hempland," a spot where hemp could be grown for household use. In Italy, it was once customary for peasant girls working on their dowries to sow a plot of hemp for this purpose every year. Hemp underwear and kitchen hempcloths can still be found at various flea markets in Central Europe, for the fabric is long-lasting. It is a little scratchy when new, which has led may people to dislike it, but becomes wonderfully soft with age. It is currently being used as an alternative for rougher fabrics such as gloves and jeans. In Romania and some parts of the former Soviet Union, it is still being grown as a fiber and oil plant, and Central European farmers are now busily experimenting with alternative uses for the versatile plant. Hemp oil is extremely valuable, and can be used as cooking oil, as well as in the preparation of soap and various cosmetics.

In Switzerland, peasants once had a piece of hempen rope, some bread, and a little salt blessed in church on the 5th of February, the day sacred to the memory of St. Agatha, and then placed the blessed objects among the newly-woven and newly-sewn clothes to protect them from mice and moths.

Cosmetic Properties

Hemp oil is an important ingredient of many household soaps and cleaning mixtures, and is characterized by a bright green color. Hemp oil is now being used like sweet almond, avocado, or jojoba oil in many cosmetic preparations. It feels very oily, and is therefore recommended for chapped, dry, or damaged skin, and is added to protective creams and cleansing mixtures for outdoor work. Hemp shampoo, hemp conditioners, and hemp facial and hand creams are all commercially available. Their only drawback is the somewhat higher price, typical of all cosmetic products made with purely natural ingredients and a limited shelf life.

Medicinal Merits

For centuries, hemp has been regarded as a loosening herb capable of expelling harmful substances from the entire body, and obstructions from the uterus. Harem-keepers in Constantinople knew how to use it to their advantage. In Germany, laboring women were laid on hemp to ease cramping pains, and its fibers were wrapped around a woman's arm or inner thigh to loosen cramps. In Bohemia, patients with fevers warmed their ears with the smoke of a hemp ball containing three pieces of many-colored cloth, three splinters, and ten lentils, burned over a coal fire. Another method of dispelling fevers was to have a woman prepare three hemp balls and then burn them. If she fanned the smoke out the window, the fever would invariably blow away as well. Hildegard von Bingen recommended the herb for those afflicted with worms. Midwives in the Lincolnshire Fens prepared birthing cakes of the seeds. Otto Brunfels used hemp to cure earaches, and Nicholas Culpeper prescribed the seeds to expel wind, to ease coughs, to remove obstructions of the liver and gall bladder, and to relieve colics.

Only the flowering tops and seeds of the female Indian hemp plant were used for medicinal purposes. Folk healers made use of hemp as a mildly hypnotic, sedative, and narcotic drug. It can aid the body in dispelling urine and mucus, and may also be taken to ease pains, and to relieve toothaches and some headaches. It acts as a mild sedative for the treatment of nervous disorders, neuralgia, infantile convulsions, and sleeplessness, as well as some cases of *delirium tremens*. A "milk" prepared from hemp seeds is still occasionally used in the treatment of gonorrhea, and the seeds are given to those suffering from liver troubles or nervous exhaustion.

Modern Medicine

Hemp is now rarely employed as a medicinal herb because of the unpredictability of its alkaloid content and legal restrictions. Individual reactions to the herb also vary dramatically, and there have been some cases of poisoning. Its effect on the hormones is not always predictable. Even sleeping in a field of Indian hemp can have unexpected results, and ingestion of the herb is often followed by a "hangover." One of the few countries to include hemp among its official medicinal herbs is Switzerland, and even here, it is not recommended for internal use, except as a nutritional oil. Despite all these drawbacks, hemp keeps being recommended for a number of possible applications and for pain relief. It can help to increase the appetite of cancer patients and to ease their pain, and has also been used in the treatment of such serious diseases as multiple sclerosis, AIDS, Hepatitis C, Crohn's disease, and glaucoma.

Hemp extract is administered in minute doses to treat headaches. A tincture of the herb is given to patients with urinary afflictions and cystitis, and to aid in childbirth. Indian hemp seeds are added in small amounts to cough mixtures, especially if the cough is spasmodic. Poultices of hemp leaves or crushed seeds are applied to the genital region, or to rheumatic pains, or to corns. A homeopathic tincture is prepared from hemp for the urogenital system and Indian hemp for the nervous system. Homeopathic *Cannabis sativa* can be useful in the treatment of sexually transmitted diseases, especially gonorrhea, cystitis, impotence, leucorrhea, and other sexual disorders.

In Chinese medicine, hemp is considered an excellent medicine for constipation, especially in the elderly, and also for sores and ulcerations that are healing poorly. Chinese doctors warn about taking too much of the herb, and caution that its overuse can lead to nausea, vomiting, coma and even death.

Uses in Husbandry

Thin hemp stalks can be added to other dried plants to serve as emergency bedding material for animals. Hemp oil is pressed from ripe seeds, and the residue used as fodder. Birds of all kinds eat hemp seeds greedily, and they are often included in commercial bird food. Canaries are said to sing better if given some hemp, and chickens will lay longer in winter and gain weight faster if hemp seeds are added to their diet. Field mice have an aversion to the plant's resiny smell, and will leave a burrow if hemp seeds are poured down the opening. This may be worth a try with various persistent rodent pests such as voles and gophers.

Pressed hemp oil can, if necessary, be used as burning oil, although the results are not always satisfactory. An excellent varnish that dries fairly fast is prepared from hemp oil. It is also occasionally added to detergents. There is now discussion about using hemp for the production of biodiesel.

Hemp fibers are not only woven to produce cloth, but they are also twisted to form rope and string, or roughly woven for sturdy sacks and sail cloth or packing material. The best hemp quality is said to come from Italy and Russia. Hemp fibers were once used to produce a very high quality and extremely durable paper. Many ancient manuscripts were printed on hemp paper and are still in very good condition, considering their age. The Gutenberg Bible was, for example, printed on hemp paper.

Shredded hemp stalks are sold as litter for house pets, and the fibers are now used in many building and insulation materials. Heating pellets have even been produced from hemp.

But the most famous (and profitable) commercial use of Indian hemp is as an intoxicant. The sale of hemp leaves, resin, and seeds has become big, if illegal, business in many countries. Hemp leaves can be smoked, or a tea is prepared from the female leaves, flowers, and seeds. The resin is often gathered separately as *hashish* or *churras*, and a drink named *bhang* made from the leaves and seeds of the female plants. The seeds can also be roasted and eaten as an intoxicating delicacy. The best hemp for these purposes is grown from Indian hemp in hot climates in wooded areas. Northern *Cannabis sativa ssp. sativa* plants are almost devoid of narcotic substances (THC), but the flowering tops of female *Cannabis sativa ssp. indica* plants grown in warm regions are often potent enough to cause poisoning and delirium. When moderately used, hemp can have an effect similar to that described by Robert Burton in his *Anatomy of Melancholy*:

> Gracias ab Horto makes mention of another herb called bang, like in effect to Opium, which puts them for a time into a kind of Extasis, and makes them gently to laugh.[51]

Veterinary Values

Indian hemp is sometimes given to cattle to ease stomach complaints, flatulence, and colics. Hemp oil is also rubbed onto cows' udders to decrease excessive milk production.

Miscellaneous Wisdom

Hemp has been regarded as an "uncanny" plant for centuries because of its ability to cause hallucinations, and to set its users in a trance, occasionally favoring them with the gift of second sight. Witches and sorcerers practicing both white and black magic

---

51. Burton, *The Anatomy of Melancholy* (1621) (London: Tudor, 1977), 593.

have therefore used it extensively. The expressed juice of the fresh plant was also once thought to make water freeze on impact, and people who slept in a hemp field were supposed to turn mad or die. Pregnant women were warned against urinating on the herb, and hemp rope was used to hang criminals. In the Lincolnshire Fens, neighbors warned criminals that their uncouth behavior would lead them to the gallows by drawing a willow stake and hemp rope on their doors at night. This was supposed to mean that the offender would soon be hanged, his body buried at a crossroads, and a willow stake driven through his body. His restless soul would have to haunt the crossing until laid to rest by a merciful good Samaritan.

One of the most notorious hemp products is hashish, which owes its name to Hassan-i-Saban, otherwise known as the "Old Man of the Mountain." In the eleventh and twelfth centuries, he gathered a group of insurgents around him, and instigated many political intrigues, acts of violence and Hassan-ssinations, or assassinations. His followers smoked large quantities of hashish to build up their courage and induce a state of unnatural sensibility.

A campaign to eradicate hemp has taken place in this century, which has led to its being outlawed in most countries. This is not just a paranoid idea of some potheads, but began as sorry mercenary reality. The paper industry was not interested in paper that could outlast its products, especially cheap newsprint, and went to work to give hemp a bad name. In the 1930s, the campaign against hemp took on an almost hysterical tone, thanks to the undifferentiated speeches of Harry J. Anslinger of the FBI.

Today, hemp has been rehabilitated, and it has become a profitable crop. Forty thousand different commercial products can be produced from hemp. In Berlin, a hemp museum has opened its doors, and the plant is praised to the skies on hundreds of websites. There have been repeated attempts to legalize cannabis for medicinal uses, up to now with only moderate success. In the United States, some states make exceptions to its general prohibition as a medicinal drug, while it is still forbidden on a national level.

Oracular Worth

In the British Isles, hemp was often consulted as a love oracle on such important dates as Valentine's Day, Midsummer's Day, Halloween, and St. Martin's night. The diviner went directly home from church on St. Valentine's Day, and then, at precisely 12:30 PM, scattered hemp seeds and called out:

> Hempseed I sow, hempseed I grow,
> She (or he) that will my true love be,
> Come rake this hempseed after me.

The promised one would then follow the chanter, raking the hemp seed into a winding sheet.[52]

On Midsummer's Day, the procedure is similar. A girl should go through her garden with a rake on her left shoulder and throw hemp seed over her right shoulder, repeating the following rhyme:

Hempseed I set, hempseed I sow,
The man that is my true love
Come after me and mow.[53]

or

Hempseed I scatter
Hempseed I sow
He that is my true love come after me and mow.[54]

The loved one will take on the appearance of Death and follow the girl with a scythe, reaping her hempen seed crop.

On Hallowe'en, girls and boys sow and harrow hemp seed, and then say:

Hemp-seed, I saw thee;
And him that is to be my true love,
Come after me and pou thee.[55]

The person who has the courage to look over his or her left shoulder will see someone following, pulling up the hemp.

Girls in Norfolk scatter hemp seeds around the table at midnight on St. Martin's Eve (the 11th of November), and then chant:

Hemp-seed I sow, hemp-seed I grow,
If you be my true love came after me and mow.[56]

---

52.   G. F. Northall, *English Folk-Rhymes* (1892) (Detroit, MI: Singing Tree Press, 1968), 111.

53.   Ibid., 110.

54.   Ruth L. Tongue, *Somerset Folklore* (London: The Folk-Lore Society, 1965), 91.

55.   John Brand and Sir Henry Ellis, *Observations on the Popular Antiquities of Great Britain* (1849), vol. 1 (Detroit, MI: Singing Tree Press, 1969), 383.

56.   William Henderson, *Notes on the Folk-Lore of the Northern Counties of England and the Borders* (London: The Folk-Lore Society, 1897), 104.

Literary Flowers

Come you fatall Sisters three,
Whose excercise is spinning:
And helpe us to pull out these thrids,
For heer's but a harsh beginning.
Oh hemp, and flax, and tow to to to
Tow to to to, tow tero.
Oh hemp, and flax, and tow to to to
Tow to to to, tow tero.
If the Millers art you like it not,
To the hempe blocke packee yee:
Thumpe, and thumpe, and thump apace.
For fear the whipper take yee.
Oh hemp, and flax, and tow to to to
Tow to to to to tero.
Oh hemp, and flax, and tow to to to
Tow to to to to tero.

—AN ELIZABETHAN BROADSIDE BALLAD,
IN MATTHEW HODGART'S *THE FABER BOOK OF BALLADS*

Flowers have an expression of countenance as much as men and animals.
Some seem to smile; some have a sad expression; some are pensive and diffident;
others again are plain, honest and upright, like the broad-faced sunflower and the hollyhock.

—Henry Ward Beecher

HOLLYHOCK & MARSHMALLOW

Name

Hollyhocks, marshmallows, and common mallows are all members of the **Mallow** family, which is quite varied. Because of the similarities between species, herbalists and authors have confused and exchanged the names of the members of this family for centuries. For the sake of clarity, the **Mallows** are divided, in this book, into two chapters due to their distinct healing properties. This chapter focuses on hollyhocks and marshmallows; a chapter on the common mallow can be found within the Lunar Herbs section.

The marshmallow, *Althaea officinalis*, is usually a perennial plant. *Althaea* is derived from the Greek word *altheo*, meaning "to cure"; the term *officinalis* designates the plant's official use in medicine and its listing in pharmacopeias. It is a member of the **Mallow** or *Malvaceae* family, as is the beloved hollyhock (*Alcea rosea*). Hollyhocks are usually biennial, but may also be annuals or even perennials.

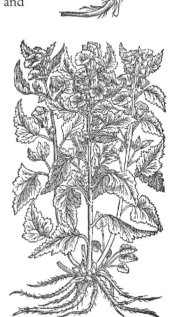

Folk Names

Marshmallow is also known as white mallow, moorish mallow, mallards, mauls, althaea, sweet weed, schloss tea, wynote, and mortification root. German names are *Eibisch* (derived from hibiscus), *Althee, alter Thee, alte Eh, Stockmalve, Kindsbetttee, Heilwurz, Schleimwurzel,* and *Samtpappel.* The French call it *guimauve sauvage* and *bourdon de Saint Jacques;* the Italians, *altèa, bismalva, benefischi, malvavisco,* and *malvaccioni;* the Russians, *altej lekarstvennyj.*

Hollyhock is also called hibiscus in English; in German, it is named *Stockrose, Stock-malve, schwarze Stockrose, Gartenmalve, Baummalve, auf und auf Rose, Pappelrose, Rosenei-bisch*, and *Herbstrose*. The French call the plant *rose trémière*; the Italians, *malva rosa* and *rosoni*; the Russians, *štokroza*; the Turks, *khatmi*; and the Arabians, *khatmae*.

Appearance

The marshmallow plant can grow to a maximum height of 6 ft., although its normal height usually varies between 2 and 5 ft. Its thick, perennial rootstock is yellowish-white and of a corky texture on the outside, and white and fleshy on the inside. It branches and grows several feet down into the ground or sideways. According to Nicholas Culpeper,

> The roots are many and long, shooting from one head, of the size of a thumb or finger, very pliant, tough, like Liquorice, of a whitish yellow color on the outside, and white within, full of a slimy juice, which if laid in water will thicken, as if it were a jelly.[57]

Marshmallow stalks are upright, and both stem and leaves are cloaked with a silvery-gray-green sheen. Marshmallow leaves are soft, hairy, felty in texture, and smaller and more pointed than the leaves of the common mallow. They are heart-shaped at the bottom of the stalk, but their form becomes more irregular and they become softer higher up the stalk. Marshmallow flowers can be as large as 2 in. across, and their color ranges from white to a pale purplish pink. Their texture is silky, and the stems of the single flowers are short. Marshmallow fruits look like the characteristic mallow "cheeses," with the seeds pressed up close to one another in rings.

The hollyhock is common enough not to need a detailed description. Its flowers vary more widely in color than those of the marshmallow: they may be single, filled or double, frilled, reddish, yellow, pinkish, apricot, dark violet, or any shade in between. Some flowers are described as being black, but they are usually a very dark violet. For medicinal purposes, the single dark red flowers are the best.

Place, Season, and Useful Parts

The marshmallow is a native of Europe, and can be found from Siberia to southern Denmark and England on down to the western Mediterranean. It is occasionally grown in the northeastern United States, and was once commercially cultivated in Europe. The marshmallow can be encountered wild on the banks of tidal rivers or in salt marshes,

---

57. Culpeper, *Culpeper's Complete Herbal* (1653) (London: Foulsham, undated), 223.

on beaches, in ditches, or on damp ground. It can occasionally be found on the edge of woods or in moist pastures, or as an escape from neighboring gardens.

Marshmallow blossoms from July to August, and blooms in some cases in June and September as well. The plant's stem dies down each fall, but new sprouts shoot up in great numbers from the roots in spring. The roots of two-year-old plants can be gathered in the spring, or again in the fall. The leaves are gathered shortly before the blossom, and the flowers are harvested as they appear.

The hollyhock can occasionally be found growing wild in the Middle East and southeastern Europe, and where it has escaped from garden culture. It blossoms from July to October of the second year, and the flowers should be gathered just before they open completely.

Gathering, Drying, and Storage

Two-year-old marshmallow roots are usually gathered after the plant has flowered in the fall, but can also be harvested in early spring. The leaves, and especially the marshmallow flowers, must be picked carefully and handled as little as possible to avoid bruising. Hollyhock flowers should only be gathered on clear, sunny days after the dew has dried.

Marshmallow roots should only be washed if absolutely necessary. It is best to rub them clean with a soft cloth, and then dice them. They are dried in the dark at an ideal temperature of 95° F, and must be turned often. Marshmallow flowers and leaves should be dried quickly in dark, airy rooms. Hollyhock flowers must be dried very quickly in thin layers in the shade, or they will mildew. If dried too long, they tend to crumble.

Seed Saving and Germination

There is relatively little variation between marshmallow varieties, and the plants can easily be propagated true-to-type by root division. Each piece of root with a pointed eye will form a new plant. To harvest the seeds, it is best to pick the single fruits, and then to separate the seeds by hand, or to press the fruits through a coarse sieve. Harvesting the entire seed-bearing stalk is not usually advisable, for it is difficult to separate the light seeds from the felty leaves. Winnowing will not work well, for they are the same weight.

Hollyhocks will cross with each other, and must be isolated if the various varieties are to be kept separate. It is easy to grow out two varieties by raising one from seed each year, and preventing the plants from blossoming the first year. This way, only one variety will blossom each year, and the seed harvest will be of only one variety. Dried seeds keep well in a cool, dark, airy place.

Gardening Hints

Marshmallows are propagated by the root division of two-year-old plants in fall, or by sowing seeds in spring, and then transplanting the small plants to their final position in summer. The plants are relatively easy to propagate, for each piece of root with an eye will quickly produce a new plant. Excess plants should be removed from the garden as soon as possible, and larger plants divided, or they will send down long roots and become extremely hard to transplant. Each plant should be allowed at least 2 ft. clearance on each side to ensure luxuriant growth. Marshmallows have been cultivated in gardens since the ninth century, when they were recommended to gardeners by an ordinance of Charlemagne. They grow best on damp, sandy soil, but will also thrive on loam or clay.

The garden hollyhock with its showy flowers and tall stems is a familiar plant to most gardeners and is very popular in the British Isles as a cottage flower. It thrives in a sunny condition, and often self-seeds in the sunniest part of the garden, or up against a warm wall. It needs rich, but not freshly fertilized, well-drained soil, and will do well in sandy, limestone-rich areas (near walls or buildings). Some organic farmers suggest planting mallows or hollyhocks as a regenerating crop after potatoes or grain.

Since hollyhocks are normally biennial, the seeds are sown in the summer, and will flower the following year. It is also possible to separate and plant new shoots in a rooting medium in late summer or fall. Sturdy plants can be left out to overwinter, and will send up flower stalks in spring. Weaker plants should be overwintered in a cold greenhouse or a cold frame. When planting hollyhocks in their final position, allow at least 1 ft. between plants, and remember that they will grow to a great height and can overshadow other plants. Short herbs such as chamomile can be planted between hollyhocks if space is limited in the garden. The major disease problem is rust, which will quickly spread from plant to plant, and may be transmitted from neighboring gardens. Good garden hygiene is essential if any headway is to be made against rust. Diseased plants must be immediately thrown away (not onto the compost heap!).

Culinary Virtues

The very tender leaves and tops of young marshmallow plants are eaten raw in salads or cooked as a vegetable, just like those of the common mallow. The roots of the marshmallow are large and fleshy, and are therefore preferred to the roots of the common mallow as a vegetable. Marshmallow roots were once considered a great delicacy in ancient Rome and China, and have been used by the Egyptians, Syrians, Armenians, and Greeks as famine food. The roots are peeled, boiled, and then sliced into salads. They can also be peeled, sliced, cooked in boiling water until softened, and then browned with onion in butter. A decoction of marshmallow roots can be beaten like egg white, or employed in the preparation of marshmallow sweets. Marshmallow sweets were once considered to have great medicinal properties, and were prescribed against coughs. Needless to say, the modern sweets sold under the same name have no medicinal value, and have never seen a marshmallow plant.

There are a number of vegetable mallows raised for their soft leaves. These tender greens are often added to salads, but usually are cooked as spinach substitutes. In Arab countries, a traditional soup is prepared with mallow leaves (see the common mallow chapter).

The dark red, almost black flowers of some hollyhocks have occasionally been used alone or together with elderberry or poke root berries to color wine that is too pale.

Household Applications

Red or reddish-black hollyhock flowers are often added to potpourri because of their strong color. The large red flowers of another member of the mallow family, *Hibiscus sabdariffa,* or Roselle, are in particular demand for this purpose because of their brilliant red flowers. They are also sold as a decorative red tea. At one time, fibers of the hollyhock were used experimentally in paper and cloth production.

Cosmetic Properties

Like the common mallow, marshmallow is employed in the preparation of moisturizing creams and lotions to soften chapped hands or lips and dry skin. Marshmallow roots can be chewed like mallow roots to whiten and cleanse the teeth. Marshmallow roots are taken internally, and also applied externally to the scalp to induce hair growth. The viscous mixture produced by boiling marshmallow roots down to a paste is sometimes used to set hair, in the same manner as Irish moss.

Noteworthy Recipes

Hair Growth Lotion: This antiquated remedy will hardly appeal to modern readers, but may point the way to more contemporary applications:

> If Hair, that comely Ornament of your Sex, be wanting, occasioned by Sickness or defect of moisture, & c. To recover it, Take the Ashes of Hysop-roots, the Juyce of Marshmallows, and the Powder of Elicampane-Roots, of each an ounce: boil them in half a pint of White-wine, with a dram of Oyl of Tartar, till half be consumed, and with the remainder, anoint the bald pate, and the hair will be restored.[58]

A Moisturizing and Softening Body Lotion: Prepare ½ pint of a concentrated comfrey-leaf or marigold-petal infusion. Add 2 Tbsp. of powdered marshmallow roots to

---

58. John Shirley, *The Accomplished Ladies Rich Closet of Rarities* (London: N. Bodington, 1688), 56.

the infusion, and boil gently over a low flame until the mixture begins to thicken. Pass through a strainer while still warm, and then add 1 Tbsp. of honey and 1 oz. of melted lanolin. Stir the mixture continuously until cooled, adding a few drops of warm comfrey or marigold infusion if the consistency becomes too stiff. Store in wide-necked jars in a cool place and use generously.

Medicinal Merits

Dioscurides' herbal was recognized as a major authority in the field of herbal medicine for many centuries. The following passage deals with the medicinal merits of the marshmallow:

> It is called Althea for ye much vertue and divers use of it. For being sod in Melicrate or wine, or beaten of itself, it is good for wounds, ye Parodites, ye struma, Suppurations, enflamed duggs, ye griefs of the seats, bruises, flatulent humors, ye distensions of ye nerves, For it dissolves, & ripens, or breaks and brings to a Cicatrix. But being sodden as is said and kneaded together with swines grease or goose grease, or turpentine, it is good in a Pessum for ye inflammations & preclusions of ye matrix, and the decoction of it performes the same, expelling also ye so-called after-purgaments. And the decoction of ye root being drank with wine doth help ye dysentericall, ye ischiaticall, ye tremblers, ye troubled with ruptures and assuageth ye pains of ye teeth, being sodden with vinegar, & ye mouth washed with it.[59]

In the ninth century, *The School of Salernum* stated the matter more succinctly:

> In Physicke Mallowes have much reputation,
> The very name of Mallow seems to found,
> The roote thereof will give a kind purgation,
> By them both men and women good have found,
> To womens monthly flowers they give laxation,
> They make men soluble that have been bound.[60]

Modern Medicine

The leaves of the marshmallow are used by modern herbalists for their softening, dissolving, soothing, healing, coating, and protective properties. Common mallow leaves are somewhat astringent; marshmallow leaves have almost no astringent qualities.

---

59. Robert T. Gunther, ed., *The Greek Herbal of Dioscurides* (New York: Hafner, 1959), 388.

60. Sir John Harrington, trans., *The School of Salernum* (Salerno, Italy: Ente Provinciale per il Turismo, 1953), 52.

Marshmallow leaves can be rubbed onto bee or wasp stings to lessen the swelling and itching. A tea of the leaves can be used as a gargle to wash out a mouth dry with fever, or to ease a sore throat. The leaves of the hollyhock are used in steaming and inhaling mixtures for sore throats, sinus problems, or earaches.

Marshmallow roots are stronger in their softening action than either marshmallow leaves or the common mallow. If marshmallow roots are unavailable, hollyhock roots can be substituted. A strong decoction of marshmallow roots has approximately the same consistency as mucus, and it will help to dissolve it, without irritating or infecting the mucous membranes as it passes through the digestive system. On the contrary, it can also help to heal and to disinfect. Because of this, marshmallow-root tea is an excellent medicine for those suffering from sore throats, colds, coughs, from irritations in the alimentary canal or the urinary and respiratory tracts, from intestinal infections, stomach upsets, dysentery, some forms of venereal disease, or from "the whites" *(fluor albus)*. It can be recommended to patients recovering from bouts with urinary stones or gravel or cystitis. Marshmallow-root tea is administered by some midwives before delivery to soften the genital area, and is drunk regularly for several weeks before birth to lubricate the membranes.

Poultices of scraped fresh marshmallow roots thickened with honey or bread are used externally to ripen carbuncles or boils, and to draw out infections. A hot poultice of marshmallow roots and slippery elm bark *(Ulmus americana var. rubra)* can help to keep a large wound from "mortifying," or becoming gangrenous, until medical attention can be attained—hence its folk name, mortification root. Marshmallow-root poultices are sometimes applied to the bladder region to ease infections. Marshmallow-root powder is used in the commercial production of pills.

The pink flowers of the marshmallow, as well as single red hollyhock flowers, can be used like the flowers of the common mallow to ease the pains of sore throats, coughs, chest troubles, and hoarseness. They can also be employed in the preparation of eye-washes. Because of their pretty purple color, mallow flowers are often added to electuaries, syrups, and confections. The dark purple flowers of *Alcea rosea var. nigra* are employed specifically for children's coughs. The commercial herbal tea sold under the name of Hibiscus or Karkadé has mild diuretic properties, and consists of the bright red flowers of roselle, a related mallow species.

Special Cures

Marshmallow Root Tea: The best method of preparing marshmallow root tea is by the cold extraction method. Place ½ oz. of the roots in a pot with 1 pint of cold water, cover, and leave overnight. The next morning, heat the mixture gently over a low flame until a somewhat viscous consistency is obtained. If the tea is allowed to cook for too long, it may jell into a rubbery mass when cooled. The hot tea can be strained into a thermos bottle, and drunk in small amounts every few hours. Marshmallow-root tea should not be kept for more than a day.

Tea Mixture for Bladder and Kidney Problems: This bladder and kidney tea can be taken when a burning sensation or a kidney or bladder irritation is present. It can be mixed from the following ingredients: finely cut marshmallow roots, marshmallow leaves, sage leaves, and oat straw (obtained after the harvest from unsprayed fields). The tea is prepared daily as an infusion, and drunk regularly for at least 4 weeks. It is not recommended for pregnant women.

Marshmallow Syrup: Marshmallow syrup cleanses the entire respiratory system, and is especially effective in the treatment of children's coughs. It has been a treasured home remedy for many centuries. In acute cases, it is advisable to administer the syrup in small amounts every hour.

Marshmallow syrup is often made with sugar syrup, but the most effective preparation is made with honey. Boil ½ oz. of marshmallow roots in 1 pint of water for 10 minutes, or use the cold extraction method overnight. Then add ½ oz. of mullein flowers and heat for 5 minutes. Strain and add 2 lb. of thick honey. Heat very gently (at best on the back of a wood stove) until a syrupy mass is reached, and then pour into sterilized containers. Seal and store in a cool place.

Marshmallow Sweets: The first "marshmallows" were pleasantly sugarcoated medicinal sweets for children, and were prepared from marshmallow roots, sugar, gum arabic, and egg whites. The French named these sweets *"pâte de Guimauve."* Another kind of marshmallow sweet, which can be eaten as a treat or taken as cough drops, can be prepared from 3½ oz. of finely-powdered marshmallow roots, 2 lb. of confectioner's sugar, and rose water. Add the rose water slowly to the dry ingredients to form a stiff dough, and then roll very thin. Cut out small, tablet-shaped circles, and let them dry in a very slow oven or in a warm place. Store in airtight and moisture-proof containers.

Here is a modern recipe for marshmallows:

4 Tbsp. marshmallow roots

1 ¾ cup refined sugar

1 ¼ cup gum arabic

Water of orange flowers (for aroma)

2 cups water

1–2 egg whites, well beaten

Make sure the mallow roots aren't moldy or too woody. Make a tea of marshmallow roots by simmering in a pint of water for 20 to 30 minutes, or letting the roots steep in the water overnight. Add additional water if it evaporates during cooking. Strain out the roots. Heat the gum and marshmallow decoction in a double boiler until they are dissolved together. Strain with pressure. Stir in the sugar as quickly as possible. When dissolved, remove from the fire and add the well beaten egg whites, stirring constantly. Pour out on a flat surface such as marble, let cool, and cut into smaller pieces.

Uses in Husbandry

Goats are fond of mallow leaves, and bees visit the plants' blossoms. Marshmallow fibers have on occasion been used to manufacture paper and cloth. *Althaea cannabina* has also been grown as a fiber plant in southern Europe. The dark red, almost black flowers of *Alcea rosea var. nigra* are highly prized by husbandmen. The beautiful red color they produce is employed to color syrups, liqueurs, and particularly red wine.

Veterinary Values

Poultices prepared from the entire marshmallow plant, including the roots, are applied to abscesses to ripen them, to swollen udders to lessen the chance of infection and to relieve pain, and also to wounds and inflamed eyes. Warm marshmallow-root tea can be given to animals with intestinal colds, or to increase the flow of milk. Dogs, cats, and whelps profit from the addition of a small amount of chopped marshmallow, or common mallow leaves, to the diet. Puppies that chew on every- and anything can be distracted from doing real damage by giving them a dried marshmallow root to gnaw on.

Miscellaneous Wisdom

According to the ancient Greek physician Dioscurides, marshmallow juice

> is available for ye stingings of bees and waspes, and if a man beforehand be anointed therewith raw, beaten small with oyle, he remaines unstrikable.[61]

A marshmallow salve has, similarly, been used in Germany to protect its user against evil and in particular against the Evil Eye.

Literary Flowers

For want and famine they were solitary;
fleeing into the wilderness in former time desolate and waste.
Who cut up mallows by the bushes, and juniper roots for their meat. ...
Among the bushes they brayed; under the nettles they were gathered together.

—JOB 30:3–4, 7

---

61. Robert T. Gunther, ed., *The Greek Herbal of Dioscurides* (New York: Hafner, 1959), 157.

Tiny telescoping towers of Babel,
able to bend in the wind, yet as strong as a skeleton.
—Sister Clarissa

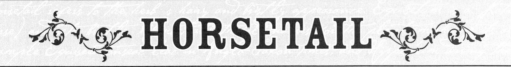

HORSETAIL

Name

The name "horsetail" refers to the herb's hairy and bristly appearance. The botanical name, *Equisetum,* is a Latin word composite of *equus* (horse) and *seta* (bristle). Almost all the old names for the plant emphasize its association with the horse, such as *Equiseia tonseac leac* in Anglo-Saxon times and *Hippurium* during the Middle Ages.

The coal-age predecessors of the present-day **Equisetaceae** family were giant, tree-like plants. The horsetails of medicinal fame are *Equisetum arvense* (field horsetail) and occasionally *Equisetum sylvaticum* (wood horsetail). Other members of this family, such as *Equisetum palustre* (also known as *Equisetum fluviatile*) and *Equisetum hyemale* can be of value in the household.

Folk Names

Horsetail has many descriptive names: horsetail rush, bottle-brush, paddock pipes, joint grass, foxtail, scrub grass, shavegrass, pewterwort, dutch rushes, scouring rush, scone scouring rush, mare's tail, and meadow pine. Germans call the plant *Schachtelhalm, Zinnkraut, Katzenschwanz, Hexenbesen,* and *Tannenkraut;* the French, *prêle des champs* and *équisette;* the Italians, *coda di cavallo, setolini,* and *rasparella;* the Spaniards, *equiseto* and *cols de caballo;* the Japanese, *tsukushi;* and the Irish, *eireaball capaill.*

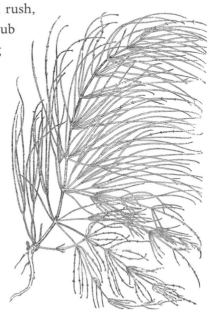

Appearance

The most characteristic features of horsetails are that they do not flower, they do not have proper leaves, and their barren summer shoots closely resemble miniature pine trees. The spring shoots are pinkish, and unbranched. They end in an elongated spore capsule, and are *not* suitable for medicinal purposes. They wilt quickly and turn brown, and are replaced in May by large, green, branched summer shoots. The shoots of field horsetail are barren and grow to a maximum height of 2 ft. Shoots of *Equisetum giganteum* have been known to grow a little taller in South America. Each hollow stem and branch is divided into tiny segments, joined together by telescoping joints. The famous German plant photographer, Karl Blossfeld, was fascinated by the plant, and made several portraits in which the architectural structure of the plant resembles the Tower of Babel. Children are also fascinated by the ease with which the joints of the plant can be pulled apart, like horticultural Tinker Toys. The entire plant is brittle, and the branch whorls become progressively smaller up the stalk.

Horsetail has no particular smell, but tastes bitter, gritty, and even somewhat salty. The shoots grow from knots in a perennial rootstock, which is branching, and brown or black in color, and goes deeply down into the soil.

A local botanical guide is invaluable when learning to identify the different horsetails. As a rule, the marsh horsetail *(Equisetum palustre)*, which is not used for medicinal purposes, has thicker, shorter branches. Field and wood horsetails *(Equisetum arvense* and *Equisetum sylvaticum)* are medicinally valuable and have longer, thinner branches set more noticeably in whorls and ending in a point.

Place, Season, and Useful Parts

Horsetails grow throughout the Northern Hemisphere on sandy, loamy, or damp soil, in fields, ditches, underbrush, on roadsides, rubble, ruins, and railroad embankments, from the flatlands to alpine heights. Giant horsetail can be found in South America. Marsh horsetails grow only on damp or swampy ground, but field and wood horsetails can be found in dry meadows or on the edges of woods. The spores ripen between March and May, and the barren shoots appear shortly after that.

Gathering, Drying, and Storage

It is difficult to correctly identify the various horsetails. Only the field horsetail and the wood horsetail are suitable for medicinal purposes, and of these two plants, only the sterile summer shoots are gathered from unsprayed stands. The plants should be harvested no later than July, and rust-colored stems must be avoided, for they are infested by a fungus. The best horsetails grow on moist, loamy, but not swampy soil. Horsetails are gathered by cutting the plant carefully above the ground from May to July. The fronds must retain their pale green color when dried. This can be done outdoors in an airy place, or in well-ventilated attics in thin layers. The horsetail root should never be included with the dried drug.

Seed Saving and Germination

Where the perennial horsetail occurs, it will often attempt to take over suitable areas, becoming something of a garden pest. It is almost always propagated by plant and root division.

Gardening Hints

It is fortunate for gardeners that the horsetails prefer warm, shady, and very damp soil, or they would be even greater pests than they are in gardens. They can spread with alarming rapidity wherever they do put down roots, for they propagate themselves by spores as well as roots. Despite the fact that they are a very useful plant in the garden as liquid fertilizer, they should be banished to an unused part of the yard where they will not interfere with more sensitive garden plants.

French or African marigolds *(Tagetes tenuifolia)* are said to inhibit horsetails' growth, and can be planted in masses next to an existing stand of the herb to keep it from spreading into the garden. Solarization will also kill off the herb: the soil is cleared, and heavy black plastic is laid down and weighted with rocks. The soil heats up to such a degree under the plastic that the plants and roots are scorched. The plastic must be left in place for at least a month or two, or for the entire growing season.

Culinary Virtues

The starch found in the tubers of the larger members of this family is said to be nutritious, and can be eaten in times of need. Ancient Romans cooked the young heads of *Equisetum maximum*, preparing them as we do asparagus, or dredging them in flour and then frying them. The pithy inner part of horsetail stems can be eaten as survival food. The whole plant has been used as a vegetable by the Japanese.

Household Applications

Because the members of this family contain so much silica, they have excellent abrasive properties, and are often used as scouring rushes. Horsetail is an inexpensive and particularly effective pewter polisher, hence the name Pewterwort. The pewter pieces are scrubbed with a tuft of fresh or dried horsetail until they begin to shine, and then rinsed in clear water to remove the green stains that have rubbed off onto the metal. Watchmakers use the herb to smooth off watch parts after filing. Arrowsmiths once finished the shafts of their arrows with horsetail, and knights' squires made their masters' armor shine with the herb. Weavers cleaned and smoothed their shuttles with horsetail, and dairymaids scoured their milk pails with the plant. Combs were polished with horsetail, and pieces of wood flooring scrubbed with the herb, and then rinsed well. A handy tuft of horsetail can always be used as an emergency scrubbing brush for pots and pans, especially on camping trips. Together with the mordants ferrous or copper sulphate, it is possible to create a dark green dye from horsetail. Chrome or alum will produce yellow hues.

Cosmetic Properties

Horsetail is one of the most important cosmetic herbs. It can be taken internally or applied externally. Drinking horsetail tea regularly helps to cleanse the body of impurities and excess water, and therefore improves facial color and reduces swelling and puffiness. This treatment is especially effective after prolonged illness or great exertion. The body can readily absorb the silica in horsetail, and horsetail tea will help to keep nails from breaking and hair from splitting.

Horsetail rinses can strengthen hair, improve the general condition of the scalp, discourage dandruff, and restore the scalp oil glands to their proper working condition. It can make oily hair less greasy, and hasten the scalp's recovery from rashes, fungal diseases, allergic reactions, and wounds, as well as preventing hair loss.

Horsetail tea can heal skin damaged by a rash, irritated from shaving, or disfigured by blemishes and acne. It can be combined with a thickening agent such as honey, oatmeal, Bentonite or French green clay, Irish moss, or almond meal and used as a facial mask to cleanse large pores and remove blackheads. Horsetail compresses can further relieve the discomfort of swollen or puffy eyes. Skin damaged by fungal diseases or allergies is washed with horsetail tea or dusted with horsetail powder. Brittle fingernails and damaged cuticles should be bathed as often as possible in horsetail infusion.

- The best way to take a cosmetic horsetail cure is to drink a cup of tea 2–3 times a day for at least 4 weeks. Treat the damaged body part once or twice a day for the same amount of time with horsetail tea or horsetail powder. After 6–8 weeks, take a pause to allow the body to recover from the cure.

Horsetail capsules are also effective. As a general rule, horsetail tea should be used on dry rashes or eczema, and horsetail powder on sores.

Medicinal Merits

Horsetail contains more silica than most medicinal herbs. This can be tested by burning a plant: each shoot will burn to a white silica skeleton before dissolving into ash.

Weakened kidneys and the resulting faulty elimination of water from the body can be the cause of many complaints and diseases, especially among the elderly or menopausal women. Drinking horsetail tea can stimulate the kidneys and rid the body of excess fluids, toxins, and impurities. A horsetail tea cure will act to strengthen the kidneys and prevent water retention, and is particularly effective if taken regularly in small amounts. Malfunctioning kidneys, kidney stones and gravel, water on the lungs, swollen legs, glandular disorders, eczema, excessive perspiration, prostate troubles, mild forms of rheumatism and gout, as well as nervous irritability can all be relieved to some extent with the help of horsetail tea. A horsetail tea cure can be taken to support a reducing diet, and is so mild that it can also be taken when growths or ulcers are present.

The herb is a purifying as well as a blood-staunching medicine. It is taken to lessen bleeding from the lungs or uterus, to dry out ulcers, and to help heal internal wounds. Inserting the juice of the fresh plant into a nostril can stop nosebleeds. Some herbalists also prescribe the juice of the fresh plant as a sanguinary tonic.

Modern Medicine

Horsetail is one of the best herbs for the external treatment of skin diseases and is one of very few herbs with recognizable fungicidal properties. Eczema, rashes, fungal diseases, badly healing or even festering wounds as well as genital sores are dusted with horsetail powder. Dry rashes, flaky eczema, or open wounds are washed with horsetail infusion. Horsetail baths are also used to wash sores and open wounds, sore feet and diseased skin. Steam baths alleviate painful water retention, bladder cramps, or colds. Gargling with horsetail can cleanse and strengthen the gums, and help prevent infections of the mouth or tonsils. It is often prescribed to strengthen the bronchia and lungs against further infection. A horsetail tea cure is also effective in strengthening connective tissue throughout the body. The ashes of burned horsetail are employed in the treatment of excessive stomach acidity, and homeopaths prescribe plant preparations for irritations or infections of the bladder and kidneys, as well as prostate problems. *Equisetum hyemale* is used for many of the same complaints as the fresh herb, as a homeopathic kidney tonic for cystitis, dropsy, gravel, and bedwetting, and for patients with a constant desire to urinate.

Chinese medicine employs *Equisetum hyemale* to treat red and painful eyes with blurred vision, and also to help stop bleeding. It is contraindicated in pregnancy and dehydration.

Special Cures

Diuretic Tea: A simple yet effective tea for the elimination of excess water from the body can be prepared from a mixture of equal amounts of goldenrod *(Solidago virgaurea)* and horsetail. One heaping teaspoon of the herb mixture is taken for every ½ pint of boiling water, and then allowed to steep for 10–15 minutes. Herbalists suggest that this tea should be taken in small sips for 4–8 weeks at a time. Then, it is highly advisable to change to another diuretic herb, or to take a pause, to avoid damaging the kidneys. The easy availability of herbs in supermarket shelves or across the counter seduces many people into thinking herbs are completely harmless, and can be taken indefinitely. Legislation in the United States forbids making any unproven statements about the efficacy of herbs, but it also limits the cautionary advice that should be passed on with the herbs for proper use. The constant use of diuretics, herbal or non-herbal, can leach essential nutrients out of the body. They should therefore never be taken as an excuse to lose weight or to avoid a bothersome diet. The point of diuretics is to rid the body of excess water, to strengthen the kidneys, and train them to resume their natural functions. Constant use of diuretics is like the constant use of a girdle: the body gets used to it, and stops trying to solve the problem on its own.

Uses in Husbandry

Meadows, pastures, and gardens infested with horsetail pose a problem, since the plant is extremely difficult to eradicate once it has established itself. Reindeer thrive on some horsetails, but cattle and horses can be poisoned by *Equisetum palustre*.

Veterinary Values

Veterinarians use horsetail tea and horsetail powder in much the same manner as herbalists, to heal and strengthen animals' skin, and to treat rashes and fungal diseases.

Miscellaneous Wisdom

In Germany, a girl who can be made to drink a tea prepared from the giant horsetail, *Equisetum giganteum*, is considered easy prey for would-be lovers. A treasure is also believed to be buried under each and every horsetail plant. The treasure can only be obtained by anyone who manages to dig out each and every one of the plant's roots. This sounds suspiciously like an old wives' tale invented by people who wanted to get rid of the horsetail in their garden, one of those tales children fall for until they know better. Children also use the herb in their games: they make excellent bottle cleaners and shaving brushes, and the telescoping joints are a constant source of wonderment.

Legends

Russian, Czech, Slovakian, and German forest sprites are said to be able to change their size and height at will: they can shrink to be as small as the smallest "tree" in the forest, the horsetail, or they can grow and expand to the size of the largest oak in the wood.

Be thou the marigold, and I will be the sun
Be thou the friar, and I will be the nun.

—Robert Burton, *Anatomy of Melancholy*

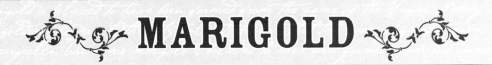

MARIGOLD

Name

The name "marigold" is believed to have been formed from combining the name of the Virgin Mary with "gold," referring to the marigold's golden flowers. Other etymologists believe that the name originated from the Anglo-Saxon word *merso-meargealla*.

The Latin name of the plant, *Calendula*, is a diminutive form of the word *calendae*, and means "little calendar" or "little clock." This points to the marigold's habit of rising and setting with the sun, and of blooming during most of the months of the calendar. Other ancient names are *Solis sponsa*, *Caput monarchi*, and *Oculus Christi*.

The marigold is known under the botanical name *Calendula officinalis*, and was once called *Caltha officinalis*. It is a member of the widespread **Daisy**, *Asteraceae* or *Compositae*, family. Marigolds are usually annuals, although they have been known to live through the winter and seed in their second year.

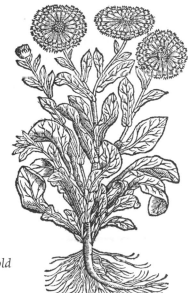

Folk Names

Calendula, summer's bride, golden golds, golds, marygold, mary goolds, mary bud, pot marigold, European marigold, Scotch marigold, ruddes, drunkards, jackanapes, horseback, jackanapes-on-horseback, and poor man's saffron. The most common German names *Ringelblume*, *Ringelröschen*, *Totenblume*, *Wucherblume*, *Krebsblume*, *Sonnwendblume*, *Marienrose*, *Studentenblume*, and *Regenblume*. In French, the plant is called *souci des jardins* and *fleur de tous les mois*; in Italian, *calendula*, *calta*, *fiorrancio*, and *fior d'ogni mese*; in Spanish, *flemeniquillo*, *maravilla*, and *mercadela*; in Welsh, *gold mair*; in Russian, *nogotki lekarstvennye*.

Appearance

The two most characteristic features of marigolds are their brilliant orange or yellow sun-like flowers, and the resiny, pungent, and even unpleasantly balsamic odor of the plants. The flowers are heliotropic, like the sunflower, and follow the sun in its movements. The petals usually open between 7 and 9 AM, and close between 3 and 5 in the afternoon. Marigolds and arnica can be confused with each other, although arnica's smell is more aromatic, and its flowers stragglier in appearance than those of the marigold.

Marigolds grow to a height of 2 ft. Their tap roots have many rootlets. The leaves are pale green, elongated, rounded, and fleshy on upright, downy stems. The leaves decrease in size and become narrower further up the stalk. They have a plastic, flexible, somewhat sticky consistency, and are covered with almost invisible soft hairs. They taste bitter. Marigold flowers taste aromatic, and the single petals are papery and somewhat shiny, and even a little phosphorescent. Wild marigolds have single blossoms, but most cultivated varieties have double or filled flower heads. All forms are medicinally potent, and can be used interchangeably. Marigold fruits resemble tiny rolled-up worms, hence the German name for the plant, Ringelblume.

Place, Season, and Useful Parts

Marigolds were originally a southern European plant, but are now sown in gardens the world over. Early settlers brought the plant to America. Marigolds sometimes escape from gardens to grow on rubble, roadsides, vineyards, meadows, fields, and next to fences. Under favorable circumstances, the plants will blossom from May until the first frost. The flower heads are the most widely employed part of the plant.

Gathering, Drying, and Storage

Marigold leaves are gathered before the plant blossoms. The entire plant is cut when the plant is flowering, and the single flowers are harvested when fully opened. Marigold flowers can be picked with or without the calyx, or flower receptacle. Drying proceeds easier and faster without the calyx, but picking takes longer. The best time to pick marigolds is after a spell of sunny weather, as soon as the dew has dried in the morning.

All parts of the marigold plant should be dried in thin layers in a shady, airy place. The flowers dry best if the petals are separated from the green calyx and then spread out thinly on paper in a dry room. The flower petals must retain their characteristic color on drying. Because of the disconcerting wormlike appearance of the fruits, it is best to check the flowers after drying to make sure that no fruits are present. Commercial marigold flowers are sometimes treated with a red dye to make them appear fresher than they actually are. Marigold salve should be refrigerated, or stored in a cool, dry place.

Seed Saving and Germination

Single marigold varieties are usually maintained through selection. Select repeatedly for the desired characteristics, ruthlessly ripping out any plants with undesirable traits. When an acceptable selection has been made, only grow this one variety to avoid crossing, continuing to rogue out undesirable plants. Marigold plants tend to revert to single blossoms if left to their own devices, and will need careful selection if filled varieties are desired. Gather the seeds when the seed heads have turned light brown, and the single, clawlike seeds can be seen. The best way to clean the seeds is by hand, carefully picking through and removing leaf parts and the calyxes. The seeds are bulky, but they keep well in a dry, cool place, or they can be dried with silica gel and then frozen.

Gardening Hints

Marigolds are very easy to grow, and should pose few problems, even for children or beginning gardeners. They bloom quickly, are offered in many varieties, grow lushly, and are a sunny addition to any garden. The major drawback with marigolds is that so many of them will come up the next year, and then they have to be ripped out. Many beginning, or hesitant, gardeners cannot bear to remove them, and their soil is leached of nutrients as a result. Marigolds are heavy and aggressive feeders, and will take essential minerals away from other plants.

Marigolds prefer a sunny position, but will grow in almost any soil, and tolerate a good deal of drought. They only need to be sown once, and will then self-seed very happily. The usual practice is to sow them outdoors in March or April in their final position, and to cover the seeds well. They will begin to blossom a few months later, and will continue to bloom on into the fall or even winter if the flower heads are cut or picked out regularly, and the weather does not turn extremely hot. There is often a second blossom in the fall. A few heads can be allowed to go to seed to ensure fresh plants for the following spring. These can then be transplanted where they are needed and the surplus plants thrown on the compost or included in a herbal fertilizer brew. For bushy plants, 9–10 in. should be allowed between plants.

Marigolds are often confused with French marigolds (*Tagetes patula, T. lucida, T. tenuifolia*), also known as Indian buttonholes. Any marigold is a useful addition to the garden, for its strong-smelling flowers discourage insects, aiding the growth of many plants. Nematodes can be killed if large amounts of French marigolds are turned into the soil as green manure. French marigolds can help to repel melon, pumpkin, squash, cucumber, potato, or bean beetles as well as white flies. The growth of tomatoes and potatoes can be positively influenced by *Tagetes* plants, and the growth of such persistent garden weeds as ground ivy and ground elder inhibited. The plants are also used in commercial insect repellents. Unfortunately, marigold plants do not have the same properties, although this misunderstanding has been widely published in literature on organic gardening. Too many marigold plants can have an extremely negative effect on the growth of neighboring plants and even stunt them, for marigolds are aggressive in their search for nutrients.

According to a Franconian tradition, all the crumbs from the Christmas table must be gathered carefully together. In spring, the crumbs are planted in the firm belief that they will bring forth marigold flowers.

Culinary Virtues

According to John Gerard, "no broth is well made without dried Marigolds." Fuller (*Antheologie*, 1655) seconded his opinion, calling marigolds the "Herbe generalle in all pottage."[62] In the Middle Ages, both the leaves and the flowers were held in high esteem as salad herbs and also as potherbs. It seems surprising that the herb is as little used today as it is in the kitchen.

Marigold petals impart a light golden color and a mildly aromatic, bitter taste to foods. They can be substituted for saffron in most recipes, and are a welcome addition to sweet-sour dishes. Commercial saffron has been adulterated with marigold petals on occasion, and it was once accepted as a cheap substitute for the much more expensive herb.

Well-chopped marigold flower petals can be added to herbal butters, to jellies, summer drinks, cheese dishes, and to salads to liven their color. They make unusually bright garnishes, candied or fresh. Deviled eggs, cheese dips, broths, soups, omelets, rice dishes, boiled potatoes, biscuits, and bread puddings can all be improved by the addition of a few marigold flower petals. Bakers sometimes boil the petals in water or milk, and then let the mixture steep before straining and mixing it with the yeast, and the rest of the dough. The resulting loaves of bread have a refreshing yellow color and an unusual taste. Marigold petals are further used in the preparation of marigold wine, marigold syrup, marigold cordials, and marigold conserves.

Noteworthy Recipes

Marigold Cordial: Mrs. C. F. Leyel, the English herbalist and writer, offers this recipe:

> Take a peck of Marigold flowers and put them in an earthenware bowl with ½ pounds of stoned raisins. Pour over them a liquid made with 7 pounds of sugar, 2 pounds of honey and 3 gallons of water. Clear this liquid while it is boiling with the whites and shells of 3 eggs, and strain before putting in

---

62. Qtd. in Mrs. Maude Grieve, *A Modern Herbal* (1931) (London: Penguin, 1976), 517.

the flowers. Cover up the bowl and leave it for two days and nights. Stir it well and leave it for another day and night. Then strain it and put it into a 6-gallon cask which has been well cleansed, and put to it 1 pound of sugar candy (or brown sugar) and the rinds of 6 oranges (unsprayed), which have been peeled and stripped of all white pith.

Stir into it 4 tablespoons of German yeast and cover up the bung-hole. Leave it to work until it froths out; when the fermentation is over pour in a pint of brandy and 2 ounce of dissolved gelatine. Stop[per] the cask and leave it for several months before bottling.[63]

Marigold Rice: In a saucepan, brown ½ onion in a little butter, and then add 4 cups of stock or bouillon. Add ½ tsp. of salt, and ½ cup of finely chopped calendula petals together with 2 cups of rice. Bring to a boil, cover, and simmer for 20 minutes for white rice, and up to 45 minutes for brown rice. White rice will have a pleasant golden color, and a mildly bitter aftertaste.

Scrambled Eggs with Marigold Flower Petals: Beat 4 eggs well in a bowl, adding a little milk if desired. Season with salt and pepper and a pinch of paprika. Melt 1 Tbsp. of butter in a pan, and then scramble the eggs, adding the chopped flower petals of 4 small calendula flowers at the last minute. Serve the eggs on buttered rolls, tortillas, or muffins immediately.

Household Applications

Golden-yellow marigold flower petals are added to sachets and to potpourri, and the flower heads are colorful in garlands and wreaths. Alum-mordanted wool will turn a light, sunny shade of yellow if dyed in a strained decoction of marigold petals, or a mixture of marigold and other members of the **Daisy** family, such as *Anthemis tinctoria*. Together with the mordant copper sulphate, a green tinge can be produced, or an orange hue with bichromate of potash, and yellowish-beige with chrome. Marigold petals are often used as strewing herbs, especially in Indian temples.

Cosmetic Properties

Marigold's most important cosmetic property is its soothing and gentle, yet thoroughly healing, effect on skin damaged by acne, scars, chapping, sunburn, or thread and varicose veins. The leaves and the flower petals are added to acne creams and lotions, to sunburn lotions, to baby oils, to lotions suited for those with thread-vein complexions, or to healing creams for chapped or work-roughened skin. Marigold compresses can

---

63. Leyel, *Herbal Delights* (London: Faber & Faber, 1937), 72.

help to hasten scar formation, and promote the healing of rough skin or acne scars. A marigold infusion can be used as an eyewash or included in facial steaming mixtures, although it should never be used on thread veins. Marigold footbaths, handbaths, and hot baths are healing and stimulating. Marigold petals are often used as coloring agents for hair waters or hair oils. They will also tinge hair golden red if applied in massive quantities.

Medicinal Merits

Since at least the year 1100, Western medicine has recognized the marigold as a mildly strengthening and diuretic herb with a positive effect on uterine, intestinal, and stomachic disorders. According to the doctrine of signatures (the orange-yellow color of the flowers), it was once prescribed as one of the few available treatments for jaundice. Some early herbalists recommended the herb to provoke menstruation and the afterbirth, as well as expelling stillborn children. It was valued as a medicine for eye inflammations and as a treatment for typhus, plague, and cancer, and was also prescribed for tremblings of the heart and melancholy. According to Robert Burton, "Marigold is much approved against Melancholy, and often used therefore in our ordinary broth, as good against this and many other diseases."[64]

Modern Medicine

Modern medicine recommends two major uses for marigold: external application as a wound herb, and internal use as a bitter herb, with healing effects on the intestinal and digestive organs.

Marigold salve is a gentle yet very effective vulnerary medicine. It can help to regenerate damaged tissue, to aid scar formation and hasten the growth of new cells. Marigold salve can soften old, hardened scars, and cleanse, heal, and draw wounds together. Modern scientific experiments have corroborated the widely held folk belief that marigold salve, regularly applied, can exert a positive effect on some types of skin disorders and even skin cancer. It can also be applied to cysts, scrofula, syphilitic sores, varicose veins, chapped skin, burns, chilblains, operation wounds, and abscesses. The main word to remember when using marigold salve is "perseverance." No results will be achieved with an occasional slathering with the salve, but steady applications, day after day, can bring results verging on the miraculous. If the skin is not wounded or irritated, marigold tincture or compresses of the fresh plant can be substituted for the salve. Fresh marigold leaves or flowers can be applied as first-aid bandages to cuts or wounds until they can be treated. The fresh leaves are often rubbed onto wasp or bee stings, and a marigold eye-

---

64. Burton, *The Anatomy of Melancholy* (1621) (London: Tudor, 1977), 566.

wash is a good solution to cleanse and soothe the eye if it has been hurt, lessening the chance of infection until a doctor can be reached.

Marigold is a plant that does not have to be taken alone: it mixes well with other herbs, and supports their medicinal action. Its slightly bitter, stimulating properties are increased in combination with other bitter herbs, or it can impart a pleasing color and flavor to otherwise insipid teas. Few allergic reactions to marigold have been noted. Marigold leaves and flower petals have a mildly stimulating, cleansing, and purifying effect on the blood. They also help to stimulate the kidneys and therefore to free the body of impurities. Because of these qualities, marigolds are added to tea mixtures for the treatment of allergic rashes, gout, and rheumatism, as well as to teas to help regulate glandular systems. This gentle cleansing action is so pronounced that marigolds can be used in the preventive or supportive treatment of cancer of the liver, stomach, intestines, or uterus. They can further help to alleviate some of the symptoms of incurable cases.

The combination of cleansing qualities and bitter principles in a medicinal herb that will not irritate the mucous membranes makes marigold one of the best herbs for a hardened liver, spleen, or uterus. A tea of the herb is effective in the treatment of stomach cramps, hepatitis, or gastritis, and for infections of the intestines, stomach, spleen, liver, or gall bladder. It is also a mild laxative, and can help to expel worms.

Marigold tea or a tea mixture prepared from marigold and English chamomile, taken for one week before menstruation, can help to regulate bleeding and lessen cramps. It is also efficacious in the treatment of menopausal disorders, and the supportive treatment of cancer of the uterus. Women weakened by excessive bleeding or anemics can also profit from the herb. Pregnant women, on the other hand, should make little or no use of marigold.

Marigold flower tea can help to promote perspiration, especially when used in combination with lime tree flowers *(Tilia cordata)* or elder flowers *(Sambucus nigra)*. This tea can be given to children to help "bring out" chicken pox or the measles.

Homeopathy makes use of marigold salve and tincture for the treatment of wounds. Calendula is taken internally as an important vulnerary remedy. It can be given to speed the recovery of damaged tissue, and promote granulation, and can be used for such diverse conditions as chilblains, perineum tears, cervical warts, breast infections, gunshot wounds, knife and scalp wounds, chilblains, ulcers, or postsurgical recovery.

Special Cures

Marigold Salve: Marigold tincture is prepared in the same manner as arnica tincture (see the arnica chapter). Marigold salve is usually made with lard, butter, or goat's butter because of the easy availability and cheapness of the ingredients. Lard keeps longer, and is therefore used more often than butter. It is also possible to make a beeswax, or lanolin and beeswax salve with good keeping qualities and a more pleasant smell.

For the lard salve, melt 1 lb. of lard, and bring it almost to a boil. Add 2 heaping handfuls of marigold flowers, leaves and stems (no roots). Let the mixture simmer for a short time, cover it, and let it cool away from the stove until the lard begins to harden. Melt the lard again, and strain immediately through cheesecloth or a fine strainer into clean containers. Cool and store in a cool place such as a refrigerator.

The preparation of a wax and oil salve takes a little more practice than the lard salve. It is especially important to add the ingredients in the proper order, and to make sure everything stays scrupulously clean. The main problem with salve preparation is the cleanup afterward—salves are sticky and very oily.

A Wax-Oil Marigold Salve: This salve is relatively easy to prepare, and can be used as a recipe for other herbal salves. Two handfuls of marigold flowers are heated carefully in 1 cup high-quality oil such as olive oil, grapeseed oil, avocado or almond oil on the lowest flame possible until the herbs start to wilt. They are then covered, and allowed to steep in the oil overnight. The next day, heat them again carefully, and then pour off the oil, straining through a strainer and then filter paper or cheesecloth to remove all herb residue.

Now heat 1½–2 oz. of beeswax carefully in a double boiler and then slowly add the herbal oil while mixing continuously—a handheld immersion blender is ideal for this job. The temperature should not rise above 150° F. Pour the salve into clean containers, close them, and store in a cold place. If the salve is too oily or has too much wax in it, reheat the mixture, and add oil or wax as needed, and continue to mix until the proper consistency has been reached.

If a softer salve is desired, use 1¼ oz. of beeswax and ½ oz. of lanolin. Several drops of benzoin tincture or grapefruitseed extract can be used to enhance the salve's keeping qualities.

Marigold Herbal Tea Salve: Once you have become proficient in preparing a lard or wax-oil salve, you can go on to the next, more difficult herbal preparation. It's not that easy to successfully mix the ingredients so that the consistency is just right. This salve variant also does not keep as well.

Prepare ½ cup marigold flower tea, and strain and filter it carefully, making sure to remove all plant residue. Warm 1½–2 oz. of beeswax and ¾ oz. of cocoa butter in a double boiler. Mix in 1 cup of oil, and heat everything to at most 150° F. In another pan, heat the marigold tea, and add it carefully to the mixture, mixing all the while with a handheld blender. Add 1 tsp. of lecithin, and pour the salve into clean containers. The salve shoud be stored in a cold place, and used quickly.

A Healing Tea for Cancer Patients: Cancer should of course be treated by a specialist. But if the doctor has no objections, the treatment can be supported by herbal teas. High-risk patients with a family history of cancer can also take the tea as preventive medicine. For cancer of the stomach, liver, gall bladder, intestines, or spleen, a mixture of marigold petals and Holy thistle *(Cnicus benedictus)* is prepared in tea form. It is taken in small amounts lukewarm, half an hour before each and every meal over a period of several months. For prevention of uterine cancer, a mixture of marigold flowers, violet leaves, red clover blossoms, and garden sorrel leaves should be infused and taken in small amounts several times a day between meals.

Uses in Husbandry

Veterinary Values

Marigold salve should always be kept on hand if there are animals around. Almost all animals accept its mild odor, and will consent to be rubbed with the salve, especially if it has been prepared with lard. The part that is licked off by the animals will not harm them. On the contrary, it can also aid the healing process.

- The easiest way to prepare marigold salve for animals is to heat fresh lard over a very low flame until it begins to melt, and then add 1–2 handfuls of marigold flower petals and leaves. Continue heating until the lard is liquid, and then let stand for 5–10 minutes before straining into sterile jars. If the fat begins to smell rancid, throw it out, and begin all over again. Cuts, sprains, scars, and even poorly healing wounds can be treated with marigold salve.

Miscellaneous Wisdom

Marigold flowers are often used in love potions, love magic, and love oracles. Girls who plant marigold flowers in the footsteps of their lovers think that this will ensure the men's constancy. In Slavic countries, boys carry marigold roots wrapped in violet-colored silk in the firm belief that this will make them more attractive to the opposite sex. Some French people think that married men who have an unusual liking for the plant will become cuckolds. Devonshire men who pick a marigold, or even look at it, will become drunkards. Another belief associated with the plant is also of British origin: the flower should be picked while the moon is in Virgo, and Jupiter in the ascendant while saying three Pater Nosters and three Ave Marias. The flower will then be useful in solving robberies.

Oracular Worth

Marigolds are sometimes consulted as miniature rain oracles. If the flowers have not opened by 7–9 AM, then it will certainly rain that day.

Literary Flowers

Here's flowers for you.
Hot lavender, mints, savory, marjoram;
The marigold, that goes to bed wi' the sun,
And with him rises weeping: these are flowers
Of middle summer and, I think, they are given
To men of middle age.

—WILLIAM SHAKESPEARE, *THE WINTER'S TALE*, IV.III

MARJORAM & ORGANY

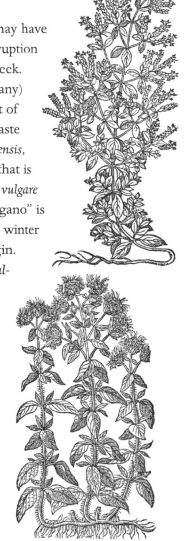

Name

The final origin of the word "marjoram" is uncertain. It may have evolved from the *amaracu* of the ancients. "Organy" is a corruption of the Latin word *origanum*, which in turn comes from the Greek.

Origanum majorana (marjoram) and *Origanum vulgare* (organy) are members of the **Mint** (***Lamiaceae*** or ***Labiatae***) family. Most of the family members can be used in cookery, providing their taste is pleasant and aromatic. *Origanum majorana* (or *Majorana hortensis*, as it is sometimes also called) is a biennial to perennial herb that is usually treated as an annual in northern climates. *Origanum vulgare* is a wild perennial herb. The seasoning generally called "oregano" is harvested from southern forms such as *Origanum onites* (pot or winter marjoram), a perennial plant of southern Mediterranean origin. *Origanum vulgare ssp. viride (Origanum heracleoticum, Origanum vulgare ssp. hirtum)*, winter sweet marjoram, was once widely cultivated but has since gone out of general favor, as has *Origanum syriacum*. *Origanum syriacum* was mentioned in the Bible, and is known as Bible hyssop, syrian oregano, zaatar, or wild oregano.

Folk Names

An old Anglo-Saxon name for marjoram was *curmelle elene*. Old English forms were *magerym* and *marjolame*. It is now called English marjoram, fine marjoram, marjoram gentle, sweet marjoram, knotted marjoram, garden marjoram, and marjory. Germans call the herb *Majoran, Maigram, Maraun, Maran, Moseran*, and *Wurstkraut*; the French have given it the name *marjolaine*; Italians call it *maggiorana*, *amaraco*, and *persia*. In Spanish it is called *mejorana*; in Portuguese, *mangeroma* and *mariorana*; in Romanian, *magheran*; in Dutch, *marjolein*; in Danish, *merian*; and in Irish, *máirtíu* and *fiáin*.

Wild marjoram or organy is also known as Spanish organy, organ, organy, oregano, origanum, joy of the mountain, common wild marjoram, field marjoram, and eastward marjoram. Antiquated forms are wilde marjerome, bastard marjerome, grove marjoram, origane, and organye. German names are *Dost, Wohlgemut, brauner Dorant, wilder Marjoram, Kolerakraut, Frauendosten,* and *Altweiberschmeckata*. French names are *marjolaine sauvage, marjolaine bâtarde, origan,* and *thym de berger*. Italians call it *maggiorana selvatica, maggiorana salvadegha, regamo,* and *acciugher*; Russians, *dušica obyknovennaja*; Spaniards, *oregano*. A Danish name is *vild merian*; Norwegian terms are *bergmynte* and *kung*; and a Swedish appelation is *lund mejran*.

Appearance

Marjoram is a small plant, usually only growing to a height of 1 ft. It has a pleasant spicy smell and taste, and is characterized by rounded, tiny, felty gray-green leaves, and tiny green flower "knots" or buds. The root of the marjoram plant is thin and black and woody; its stalk is square, woody at the base, and often veined with red and covered with fine down. The oval leaves, on opposite sides of the stalk, are soft and fragile-looking. The plant's flowers look like tiny green balls when they first appear, before they begin to take on a pale pink or purple color.

Organy plants grow to a greater height (2 ft.) on tough, upright, woody stems. They have creeping roots and a very aromatic smell. Their most characteristic features are the flowers, which are grouped together in broad lavender tufts and are usually surrounded by butterflies. The shape of the plant is similar to St. John's wort, with leaves that crowd close together. Organy leaves can also, like those of St. John's wort, be punctured with tiny holes. The leaves are somewhat larger than those of cultivated marjoram, downy on both sides, and more pointed. They, and the stalk, are a dusky green color tinged with red or purple and dotted with oil glands. Organy flowers range in color from white to purple to pink to reddish brown.

Place, Season, and Useful Parts

Marjoram is cultivated the world over. It often escapes from cultivated areas, and can be found growing wild on sunny hillsides in warm climates such as those of Egypt, India, or the southern Mediterranean, to an altitude of 6,000 ft. In the north, it dies back each year. It blossoms from July on into September.

Organy grows on grassy slopes and field borders, in poor meadows or among underbrush, on stony places and newly forested areas. It does not do well on freshly fertilized soil, and prefers limestone regions and a sunny position. It will grow as a perennial to an altitude of 6,000 ft. Organy can be found in most of Eurasia, northern Africa, and in North America. It adapts easily to new surroundings, and usually blooms from July on into October.

Gathering, Drying, and Storage

In good years, it is possible to harvest marjoram three times, from July on into autumn. The first harvest should take place when the plant begins to blossom, just before the "knots" turn into flowers. The second cut can be made before the plant blossoms again, and the third cut just before the first frost. It is worth a try to overwinter marjoram in warmer areas, or on a sunny windowsill indoors in cooler regions. Otherwise, the plants should be harvested rigorously before the first frost.

Marjoram and oregano must be dried quickly in dark airy places at a temperature not exceeding 95° F. Marjoram leaves with brown spots are not suitable for drying. Otherwise, the plants dry very well, retaining or even improving on their fresh, intensive aroma.

Organy is gathered before the plant flowers. It has a shallow, matted root that may be damaged if the plant is harvested carelessly, and not cut. Organy should be dried in loose bundles in an airy place, but does not retain its aromatic qualities as well as marjoram.

Seed Saving and Germination

Marjoram seeds remain fertile for 2–3 years. The herb will only produce seeds in warmer areas, and is often propagated by cuttings. An even easier method is to force one stem down, and cover it with earth and a rock so that new roots will form. The new plant can then be separated from the mother plant and replanted. This process is called layering. There are many variations of oil content and medicinal potency between different marjoram varieties, and these qualities can best be preserved through vegetative propagation methods. If seed is saved, the plants must be isolated to ensure varietal purity.

Gardening Hints

Marjoram was cultivated in ancient Egyptian, Greek, and Roman gardens, and has been planted in England since the end of the sixteenth century. Garden marjoram was originally a Mediterranean plant, and therefore seldom produces seeds in the north, and often suffers from cold. It prefers a sunny, warm position, and does best in rich but not freshly fertilized soil loosened with sand or gravel, and enriched with limestone. Because birds do not usually eat marjoram seeds, they can be sown directly outdoors after the last killing frost without danger of loss. Marjoram seeds are so tiny and slow to germinate that it is best to mix them with quickly germinating seeds such as radishes to mark the rows when sowing. Those who want an earlier crop should sow the seeds indoors on a sunny windowsill, or outdoors in a cold frame in early spring. The seedlings can, after several transplantations into larger pots, be set out in May after all danger of frost is past. Plants in peat pots will withstand transplantation better. Once established, the plants grow easily, and aid the growth of nearby vegetables. They may then be propagated by cuttings, plant division, or layering. Cats often destroy marjoram beds by rolling in the herbs and biting the tender tips, and should be discouraged, or decoyed with catnip plants. For kitchen use in winter, a marjoram plant can be potted and kept indoors with good results.

Oregano prefers chalky soil. It is grown in much the same manner as marjoram, but is hardier, and will tolerate a less sunny position. It is usually sown in dry, warm, airy soil outdoors in the spring. The seeds are not covered with earth, but simply pressed into damp and fairly firm soil. Mature plants can be divided in the fall.

Wild organy is easily grown from seed, or by plant division. It does not die back in winter and self-seeds so readily that it can become something of a pest in the garden. It is best to let it flower for the butterflies, who love it dearly, but then to cut it back rigorously before seeds form.

Culinary Virtues

In Germany, marjoram is called the "sausage herb," and the best sausages owe their delicate flavor to painstaking preparation, quality ingredients, and the seasoning qualities of marjoram. Forcemeat stuffings, patés, liver dumplings, veal, beef, lamb, turkey, duck, chicken, goose, liver, turtle, and eel can all be improved by the addition of minute quantities of marjoram, and roasts are rubbed with the herb before roasting. Since it is a very pungent, warming herb, marjoram should always be used sparingly. Browning fresh marjoram lightly in butter helps to intensify its taste. It mixes well with basil, savory, and thyme, the traditional herbs for turtle soup. Although primarily a seasoning for meat, marjoram is also used by the practiced cook to flavor legumes, eggs, onions, potato and farinaceous dishes, mushrooms, avocados, cooked wheat and buckwheat, stuffed vegetables, carrots, and zucchini, and it can be served as an accompaniment to meat in jelly form. Turkish coffee is sometimes prepared with finely ground coffee, sugar, and very few marjoram leaves to give it an unusually pungent taste.

Southern oregano varieties are excellent seasoning herbs for tomato sauces and are used to great advantage by Italian and Greek cooks. Unfortunately, some herb dealers sell organy as "oregano." Dried organy is worthless as a dried culinary herb, and must be used fresh. True southern oregano is always preferable to organy as a seasoning agent.

Pizzas, spaghetti sauces, and moussakas would be unthinkable without the seasoning qualities of this herb. Oregano is often used together with thyme, basil, and garlic as a general seasoning for soups, sauces, stews, and tomato dishes. It combines well with most herbs, especially plants of the Mint family, giving the dishes a zesty taste.

In Lebanon, a bread named Zaatar is prepared from dough, and spread with crushed Syrian oregano in much the same manner as Italians prepare pizza.

Marjoram or oregano can be frozen for use in winter. The fresh herb is chopped, and frozen in ice cube trays, or short stalks of the herb are placed in plastic bags and frozen for later addition to hearty soups and stews.

Noteworthy Recipes

Fricasie of Chickens: John Shirley's seventeenth-century recipe for a "Fricasie of Chickens" can be made acceptable to modern taste if the quantity of capers (and chickens) is reduced:

> To make a Fricasie of Chickens, the best way. Take four or five chickens about 2 months old, scald and sea (slay) them; put (and cook) them in Water and White-wine; then take a large onion, ten or 12 blades of Mace, and the quantity of Nutmeg grated: tye them up in a cloth, with a bundle of sweet Herbs and Salt; put them in an Earthen-pan, and let them simper a while; then take 3 or 4 Anchoveys, 5 or 6 Eggs, half a pound of the best Butter dissolved in a pint of (hot) Mutton-broth; shread the Spices small, with a quarter of a pound of Capers: mix them with the other sawce, and laying the Chickens upon it, serve them up with Sippits, garnished with sliced Lemon. Thus you may dress and dish up Partridges or Pigeons, with only the abatement of the Eggs.[65]

According to Shirley, the best sauce for a roast hare consists of:

> Marjorum, Thyme, Winter-savory, Beef-suet, hard yolks of Eggs, sweet Butter, Sugar, Nutmeg, Water and Vinegar; minced and boiled up to a Sawce, serving your Hare up whole.[66]

Cold Savoury Pie: In 1861, Mrs. Isabella Beeton provided this recipe for a Cold Savoury Pie:

> Ingredients. 1 lb. of veal, 1 lb. of fat bacon; salt, cayenne pepper, and pounded mace to taste; a very little nutmeg, the same of chopped lemon-peel, ½ teaspoonful of chopped parsley, ½ teaspoonful of minced savoury herbs, 1 or 2 eggs.

---

65.   Shirley, *The Accomplished Ladies Rich Closet of Rarities* (London: N. Bodington, 1688), 109.

66.   Shirley, *The Accomplished Ladies Rich Closet of Rarities* (London: N. Bodington, 1688), 102.

Mode. Chop the veal and bacon together, and put them in a mortar (or through a meat grinder) with the other ingredients mentioned above. Pound well, and bind with 1 or 2 eggs which have been previously beaten and strained. Work the whole well together, and the fors'cemeat will be ready for use. If the pie is not to be eaten immediately, omit the herbs and parsley, as these would prevent it from keeping. Mushrooms or truffles may be added.[67]

Italian Tomato Sauce: In a deep and heavy saucepan (the sauce will splatter if cooked in a pot that is too small), heat 2 Tbsp. of olive oil, and add ¼ diced onion, a small carrot, and a small amount of ham. If you want a meatier sauce, also fry some ground beef in the oil. Heat at medium heat until the vegetables turn glassy, and then add a wineglass full of wine. Stir until most of it has evaporated. Add peeled and diced Italian plum tomatoes, or canned and unsweetened diced tomatoes (do not use tomato sauce or paste, which will make a boring, mushy, sweet sauce) to fill half of the pan. Season with generous amounts of fresh basil, oregano, and several cloves of garlic, as well as salt and pepper. Let cook, uncovered, for at least ½ hour to evaporate the excess water. Tomato sauce improves with cooking, and can be reheated several times. If it is too watery, a few tablespoons of tomato paste can be added to thicken the sauce. Serve with freshly cooked pasta, freshly grated Parmesan, and freshly ground black pepper.

Household Applications

Marjoram oil or the expressed juice of the fresh plant can be added to furniture polishes as a scenting agent. Marjoram and organy leaves are also included in moth-repelling herbal sachets.

Pliny believed that the smell of organy could drive away ants, and Gerard thought that snakes would avoid any place strewn with organy. Organy is, in fact, one of the best air fresheners, and a bundle of the fresh herb hung in a corner of the room can disperse unpleasant odors and sweeten the air. Organy is added to potpourri, sachet, and sleeping cushion mixtures, and its pliable stems can be woven, together with hyssop and rosemary, into fragrant herbal scenting wreaths. A somewhat unstable, brownish-red dye is also prepared from organy. With alum as a fixative, green hues can be obtained, or olive green with bichromate of potash.

---

67.   Beeton, *The Book of Household Management* (1861) (New York: Farrar, Straus & Giroux, 1977), 199.

Cosmetic Properties

Before the era of commercial deodorants, organy was considered a priceless deodorizing herb and held in great esteem. Roman women employed a marjoram salve to help smooth away wrinkles. Marjoram leaves were also used as incense, and organy and marjoram baths were recommended for those in need of stimulation, or suffering from weak nerves. Young Afghani brides were washed in baths of fresh mint and marjoram before their weddings. Aristocratic ladies of the non-bathing era of European history, the eighteenth century, wore precious ornaments called smelling-apples filled with scent balls perfumed with ambergris, musk, and other exotic perfumes as well as aromatic herbs such as marjoram.

Marjoram is still a favorite bath herb. Powdered marjoram leaves are added to talcum powders, and marjoram oil is used in toothpastes and added to hair tonics and perfumes. Marjoram darkens hair, and marjoram tea can be used as a hair rinse to soften, strengthen, and scent dark or graying hair. Marjoram tea or compresses made from fresh marjoram leaves can also help to cleanse and strengthen the eyes. Marjoram oil is still used in the perfume industry.

Oregano oil is often used together with tea tree oil to treat dandruff, diaper rash, and other skin irritations. The pure ethereal oil should always be diluted with neutral oils such as almond, jojoba, or sesame to avoid burning the skin.

Noteworthy Recipes

Scent Balls: An approximate equivalent of the scent balls once used to fill "smelling apples" can be prepared by pounding mucilage of gum tragacanth with sweet marjoram leaves, and then moistening the mixture with rose water until it is possible to form small balls. Any potpourri mixture can be substituted for the marjoram leaves, and amateur perfumers may want to add essential flower oils, vanilla powder, musk, ground cloves, and gum benzoin or benzoin tincture to enhance the odor and keeping abilities of the scent balls. They should be left to dry for at least 12 hours in a warm dry place, and stored in loosely covered containers. They make an unusual conversation piece if placed in a pretty goblet on a mantelpiece or in the center of a festive table.

Medicinal Merits

In his writings on marjoram, Otto Brunfels aired his grievance against a prevalent belief of the sixteenth century: that exotic and expensive medicines were preferable to simple home remedies:

> Then we Germans are so foolish that we do not have a high opinion of the precious sweet-smelling herbs and flowers which we have growing in our own land, but as soon as we sicken, go searching for strengthening tonics at the apothecary's, tonics which must come from India or Arabia if we are to believe in them.[68]

What would the old herbalist Brunfels think of us now? The remedies of the most remote tribes or peoples are still considered the best medicines. Europeans are crazy about Native American remedies, Americans use European herbs to the exclusion of their own, and Chinese remedies are popular throughout the world, while often neglected in their own country.

Marjoram is not a plant blessed with major medicinal properties but, nonetheless, it has enjoyed quiet respect over the centuries as a gentle and effective medicine. In Bosnia, epilepsy patients were given crushed marjoram leaves to sniff after a seizure, and northern Italian herbalists administered marjoram snuff for a cold, or heaviness of the head. Pliny praised the herb's properties against snakebite. Greeks prepared a warming wound salve from marjoram and other herbs, and Arabian physicians prescribed marjoram against the effects of alcohol misuse. Otto Brunfels and Nicholas Culpeper encouraged women to use sweet marjoram in pessary form. According to Brunfels, marjoram is so warming that it can loosen a paralyzed tongue, quicken the spirits, improve loss of memory, strengthen the nerves, and restore feeling to deadened limbs. Culpeper recommended the herb as "warming and comforting for cold diseases of the head, stomach, sinews, and other parts."[69] Adherents of the theory of signatures found that the plant's knotted leaves suited it for the treatment of milk knots.

Wild marjoram or organy was held in even greater esteem than cultivated marjoram as a medicinal herb. Dioscurides praised it as an intestinal and diuretic herb; Gerard listed it as a possible antidote for the poison of hemlock and the opium poppy, as well as for the bites of venomous beasts. The juice of wild marjoram was believed to stop earaches when mixed with the milk of a nursing woman. Women were also advised to drink wild marjoram to cleanse themselves after the ardors of birth. A Swiss recipe from the seven-

---

68.   Brunfels, *Contrafayt Kräuterbuch* (1532), facsimile (Munich: Konrad Kölbl, 1964).

69.   Culpeper, *Culpeper's Complete Herbal* (1653) (London: Foulsham, undated), 227.

teenth century recommends a pancake made from organy powder and eggs as a sovereign remedy for stomachaches. A medicinal stomachic beer was prepared from wild organy.

Modern Medicine

Modern herbalists rarely prescribe marjoram for internal use, but are staunch advocates of its great value as external medicine. Taken internally in small amounts for a short period only, it is a strong relaxant, and can help to ease flatulence, stomach and uterine cramps, spasms, the breathing difficulties of newborn children, and even to calm the patient after epileptic seizures. Some herbalists extol its blood-building properties, and others praise its beneficial and strengthening action on the nerves. It can induce menstruation, and some singers believe that a marjoram electuary will keep their voices clear and pure.

Ethereal marjoram oil has stomachic, antiseptic, and calming qualities. Marjoram salve is drying and astringent, and can be rubbed onto children's chests or inserted in small amounts into their nostrils to treat colds. Marjoram can be smoked, gargled, inhaled, or sniffed by adults with colds or sinus complaints. Marjoram tea is also used as a mouth rinse to combat infections and bad breath and to calm toothaches. Marjoram oil can be dropped onto cotton and placed in a hollow tooth to ease the pain. It can also be inhaled to relieve headaches, or it may be rubbed on the skin to loosen the twinges of rheumatism and uterine cramps, as well as to strengthen the nerves and refresh paralyzed limbs. Stiff limbs and stomach or muscle cramps, as well as chilled kidneys can be warmed with marjoram poultices or the application of hot marjoram pillows. The patient can also be soaked in a hot marjoram bath. Hardened, tense breasts or milk knots can be loosened with poultices of fresh marjoram leaves. Marjoram salve is prepared in the same manner as marigold or comfrey salve (see these chapters), and can be strengthened by adding mint and sage leaves.

Marjoram, *Origanum majorana,* has been found by homeopaths to strongly influence the female sexual organs, and is rumored to enhance the sex drive. It is used as a remedy for wild sexual dreams and mania.

Marjoram is used in Chinese medicine to counteract water retention, and bad breath due to the accumulation of food. A tea of the herb can be taken to promote sweating, and also enjoyed in summer to counteract the ill effects of excessive summer heat.

Pure ethereal oregano oil is prescribed as a relatively gentle remedy for worms and other parasites. It is one of the most effective ethereal oils and is used for infections of all kinds, *Candida* overgrowth, dental inflammation, as well as chronic fatigue syndrome, fibromyalgia, irritable bowel syndrome, leaky gut, intestinal parasites, and bacterial infection. Because of these modern applications, it has become a fashionable drug among alternative health practitioners.

Wild marjoram has many of the same properties as cultivated marjoram, but is more potent if used fresh. Organy oil can help to ease toothache, and organy poultices are effective against rheumatic pains, lumbago, and menstrual disorders. Organy tea and organy oil, and inhaling mixtures of the herb, are effective in the treatment of coughs and colds. Organy is an excellent nervine and cordial medicine, and has been known to ease the queasiness experienced by sea-travelers. Homeopathy employs an essence of organy to treat hysteria and sexual disorders.

Uses In Husbandry

Marjoram and wild organy are favorite bee plants. Goats and sheep are very fond of organy, but horses and cows generally avoid the plant. Dairy keepers prize the marjorams because of their ability to keep milk from "turning". Milk pails are washed out with marjoram or organy infusions. The milk will stay sweet and fresh longer if rue, thyme, and marjoram are hung next to the milk containers. Marjoram and wild thyme are also believed to keep milk from "turning" when there is thunder in the air, and milk spoils easily. Marjoram is occasionally hung over a beer barrel to keep the contents from souring. This is attributed to its antiseptic, but also to its antidemonic, properties. Wild and domesticated marjoram are added to herbal tobacco mixtures, or the dried herbs can be used directly as snuff.

Veterinary Values

Marjoram tea or marjoram powder is given to cows to prevent them from miscarrying, and marjoram and lemon balm tea is considered an appropriate antidemonic and health-giving drink for cows after they have calved. Sheep are often given powdered organy as a corrective medicine against diarrhea, and minor mouth infections can be treated by rinsing the mouth with chamomile and marjoram tea. Dogs and cats are given marjoram tea when they are ill, and the herb can be added to flea-repelling mixtures.

Miscellaneous Wisdom

Pliny believed that tortoises rubbed themselves with marjoram before fighting with serpents, and later authors claimed that storks also protected themselves with organy when going to battle snakes. Similarly, humans were enjoined to make use of marjoram, and especially organy, before fighting with the Serpent of Evil. The *Malleus Maleficarum* mentions marjoram as an effective herb used for smoking out demons. In Dalmatia (Croatia), children suffering from fright or shock were washed down with the herb. Bavarians laid it in their beds to drive away ghosts and hung it in their rooms to expel witches. Children who would not talk were given a spoonful of marjoram water to loosen the magical bonds placed on their tongues.

Organy was considered one of the very best and most effective antidemonic herbs. As the Franconian saying goes, "Organy, hard hay and white heather / Keep the Devil from much pleasure."[70]

In ancient Egypt, girls and women were only allowed to enter certain temples if they were wearing oregano wreaths. Wild marjoram was used in purification and cleansing ceremonies in ancient Greece. Syrian oregano was also used in sacrificial ceremonies for keeping the blood of sacrificed animals from curdling. Young couples were crowned with oregano, and it was taken as a positive omen if wild marjoram grew on a grave. The herb originally known as *Origanum heracleoticum* was thought, like Heracles, to keep snakes from the house and cradle. Italians use organy, and especially organy blessed on Assumption Day (August 15th) as a preventive herb against the wiles of Satan, the influence of the Evil Eye, and any kind of "bad" magic. Germans consider Assumption Day organy to be the best protection against witches. It is hung in the stall or house, or burned in a room together with other antidemonic herbs such as St. John's wort, white heather, valerian, dill, and black cumin *(Nigella sativa)*. Organy is laid in the beds of new mothers and also in babies' cradles to protect them from harm. Hunters use St. George's Day organy to improve their shooting abilities. All the hunter has to do is to hang the herb from a bird-frequented tree, and from that day on, he will never miss a shot. White organy is thought to be particularly potent for magical reasons, and is usually gathered while repeating a spell.

Oracular Worth

In England, any girl wishing to consult the St. Luke's Day oracle had to take marigold flowers, marjoram, thyme, and wormwood leaves, dry them and rub them to a powder, and then mix them with vinegar and virgin honey. She would anoint herself with the mixture before going to bed, and invoke St. Luke:

> St. Luke, St. Luke, be kind to me,
> In dreams let me my true love see.

In order to make the spell work, she would also have to find a pea pod with nine peas in it. Then, before going to bed, she would write the words

> Come in, my dear,
> And do not fear.

on a piece of paper, tuck the paper into the pea pod, and place the pea pod under the door. The first male to enter the room would be her future husband.

---

70. Hanns Bächtold-Stäubli, ed., *Handwörterbuch des deutschen Aberglaubens* (1927–42), vol. II (Berlin: Walter de Gruyter & Co., 1987), 362.

Legends

Marjoram is sacred to the Indian gods Shiva and Vishnu, and was used as a garland of the gods Hymen and Aphrodite in ancient Greece. According to legend, Amarakos was once a companion of the King of Cyprus. One day, he let an alabaster container filled with a precious salve fall. He was so ashamed of his misdeed that he sickened and died. Aphrodite took pity on him, and transformed him into a sweet-smelling salve plant that bears his name to this very day.

In another version of this story, Aphrodite was angry with Amarakos because of his clumsiness, and in her rage transformed him into a plant. From that day on, offerings of marjoram have been given to the goddess to appease her wrath and fancy her humor.

Literary Flowers

> *And marjoram notts sweet briar and ribbon grass*
> *And lavender the choice of every lass*
> *And sprigs of lads love all familiar names*
> *Which every garden thro the village claims*
> *These the maid gathers wi a coy delight.*

—JOHN CLARE, *THE SHEPHERD'S CALENDAR*, "MAY"

When you have done, and finished your work,
Parsley, sage, rosemary and thyme
Then ... you shall be a true love of mine.

—"The Elfin Night," an English ballad

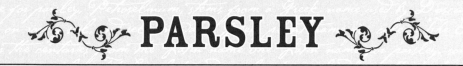

PARSLEY

Name

The Latin name for parsley, *Petroselinum*, stems from a Greek name used by Dioscurides. *Petro* specified a plant growing on rocky soil, and *selinon* was a Greek plant name for celery. The English word "parsley" has evolved over the centuries from the Latin name. *Petroselinum crispum* is the current botanical name, but other botanical synonyms may also be in use: *Apium petroselinum, Petroselinum vulgare, P. hortense, P. sativum, P. petroselinum, Carum petroselinum.*

Parsley is a biennial member of the **Apiaceae** or **Umbelliferae** family. It is divided, botanically, into two groups: leaf parsley (*Petroselinum crispum ssp. crispum*) and root parsley (*Petroselinum crispum ssp. tuberosum*, or *P. crispum convar. radicosum*). There are several kinds of leaf parsleys: plain-leaved parsley, curled parsley, fern-leaved parsley, and Neapolitan parsley. Root parsley is also known as turnip-rooted, or Hamburg, or Dutch parsley, and is grown primarily for its thick, succulent roots.

Folk Names

In ancient herbals, parsley was called *apium* or *selinon*, and was later known as petersylinge and persely. The Anglo-Saxon name was *marish*; Old French names were *jauver, juver*, and *gimbert*.

Modern German appellations are *Petersilie, Peterli, Bittersilche*, and *Kräutel*; French names are *persil* and *jauvert*. Italians call the herb *prezzemolo, petrosello, apio ortense, erbetta*, and *erborina*. In Friuli (Italy), it is known as *savòrs*; in some parts of south Tyrol, *kraitles* and *petersimbl*. Spaniards call the plant *perejil*; Russians, *petruška*; Dutch, *peterselie*; Irish, *peirsil*; and the Welsh, *persli*.

Appearance

According to Nicholas Culpeper, parsley roots

> are long, thick, and white, having a wrinkled bark; from which spring many
> shining, green, winged leaves, growing on long footstalks; which are divided
> into three sections, and each of these subdivided into three more, which are tri-
> angular and cut in at the ends. The stalks grow to be 2 ft. high, much branched
> and divided.[71]

The most important thing to remember about plain-leaved parsley is that young plants
can easily be confused with poison hemlock *(Conium maculatum)* or fool's parsley *(Aeth-
usa cynapium)*. Because of this, it is wise to rub a leaf of the supposed parsley plant
between one's fingers before gathering it. True parsley is betrayed by its spicy, fresh,
crisp, clean, and somewhat sour smell, as well as a pleasant, lightly spicy taste. Hemlock's smell is reminiscent of tomcat's urine. Gerard classified this odor as "naughty."
Parsley leaves are shiny and dark green on top, but hemlock leaves are shiny underneath, and much more finely divided.

The parsley plant only produces tender leaves during the first and at the beginning
of its second year of growth. The second-year root is white and fleshy, like a parsnip,
with an aromatic, sweet taste. The plant soon sends up smooth, but striated flower stalks
that produce umbels of green-yellow flowers, and brown-gray fruits that divide to reveal
two seeds.

Curled-leaved varieties are not as aromatic as the plain-leaved forms, and have dark
green, deeply divided and very wrinkled leaves. Root parsley resembles leaf parsley,
except for the fact that the roots are much larger and fleshier.

Place, Season, and Useful Parts

Parsley has been cultivated in gardens for more than 2,000 years the world over, but it
also grows wild in the Middle East, in northern Africa, Sardinia, and southern Europe.
It has naturalized itself in some parts of England and Scotland, and readily escapes
from cultivated areas. It will grow to an altitude of 6,000 ft. on cultivated soil, or on
rubble, walls, and cliffs. The plant is biennial: it usually flowers in June or July of its
second year, and produces fruits in August and September. Parsley roots can be dug in
the fall or the early spring. The leaves can be cut several times during the first growing
season, and again in the winter if the plants are offered some protection.

---

71. Culpeper, *Culpeper's Complete Herbal* (1653) (London: Foulsham, undated), 257.

Gathering, Drying, and Storage

Parsley leaves are gathered for kitchen and medicinal use from early spring until the first snowfall. They are harvested from the outside of the plant toward the inside, or the entire plant is cut well above the root. In a greenhouse or frame, the harvest can continue into the winter. Some gardeners prefer to grow curled varieties because they cannot be as easily confused with other poisonous plants.

- Parsley leaves should be as fresh as possible for kitchen use. Very fresh parsley stalks keep like flowers for a few days in a glass with fresh water. Parsley leaves can be dried in a heated room, or on a cloth-covered tray in a very slow oven until crisp. Dehydrators are also good if the temperature is set very low. The dried leaves are rubbed through a rough sieve or crumbled until fine, and then stored in airtight bottles in a dark place. A layer of dry salt is strewn on top of the parsley to absorb any excess moisture. A simpler storage method is to mince the leaves and freeze them in ice cube trays. The single cubes are stored in plastic bags: one is just the right size for a pot of winter soup or stew.

Parsley roots are dug in October or November, before the first hard frost, or again in spring, as soon as the soil thaws. The best and most uniform roots are saved for seed production, and the rest of the roots stored in a root cellar for kitchen use. They can also be cleaned, diced, or sliced, and then frozen or dried.

- Roots should be gathered in the fall of the plants' second year, just after they have flowered. The roots of the second-year parsley are dug up, and the leaves cut off to within 1 in. of the crown. The roots are cured for a few days in a cool, shady place. They are then cleaned of earth, and stored in dampened sand or sawdust in a root cellar or a cool, damp place. Parsley roots keep well for several weeks in the refrigerator. They can also be cut into fine slices and dried for winter use.

Parsley seeds must be harvested just before they fully ripen, or they will shatter. Parsley fruit umbels are tied together in bundles, and hung up to dry over a cloth, or they are spread out on cloth or paper in a shady, airy place to dry. As the seeds ripen, they fall off the stalks and are collected on the cloths. With a little rubbing, the remaining seeds can be removed and the chaff sieved out. Like all garden seeds, parsley seeds should be stored in a cool, dry, and dark place.

Seed Saving and Germination

Parsley seeds are notorious for their poor germination, especially after a couple of years of storage. Gardeners who complain about their parsley not germinating should throw out their old packets, and try again with fresh seed. If only for this reason, it is a wise move to save your own parsley seed. Seed saving is much easier than most people believe, and is the same for root or leaf parsley. Parsley plants set seed in their second year, and the roots have to be overwintered. In mild climates, or areas with a reliable snow cover, the plants are simply left in the garden over the winter, and will seed themselves. There will be some loss to frost, but the plants that come through will be strong and vigorous.

Weaker plants must be ripped out vigorously. If weak plants are allowed to go to seed, the weaker characteristics will be passed on to the next generation. At least twelve plants should be left for seed production in order to guarantee genetic diversity within the variety. In areas with strong frosts without sufficient snow cover, or where voles are a menace, it is advisable to dig out the roots, to cut off the leaves to within 1 in. of the crown, to select the best roots for seed production, and to store them in a cool, damp cellar in damp sand or sawdust over winter.

As soon as the ground can be worked, the best roots are planted out at a distance of 20 in. between plants, and staked well. Only one variety can be grown for seed at a time, or the varieties will cross. The stalks will usually grow to a height of 40 in., branch out, and fall over or break easily. Because of this, the plants must be supported, or the damp soil will damage the seeds. In very wet summers, some protection against damp (such as an awning) is advisable. The best seed is produced in the first umbel, and this should be gathered separately and dried carefully. Dry well using silica gel and store in a cool, dark, and dry place or store in sealed containers in a refrigerator or freezer during the winter. The seeds should be removed from cold storage shortly before sowing in the spring, and gradually thawed. Frozen parsley seed will keep well for several years if dried properly before storage.

Gardening Hints

Because of its poor and erratic germination rate, many gardeners think parsley is the most difficult of all herbs to grow. According to folk belief, parsley must be sown by a fool (France), by a liar (also France), by a woman who enjoys the mastery of the house (Cambridgeshire), or by an angry (Franconia) or a laughing (Swabia) person. Americans once believed that parsley grew better if the planting rills were watered with urine. It is thought best to sow parsley by the waxing moon if a leaf crop is desired, and by the waning moon if the roots are to be harvested. In Cambridgeshire, people believe that parsley should be sown at night by the light of the stars, in rows running from north to south. German Swabians and Franconians who want unforked roots sow parsley seeds between noon and 1:00 PM. In Somerset, parsley is sown on holidays to keep the faeries from the seeds. Good Friday, Midsummer's Day, June 29th (St. Peter's Day), and July 26th (St. Anna's Day) are thought to be auspicious sowing dates. In some areas, Wednesdays are also recommended. Parsley sown on Good Friday is expected to "come double" in Suffolk. In Germany, St. Peter's or Midsummer parsley will stay green the whole year through. In Swabia, it is believed that St. Anna's Day parsley won't "shoot" in the spring and will produce longer leaves than parsley sown at another date.

The problems the parsley gardener faces are not limited to sowing. Once in the ground, the seeds have to germinate, and that often takes up to a month or more. The Silesian explanation for this phenomenon is that the seeds have to go to Rome for St. Peter's approval before they can sprout, a journey of six or seven weeks. In Shropshire, the devil is entitled to the first eight sowings of the plant, and will only allow the ninth to germinate. According to an English saying, "It goes to the Devil nine times, and very often forgets to come back again."[72] Parsley seeds will keep for up to 2–3 years if stored properly, but quickly lose their viability if kept in a warm or damp place. Germination results can be improved by freezing old, dry seeds for two weeks, or by soaking them overnight before sowing. It is very important that the sowing rills are kept damp during the entire germination process (it may be helpful to strew sawdust thinly over the seed rows, since it retains moisture better than earth). Since the seeds need warmth to germinate well, sowing them later in the year, as late as August, may also help. If nematodes are a problem in the garden, parsley plants will not thrive, and the roots may be subject to root rot.

Leaf parsley seeds should be sown in deeply cultivated, rich soil in a shady spot, pressed down, and then covered with a thin layer of fine soil or a mixture of soil and sawdust. Parsley plants do not grow well if fertilized with fresh manure, but will thrive if dressed regularly with compost and some wood ashes. The plants should not be crowded: 8 in. spacing is ideal for stronger plants. Parsley also responds well to watering and weeding on a regular basis. Although the plants are biennial, it is advisable to sow leaf parsley from March through August at regular intervals to ensure a continual supply. Some plants can be left outdoors or in an unheated glasshouse over the winter. If the winter is not too cold, the leaves will develop early in the spring. The first February or March sowing can be harvested before the second sowing reaches harvest size. August-sown plants should not be cut back at all, but allowed to gather strength for the coming winter, and then harvested the following spring. Soon afterwards, the plants send up flower stalks and produce seed.

Root parsley is sown in March or April, in deeply dug or tilled soil. The plants are usually kept for 2 years. During the first year, the leaves can be harvested conservatively until summer. The roots should then be allowed to gather strength, and are harvested in

---

72.   Charlotte Sophia Burne, *Shropshire Folk-Lore* (1883), 2 vol. (Wakefield, England: E. P. Publishing, 1973), 248.

late fall or early spring. A few of the best plants can be allowed to set viable seeds for the coming year.

Organic gardeners often sow parsley seed between summer onions. The onions mark the rows of the slowly germinating parsley, and are harvested long before the parsley roots reach maturity. Tomatoes and asparagus are also good companion plants for parsley. Roses grown next to parsley smell sweeter, and are less prone to greenfly attack. Leaf parsley can be planted in decorative borders, or transferred to pots and taken indoors during the winter.

Traditional, superstitious gardeners would of course be horrified at the idea of transplanting parsley to a flowerpot. As the Franconian saying goes, transplanting parsley is tantamount to planting a friend in his or her grave. A spouse, or the gardener himself, may also die. Women who transplant parsley are expected to have trouble finding husbands and lovers. The Hereford saying is, "To transplant parsley puts the whole of one's garden in the hands of the Evil One, and the crops will fail."[73] In Somerset, it is also considered very unlucky to transplant parsley, except on a Good Friday. In the United States, it was once believed that anyone who transplants parsley courts misfortune.

Gardening Legends

One Devonshire legend tells of a woman whose tulips were especially beautiful. The pixies were very fond of the woman and her tulips. But then one day she died, and her son dug up the flowers she had so loved. He planted parsley in their place. Angry at the loss of the tulips and at the lack of filial piety, the pixies withered the parsley plants and destroyed the garden for several years. The flowers planted on the mother's grave, however, grew and flourished, thanks to the pixies' diligent care.

In Condover, in Shropshire, a little girl named Annie was once playing gardener by herself. She dug up the parsley plants and moved them from one part of the garden to another. Annie's aunt and mother were horrified when they saw what had happened. The aunt began to cry and prophesy that someone in the house would die as a result of Annie's game. Shortly afterward, Annie sickened and died. As soon as the funeral was over, the gardener bought some parsley roots to replace those that Annie had transplanted. Annie's mother tried to stop him, but he just laughed at her fears. In a few weeks, Annie's father followed the little girl to the grave.[74]

---

73. E. Radford and M. A. Radford, *Encyclopaedia of Superstitions* (London: Rider, 1947), 186.

74. Charlotte Sophia Burne, *Shropshire Folk-Lore* (1883), 2 vol. (Wakefield, England: E. P. Publishing, 1973), 248.

Culinary Virtues

Parsley is a very versatile culinary herb that emphasizes the inherent flavor of the foods it seasons without overpowering them. In the herbalist John Gerard's words, it is "delightful to the taste and agreeable to the stomach."[75] In Italy, a person met repeatedly is said to be "like parsley—he's found in every sauce." In fact, Italians are inordinately fond of parsley sauces. Parsley has steadily gained in popularity since its introduction to Central Europe during the reign of Charlemagne, and to the British Isles in the middle of the sixteenth century. In Germany, parsley is considered to be one of the best kitchen herbs, and is included among the cleansing Lenten herbs eaten in traditional Maundy Thursday herb cakes.

The ancient Romans made liberal use of parsley because it was supposed to counteract the noxious effects of intoxicating beverages. French and Italian cooks have continued this culinary tradition to the present day. The fancy French term *aux fines herbes* often only means that parsley has been added to a dish.

Because of its pronounced flavor, plain-leaved parsley is usually used fresh for seasoning purposes. Curled parsley is widely employed for its decorative properties, but has little taste, and the prickly leaves tend to get caught in the throat. Plain-leaved parsley can be added to soups, stews, salads, cooked grains, vegetables, and buckwheat dishes in large quantities. The fresh leaves help to lessen the overpowering taste of onions or garlic, especially when used together with olive oil.

Parsley leaves should be washed, dried with a clean dishtowel or paper towels, removed from the stem, chopped fine (or put through a food processor), and added to food just before serving. This helps to preserve vitamins and maintain parsley's fresh green color. Chopping parsley when the leaves are still wet will result in an unappetizing and watery green paste. Some cooks blanch parsley leaves in boiling salt water and then sautée them in butter. A *bouquet garni* usually consists of a bay leaf, some sprigs of thyme, and several stalks of parsley tied together with a thread. To do the term justice, basil, celery, chervil, salad burnet, rosemary, tarragon, or savory may also be included. Parsley sauces and parsley butters are used extensively in France and Germany. Snails are fed parsley before they are boiled, and snail dishes are flavored with the herb as well. English cooks have perfected the art of making parsley pies, and German cooks prepare excellent herb and parsley *Strudels*.

Parsley freezes well, especially if the dry herb is chopped fine and frozen loose in plastic bags. The herb can then be removed as needed, and the plastic bag resealed. For short-term storage, place cut parsley in a glass of water on the kitchen counter, changing the water daily.

---

75. Gerard, *Gerard's Herball* [1597]: *The essence thereof distilled by Marcus Woodward from the edition of Th. Johnson, 1636*. Ed. Marcus Woodward (London: Gerald How, 1927).

One of the most dangerous culinary myths associated with parsley is that the herb will turn yellow if it is cooked with poisonous mushrooms. This has, unfortunately, been the death of a number of well-meaning mushroom enthusiasts.

Curled-leaved parsley is a very popular garnishing herb. Butchers and fishmongers display the attractive herb between their wares, and it has even found its way into supermarket displays. Meat and fish are often served with garnishes of fresh or fried curled parsley.

The roots of Hamburg parsley are boiled and served as a vegetable, or the raw roots are grated finely into salads. Soups, stews, sauces, millet and grain stews, or bean dishes also benefit from the addition of well-washed, scraped, and diced roots. Because of their diuretic properties and unusual taste, parsley roots are a healthy addition to the often monotonous winter diet of northern countries. Many German and Scandinavian recipes call for parsley roots.

Noteworthy Recipes

A Traditional Parsley and Butter Sauce: William Kitchiner offers this recipe:

> Wash some Parsley very clean, and pick it carefully leaf by leaf; put a teaspoonful of salt into half a pint of boiling water; boil the Parsley about ten minutes; drain it on a sieve; mince it quite fine, and then bruise it to a pulp.
>
> The delicacy and excellence of this elegant and innocent Relish depends upon the Parsley being minced very fine: put it in a sauce-boat, and mix with it, by degrees, about half a pint of good melted butter—only do not put so much flour to it, as the Parsley will add to its thickness: never pour Parsley and Butter over Boiled things, but send it up in a Boat.
>
> Obs. In French Cookery Books this is called "Melted Butter, English Fashion"; and, with the addition of a slice of lemon cut into dice, a little Allspice and Vinegar, "Dutch Sauce."[76]

Modern cooks will want to omit the flour, and avoid boiling the parsley in order to preserve vitamins. A food processor can be used to mince the parsley. The sauce is served with boiled poultry, rabbit, braised veal, or calf's head, or the first potatoes of the year boiled in their skins.

Mâitre d'hotel butter can be prepared in much the same manner by mixing melted and cooled butter with pounded parsley, a little salt, a pinch of pepper, and a few drops of lemon juice until it forms a smooth paste. Serve with grilled meat or fish or with steamed vegetables.

Parsley Juice, for Colouring various Dishes: This one comes to us from Mrs. Isabella Beeton:

---

76.   Kitchiner, *The Cook's Oracle* (1817) (London: Samuel Bagster, 1860), 227.

Procure some nice young parsley, wash it and dry it thoroughly in a cloth; pound the leaves in a mortar till all the juice is extracted, and put the juice in a teacup or small jar; place this in a saucepan of boiling water, and warm it on the bain marie principle just long enough to take off its rawness; let it drain, and it will be ready for colouring.[77]

Modern cooks will find it much easier to use a vegetable juicer to extract the juice.

Fried Parsley for Garnishing: Also from Mrs. Beeton:

Ingredients. Parsley, hot lard or clarified dripping.

Mode. Gather some young parsley; wash, pick, and dry it thoroughly in a cloth; put it into the wire basket ... , and hold it in boiling lard or dripping for a minute or two. Directly it is done, lift out the basket, and let it stand before the fire, that the parsley may become thoroughly crisp, and the quicker it is fried the better. Should the kitchen not be furnished with the above article, throw the parsley into the frying-pan, and when crisp, lift it out with a slice, dry before the fire, and when thoroughly crisp, it will be ready for use.[78]

Here, a deep-fat fryer can be used with good results.

Wow Wow Sauce for stewed or Bouilli Beef: Kitchiner gives a not-quite-so-usual recipe for a spicy parsley sauce:

Chop some Parsley-leaves very finely, quarter two or three pickled Cucumbers, or Walnuts, and divide them into small squares, and set them by ready; put into a sauce-pan a bit of Butter as big as an egg; when it is melted, stir to it a table-spoonful of fine flour, and about half a pint of the broth in which the Beef was boiled; and add a table-spoonful of Vinegar, the like quantity of Mushroom Catchup, or Port Wine, or both, and a tea-spoonful of made Mustard; let it simmer together until it is as thick as you wish it, put in the Parsley and Pickles to get warm, and pour it over the Beef, or rather send it up in a Sauce-tureen.

Obs. If you think the above not sufficiently piquante, add to it some Capers, or a minced Eschalot, or one or two teaspoonsful of Eschalot Wine, or Essence of Anchovy, or Basil, Elder, or Tarragon, or Horseradish, or Burnet

---

77. Beeton, *The Book of Household Management* (1861) (New York: Farrar, Straus & Giroux, 1977), 237.

78. Ibid.

Vinegar; or strew over the Meat Carrots and Turnips cut into dice, minced Capers, Walnuts, Red Cabbage, pickled Cucumbers or French Beans, &c.[79]

Green Sauce: A very simple, but pleasing green sauce can be prepared by melting some butter, and thickening it with a small amount of flour or cornstarch, and stirring constantly until the flour is mixed well with the butter. Add cold soup stock slowly over a low flame, stirring all the while, until the right sauce consistency is reached. Just before serving, add a generous mixture of finely chopped parsley, chervil, chives, salad burnet, and a few leaves of fresh tarragon.

In Italian cooking, parsley is usually used together with olive oil and garlic. A cold savory sauce for boiled meat or tongue can be prepared from a few simple ingredients. Take 2 salted and tinned anchovies, wash them and remove any fish bones. Add 1¾ oz. of drained capers, a handful of parsley, a very small onion, half a cooked carrot, half a clove of garlic, as well as a piece of soft bread as big as a hen's egg. Process in a food processor together with the juice of half a lemon and enough extra virgin olive oil to make a smooth mixture. Add salt and pepper to taste and serve cold with meat.

Herb Strudel: Some cooks like to make herb bread by spreading herb fillings made of chopped parsley and sautéed scallions onto raised bread dough, rolling up the dough, and then letting it rise again before baking. An unusual southern German recipe makes use of the same principles to produce parsley Strudel.

First make the filling by finely chopping several handfuls of shallots and sautéeing them lightly in a small amount of butter. Remove from the fire. Add several generous handfuls of finely-chopped parsley and chervil leaves, and then mix in a few tablespoons of bread crumbs, just enough to soak up the liquid. In another bowl, beat 2 eggs with a small amount of butter until creamy and then stir in several tablespoons of thick sour cream.

The strudel dough is made with 2 cups of finely sifted white flour mounded up on a breadboard. Make a well in the middle of the flour, and break one large egg in the well. Add a pinch of salt, and then sprinkle the mound with lukewarm water. Fold the egg and water in by hand, adding warm water as needed, until a sticky, soft dough is formed. Work the dough until it stiffens somewhat, and then knead vigorously on a floured board until bubbles rise. Form the dough into a ball, brush it with some warm water, and then cover with a bowl. The bowl should be chilled if the dough is too soft, and warmed if the dough is too stiff. Let rest for 15–20 minutes.

---

79. Kitchiner, *The Cook's Oracle* (1817) (London: Samuel Bagster, 1860), 244.

Place a large clean cloth on the table, flour it, and roll the dough out on the cloth until very thin. Then tug gently at the dough from the edges until it is so thin that you can theoretically read a newspaper placed under it. Cut off the thick outer edges, spread the butter and cream paste on half of the wide side of the dough, and then spread the parsley mixture on top. Pick up the cloth and shake it until the dough starts to roll up like a jellyroll. Fold the sides of the dough in to keep the filling from oozing out, and continue rolling it up. Form the rolled strudel into a coiled shape similar to a snail, and place in a well-oiled baking pan.

Bake in a moderately hot oven for at least an hour, until the top of the strudel begins to turn golden brown, basting with butter as needed. The cooked strudel should be served piping hot with breadcrumbs browned in butter. The recipe can be varied to include other herbs such as tarragon, marjoram, sweet cicely, lemon balm, or chervil.

Household Applications

The fresh juice of the parsley plant has deodorant properties and is an effective insectifuge. In ancient Greece and Rome, festive parsley wreaths and garlands were plaited and given to partygoers. The belief was that they would then be able hold their liquor better.

Cutting boards that have taken on the unpleasantly pungent odor of garlic or onions can be rubbed down with parsley leaves. Dried and powdered parsley stalks, or the juice of fresh leaves, can also be used as a nontoxic dye for Easter eggs or as green food coloring. A greenish-yellow dye for woolens can be produced with the fresh leaves, with chrome as a mordant.

Cosmetic Properties

In the Palatine in Germany, folk healers counsel women to wash their faces regularly with parsley water or parsley tea. Professional beauticians may laugh at such simple-minded advice, but they do agree that parsley has a healing and strengthening effect on the skin. This is due in part to the great amounts of vitamin A that it contains.

Parsley leaf tea is often added to facial creams and lotions; it has a bleaching effect, and, if used repeatedly, helps to lighten unwanted freckles and make moles less prominent. Parsley leaf tea can be brewed from ½ pint of boiling water poured over a small handful of the fresh green leaves.

Parsley leaves can also be added to facial masks for oily skin:

- Brew the leaves with some boiling water and then allow them to steep in a closed container for 15 minutes. The strained tea can be thickened with honey, whole-wheat flour, yogurt, buttermilk, or Bentonite or French green clay, and applied fresh as a mask. Remove the mixture when it begins to dry and crumble.

Parsley can also be taken internally and externally as an eye-strengthening tea. Ethereal parsley oil is often added in small amounts to commercial perfumes.

People on a diet or beauty cure are told to eat as much parsley as possible because of its high vitamin content and extraordinary cleansing abilities. Eating parsley can also help to regulate perspiration and its unpleasant odors, and to sweeten the breath.

Some Italians vow that their thick hair is not due to Mediterranean genes, but to the cosmetic properties of the parsley plant. They go into the garden on the morning of Midsummer's Day on an empty stomach, without having told anyone of their venture, and bury their head in dew-dampened parsley. The seeds of the parsley plant are also used to stimulate hair growth: the seeds are crushed and then applied, dry or as a paste, to the scalp in the evening, and brushed out again in the morning. This is repeated once a month.

When parsley leaves are boiled in water, the resulting infusion can be applied as a rinse to dark hair to make it shinier and more manageable. In the days when lice were a cosmetic problem, a salve was prepared from lard and powdered parsley seeds and applied to the scalp. Cambridgeshire women once concocted a salve made from pounded parsley and hen's fat to heal chapped hands.

Medicinal Merits

In the past, parsley was held in higher consideration as a medicinal herb than as a seasoning herb. It was classified as warming and drying and used to treat a variety of diseases. Hippocrates praised its diuretic properties, and it was subsequently used to treat kidney and bladder stones, genital pains, syphilis, gonorrhea, and uterine disorders. The seeds were given to women in large amounts to induce abortions. The juice of the fresh plant was, on the other hand, supposed to prevent miscarriage, and the root was highly valued as an aphrodisiac. Women who bled strongly after a birth were told to hold on to parsley stems to stem the flow of blood.

Parsley leaves and parsley seeds were boiled in ale as an antidote to poison, and applied as plasters to the bites of rabid dogs. Parsley leaves and snails were pounded into a salve for the treatment of crop (thyroid disorders), and the herb was prescribed for "pains in the side" (which could mean anything from a stitch in the side to flatulence, or even appendicitis). Parsley water was prescribed for epileptics and paralytics, and parsley leaf poultices were applied to loosen knots in the breast and to stop the milk flow of nursing mothers. Parsley comforted the stomach, relieved flatulence, and was used in the treatment of intermittent fevers.

Modern Medicine

Modern medicine has discovered that parsley leaves are rich in the vitamins A, B, and C, iron, calcium, phosphorous, manganese, and potassium. They can help to stimulate the appetite and the digestive system, and are therefore a good dietary supplement for convalescents and anemics. Parsley leaves are carminative (i.e., they counteract flatulence), antispasmodic, and diuretic. Parsley roots and parsley seeds can be taken in various forms to cleanse the blood, the kidneys, and the bladder. They can also help to dissolve kidney stones and gravel, expel excess water from the body, and, taken for several months together with other herbs, relieve gout and rheumatism.

- Parsley root tea can be prepared by bringing ½ pint of water and one tsp. of the chopped root to a boil, and then letting the mixture steep, covered, for 15 minutes. No more than 1 tsp. of parsley seeds should be taken for each cup of parsley seed tea, which is prepared like parsley leaf tea.

Parsley roots are considered more effective than parsley leaves. Parsley seeds are stronger than parsley roots, and the oil pressed from fresh parsley seeds is the most potent medicine of all. A massive dose of parsley oil can have dangerous side effects, and cause headaches, dizziness, humming in the ears, and in some cases, even death. People with kidney disorders and acute infections must avoid parsley unless a competent herbalist, homeopath, or doctor has prescribed it.

Parsley oil has a stimulating effect on the uterus, and is therefore still used to induce abortions, often with disastrous results. But it can be prescribed by an experienced herbalist after an exhausting birth to help tone the uterus. Parsley tea is given to the nursing mother trying to wean her child and stop the flow of milk.

Parsley may also be used externally. Fresh bruised parsley leaves are applied to mosquito, wasp, and bee stings to lessen the immediate pain. They can also be used as poultices on light burns, milk knots, and scrofulous swellings. Swollen eyes can be rinsed with lightly salted lukewarm parsley leaf tea. Parsley packs are applied to the breasts of nursing mothers at weaning time.

Homeopathically, parsley treats those who have the constant urge to urinate, or have a deep and burning itch in the urethra or chronic urinary complaints. Itching hemorrhoids have also been treated with parsley.

Uses in Husbandry

Parsley is endangered in every country garden because hares, rabbits, and voles love it so dearly. Sheep and cows will also eat it, but it should not be fed to chickens and under no conditions given to parrots or ferrets. Blossoming parsley encourages bees to visit a garden, and the leaves are said to have a healing effect on sick fish if thrown into a fishpond. Cats and dogs profit from a little finely chopped parsley added to their diet on a regular basis.

In Galicia and Moravia in eastern Europe, cows were once fed parsley on June 24th, 25th, and 26th to protect them from witches. In Silesia (Germany), hunters made use of a mixture of parsley seeds and leaves, fennel seeds, and breadcrumbs to lure rabbits and hares to their death.

Veterinary Values

Parsley is widely used by veterinarians. The seeds are administered to dogs to expel worms, and large quantities of the leaves are given to sheep as a preventive against foot rot. Parsley leaves, finely chopped, are administered to dogs suffering from rickets, arthritis, rheumatism, obesity, glandular troubles, bad breath, kidney and bladder troubles, and water retention. Parsley leaves and roots, or parsley tea, can be given to cows having trouble calving or expelling the afterbirth. Parsley oil has been administered as a sedative to skittish mares during breeding, and a concoction of parsley water and oil is rubbed onto barnyard fowl plagued with lice and other parasites. Parsley seeds are supposed to discourage fleas.

Miscellaneous Wisdom

Parsley is associated with three of the most important events in human life: marriage, birth, and death. Bride and bridegroom wear it at marriage ceremonies, and singers and dancers are often garlanded with parsley, rosemary, and myrtle. In Galicia (Spain), the bride traditionally carried bread and parsley under her arm to drive away evil spirits. In Germany, lovers once sowed their names with parsley seeds as growing proof of their affection.

Parsley is not only associated with the ceremonial side of marriage, but also with sexuality and procreation. In Limburg, Germany, the door of a girl who "isn't better than she ought to be" is decorated with parsley on May 1st. The red-light districts in France and Germany are sometimes called "parsley alleys." The term "parsley bed" has sexual connotations, and Calypso's island was supposed to have been covered with parsley. According to how one feels toward sexuality, parsley is "poison to men and salvation to women" or a parsley field can "bring a man to his saddle and a woman to her grave."[80] The English say that babies come out of the parsley bed. In the Slavic countries, parsley

---

80. Hanns Bächtold-Stäubli, ed., *Handwörterbuch des deutschen Aberglaubens* (1927–42), vol. VI (Berlin: Walter de Gruyter & Co., 1987), 1529.

and garlic were once tied into the sheet of a laboring woman to protect her from evil spirits. In Cambridgeshire, newborn babies' eyes were washed with an infusion of parsley and storm rainwater to improve their eyesight.

Parsley was widely used in ancient Greek funeral ceremonies, and considered sacred to Persephone. It was planted or strewn on graves, and was so closely connected to funeral practices that it was rarely brought to the table. If a man was in need of parsley, then that meant that he was either impotent or close to death. Victors at ancient funeral games or at the Isthmian and Nemean games were garlanded with wreaths of parsley. Roman gladiators were fed parsley to enlarge their biceps and enhance their chances of victory. Warhorses were fed parsley to make them strong and swift-footed. In later years, the herb came to be associated with St. Peter, but still retained its reputation as an effective antidemonic and funereal herb.

The English saying "we are at the parsley and the rue" also has its origins in antiquity. Greek gardens were often bordered with parsley and rue. A person beginning an undertaking begins figuratively at the beginning of the garden, or at the parsley and the rue. The Victorians believed that cutting down parsley would also cut down one's luck in love, and that to give away parsley was equivalent to giving away luck. The only possible method of regaining good fortune was to steal the plant back. Another curious belief comes from Cambridgeshire: eating chopped parsley meal and boiled pig's brains is believed to make a person wise.

Legends

In Greek mythology, the little boy Archemorus was once left untended by his nurse. When the nurse returned, she was horrified to see that a snake had bitten the boy. Archemorus died from the serpent's poison, but his death was not in vain: parsley plants sprang from his blood. The Nemean games were held in his honor, and the victors garlanded with wreaths of parsley.

Oracular Worth

In southern Germany and the United States, it is taken as a sign that someone in the house will die during the year if parsley consistently refuses to germinate in the garden. If the plants are spindly, or produce white stalks, it is also taken as a sign that someone must die. As an extension of this belief, some Americans believe that a child will be born if the parsley grows exceptionally well. In Cambridgeshire, tall parsley in the garden is taken as a sure sign that the lady of the house will give birth to a baby girl. In Shropshire, a good crop of parsley shows that "the missis is master." In Germany, a good stand of parsley promises good health and long life for the gardener. If the plants grow poorly, they were certainly sown by a blabbermouth. In Transylvania, long-rooted parsley is thought to presage a long winter.

Literary Flowers

Can you make me a cambrick shirt,
Parsley, sage, rosemary and thyme
Without any seam or needle work?
And you shall be a true love of mine.

Can you wash it in yonder well
Parsley, sage, rosemary and thyme
Where never sprung water nor rain ever fell?
And you shall be a true love of mine.

Can you dry it on yonder thorn,
Parsley, sage, rosemary and thyme
Which never bore blossom since Adam was born?
And you shall be a true love of mine.

Now you have asked me questions three,
I hope you'll answer as many for me.

Can you find me an acre of land
Parsley, sage, rosemary and thyme
Between the salt water and the sea sand?
And you shall be a true love of mine.

Can you plow it with a ram's horn,
Parsley, sage, rosemary and thyme
And sow it all over with one pepper corn?
And you shall be a true love of mine.

Can you reap it with a sickle of leather,
Parsley, sage, rosemary and thyme
And bind it up with a peacock's feather?
And you shall be a true love of mine.

When you have done, and finished your work,
Parsley, sage, rosemary and thyme
Then come to me for your cambrick shirt.
And you shall be a true love of mine.

—"THE ELFIN KNIGHT,"

FRANCIS CHILD'S *THE ENGLISH AND SCOTTISH POPULAR BALLADS*

Who passeth by the rosemarie, And careth not to take a spraye,
For woman's love no care has he, Nor shall he though he live for aye.

—A Spanish saying

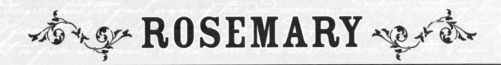

ROSEMARY

Name

Etymologists disagree about the final origins of the word "rosemary," and it is a matter of learned dispute whether the name evolved from the Greek *rhops myrinos* (meaning "odoriferous shrub"), from *ros* (the Latin name for an aromatic plant), or from *ros marinus* (meaning "sea dew"). It is believed that the Virgin Mary did not give her name to the plant.

Rosmarinus officinalis is a perennial member of the **Labiatae** or **Lamiaceae** family, and is synonymous with the older term *Salvia rosmarinus*.

Folk Names

Ancient terms for the shrub were *rosmarinus coronarium*, *incensier*, and *gardrobe*. Modern English names are rose mary, polar plant, compass-weed, and compass plant. German designations are *Rosmarin*, *Kranzenkraut*, *Meertau*, *Weihrauchkraut*, and *Brautkraut*. French names are *rosmarin* and *romarin*; Italian, *rosmarino, rosmarín,* and *ramerino*; Spanish, *romero*; Portuguese, *rosmaninho*; and Greek, *anthos*. In Denmark and Sweden, the herb is called *rosmarin*; in Ireland, *rós mhuire*.

Appearance

Some English gardeners believe that rosemary plants will continue to grow very slowly for thirty-three years until they attain the height of Jesus of Nazareth. Then they will stop growing upward, but will continue to expand outward. Although this theory is charming, it can only hold true in very mild climates, where rosemary does occasionally grow to be 6 ft. high. In the north, rosemary plants have to be protected in the winter, and often succumb to frost.

Rosemary grows from a long, woody root. As Nicholas Culpeper explains,

> The shrub is covered with a brown tough bark; and the young shoots are of a greyish green. The leaves are numerous, and of a firm substance; they are oblong, narrow, sharp-pointed, not at all indented at the edges, and of a very fragrant smell: they are of a beautiful green on the upper side, and silvery grey underneath. The flowers rise in great numbers from the bosom of the leaves toward the upper part of the branches; they are large, and of a pale blue, variegated with white. The seeds are small and oblong. The whole plant has a fragrant and aromatic smell, it is lighter and more delicate in the flower, and stronger in the leaves. The taste is pleasant, warm, and aromatic.[81]

It should be added that the herb's fragrance is reminiscent of camphor, pine needles, and nutmeg. The elongated leaves of the rosemary plant are often rolled down at the edges, which gives them an even more needle-like appearance. Rosemary flowers are similar to the flowers of the sage plant, and may vary between purple, blue, and white, but are quite small and often hidden along the stem. In warm climates, the plant spreads outward and can be used as a ground cover or a covering for low walls.

Place, Season, and Useful Parts

Rosemary was originally a native of southern Europe, but has been cultivated for a long time in central and northern Europe. In more recent times, it is grown as a cash crop in other parts of the world as well, such as the southern United States, South Africa, and Australia. It still grows wild on sunny slopes in the Orient, in Spain, Italy, Dalmatia, southern France, and northern Africa, to a height of 4,500 ft. It blooms from March to September, depending on the climate, and is usually cut above the roots or main stems just as the plant begins to blossom.

Gathering, Drying, and Storage

Rosemary leaves can be harvested from April to October, just before the flowers begin to open. The flowers can also be gathered separately after they open, usually in April or May, and then again in the fall according to location. Rosemary oil is usually distilled from the flowering tops of rosemary plants, but may also be obtained from rosemary leaves and stems.

Rosemary leaves dry easily, either on the branch or singly. The best drying method is to strip them from the stalks as soon as possible after harvesting, and then spread them

---

81.   Culpeper, *Culpeper's Complete Herbal* (1653) (London: Foulsham, undated), 302.

in thin layers on a cloth in a dark, dry, and airy place, and dry them quickly. They should be stored in airtight containers, but can also be preserved while still fresh under (olive) oil or in vinegar.

Seed Saving and Germination

Rosemary plants vary according to location, and great differences in height and frost-sensitivity between varieties have been recorded. It is common to propagate the plants by division in fall, or by layering or cuttings. Plants reproduced by cuttings will be identical to the parent plants, and there is no need to isolate them in order to keep different varieties from crossing. Seeds are only rarely set in colder climates, and germination can be erratic. This is another reason to use layering or cuttings for propagating the herb.

Gardening Hints

Rosemary grows wild in great quantities in Mediterranean and other southern countries, but has also been cultivated in less clement climates since ancient times. The plant is frost-sensitive, and often dies down in the winter in the north, or is so damaged by the frost that it takes most of the following year to recover. It prefers dry, yet sandy and humus-rich, soil, and a wind-sheltered position in full sunlight. Rosemary seeds are sown indoors in the spring, or in a warm, sheltered place outdoors after all danger of frost. Rosemary seeds do not germinate easily, and it may be necessary to re-sow. Rosemary seedlings can be planted in their final position as soon as they have four true leaves.

Cuttings are usually taken in July through August, and pushed deep into the soil under a hand glass. An even easier method is to layer the growing plant. To do this, take a branch and weigh it down with a rock, covering the place where the plant connects with the soil. After a few weeks, roots should have formed, and the new plant can then be cut off from the mother plant and replanted. Plants should be set out approximately 10 in. apart. In warmer climates, rosemary plants can also be divided in the fall. In northern countries, it is advisable to bring the plants indoors each winter, and then to divide them if desired in the spring. Many gardeners have problems with overwintering rosemary plants indoors, and should remember that they do not like to be waterlogged, but prefer light, sandy soil and a sunny position.

With proper care, rosemary plants can grow to be twenty years old. It is advisable to trim them a little in summer to discourage spindly growth and encourage bushiness. Trimming too late in the season will weaken the plants, and make them more susceptible to frost. In warmer climates, they can be planted to form a large garden hedge to discourage such garden pests as carrot fly, cabbage moths, and bean beetles. Single smaller plants can also be set throughout the garden for the same purpose. Cabbages grow better in the vicinity of rosemary plants, and sage and rosemary will both thrive if planted next to each other. Grains do not tolerate rosemary in their vicinity, and may even be stunted if subjected to smoke from a rosemary wood fire.

Many gardening superstitions surround the rosemary plant. The most popular belief about it in Herefordshire is that "rosemary only grows where the missis is master."[82] This belief, and the fear of becoming the butt of nasty jokes, has led some men to undertake nightly raids on the rosemary plants in the garden. Westfalians are of the opinion that a rosemary shrub will die if a pregnant woman touches it, and some Austrians believe that sick people can transfer their illness to the plant. Strips of red cloth are tied to the rosemary to protect it from harm and magical interference. In Switzerland, the rosemary plant is always informed when the master of the house dies, and is "knocked upon." If this ritual is overlooked, the plant will die, and visit misfortune on the house. English gardeners believe in the animosity and jealousy felt by the rosemary plant for the laurel tree, and vice versa. If the gardener tends the one to the exclusion of the other, then the neglected plant is sure to die.

Culinary Virtues

Rosemary was well known to the ancient Greeks, Arabs, and Saxons as a culinary herb. In medieval England, a boar's head was traditionally garnished with bay leaves and rosemary at the Christmas feast. Rosemary is now primarily used in Mediterranean cookery, and northern cooks tend to distrust its pungently aromatic taste. Honey produced in southern countries often owes its delicate flavor to rosemary flowers. The herbal seasoning mixture *Herbes de Provence* contains large amounts of the herb. In most southern countries, lamb, kid, sucking pig, and veal are seasoned with fresh sprigs of the plant before roasting or grilling. Rosemary can also be added to sauces, soups, egg dishes, fresh goat's cheese, casseroles, fish, roast potatoes, spinach, squash, peas, rye, and wheat dishes. Rosemary is available in powdered form, but this seasoning tends to have little flavor and dry out quickly. It is usually better to add a sprig of the fresh plant to the dish, and remove it before serving, since cooking does not reduce the spikiness of the leaves.

Pork, lamb, kid, beef, veal and venison roasts are often rubbed with rosemary and garlic before putting them in the oven, or they are served with rosemary jelly. Fish can be seasoned before grilling with a mixture of olive oil and herbal vinegar brushed on with a rosemary twig. Rosemary is an aromatic addition to herbal butters and vinegars. Even fruit cups and puddings can be flavored with minute amounts of powdered rose-

---

82. *Choice Notes from Notes and Queries* (London: The Folk-Lore Society, 1859), 242.

mary, or garnished with a sprig of the fresh herb. A sprig of rosemary in the fruit bowl will impart a delicate flavor to apples and pears.

Both rosemary wine and rosemary beer are heartening and heart-strengthening drinks that keep well, for the rosemary acts as a preserving agent. Simple rosemary tea can be prepared in quantity and served as a pleasant, refreshing, cool drink.

Noteworthy Recipes

Sawce for Red Deer: The following recipe is from the seventeenth century:

> Sweet Herbs chopped small, the Gravy, with the Juyce of an Orange or Lemon, and grated Bread or Vinegar, Claret-wine, Ginger, Cinnamon and Sugar, boiled up with a sprig of Rosemary, some whole Cloves and grated Bread; and if you stuff or farce your Venison, let it be with whole Cloves, sweet Herbs and Beef-suet, the two latter cut very small.[83]

In this recipe, sweet marjoram, savory, thyme, parsley, basil, and even small amounts of chervil could be used as "sweet" herbs. For clarity's sake, the recipe should probably read: "with the juice of an orange, or a lemon, or a little vinegar, and some grated bread."

Italian Roast Lamb with Rosemary: This dish is traditionally served at Easter and prepared with lamb only a few months old. Take 1 leg of lamb, and rub it with a cut clove of garlic, tucking pieces of garlic into any cut or fold of the meat available, or cutting a few slits. Tear the rosemary into smaller pieces, and tuck it under the roast in a roasting pan. Baste the roast with olive oil applied with a large sprig of rosemary or a basting brush. Salt the roast. Brown it in the oven on both sides at highest temperatures, taking care not to burn the rosemary. When the outside of the roast is browned, turn the heat down to medium to finish roasting, basting occasionally with the olive oil and juices from the roast. Modern cooks will probably want to use a meat thermometer to test the meat, but should avoid overcooking lamb. Lamb roasts should still be a little rosy inside, with a crunchy and aromatic crust on the outside. Let the roast rest for 10 minutes before carving, and serve with parsley potatoes.

Household Applications

It was once common practice to place pots of rosemary in and around the house as living incense, or to strew the floor with the fresh herb. The Greeks even went so far as to gild rosemary wreaths. In the Middle Ages, rosemary was fashioned into chaplets and presented to the Virgin Mary, and rosemary stalks were burned as a substitute for

---

83. John Shirley, *The Accomplished Ladies Rich Closet of Rarities* (London: N. Bodington, 1688), 134.

exorbitantly expensive frankincense. Even after the invention of the printing press, books were so valuable that they were protected from worms and moths by placing sprigs of dried rosemary between the pages. Rosemary is now added to moth-repellent herbal mixtures, to potpourris and sachets as well as to herbal sleeping pillows. The Welsh say that rosemary can keep snakes and adders from entering the house if it is placed under the doorpost. In France, large, aromatic rosemary branches are often burnt with the firewood. Modern housekeepers spray rooms with a freshening mixture of water and ethereal rosemary oil to freshen them.

Cosmetic Properties

Rosemary is best known to cosmeticians as the hair herb *par excellence*. A hair rinse made of rosemary can encourage the growth of hair and help prevent baldness by increasing circulation in the scalp. It may also prevent premature graying. Rosemary will darken existing gray hairs, especially if used together with sage as a hair tonic. It helps to prevent dandruff, revitalize damaged hair, keep curled hair from uncurling in damp weather, and drive away parasites. Some rosemary tea can be added to a neutral or Castile shampoo (those with dry hair may want to add a few drops of burdock root hair oil as well), or a strong rosemary infusion can be used directly as a rinse after shampooing.

Not only does the scalp react positively to treatment with rosemary, but the skin can also benefit from the herb. Rosemary baths, prepared either from rosemary infusions or a few drops of rosemary oil added to the bath water, help to increase the circulation, and are therefore warming, stimulating, and healing. Rosemary baths should not be taken by pregnant women or directly before going to bed.

Rosemary footbaths and steaming mixtures also help to improve the circulation. Rosemary is often an ingredient of after-bath lotions and tonics, and is occasionally powdered and added to talcum powders. Rosemary oil is an aromatic ingredient of many massage oils. Participants in the ancient Greek Olympic Games were once rubbed down with sweet-smelling oils containing rosemary to improve skin tone and ease muscle pains.

Rosemary oil is highly valued by the perfume industry, and is usually added to eau de cologne. At one time, rosemary was a favorite ingredient of those perfumed balls known as scented apples (see the marjoram chapter for a recipe). John Gerard suggested that a distilled water of rosemary, cloves, mace, anise, and cinnamon be used to sweeten bad breath, which was probably a good idea in his day and age, seeing that visits to the dentist were few and far between. The ashes of burned rosemary branches were also used to clean teeth before commercial toothpastes were invented. Rosemary ashes helped to whiten fingernails, and toothpicks of aromatic rosemary wood were once preferred above all others.

Noteworthy Recipes

Hungary Water: The most famous of all rosemary preparations was Hungary water, once the cosmetic secret of Elizabeth, Queen of Hungary. According to legend, the seventy-two-year-old queen was freed from all rheumatic complaints, and so rejuvenated by repeated use of this water that the King of Poland asked for her hand in marriage. The Queen's recipe is no longer a secret: it can be prepared by steeping three parts of rosemary leaves and one part of lavender flowers for four days in spirits of wine, and then distilling the liquid.

Rosemary Water: Another recipe for rosemary water comes to us from John Shirley's book of cosmetic advice and recipes, *The Accomplished Ladies Rich Closet of Rarities*:

> To make Rosemary Water Take the Flowers and Leaves of Rosemary in their prime, half a pound, and four ounces of Elicampane roots [elecampane, *Inula helenium*], a handful of Red-Sage [as this is difficult to find, normal sage, *Salvia officinalis*, or Clary, *Salvia sclarea*, can be substituted], three ounces of Cloves, the same quantity of Mace, and twelve ounces of Annisseeds: beate the Herbs together, and the Spices seperately, putting to them four gallons of white wine; and after a Weeks standing, Distil them over a gentle fire.[84]

Rosemary Hair Water: One other antiquated rosemary recipe that may interest modern readers is from *The Art of Cookery Made Plain and Easy* (1760). It is "An Approved Method Practised by Mrs. Dukeley, The Queen's Tyre Woman, to Preserve Hair and Make it Grow Thick":

> Take one quart of white wine, put in one handful of rosemary flowers, half a pound of honey, distill together, then add a quarter of a pint of oil of sweet almonds, shake it very well together, put a little of it into a cup, warm it blood warm, rub it well into your hair and comb it dry.[85]

Rosemary Oil: A more modern method of using rosemary is to prepare an infused oil of the herb, and then to use it as a base for massage oils, skin creams, and bath oils. First take a wide-mouthed jar with a tightly-fitting lid, wash it carefully with baking or washing soda to remove all odors, fill loosely with rosemary leaves, and cover with sweet almond oil. Other oils such as sesame or jojoba may also be used, but care should be taken to obtain only the very best and freshest oils. Close the jar carefully, and put it in a sunny place. Let stand for two days, or until the oil begins to change color. Strain and then filter through filter paper, and add a tenth

---

84. Shirley, *The Accomplished Ladies Rich Closet of Rarities* (London: N. Bodington, 1688), 11.

85. Hannah Glasse, *The Art of Cookery Made Plain and Easy* (London: Millar, Tonsan, et al., 1760).

part of wheat germ oil or vitamin E oil to the liquid to improve its keeping qualities. If a stronger-smelling oil is desired, a few drops of essential rosemary oil can
be added in place of the wheat germ oil.

Medicinal Merits

Rosemary has been put to so many uses over the centuries that it is not surprising that
people once swore by the herb. As Eachand notes in his *Observations* (1671):

> I cannot forget him, who having at some time or other been suddenly cur'd of
> a little head-ach with a rosemary posset, would scarce drink out of anything but
> rosemary cans, cut his meat with a rosemary knife, and pick his teeth with a
> rosemary sprig. Nay, sir, he was so strangely taken up with the excellencies of
> rosemary, that he would needs have the Bible cleared of all other herbs, and
> only rosemary be inserted.[86]

It may be that rosemary had not only cured this man of his headache, but also of a hangover. Because of this, many thoughtful women tried to slip the herb secretly into their
husbands' beer.

Because of its warming properties, rosemary was also thought to comfort the brain
and to restore memory, to drive away melancholy and damp brain vapors, to keep a man
young and active and a woman lusty, to drive old age from the doorstep and Death from
the door, to warm cold blood marrow, to loosen a palsied tongue, to purify the air in hospitals and jails, and to quicken the spirits and ease the mind of cares. Patients with colds
or influenza were carefully wrapped in warm woolen sheets smoked with rosemary,
elderly people were given smelling-boxes made of rosemary wood to preserve their van-
ishing youth, and rosemary leaves were placed under beds to prevent nightmares and
on the stomachs of women in labor to ease their pains. Nursing women's breasts were
rubbed with rosemary to make their babies' hair grow faster, and gouty patients were
told to eat a great quantity of the leaves every morning on an empty stomach. Greek students wore rosemary wreaths at examination time to improve their memory, and those
troubled with shortness of breath were given bread baked over a rosemary fire.

Special Cures

Rosemary Cordial: Rosemary was once considered such an excellent cordial and
  nerve-strengthening herb that it was prescribed as follows:

> To remove the humour that occasions the Greensickness in Virgins and
> young Widows ake a quart of Claret, a pound of blue Currans, a handful

---

86. Qtd. in John Brand and Sir Henry Ellis, *Observations on the Popular Antiquities of Great Britain* (1849). 3
vol. (Detroit, MI: Singing Tree Press, 1969), 122.

of young Rosemary-tops, with half an ounce of Mace; bruise them, and boil the liquid part to a pint, and let the party afflicted drink half a pint hot morning and evening for a Week together.[87]

Another famous rosemary preparation was white arquebusade, a disinfectant vulnerary, or wound-herb, concocted from rosemary, sage, rue, and lavender.

Modern Medicine

Most people consider rosemary a harmless culinary herb, but this is far from the truth. Rosemary is so potent that it can cause poisoning if taken in large amounts for a long time, or in massive doses. It is an especially effective tonic stimulant for patients with weak hearts, poor circulation, low blood pressure, anemia, mental exhaustion, paralysis, tension headaches, or cardiac insufficiency. Herbalists recommended rosemary wine for centuries as a heart-strengthening drink. Rosemary tea is a gentle stimulant for the digestive tract, the female organs, and the kidneys. Seasoning foods with rosemary aids the digestion. Furthermore, the herb can help to bring on menstruation and has even been known to cause miscarriages. It can eliminate excess water from the body, especially if the patient's circulation is poor. A homeopathic tincture of the herb is considered effective for the treatment of headaches, poor memory, mental exhaustion, and dizziness. It can help to alleviate drowsiness.

Chinese doctors use rosemary to disperse cold and to treat the common cold, headache, indigestion, and menstrual pain. It can also be used to speed up the menstrual flow, especially in menopause.

Externally applied, rosemary is equally efficacious. It has astringent and mildly disinfectant properties and is therefore useful in the treatment of wounds. It can ease the stiffness of strained ligaments and partially paralyzed or rheumatic limbs. Rosemary baths are very stimulating, and are recommended for those suffering from circulatory complaints, rheumatic disorders, or nervous exhaustion. Rubbing one's temples with rosemary oil, or washing one's face and head with a rosemary infusion can help to relieve certain kinds of headaches. Rosemary oil is often employed as a counterirritant for the skin, for example as a treatment for rheumatism. Weak rosemary tea is an effective eyewash.

Special Cures

Rosemary Wine: Modern herbalists recommend rosemary wine for those suffering from chronic headaches, poor circulation, or a weakened heart. Rosemary wine can be prepared at home by simply placing 2 oz. of dried, or three times that

---

87. John Shirley, *The Accomplished Ladies Rich Closet of Rarities* (London: N. Bodington, 1688), 71.

amount of fresh rosemary leaves in a wide-necked bottle and covering them with good red wine. Leave the firmly stoppered bottle in a warm place, and strain after 3 days. Rosemary wine can also be prepared from white wine, although it tends to be more astringent than red wine. This medicine should be taken in very small doses (1–2 Tbsp.) every day for several weeks for best results.

Uses in Husbandry

The aromatic herb is a favorite plant of bees as well as sheep. Rosemary is used commercially to denature spirits and oils, and is one of the principal ingredients of herbal tobaccos. Smoking rosemary oil is said to relieve asthma and bronchial complaints. One old name for the rosemary plant, "compass plant," points to the use of its needles as primitive compasses. An infusion of rosemary, or water and rosemary oil, can help to deter fleas if it is used to wash animals' sleeping places.

Veterinary Values

Dogs with bald spots, scurf, or mange can be bathed with a rosemary or marigold infusion. It is an excellent heart-strengthening herb, and can be administered together with honey as a cordial. Bruises, cuts, sprains, infected or irritated gums, arthritis, and rheumatism heal better if washed regularly with a rosemary infusion. Rosemary can also be used externally to increase the flow of blood to the wounded area.

Miscellaneous Wisdom

Rosemary is a plant that can influence the heart. It is used in love magic throughout Europe, and is often associated with marriages as well as funerals. In ancient Greece, it was declared sacred to Aphrodite and employed in marriage ceremonies. In seventeenth-century England, it was considered to be a man's flower, and worn at weddings and used to decorate the bridal bed. Sprigs of rosemary were gilded and presented to the marriage guests. In the German Hessian province, the bridal couple is often garlanded with the herb, and the path to church strewn with it. In Baden, it is customary for the bride to tuck a sprig of rosemary under the groom's hatband and in the tip of her own shoe to ensure his fidelity. At the doorstep of her new home, she then slips the herb from her shoe, and crosses herself three times with it before stepping into her new life.

In northern Italy, men wishing to obtain great sexual prowess are told find a rosemary bush and then to urinate on it precisely at midnight on Midsummer's Eve. In Poland, girls wishing to win the affections of a young man are told to sew the tip of a rosemary plant into his shirt without his knowledge. Some French and Belgian mothers tell their curious children that babies are found in a rosemary bush, and are not brought by the stork.

Rosemary has also been thought to symbolize remembrance and fidelity. Greek girls present their departing lovers with sprigs of rosemary "to remember them." According to English lore, a man wanting success and a good memory should always wear rosemary in his lapel. A dream in which rosemary figures centrally is interpreted as being a dream about honor. The Welsh are of the opinion that everything eaten with a rosemary spoon has to be nutritious, and that the fumes of the burning plant can help to release a man from jail.

In Spain and Italy, rosemary was used to drive away witches, and in Great Britain, the plant was placed on the lintel to keep witches and other "uncanny" people from entering the house. Hung from the rafters, it is supposed to improve the memory of those living in the house. In Franconia, Germany, rosemary twigs were placed in the cradle to protect babies from harm. Sicilians believed that young elves, or *fate*, hid under rosemary bushes in the guise of snakes. Northern Italians believed that these snakes were in truth maidens enchanted by evil witches.

Because of its reputation as a love herb, rosemary is an important part of many ceremonies, especially Christmas season celebrations. In Germany, it is used as a *Lebensrute*, or wand of life, on certain days that vary according to region. Young women are beaten or "peppered" publicly with rosemary, birch, or juniper branches to render them fertile. After a christening, it is customary for the child's godmother and godfather to stroke each other with rosemary branches dipped in holy water. In another part of Germany, boys once ceremoniously washed the feet of the village women with rosemary water to ensure their prosperity and fertility. Bakers' apprentices in Hildesheim were in the habit of beating their customers with rosemary branches on Shrove Tuesday (the Tuesday before Ash Wednesday). They were rewarded for this unaccustomed show of good spirits with gifts and baked goods. Until about 1650, a rosemary plant also figured in the ceremony by which a journeyman baker was elevated to the position of master in France. He had to present a pot of rosemary decorated with sugared fruits to the Grand Pantler and the other judges.

In England, the belief is still prevalent that rosemary blooms at midnight on Christmas Eve and that it should be used to decorate the house, along with holly, ivy, mistletoe, and laurel. According to a German saying, "On midnight on Christmas Eve, all that is water turns to wine, and all the trees to rose-mary."[88]

Oracular Worth

In keeping with its aphrodisiacal properties, rosemary is often consulted as an oracle during the marriage ceremony. In Bohemia, a bridesmaid may place a rosemary wreath

---

88. Hanns Bächtold-Stäubli, ed., *Handwörterbuch des deutschen Aberglaubens* (1927–42), vol. VII (Berlin: Walter de Gruyter & Co., 1987).

on the groom's head before the wedding. If she or the best man can wrest it from him as soon as the ceremony is completed, then it is taken as a sure sign that she, or the best man, will marry soon. If unsuccessful, both the bridesmaid and the best man have to pay a fine to the newly wedded couple. In southern Germany, it is taken as a particularly bad sign if the groom's rosemary wreath falls off during the marriage ceremony, or if it begins to wilt. If the ends dip downward, then the marriage will soon deteriorate. If the bride can manage to take the wreath off her husband's head after the ceremony, then she will have the mastery in the house. In certain parts of Austria, it is customary to stick a branch of rosemary in the ground directly after the ceremony. If it strikes roots, then the marriage will be harmonious and prosper. Maybe this is one reason why May weddings are so popular.

After all the wedding festivities are over, careful watch is kept on the rosemary bush in the garden. If it grows upward and outward, it is taken as a sign that the woman is master in the house. Others believe that the wife will soon produce a child, and most likely a baby girl. If the bush blossoms shortly before birth, then the child will be a boy.

Rosemary is also consulted as an oracle of death. If it blossoms while a member of the house is death-ridden, then that person will undoubtedly recover. If it dies, then the patient has little chance of recovery. The sudden death of a rosemary plant can also presage a sudden death in the house. In many countries, it is customary to throw sprigs of rosemary into new graves. The bush from which the cuttings were taken will slowly wilt and die, just like the sprigs under the earth.

Legends

The rosemary plant is considered sacred in Spain because Mary once supposedly dried Jesus' clothes on the bush. Since that time, rosemary plants have flowered every Friday, and retain their green color and fresh fragrance the whole year through.

The herb rue
Every evil eschews.

—Italian folk saying

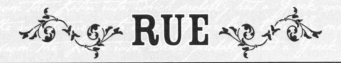

RUE

Name

The name "rue" is derived from the Latin *ruta*, which probably had a Greek source. Despite all puns, it has no common origin with the verb "to rue" (to regret).

Garden rue, or *Ruta graveolens* (*graveolens* literally means "heavy-smelling" or "fetid") is also known as *Ruta hortensis* and *Ruta officinalis*. It is a perennial member of the **Rutaceae** family. Also included in this family are several wild rues, including the strongest-smelling, *Ruta montana*.

Folk Names

Rue is also called herb of grace, herbe grace, herbygrass, garden rue, common rue, and German rue. German names are *Raute*, *Weinraute*, *Gartenraute*, *Hexenkraut*, *Rute*, and *Frauenkraut*; French names are *rue*, *rue des jardins*, *rue puante*, and *rue fetide*. Italian names are *ruta* or *ruda*. In Persia, the plant is called *aspand*.

Appearance

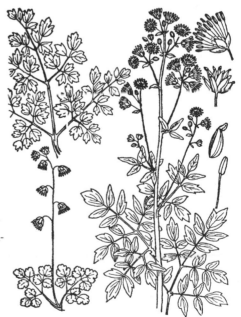

Rue is easily confused with other strong-smelling plants until the harvester becomes better acquainted with its unique odor. It is evergreen, and bushy, but not too large, only growing to a maximum height of 3 ft. It gives off a somewhat fruity smell when only lightly disturbed, but when crushed or agitated exudes a powerful musk similar to that of a tomcat, and the odor remains on the skin. Its taste is bitter, biting and unpleasant, to some people even nauseous. Rue has woody, fibrous roots, and a round, hard, upright stem. Its leaves do not grow in pairs, but are staggered on the stalk. They are an unusual gray-green or blue-green color, and tough and fleshy in texture, but relatively small. They resemble the clubs of a pack of playing cards, three-lobed. Rue leaves and flowers are dotted with oil glands. Rue flowers are small, and yellow, golden, or greenish-yellow in color.

Place, Season, and Useful Parts

Rue has been cultivated for centuries in most of Europe. Garden rue originally came from the Mediterranean region, and still grows wild there on rocky hillsides. It can also be found growing wild as a garden escape in vineyards and gravel pits, on rough, stony ground, or on ash heaps. Rue blossoms from June on into September, and the entire plant is gathered without roots before the flowers open fully.

Gathering, Drying, and Storage

The flowering tops of the rue plant are gathered before the flowers open. Old herbals are very particular about the rituals that must be observed while gathering the plant. Rue should never be harvested by menstruating women or cut with iron. It should not be touched with bare hands, and should never, ever be brought into contact with a cat. One author recommends smearing a salve of poison hemlock on one's hands to counteract the dermatitis sometimes caused by the herb's ethereal oils. (Note: this has not been confirmed by modern research. A much better method is simply to wear gloves when working with the plant if your skin is sensitive.)

Rue should be dried rapidly in the shade in a warm, airy place. Turning the leaves helps to speed the drying process. Rue keeps well, and can be stored in wooden containers.

Seed Saving and Germination

There is much more diversity than one would expect between different rues, for many local variants exist. The plant is usually propagated by seed, which germinates readily after a cold period, especially if the soil temperature is high enough.

Gardening Hints

Rue is so easy to grow that it may become a nuisance in the garden, especially because it does not exert a beneficial influence on its neighbors, but can poison the very soil around its roots. If the seeds are allowed to ripen on the plant, it will propagate itself, and choose to germinate in the driest and stoniest part of the garden. It thrives in loose, lime-containing soil, a sheltered situation, and a warm, dry climate. The soil should be fertilized with ashes instead of fresh manure, because rue's sensitivity to frost increases in rich soil.

Rue seeds should be sown outdoors in spring, and barely covered with soil. They germinate very slowly, and may need a cold spell, or a short freeze in a freezer, to allow them to germinate. Ancient Romans believed that they would germinate better if sown with oaths and curses. The seedlings should be thinned or transplanted to allow 1 ft. space between plants, and the beds then weeded periodically. Cuttings or rooted slips can also be taken from established plants in the spring and rooted in a shady place, or a flower pot, and then transplanted. According to gardening superstition, cuttings or plants stolen from another garden will grow better than bought plants (maybe this is due to the extra care given stolen plants—bought plants can always be replaced, but stolen plants are a challenge). Rue is supposed to grow best next to figwort (*Scrophularia nodosa*) or to fig trees. Cabbage, sweet basil, and sage will grow poorly, and even die, if planted next to rue.

Culinary Virtues

Rue is not everyone's first choice of a pleasant kitchen herb. Dioscurides was of the opinion that

> Rue mountainous and wild is sharper than tame or garden Rue, & unfit for eating. And of ye garden kinde, that is fittest for eating which grows near fig trees... being chewed, it ceaseth ye rank smells which come of garlick & onions.[89]

And as Sir Thomas Browne, the seventeenth-century physician and scholar, pointed out,

> Most of the ancient sauces have a wild and poisonous savour, including privet, rue, fenugreek, green coriander and even cumin. I certainly, who think it torture to endure fat gnats and put far from my table cumin seed that is musty with bugs, would have my stomach turned by the sausages, tripe, morsels and coarse greens of Apicius. The table of the King of Ceylon I would likewise let go, or a country mess which even smells of garlic.[90]

Which goes to show how much tastes have changed, and are subject to fashions. Some people certainly do relish the herb, and add it in small amounts to soups and ragouts, and flavor beer with it. They eat it alone or in a mixture, finely chopped on bread or cottage cheese. It is also occasionally used in pickling mixtures.

Rue is one of the most important herbal ingredients of grappas. The Italian distilled spirit owes some of its unusual flavor to the herb's bitter principles.

---

89. Robert T. Gunther, ed., *The Greek Herbal of Dioscurides* (New York: Hafner, 1959), 286.

90. Browne, *The Works of Sir Thomas Browne*, vol. 3 (London: Faber & Faber, 1965), 178.

Household Applications

Rue's unpleasantly pungent smell generally makes it an unwelcome guest in the house. But it may help to drive away even more unpleasant guests: rats, cats, martens, moths, and fleas all dislike the plant's pungent aroma. Because of its antiseptic and rat-repellent properties, rue was widely used as a strewing herb during the plague years. According to some authorities, rue attracts flies; others believe that it repels them. Pliny thought that snakes also fled from the odor of burning rue. Rue can added in miniscule amounts to sachets and moth-repelling mixtures to give them an unusual touch, and can also find its way into insecticidal mixtures, soft soaps, and perfuming agents.

Cosmetic Properties

Rue has a much too pronounced aroma to be highly valued as a cosmetic plant. It can be applied in poultice or cream form as the herb of last resort for stubborn blemishes. It is also rubbed on hands to remove the obnoxious smell of onions or garlic. Rue was one of the most important ingredients of the Vinegar of the Four Thieves (see sage chapter).

Medicinal Merits

Mithridates, the greatest expert on poison in the ancient world, is reputed to be the discoverer of rue's medicinal merits. It was subsequently considered to be the universal antidote to poison. Hippocrates mentioned the plant; Dioscurides recommended a draught of rue seeds in wine to counteract the poison of mushrooms, medicines, serpents, bees, and scorpions (modern herbalists will shudder at the thought!). Pliny praised rue's healing powers against the bites of snakes, scorpions, spiders, wasps, bees, hornets, mad dogs, and salamanders, as well as the poison of Spanish fly and hemlock.

According to the ninth-century herbal, *The School of Salernum*,

> Sixe things, that here in order shall ensue,
> Against all poysons have a secret power
> Peare, garlicke, Reddish-roots, Nuts, Rape, and Rue.[91]

Wahlafridus Strabo, in his herbal, also wrote about rue's powers as an antidote:

> Touch it but gently and it yields a heavy
> Fragrance. Many a healing power it has -
> Especially, they say, to combat
> Hidden toxin and to expel from the bowels
> The invading forces of noxious poison.[92]

---

91.   Sir John Harrington, trans., *The School of Salernum* (Salerno, Italy: Ente Provinciale per il Turismo, 1953), 29.

92.   Strabo, *Hortulus* (c. 840), trans. Raef Payne (Pittsburg, PA: Hunt Botanical Library, 1966), 33.

A few centuries later, John Gerard assured his readers that rue could cure malaria and the plague. According to him, the odor of wild rue is so powerful that it raises blisters on the skin. Until recently, bunches of rue were hung next to English judges to protect them from jail fever.

Women who suffered from incontinence and menstrual obstruction, or who wanted to rid themselves of unwanted burdens, were told by ancient authorities to resort to rue. A wind-filled or badly positioned uterus was treated with plasters of honey and rue. Tyrolean peasants in southern Europe recommended placing poultices of chopped rue and hard-boiled eggs on the stomachs of women having trouble with childbirth. Rue was applied, together with laurel leaves, to infected testicles. Authorities generally agreed that rue had one unpleasant side effect: it could lessen a man's virility. The following passage from *The School of Salernum* makes that very clear:

> Rew is a noble hearbe to give it right,
> To chew it fasting, it will purge the sight,
> One quality thereof yet blame I must,
> It makes men chaste, and women fils with lust…
> Faire Ladies, if these Physicke rules be true,
> That Rew hath such strange qualities as these,
> Eat little Rew, lest your good husbands
> And breed betweene you both a shrew'd disease,
> Rew whets the wit, and more to pleasure you,
> In water boyld, it rids the roome of fleas.[93]

The medicinal employment of rue in ancient times extended even further. Rue, like celandine *(Chelidonium majus)*, was said to clear and sharpen the sight, and was applied with honey and nut paste to all manner of impurities, fungal diseases, blemishes, and pustules, even those caused by the plague. Rue oil was used to treat earaches and the tea was said to ease the chills of fever and to prevent intoxication. Vertigo and St. Anthony's fire were prevented with the help of rue ointments and amulets, and rue was prescribed for agues, sciatica, gout, and dropsy. If a patient sneezed when rue juice was put up his nose, it was taken as an infallible sign of returning good health.

Modern Medicine

Rue is used much more carefully and discriminately in our times, and its sale is restricted in many countries. In the massive doses needed to induce abortions, it is often deadly to

---

93.   Sir John Harrington, trans., *The School of Salernum* (Salerno, Italy: Ente Provinciale per il Turismo, 1953), 55.

the mother as well as the unborn child. It vies with arbor vitae *(Thuja occidentalis)* as the cause of young women's death. Rue poisoning can result in stomach, liver, or kidney damage, narcosis, and death. Because of this, it is usually used externally as a counterirritant to sciatica, chronic bronchitis, or uterine cramps, or administered in homeopathic doses. Rue plasters can help to draw out splinters and heal infections, as well as ease eye and ear afflictions. The seeds are sometimes used as a vermifuge, and minute doses of rue tincture are given to the nervous and hysterical. Rue's active principles can be extracted better with water than with alcohol. Rue tea should only be allowed to steep for five minutes, and it is better to make it too weak than too strong. Pregnant women, convalescents, and children should avoid the use of rue altogether.

A homeopathic essence of rue is given to gouty patients, or those suffering from neuralgia, rheumatism, and menstrual disorders. It is a remedy for optic nerve inflammation, but also for lumbago, and slipped or herniated discs. It has a healing effect on injured joints and tendons as well as bruised bones and fibrous tissue. Eyestrain and ganglions of wrists are also treated with rue.

Uses in Husbandry

Rue is generally used as a preventive herb to drive rats and witches away from stalls, cats away from dovecotes, and martens and rats from chicken coops. For some strange reasons, bees are very partial to the strong-smelling herb, and visit it avidly. Sweetened rue tea may be fed to the insects in winter.

Dioscurides and Pliny observed that wild goats improved their eyesight with rue, and therefore recommended the herb to gem-cutters, painters, sculptors, writers, and students for their eye complaints.

Veterinary Values

In general, modern veterinarians are somewhat reserved toward the herb because of the unreliability of individual reactions. When dealing with rue, the same caution is called for with animals as for humans. Some animals will develop an allergic reaction to it, some will react negatively to it, and pregnant animals should not be given rue at all. Marjoram and oregano can be used in place of the herb if it is too strong. If it is tolerated, though, it is a potent antiseptic that can be life-saving. It is also helpful in the treatment of hysteria and extreme nervousness, and can counteract some poisons. A rue and rosemary infusion is used externally to treat wounds and gently disinfect them. Rue is a natural worm-repellent, especially in combination with garlic, and can be included in preventive "pills." Rue is also an important insect-repellent herb. The leaves are fed to poultry to prevent croup. Pliny once prescribed rue for animals suffering from shortness of breath.

Miscellaneous Wisdom

Folk authorities are of the opinion that rue can drive away witches, demons, elves, and the devil. It can help keep cats away from chicken meat, counteract sorcery and protect against the Evil Eye, avert lightning, and even, in Greece, protect the user against the nervous indigestion caused by eating in front of uncanny strangers. The inhabitants of Friuli believe that demons can be forced into submission with rue gathered on Midsummer's Eve. In Galicia, rue is considered a dark, sad plant. Slavs prefer wild-growing mountain rue to garden rue for magical purposes. Germans included the herb in the magical *Kräuterbüschel* gathered on Assumption Day and blessed in the church. In the Germanic countries, a candle made with rue, or oak coals, and a piece of Christmas bread is buried under the threshold with a spell to protect the house against magic. Rue fruits that divide into five segments are considered the best for magical purposes.

Rue is also used in procreative magic. In Germany, the bride carries rue in her shoe when going to the altar. Rue is thrown onto the wedding table, wedding candles are covered with rue, the leader of the wedding procession carries a hazelnut staff decorated with rue, and rue is placed in the wedding bed or sewn into the four corners of the bedspread. Rue was used in love spells, and a concoction of grapes, onions, rue, and theriak was taken to counteract the effects of a love spell or charm. In his *Anatomy of Melancholy*, Robert Burton writes that "Lemnius admires Rue, and commends it to have excellent virtue, to expel vain imaginations, Devils, and to ease afflicted souls."[94]

Rue, otherwise known as the herb of grace, was also used to sprinkle holy water during exorcisms. It was placed on coffins to protect the dead, and some Austrians still believe that a sprig of rue placed on a corpse's chest will turn to gold on Judgement Day. In the Middle Ages, rue was employed as a hallucinogen capable of conferring the gift of second sight. According to Pliny, weasels eat rue before giving battle to snakes to protect themselves against poison. Bartholomaeus extended this belief to include basilisk-fighting weasels.

Legends

Some Swiss believe that the herb of grace attained its healing powers when the Virgin Mary hid the rags stained with her first monthly "flowers" under the plant.

Another legend, from Tyrol, tells of how the devil abducted a young girl, but was then robbed of his prize by the rue she carried with her. In his anger, frustration, and disappointment, he yelled, "Rue, you herb true and tried, You've robbed me of my bride!"[95]

---

94. Burton, *The Anatomy of Melancholy* (1621) (London: Tudor, 1977), 567.

95. Hanns Bächtold-Stäubli, ed., *Handwörterbuch des deutschen Aberglaubens* (1927–42), vol. VII (Berlin: Walter de Gruyter & Co., 1987), 546.

Literary Flowers

Queen: *"Gardener, for telling me this news of woe,*
Pray God the plants thou graft'st may never grow."
Gardener: *"Poor Queen! so that thy state might be no worse,*
I would my skill were subject to thy curse. -
Here did she fall a tear; here, in this place,
I'll set a bank of rue, sour herb of grace:
Rue, even for ruth, here shortly shall be seen,
In the remembrance of a weeping queen."

—William Shakespeare, *King Richard II*, III.iv

There lived a carl in Kellyburnbraes,
Hey and the rue grows bonnie wi' thyme,
And he had a wife was the plague o' his days,
And the thyme is wither'd and rue is in its prime.

—"Kellyburnbraes" (Robert Burns' version)

There's rue for you; and here's some for me: we may call it herb-grace o' Sundays:-
O, you must wear your rue with a difference.

—William Shakespeare, *Hamlet*, IV.v

Plant laurels all around, and fragrant thyme;
Set out a crop of pungent savory,
And violet beds to drink the trickling spring.

—*Virgil's Georgics*

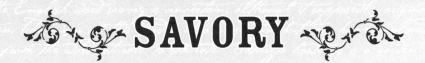

Name

The derivation of the English word "savory" is uncertain, although it supposedly originated from the plant's Latin name, *satureia*. The origin of this word is also uncertain — it may have evolved from the Greek word for satyr, but also from the word *saturare*, to saturate. *Satureja hortensis* is a garden savory, and *Satureja montana* a mountain herb.

Savories are members of the ***Lamiaceae***, or **Mint**, family. The garden (or "summer") savory, an annual, is often grown in the south where it will readily seed. The mountain (or "winter") savory, a perennial, is less aromatic but an obvious choice for more northern locations. The two are often confused in folk parlance, and some folk botanists also believe that hyssop is a savory. This is not the case, although all three do belong to the same botanical family.

Some aromatic herbs from southeastern Europe, such as *Micromeria croatica*, were once classified as savories. A Mexican savory is also cultivated in Central American gardens.

Folk Names

Germans call the summer savory *Bohnenkraut, Kuttelkraut, Kalbhyssop, Eselspfeffer, Bergminze, Wirbeldost, Hühnerfüll, Weinkraut,* or *Pfefferkraut,* occasionally confusing it with hyssop, oregano, or other members of the **Mint** family. The French know summer savory as *sarriette annuelle, savourée,* or *sadrée,* and Italians call the herb *santoreggia, coniella,* or *savoreggia.* The Spaniards call it *ajedrea;* the Dutch, *bonenkruid;* and the Irish, *sáibhre.* Summer savory is called *Čaber sadovyj* in Russian.

Winter savory is known in German as *Winterbohnenkraut*, and even more confusion about its name exists in folk parlance than is the case with summer savory. French speakers call it *sarriette vivace*, and Russians, *Čaber zimnij* or *Čaber krymskij*.

Appearance

Summer savory plants have a spiky, needle-like appearance, similar to rosemary, because the leaves often roll up when dry. They are much smaller than rosemary plants. Winter savory is smaller, more compact, and bushier, with broader, shinier, and more pointed leaves.

Summer savory reaches a height of at most 2 ft. The entire plant has a strong and spicy smell reminiscent of camphor, especially when the leaves are disturbed. This is due to the ethereal oil present in tiny oil glands on the narrow leaves. Summer savory has small, yet stringy and sturdy roots, and its stems are hairy and woody, tinged with red. The leaves are short, oblong, and pointed, resembling a spear's head, and are of a dark green or grayish color often tinged with purple or red. The plant's flowers appear in groups of five. They are usually white, pink, or blue with a pink blush, and their color may vary from one branch to another on a single plant. The seeds are gray-green to dark brown in color.

Winter savory is similar to summer savory, but generally darker in color, and much smaller, only 1 ft. high. The stems and branches are very woody and may grow to be thick. The leaves are hard and stiff, and look as if they have been pierced with a pin, like the leaves of St. John's wort. The small flowers are of a purple or white color with a yellowish cast.

Place, Season, and Useful Parts

Summer savory is a cultivated plant, and can rarely be found in the wild. It blossoms from July through September. Winter savory is often cultivated, but also escapes easily from cultivated areas. It originally came from southern and eastern Europe, and can still be encountered there and in other areas, on cliffs and railroad embankments, or in fields and graveyards, to an altitude of 3,750 ft. Winter savory flowers shortly before the summer varieties, which makes it easier to harvest viable seeds in the north.

Gathering, Drying, and Storage

It is wise to keep a few savory plants for continued cut-and-come-again kitchen use, and a few plants as harvest plants for winter use. The harvest plants are cut just before the plant begins to blossom, in June or July. The last winter savory harvest should be cut before the end of July, so that the plants will have time to recover before the first frosts. Winter savory can also be transplanted to pots for winter use.

Savory should be hung in small bundles in an airy, shady place to dry, then stripped off the stems and stored in airtight containers. It is one of the very few herbs whose aroma and flavor *increases* with drying.

Seed Saving and Germination

Savory seeds generally only remain viable for 2–3 years. There are several distinct varieties that will all cross with each other if allowed to pollinate openly. The different varieties can vary widely in oil content and aromatic properties, and there are several local varieties and species, especially in southeastern Europe. Winter savory is usually propagated through cuttings and root division, and the variety will remain true to type if the plants are not allowed to self-seed. Summer savory varieties must be isolated from one another if the seed is to remain unmixed. Isolation can be temporal, with staggered blossoming times, or it can be spatial, separating different varieties so that bees will not visit both varieties and transfer pollen. Herb growers can also isolate varieties by caging them with insect-proof row cover or very fine insect mesh over wooden or wire frameworks, and then introducing bees to pollinate the flowers.

Gardening Hints

Summer savory is an annual plant that thrives in a moist, warm places. It is sown directly outdoors in March to May, depending on the climate, and covered lightly or as little as possible, but kept moist. Germination is slow (2–3 weeks), and the plants do not respond well to transplanting. Savory prefers rich, light, but not freshly fertilized soil in full sunlight, and regular watering. It will tolerate dry, alkaline conditions. The seedlings should be thinned to a distance of 6 in. between plants. If left without thinning, the plants will be spindly and develop few leaves. Some cooks like to sow the seeds later, particularly in warmer climates, so that the savory will be ready to harvest just as beans begin to ripen. Summer savory will suffer from drought, and is also sensitive to frost, dying back after the first cold snap.

Winter savory is a perennial plant grown from seed, cuttings, or plant division. It grows best in lime-rich, stony, poor soil, or in mountainous areas. The seeds are sown in spring in trays or outdoors like those of the summer savory, and the roots are divided in March or April. Seedlings are transplanted to their final position, with at least 1 ft. between plants. Germination may be erratic. Cuttings of side shoots with a woody heel should be taken in summer, and then placed under a hand glass until roots form. Winter savory must be clipped back in late summer to prevent the stems from turning too woody, and to keep the plants bushy. Woody plants, and plants that have been cut back too late in the year, succumb much more easily to frost. A little winter protection is advisable in areas with alternate freezing and thawing, especially in spring.

Both savories grow well together with beans and aid their growth. They can also be planted as border plants around onion beds with good results.

Culinary Virtues

Winter and summer savory are both excellent peppery seasoning herbs. Summer savory is usually used fresh, although it also dries well. Winter savory's leaves are a little tougher, and less aromatic; they are usually used in well-cooked stews, soups, and other savory dishes.

Savory is the bean herb *par excellence*. The German name *Bohnenkraut* says it all: it should be included in all bean dishes. It helps to stimulate the digestive glands, warms the stomach, has a positive effect on the secretions of the gall bladder, and can ease the feelings of fullness and flatulence that often follow a bean meal. Its flavor complements beans, and it will even aid the growth of the bean plants if planted next to them.

Savory was once used in combination with onions and garlic to preserve foods that otherwise would not keep very well, such as salami or sausages. Today, it is often used in herbal salt substitute mixtures. It is an excellent addition to most legumes and pulses, and can also be used to season soups, sausages, egg dishes, stuffings, dips, and cottage cheese or cream cheese mixtures, pork pies, meatloaves, split pea soup, stuffed zucchini, salads, lentils, cooked cauliflower, eggplant, squash, tomatoes, cabbage, and turnips. The strong odors of these vegetables are tempered by savory. Savory can be rubbed onto cuts of meat before roasting, or added to chicken, fish, or lamb dishes. A mixture of juniper berries, laurel leaves, fresh sage, thyme, and savory is an excellent seasoning for game. A pinch of powdered thyme, marjoram, and savory can also be added to breadcrumbs to create an aromatic breading mixture. The ancient Romans made extensive use of savory vinegar, which is still employed as pickling vinegar.

Noteworthy Recipes

French Beans: The simplest, and tastiest method, of preparing string beans is with savory. Tail and string the beans, wash, cut into mouth-size pieces, and place in a saucepan. Add only enough slightly salted water to cover the bottom of the pan, several sprigs of fresh savory (summer savory is usually used, but winter savory is also fine), and 2–3 cloves of garlic, peeled and cut into slices. Steam under medium heat until the beans are soft, but don't fall apart. Beans prepared this way are easier to digest, and have a pleasant "beany" flavor.

Household Applications

It was once widespread practice to sprinkle rooms infested with fleas and bedbugs with savory tea, or to strew savory on the floor. Moths also dislike the smell of savory, and it is used in moth-repelling sachets for linen closets. The root latex of winter savory has been used as chewing gum in times when nothing else was available. Summer savory can be added to invigorating and aromatic herbal baths.

Medicinal Merits

According to Otto Brunfels, savory is a hot, drying medicine, very similar to thyme in its medicinal properties. Its primary use in the Middle Ages was as an aphrodisiac, to increase the sexual vigor of men, and as an effective healing herb for female complaints. Summer savory was considered a food suitable for pregnant women, and was considered capable of counteracting poison and sorcery.

Modern Medicine

Summer savory is the savory recommended in all herbals for medicinal use; winter savory is rarely mentioned, although it is medicinally very similar. Savory has a positive influence on the entire digestive system. It can help to increase the appetite, strengthen the stomach, liver, and especially the gall bladder, and remove obstructions. It counteracts stomach cramps, colics, and flatulence, lessens diarrhea and nausea, and discourages worms. Savory and bean hull tea are particularly helpful for diabetics, helping to regulate blood sugar levels. It is also the seasoning of preference for diabetics. Savory is further believed to exert a mildly stimulating influence on the bladder, to provoke perspiration, strengthen the nerves, ease breathing and help loosen a cough. Gargling with savory tea is recommended for those with swollen tonsils, or for patients recovering from having their tonsils removed. Savory is employed externally on boils and itching insect bites, and the fresh juice of the plant can be used as eardrops.

Uses in Husbandry

Savory, like lemon balm, is an excellent bee herb, avidly visited by the insects. It can also, like lemon balm, be rubbed onto bee or wasp stings to lessen the pain. In ancient times, savory was given to donkeys as an aphrodisiac. Modern veterinary medicine prescribes savory tea for animals with cramps or diarrhea.

Miscellaneous Wisdom

The ancient Greeks believed that the odor of savory was reminiscent of satyrs, and would cause all nymphs to flee. It would be interesting to see if modern-day nymphs react in the same fashion. There may even be a market for such a repellent.

Literary Flowers

Where the bees may stop to dry their moistened wings
In the Summer sun …
Plant laurels all around, and fragrant thyme;
Set out a crop of pungent savory,
And violet beds to drink the trickling spring.

— VIRGIL'S GEORGICS, BK. IV

Docken in and nettle out,
Like an auld wife's dish clout.

—AN ENGLISH SAYING

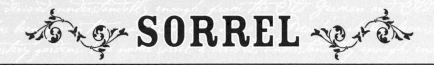

SORREL

Name

The name "sorrel" is derived, understandably enough, from the Old German and Old French words for "sour." In folk botany, little differentiation is made between the various sorrels, with a few notable exceptions. This leads to a confusion of folk names, especially since the terms "dock," "rhubarb," "spinach," and "sorrel" are used interchangeably.

The sorrels are perennial plants and members of the **Buckwheat** family *(Polygonaceae)*. Some of the most important members of this family are:

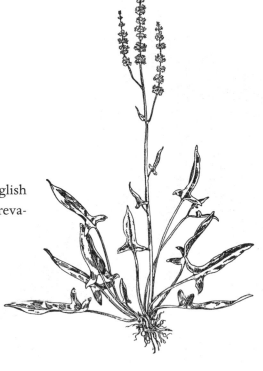

Rumex acetosa: Garden sorrel

Rumex acetosella: Sheep's sorrel

Rumex alpinus: Mountain rhubarb

Rumex crispus: Curled dock

Rumex hydrolapathum: Great water dock

Rumex hymenosepalus: Tanner's dock

Rumex obtusifolius: Dock, wild patience

Rumex patientia: Patience dock

Rumex scutatus: French sorrel

Rumex vesicarius: Bladder dock

(*Rumex alpinus* has been given the quaint English name of "monk's rhubarb" because of the prevalence of the plant in monastery gardens.)

Folk Names

The sorrels, and especially *Rumex acetosa* (garden sorrel), are also known as dock, sour dock, sour grass, sour sabs, sour sops, sour suds, sourrock, sour leaves, sour salves, sour lick, cuckoo sorrow, cuckoo's sorrel, cuckoo's meat, cock's sorrel, dock seed, donkey's oats, gypsy's baccy, green snob, lammie sourdocks, London green sauce, redshank, red sour leek, sallet, soldiers, sorrow, sow-sorrel, bread and cheese, brown sugar, green sauce, sour sauce, Tom Thumb's thousand fingers, and wood sour. German names are *Sauerampfer*, *Sauersenf, Saustompfer, Sauerkraut*, and *Sau-pompfer*. French terms are *oseille, oseille commune, grande oseoille, surelle, surette*, and *vinette*. Italians call it *acetosa, lapazio, saleggiola, pan e vin*, and *pan cúch*; the Dutch, *amper*; the Spaniards, *acedera* and *vinagrella*; and the Russians, *ščavel obyknovennyj*.

Rumex acetosella (sheep's sorrel) is also called field sorrel and sheep sorrel. It is known as *kleiner Sauerampfer* in German; *petite oseille, oseille sauvage, oseille des prés, oseille de brebis*, and *vinette sauvage* in French; *acederilla* or *cizana* in Spanish; and *acetosella* in Italian.

Rumex alpinus (mountain rhubarb) is also known as monk's rhubarb, butter leaves, alpine dock, and lapatium; *Mönchs-Rhabarber* and *Alpen-Ampfer* in German; *patience des Alpes, rhubarbe des moines*, and *rumex des Alpes* in French; *rabarbaro alpino* in Italian; and *ščavel al'pijskij* in Russian.

Rumex crispus (curled dock) is a synonym for yellow dock; it is *krauser Ampfer* in German, and *lengua de vaca* and *hualtata* in Spanish.

Rumex hydrolapathum (great water dock) is also known as gabo, wild rhubarb, and red dock; in German, *Flußampfer* and *hoher Ampfer*; and in Spanish, *paratella*.

Rumex hymenosepalus (tanner's dock) is called wild rhubarb, pie dock, sour dock, red dock, and sand dock. In Spanish, it is *canaigre*, and in Russian, *kanegra* and *ščavel severo amerikanskij*.

Rumex obtusifolius (dock) is also called common wayside dock, butter dock, and bitter dock; in German, it is *großer Ampfer, Blacke*, and *Saukraut*.

Rumex patientia (patience dock) is, to heighten the confusion, also called monk's rhubarb, garden patience, herb patience, spinach dock, or passion's dock. German names are *Gemüseampfer, ewiger Spinat, Gartenampfer, englisher Spinat*, and *Winterspinat*. French terms are *patience, épinard oseille, épinard immortel*, and *oseille d'Amerique*; in Russian, it's *ščavel špinatnyi*.

Rumex scutatus (French sorrel) is known as French garden sorrel and buckler-shaped or buckler-leaved sorrel. German names are *Schildampfer, schildblättriger Ampfer, römischer Ampfer*, and *französischer Spinat*; French, *oseille ronde* and *patience á écousson*; Italian, *erba pan e vin*; Russian, *ščavel ščitkovidnyj*.

Rumex vesicarius (bladder dock) is also called *ščavel puzyčratyj* in Russian and *chukra* or *chuka* in Hindi.

Appearance

Garden sorrel grows to a maximum height of 3 ft. It is characterized by long, dark green leaves punctured with snail holes, slender, red-tinged stalks, and reddish seed clusters in the late summer and fall. As Culpeper says,

> the leaves are smooth, succulent, and tender, long and sharp-pointed, ending next the footstalks in two sharp ears like spinach, of a very sour taste; the stalk is long and slender, set with two or three smaller leaves, and at the top a long reddish spike of small staminous flowers, succeeded by small shining three-square seed. The root is about a finger thick, branched and full of fibres, of a yellowish brown colour, abiding several years.[96]

Most of the other sorrels are large-leaved, similar to garden sorrel, with the leaves centered around the flower stalk, which sports the characteristic red sorrel flowers and seeds.

Sheep's sorrel differs somewhat from its large-leaved cousins. It grows to a maximum height of 1 ft., and the leaves are found along the stalk instead of the root. Sheep's sorrel leaves are much smaller than those of other sorrels, and they resemble barbed spearheads. French sorrel is characterized by medium-sized, fleshy, gray-blue-green leaves, which form a compact bush. The shape of the leaves is different from the other sorrels, broader, and shield-shaped.

Place, Season, and Useful Parts

The sorrels grow in temperate zones in Europe, Asia, and North and South America to an attitude of 6,000 ft. They are such persistent meadow and pasture weeds that entire landscapes can be colored red by the seeds' stalks in autumn. They prefer damp places and soils with high iron content, but will grow almost anywhere, beside brooks and burnt-out fires, among bracken, in abandoned pastures, in ditches and dry gravelly places. The only places they can never be found is in the tropics and deserts. The sorrels bloom from spring on into summer, and sometimes again in the fall.

Gathering, Drying, and Storage

A rule of thumb to follow while gathering sorrel is: always taste the leaves before gathering them. None of the sorrels are poisonous, but some are acridly and unpleasantly bitter and it is easy to confuse species and varieties. Because of the difficulty in identifying the plants, and the tedious work necessary to gather the small-leafed wild varieties, many people prefer to cultivate sorrels. Young sorrel leaves should be gathered

---

96. Culpeper, *Culpeper's Complete Herbal* (1653) (London: Foulsham, undated), 399.

singly from early spring through June, before the plant sends up flower stalks. Leaves harvested late in the year are much bitterer, and sourer, than young leaves.

Sorrel leaves can be dried in a warm, airy place for medicinal use; sorrel roots should be brushed to remove dirt and, if necessary, washed, split, and then hung up to dry.

Sorrel can be preserved for kitchen use in the same way as spinach: canned and processed, or blanched for two minutes and frozen. Some cooks preserve sorrel in crocks in the cellar, sealed with clarified beef fat and parchment paper. But freezing is preferable, since the high vitamin content is best preserved this way, and there is little danger of spoilage.

Seed Saving and Germination

In Russia, sorrel is such a favorite soup plant that breeding programs have been developed to produce varieties with soft leaves and little fiber, and with a pleasant taste. Unfortunately, these programs are now endangered, due to lack of financing.

Since most people only keep one sorrel variety for seed, it is fairly easy to maintain pure strains. Cut the plant back until all the wild sorrels of the same species have stopped blossoming, and only then let it go to seed. The resulting seed will be true-to-type. Or keep the plants in an unheated glasshouse or cold frame, and let them blossom earlier than the wild varieties. Cultivated varieties can also be propagated by plant division in fall.

Not all sorrel fruits contain seeds. It is good to look at the ripening stalks with a magnifying glass to discover the small seeds. The stalks can be gathered before the seeds ripen fully, and dried on paper or cloth. The plants must be dried in a very dry place (but not a dehydrator), because sorrel leaves absorb water and the plant parts remain damp under normal conditions.

Gardening Hints

Wild sorrel is a hated garden weed, but cultivated sorrel can be one of the most welcomed spring greens. The cultivated varieties are very frost-hardy, and produce succulent green leaves as soon as the ground begins to warm up in the spring. French garden sorrel, *Rumex scutatus*, likes light, rich, neutral soil and a sunny, fairly dry situation. Sorrel seeds can be sown outdoors in March or April, and covered lightly with soil, or the roots are divided in the spring or fall. The young seedlings should be thinned, and the mature plants spaced to allow a distance of 15 in. between plants. Flower stalks should be removed as soon as they appear to encourage the production of fresh green leaves. Other sorrels grow best in damp soil. The massive presence of sorrel or dock plants in a field is taken as an indication of the soil's acidity. Consequently, sorrels prefer slightly acid soil.

Culinary Virtues

At the beginning of this century, sorrel was dismissed as being food fit only for peasants. Now, it is considered a great delicacy, and is employed by *nouvelle cuisine* chefs. The popularity of French cooking, and the development of culinary varieties, has led to sorrel's wide acceptance in other countries. In Russia, sorrel is one of the most important vegetables because it is so widely used as a soup herb.

Sorrel is often added to drinks as a substitute for oranges and lemons. As a seasoning, it mixes well with other herbs, or may be used alone, but must always be employed in moderation because of its sour, tangy taste. Some people react to the acids present in the plant, and it may be necessary to boil the herb in two waters before serving it. Sorrel is extremely rich in vitamin A.

Sorrel has been enjoyed in China, Russia, and India for centuries. Greeks, Romans, and medieval monks cultivated monk's rhubarb as a spinach plant in the monastery gardens that served as the model for European cottage gardens. In Lapland, cheese was and still is prepared from sorrel juice and reindeer milk. In Scandinavia, sorrel seeds were ground into powder and baked in bread in times of famine, and the Hebridean peasants also made extensive use of the plant. In Ireland, sorrel was eaten with fish and milk. Breton cooks still prepare a fish soup seasoned with sorrel, chives, parsley, mint, and spring onions. In England, the herb was often cooked, mashed, and combined with sugar and vinegar to make a sweet-sour green sauce.

Today, sorrel is used for seasoning soups, stock, salads, fried eggs, omelets, fish, turnips, and spinach. It can be substituted for spinach in many recipes. Sorrel purée is served with roast goose or pork, or with lamb and veal roasts. Sorrel seeds can be ground into a flour similar to buckwheat (the plants belong to the same family), and added to bread and pancakes. Sorrel juice will curdle milk, and is sometimes substituted for commercial rennet.

French garden sorrel has very soft leaves with little fiber, and grows back quickly, making it an ideal kitchen herb. But wild sheep's sorrel is also palatable, and garden sorrel varieties have been developed with very good culinary qualities. As a general rule, the other sorrels are used as potherbs, and not eaten raw.

Noteworthy Recipes

Cold Sorrel Soup: This dish can be prepared by carefully washing and picking over 1 lb. of fresh sorrel leaves, and chopping or shredding them finely. Cook over a low flame with 1 qt. water until wilted. Season with salt and pepper to taste, remove from the heat, and strain or purée. Let cool, pour into individual bowls, add some finely chopped parsley and cucumber and a little lemon juice. Chill again and serve cold.

Those who prefer a mild soup may want to temper the sorrel's acidity by adding blander leaves such as spinach or lettuce.

Sorrel Salad: Prepare as above, but with less water. Drain the leaves after cooking, and then season with salt, parsley, pepper, a little olive oil, and lemon juice, and garnish with cucumber and hard-boiled eggs. Mild-tasting lettuce leaves combine well with cooked sorrel.

Sorrel fans will want to eat the herb without cooking it, simply adding a few shredded leaves to a normal salad, or serving a mixture of head lettuce, rucola (arugula), sorrel, and chervil.

Creamy Sorrel Soup: A heartier soup can be prepared from preserved or frozen sorrel in winter, or from the fresh leaves in spring. Carefully wash and pick over 1 lb. of fresh sorrel leaves, removing stems if necessary, and then drain and shred the leaves finely. Melt 2–3 Tbsp. of butter in a saucepan, add 3–4 Tbsp. of chopped spring onions, and the sorrel. Heat until wilted, and then add 3 cups of chicken broth. Bring to a boil, reduce the heat, and then let cool. Add a lightly beaten mixture of 2 egg yolks and 1 cup of fresh cream carefully with a whisk into the cooled broth, and then heat the soup again until hot, but not boiling. Otherwise the egg and cream will curdle. Season with salt and pepper, and garnish with chives.

Sorrel purée can be prepared in much the same manner. The onions should be omitted, and the amount of broth and cream reduced by half. Sorrel purée is usually served as a side dish with meat.

Sorrel and Potato Soup: This soup is an even thicker version of creamy sorrel soup. Wash, drain and shred the sorrel leaves as above, and peel and cube 2 lb. of potatoes. Melt 2–3 Tbsp. of butter in a saucepan, and add 3–4 Tbsp. of chopped spring onions, ¾ of the freshly washed sorrel, and the potatoes. Cook over a low flame for 20–30 minutes, adding a little water if necessary. Purée the mixture, replace it in the saucepan, and heat gently. Add 1 cup of fresh cream with a whisk, and then stir in the remaining sorrel. Season to taste. This soup can be served hot or cold.

Green, or Sorrel Sauce: Sorrel sauces are not as popular as they once were, although they deserve more attention. Here is a recipe from the nineteenth century:

Wash and clean a large Ponnet of Sorrel, put it into a Stewpan that will just hold it, with a bit of Butter the size of an Egg. Cover it close, set it over a slow fire for a quarter of an hour, pass the Sorrel with the back of a wooden spoon through a hair sieve, season with Pepper, Salt, and a small pinch of powdered Sugar, make it hot, and serve up under Lamb, Veal, Sweetbreads, &c,. &c. Cayenne, Nutmeg, and Lemon-Juice, are sometimes added.[97]

Green Sauce for Green Geese or Ducklings: Here is another nineteenth-century recipe:

Ingredients. 3 pint of sorrel-juice, 1 glass of sherry, 2 pint of green gooseberries, 1 teaspoonful of pounded sugar, 1 oz. of fresh butter.

Mode. Boil the gooseberries in water until they are quite tender; mash them and press them through a sieve; put the pulp into a saucepan with the above ingredients; simmer for 3 or 4 minutes, and serve very hot.

Time. 3 or 4 minutes.

Note. We have given this recipe as a sauce for green geese, thinking that some of our readers might sometimes require it; but, at the generality of fashionable tables, it is now seldom or ever served.[98]

Versatile Green Sauce: A recipe from the seventeenth century advises,

To make an Excellent Green-Sawce, to serve on any occasion wherein it is requisite:

Take large Sorrel, white bread grated, pared and cored Pippins [apples], some sprigs of Mint, a quantity of Verjuyce sufficient to moisten it [note: verjuice is the juice of small crab apples or green grapes]; and being stamped very small, scrape Sugar on it, and mix it well together, and so serve it up, with Pork, veal, Chickens, Kid, Lamb, Gosling, or the like, they being boiled."[99]

Sorrel Fritters: Prepare a light batter from 2 cups of whole wheat or corn flour, 1 Tbsp. of melted butter, 2 beaten eggs, ¼ tsp. salt, and enough water or milk to make a light but not runny batter, an hour beforehand. Let the washed and drained fresh leaves stand in a little oil seasoned with salt and pepper for several minutes. Press several large leaves together, dip into the batter, and deep fat fry. The sorrel leaves can also be laid out on the table with a spoonful of forcemeat or stuffing placed in the middle, rolled up, and dipped in batter and fried.

Another, sweeter version can be made by preparing a stiff dough, rolling it out thinly, and then cutting out medium-sized rounds. Place a mixture of chopped sorrel, a little lemon juice and some brown sugar on one side of the circle, fold

---

97. William Kitchiner, *The Cook's Oracle* (1817) (London: Samuel Bagster, 1860), 234.

98. Mrs. Isabella Beeton, *The Book of Household Management* (1861) (New York: Farrar, Straus & Giroux, 1977), 207.

99. John Shirley, *The Accomplished Ladies Rich Closet of Rarities* (London: N. Bodington, 1688), 137.

it over, and press a fork against the edges to seal the pouch, just like ravioli. Fry until golden brown in hot fat.

Yet another recipe, this time of a medicinal nature, calls for a mixture of finely-chopped fresh herbs such as fennel, dill, chervil, violets, watercress, sorrel, betony, spinach, and the leaves of black currant bushes combined with just enough crushed zwieback or dried bread to make a dough. Form the mixture into patties, and then fry in butter. These fritters should be eaten in quantity in the spring to cleanse the blood and sharpen the senses.[100]

> *In the making sallets [sorrel] imparts a grateful quickness to the rest*
> *as supplying the want of oranges and lemons. Together with salt,*
> *it gives both the name and rellish to sallets from the sapidity, which renders*
> *not plants and herbs only, but men themselves pleasant and agreeable.*
>
> —JOHN EVELYN, *ACETARIA: A DISCOURSE OF SALLETS*

Household Applications

The sorrels can be of great value to the housekeeper. The large leaves of many docks are good as wrapping material for butter and other perishable foods. The fleshy sorrel roots of the larger varieties can be boiled to produce red food coloring. Sorrel juice, like lemon juice, will whiten and clean hands stained from vegetable matter, and keep fresh fruits such as apples and pears from turning brown. Sorrel salt, or, as it is usually called, the essential salt of lemons, is such an effective whitener that it is used to bleach straw and remove stubborn stains from linens such as rust and ink.

The reddish seed stalks of dock, sorrel, or blood-veined dock can be gathered in late summer and autumn, before they ripen completely, hung upside down to dry, and arranged in vases and everlasting flower arrangements. Several dyes can be prepared from sorrel tops: a dark olive with ammonia or ammonia and ferrous sulphate, a dark yellow with bichromate of potash, a green with copper sulphate, a light pink with vinegar, a brown with ammonia and copper sulphate, a yellowish-beige with chrome, and a yellowish green with tin. Dock roots can be boiled as dye and the wool mordanted with iron and cream of tartar for gray, and chrome for a brownish orange. There is much room for experimentation here, since no dye batch will turn out quite like the last: a wide range of tones can be obtained using only the sorrels.

---

100. Caspar Schroeter, *Allzeit fertiges Haußverwalter rarem Kochbuch* (1712), qtd. in Eva Marie Helm, *Feld-, Wald- und Wiesenkochbuch* (Munich: Heimeran, 1978).

Cosmetic Properties

Sorrel is rarely used today as a cosmetic herb. Otto Brunfels once recommended using sorrel roots to treat leprosy sores, and sorrel baths for the "itch." John Gerard recorded a recipe for a drink made from the roots of red madder *(Rubia tinctorum)* and monk's rhubarb together with senna, anise, licorice, scabious, and agrimony infused in strong ale. This strongly-cleansing and laxative draught was supposed to make "young wenches look faire and cherry like."[101]

Medicinal Merits

In old herbals, sorrels were divided into male and female plants. They were thought to loosen the bowels and, at the same time, to counteract diarrhea. As Horace says, "If the bowels be costive, limpet and common shell-fish will dispel the trouble, or low-growing sorrel."[102] Sorrel seeds were given to dysentery victims as a strong astringent. Monk's rhubarb was used in large amounts as a purgative. The sorrels were also given to patients troubled with eczema and skin diseases, sluggish kidneys, and scurvy. In Italy, juice prepared from sheep's sorrel, radishes, angelica, carline thistle, plantain, and speedwell were considered especially effective as a scurvy cure. Sorrel was further administered to people suffering from ague and jaundice; was taken to strengthen the stomach, cure chronic catarrhs, cool feverish diseases, loosen stones, ease earaches, and stop menstrual bleeding. Sorrel salve was applied to skin eruptions, and the large leaves were warmed together with cabbage leaves and applied to abscesses, scorpion bites, and inflammations.

Modern Medicine

Today, sorrel is mainly used as a depurative, or blood-purifying herb. It is included in spring tonic mixtures, in teas to dissolve swellings and growths, for those troubled with skin diseases, and in blood-building teas for anemics. The seeds and roots of the sorrel plant are astringent and can be used to treat diarrhea; the cooked leaves are cleansing and have a laxative effect. A drink prepared from sheep's sorrel has a cooling effect on fevers, and the root of curled dock is prescribed in the treatment of skin diseases and chronic itches. Sorrel leaves contain large amounts of vitamin C, and are therefore valuable as a spring food, but they also contain large amounts of oxalic acid, which may cause stomach trouble. People with rheumatism, gout, sensitive stomachs, weak kidneys, and

---

101.   Gerard, *Gerard's Herball* [1597]: *The essence thereof distilled by Marcus Woodward from the edition of Th. Johnson, 1636.* Ed. Marcus Woodward (London: Gerald How, 1927), 100.

102.   Horace, *Satires, Epistles, and Ars Poetica*, trans. H. Rushton Fairclough (Cambridge, MA: Loeb Classical Library, 1926).

women with unborn children should avoid the use of the plant altogether. Other patients should only employ sorrel 3–4 weeks at one time, or make use of a homeopathic preparation of the herb for the treatment of colds and coughs. Homeopathic *Rumex crispus* treats enlarged lymph nodes, flatulence, diarrhea early in the morning, and tickling in the pit of the throat that causes coughing.

Uses in Husbandry

Rumex alpinus, mountain rhubarb, is gathered in large amounts in the Alpine regions. The leaves are fermented like sauerkraut and fed to pigs in winter. It should be noted that fresh sheep's sorrel can cause diarrhea and even poison animals if it is fed to them in quantity. Normal dock is also a hated weed in pastures, for it is difficult to eradicate, and robs other more profitable plants of nutrients. Curled dock is sometimes included in herbal tobacco mixtures.

Veterinary Values

According to old folk belief, sick animals should be smoked with the burning seeds of curled dock. The best seeds for this purpose are those blessed in church on Assumption Day. Other German folk veterinarians rub down maggot-infested animals with folded sorrel leaves while reciting a spell.

Miscellaneous Wisdom

The English sometimes call sorrel "cuckoo's meat" because they believe that the cuckoo uses the sour plant to clear his voice in spring. In Germany, old wives caution children not to eat sorrel or they will get lice (this superstition stems from the similarity in appearance between sorrel seeds and lice). An amulet of sorrel seeds is presented to virgins to keep them from having "improper" dreams. Children love to chew and suck on sour-tasting sorrel leaves. Sorrels may be used, like dock, to neutralize nettle stings (see nettle chapter).

The hoary-headed garden companion kisses quick and then goes,
a lasting remembrance of sweet garden days...
—Sister Clarissa

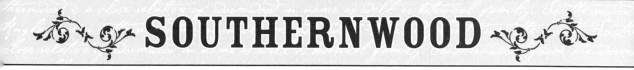

SOUTHERNWOOD

Name

"Southernwood" (from the Anglo-Saxon *sutherne vude*) originally meant "a woody-stemmed plant from the South." Also known as *Artemisia abrotanum*, it is a close relative of wormwood—both in genus *(Artemisia)* and in botanical family (the **Daisy** or **Asteraceae** family).

Although the term *Artemisia* is associated with the moon and Artemis (or Diana), old herbals consistently divide the *Artemisias* into male and female plants. The Bauhin brothers (1600) distinguished three male and fourteen female *Artemisias*. (One of wormwood's folk names was "old woman," and southernwood, correspondingly, was called "old man." The hoary leaves also support the image of the plant as an old man.)

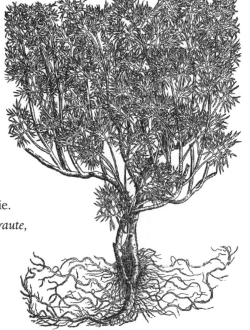

The second botanical name for southernwood, *abrotanum*, is of uncertain origin. It may have evolved from the Greek *abrós*, meaning "thin," or from *ábrotos*, "immortal." *Artemisia abrotanum* is a perennial.

Folk Names

Old man, kiss-me-quick-and-go, kiss-me-quick, boy's love, maid's love, old man's love, lad's love, maiden's ruin, old man tree, stalewort, southern wormwood, sloven wood, and appleringie. Included among the German folk names are *Eberraute*, *Eberreis*, *Gartheil*, *Herrgottskräutel*, *Stabwurz*, and *Hexenkraut*. In Middle High German, the herb was called *Eberreize*, meaning "boar's aphrodisiac." The Italians call the plant *abrotano maschio* or *abrotono*; the French, *avarone*, *aurone*, *abrotone*, *citronelle*, and *garde-robe*; the Turks, *pelina-gaci*; and the Russians, *bož'e-derevo* and *polyn lečebnaja*. Pliny and Plutarch knew the herb under the names *abrotonon* and *habrotanum*.

Appearance

Southernwood is an evergreen shrubby plant, and can grow to 3 ft. in height. The leaves are needlelike and feathery, of a light green color, and much finer than wormwood. The whole plant looks like a pale green upright brush. The plants do not often flower in the north. When they do, the flowers are so small that they are often overlooked. They are almost perfectly round, and hang downward. The odor of the plant when disturbed or bruised is very aromatic, fresh, and lemony, and vaguely reminiscent of commercial disinfectants.

Place, Season, and Useful Parts

Although no final agreement on the herb's origins has been reached, it is probable that the plant came to Europe from the Near East. It grows wild in southern Europe, temperate Asia, and North America. It is cultivated widely in eastern European gardens and to a smaller extent in central and northern Europe. It only occasionally blossoms (July to September in the south) and rarely seeds in northern Europe. The herb tips or the branches are gathered in summer, and the leaves stripped from the stalks. It is not advisable to cut the plant too late in the season, since this will increase the chance of frost damage.

Gathering, Drying, and Storage

Southernwood should be gathered, dried, and stored like wormwood (see the wormwood chapter in the "lunar herbs" section).

Seed Saving and Germination

Several different southernwood varieties exist, varying in leaf color, growth habit, fragrance, oil content, and ornamental value. These should be propagated exclusively by cuttings, root division, or layering to produce genetically identical young plants. If the plants do blossom, it is best to cut them back and avoid seed propagation in order to keep varieties pure.

Gardening Hints

Southernwood has been planted in southern European gardens since Roman times. It was popular in the cloister gardens of the ninth and tenth centuries, and was introduced into England in 1548. It rarely blossoms in northern Europe, but is nonetheless widely grown as a border plant in herb gardens. It prefers richly fertilized, dry soil and a sunny situation, and may be propagated by plant division, cuttings, or layering. Southernwood exudes a strong lemony fragrance if disturbed, and may therefore be placed on the edges of walks and garden paths with good effect. Older plants must be cut back in June or at the latest in July to keep the plants from getting too spindly and lopsided. The trimmed branches can be snipped into smaller pieces, and used as cuttings. Southernwood is not as aggressive as wormwood, but will leach the soil if it is not fertilized regularly.

Culinary Virtues

Those who are delighted with southernwood's pleasant fragrance may be disappointed by its surprisingly bitter taste. Tender southernwood leaves are occasionally used in very small amounts as kitchen herbs because of their lemony aroma. They can be added in small amounts to dip mixtures, included in salad seasonings, or used to complement the flavor of buckwheat dishes. Before refrigeration was widely used, meat that was going "off" was washed with southernwood water to keep it from spoiling completely. Southernwood was also included in breads and alcoholic drinks for its conserving qualities.

Household Applications

Southernwood was added to beer before hops became the officially preferred additive, and the famous *abronite* wine of ancient times was flavored with its leaves. Garlands of southernwood were worn to keep celebrants awake at festivals, and to scare insects away. Peasant women in the Baltic countries carried pungent bouquets of southernwood and tansy to church to combat drowsiness, and British women added lemon balm to these posies. Southernwood is still used to discourage vermin, bees, and moths, and is preferred to wormwood for linen-closet sachets because of its more agreeable odor. The French name *Garde-robe* (wardrobe) shows in what high esteem it was once held as a linen herb. A decoction of southernwood branches imparts a deep yellow hue to wool.

Cosmetic Properties

Modern research and experiments have shown that baldness and hair loss can be due to a multitude of factors: to nutritional deficiencies, hormonal imbalance, heredity, circulatory troubles, infections, fungal diseases, or as a result of serious illness or chemotherapy. A cure that works for one patient will have little or no effect on the next. But southernwood has been persistently included among the herbs thought to stimulate hair growth. It is probably effective as a corrective for nutritional deficiencies, a hormonal regulant and stimulant, and as a circulatory aid for the scalp.

Southernwood can exert a positive influence on hair appearance, and its odor is agreeably pleasant. Dark hair can be rinsed with an infusion of the herb to give it extra sheen. The herb cooked down to a pulpy mass with barley and water can be applied externally to skin impurities or pimples to "ripen" them.

Noteworthy Recipes

Hair Tonic: In the seventeenth century, Nicholas Culpeper suggested that bald men use hair oil made from the ashes of burned southernwood and salad oil to cure their condition. A more effective, and much less messy version of this cure can be prepared from the following dried herbs: 2 parts sage leaves, 1 part stinging nettle leaves, 3 parts nettle roots, and 3 parts burdock roots, 1 part rosemary leaves, 2 parts southernwood, 2 parts birch leaves, 2 parts horsetail, and 1 part coltsfoot leaves. Mix well together. 1 Tbsp. of the mixture should be infused with ½ pint of boiling water and left to cool. When cool, add 1 tsp. of mild cider vinegar, and strain. Apply sparingly and massage well into the scalp. This hair tonic can be applied in small amounts daily, and lavishly before a shampoo to stimulate hair growth and strengthen the scalp. The added vinegar acts as a mild preservative, and the mixture can therefore be kept for a few days if stored in a cool place or the refrigerator. Caution: the lotion tends to darken light hair, and is not recommended for blondes.

Medicinal Merits

The blossoming southernwood plant was once official under the name *herba abrotani* or *abrotonon*, but has recently been omitted from the pharmacopeias. It was used, like wormwood, as an antidote for snake and spider bites, to fumigate rooms, to provoke abortions and women's courses, and as a bitter liver and stomach herb with the ability to expel worms. It was considered a male *Artemisia*. Its mild diuretic properties were well known, and it was valued as an aromatic bronchial herb to relieve coughs, colds, and mild asthmatic attacks. Nicholas Culpeper was a great supporter of the herb, and recommended it for everything from sciatica to eye inflammations.

Modern Medicine

Although officially considered an obsolete drug, southernwood has retained its official position in folk medicine, especially in the eastern European countries and in Austria and Bavaria. It has many of the same medicinal merits as wormwood, and is often taken as a substitute or complement for that herb. The active principles of southernwood have not yet been studied completely, except that they have tonic and antiseptic properties. Southernwood is used to tone the stomach, liver, and intestines, and to cleanse the digestive and respiratory tract of mucus and the intestines of worms. It can help to bring down a light fever and bring on menstruation, and acts as a mild diuretic. All the warnings and restrictions that apply to wormwood also apply to southernwood. It is better to be too stingy when administering southernwood than too generous.

Homeopathically, southernwood is used in the treatment of anemia, scrofula, colic, and gout. Malnourished children who do not thrive, with emaciation of the lower limbs, benefit from *Abrotanum*, as do those with indigestion and a voracious appetite.

Uses in Husbandry

Southernwood is planted near fruit trees to protect them against fruit tree moths, and near cabbages to repel cabbage moths.

Veterinary Values

In many cases, mild southernwood can be substituted for wormwood in herbal mixtures if wormwood causes side effects. It is a strong antiseptic and insectifuge, and can be helpful in the treatment of jaundice or vomiting not related to poisoning, and is often included in worm mixtures, together with wormwood or epazote *(Chenopodium ambrosioides)*. The addition of just a pinch of southernwood to the diet helps to strengthen dogs before conception and ease pregnancy.

Miscellaneous Wisdom

Southernwood is a very important herb for love magic, as can be seen by its many "male" folk names. As Henry Lyte, a sixteenth-century botanist and antiquarian, observed, "Plinie writeth if it be layde under the bedde, pillow or bolster, it provoketh carnall copulation, and resisteth all enchantements, which may let or hinder such businesse and the encitements to the same."[103]

Young men have tried to make their beards sprout with southernwood, and also attempted to attract the opposite sex with its help. In Saxony, men believed they only had to tuck a sprig of the plant under a girl's apron without her noticing it to make her come to them. Unfortunately, the effect was only temporary and wore off quickly. According to North American folk belief, the first man met by a girl wearing southernwood next to her skin would be her husband. A Lincolnshire boy with girls on his mind was told to stick southernwood in his buttonhole when promenading and to ostensibly sniff the plant. He could then present the twig to any girl who took notice of his behavior. If she accepted it, she accepted him.

In the eighteenth century, the aromatic properties of southernwood were considered so potent that bunches of it were hung beside the dock in courtrooms to protect judge, jurors, and spectators from jail fever. The aromatic properties of southernwood are still highly prized by Slavs, who use the herb to expel witches. In the Czech Republic and Slovakia, southernwood is invoked in rituals intended to make hunters sure marksmen, and some northern Germans still believe that anyone who cannot smell a bunch of southernwood

---

103.   Geoffrey Grigson, *The Englishman's Flora* (London: Granada/Paladin, 1955), 117.

must be a witch. Milk can be prevented from spoilage by passing it through a cloth covered with southernwood, and the plant is hung on children as an amulet against worms in some parts of Italy.

Legends

In 1300, a French woman had marital troubles, and went to a witch to ask for her advice. The witch told her to break off a branch of *avarone* (southernwood), and then ask it three times why her husband had mistreated her. The southernwood would have to tell her why things were the way they were, and what she could do to win back her husband's approval.[104]

Literary Flowers

And marjoram notts sweet briar and ribbon grass
And lavender the choice of every lass
And sprigs of lads love all familiar names
Which every garden thro the village claims
These the maid gathers with coy delight
And tyes them up in readiness for the night
Giving to every swain tween love and shame
Her 'clipping poseys' as their yearly claim
And turning as he claims the custom kiss
With stifld smiles half ankering after bliss
She shrinks away and blushing calls it rude.

—JOHN CLARE, *THE SHEPHERD'S CALENDAR*, "JUNE"

---

104. Hanns Bächtold-Stäubli, *Handwörterbuch des deutschen Aberglaubens* (1927–42), vol. 2 (Berlin: Walter de Gruyter & Co., 1987), 528.

*This corner of the farmyard I like most: / As well as any bloom upon a flower
I like the dust on the nettles, never lost / Except to prove the sweetness of a shower.*

—EDWARD THOMAS, "TALL NETTLES"

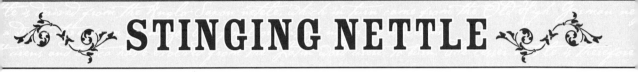

STINGING NETTLE

Name

"Nettle" is derived from the Anglo-Saxon *netele*, which in turn came from the Old High German *Nezzila*, a diminutive form of *nazza*. The final origins of *nazza* are uncertain.

Both *Urtica urens* (lesser nettle) and *Urtica dioica* (greater nettle) are members of the **Nettle (Urticaceae)** family. The terms *urens* and *urtica* both evolved from the Latin word *urere*, "to burn"; the lesser nettle is therefore a doubly burning plant. *Urtica dioica* is called *dioica* because the species possesses two "houses," or distinct male and female plants. There is little medicinal or culinary difference between the greater and lesser nettles, and they can be used interchangeably. *Urtica dioica* is a perennial in most cases; *Urtica urens*, an annual.

Another species, Siberian hemp nettle (*Urtica cannabina*), is used in the preparation of cloth, and *Urtica pilulifera*, or Roman nettle, produces oily seeds used as medicine. Dead nettle (of the *Lamiaceae* family) is discussed in a later chapter.

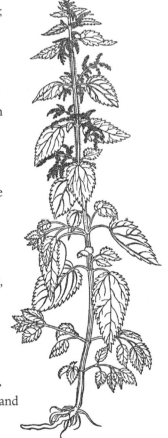

Folk Names

The common, great, or greater nettle is also known as devil's leaf, devil's plaything, hoky-poky, tanging nettle, heg-beg, hodgy-pidgy, Jenny nettle, and naughty man's plaything. German names are *Brennessel, Saunessel, Gänsenessel, Donnernessel, Hanfnessel,* and *Haarnessel*. French call it *ortie, ortie méchante,* and *grande ortie*; the Spanish, *ortiga*; the Italians, *ortica* or *urtie*; the Danish, *nedde*; the Swedes, *nässla*; the Irish, *neantóg*; and the Welsh, *danadl*. It is known in Tessin as *danadl*, and the Russian name is *krapiva dvudomnaja*.

The lesser nettle is not always differentiated from the greater nettle. It is known in German as *Eiternessel*, *Harnnettel*, *Krusenettel*, and *Hafernessel*. French call it *ortie brulante*, *ortie grièche*, and *petite ortie*. The Russian name is *krapiva žgučaja*.

Appearance

The stinging nettle is one plant that most people in temperate climates recognize at once, since they have usually had an unpleasant encounter with it. Stinging nettles can be confused with white, yellow, or red dead nettles, or motherwort *(Leonurus cardiaca)*, but these are healing herbs in their own right.

The difference between *Urtica dioica* and *Urtica urens* is of little importance to the wild food enthusiast or herbalist. The greater nettle grows to a height of 4½ ft. The rhizome is perennial, and is characterized by a deep carotin-rich yellow color. It is round, branched, and crawling or creeping, with many secondary roots. The stem is sturdy, square, and straight, and often tinged with purple. The green leaves form a cross from the stem; have 3, 5, or 7 nerves; and are serrated with jagged edges, becoming more serrated higher up on the plant. All the leaves are hairy and end in a sharp, hard point. Leaf hairs are filled with a burning juice that is released when these brittle hairs are damaged or broken. The plants produce either male or female flowers. The male flowers appear a little later than the female, and are usually larger. They stand upright instead of hanging downward like the female flowers, in an ear that resembles a cluster of millet seeds, only smaller. The seeds are tiny, dark, and oily, and fall out easily.

Urtica urens, the lesser nettle, is a petite version of the greater nettle. It rarely grows over 2 ft. in height. The plant is less hairy than the greater nettle, the leaves are smaller, and one plant can produce both male and female flowers.

Place, Season, and Useful Parts

The nettle is a cosmopolitan plant. It does not grow in the African tropics, most of South America, India, the polar regions, the desert, above 7,500 ft., or in extremely isolated areas. Both greater and lesser nettles prefer well-fertilized soil in the vicinity of human dwellings, barns, garden fences, chicken coops, graveyards, compost or manure heaps, damp woods, hedges, or ruins. The lesser nettle is usually found next to houses, and the greater nettle closer to woods and hedges. Nettles often grow where other plants will refuse to root, and have even been found growing in willows, poplars, beeches, ashes or oaks. According to popular belief, nettles grow where innocent blood has been shed or a corpse has been buried. If farmyard animals are included in this body count, it is probably true. Nettles blossom throughout most of the year in warm climates, and from May to October in northern regions. The young leaves are gathered between April and

August, the seeds from late summer on into the fall, and the roots dug in the spring or autumn.

Gathering, Drying, and Storage

The entire plant or the single leaves are gathered before the plant has attained the height of 1 ft. The harvest can be repeated three times in one year, until the nettle begins to blossom. It is cut with a gloved hand and a knife or shears well above the root, and the leaves are stripped from the stems into baskets without bruising them. The seeds are brushed from the plants with gloves onto cloths as soon as they ripen. It is hard to avoid brushing some of the seeds onto the ground during the harvesting process. The roots are dug commercially in September and October by plowing or loosening the soil and then picking out the roots. In smaller gardens, they are dug with a fork in fall or again in the spring. The fibrous stalks of the greater nettle are cut after the plant blossoms. Care should be taken not to bend the stems. The plants are then subjected to a leaching process, like flax, to lay the useful fibers bare.

Nettle seeds can be dried on paper in shady, airy rooms, and then cleaned with a sieve. The roots should be washed quickly but thoroughly, dried in the open for 10 days, and then hung up to finish drying, or parched in a very slow oven. Nettle roots tend to absorb moisture, and should be stored in airtight containers. In dry climates, the leafy plant can be tied in bundles, spread out fan-wise, and then hung up to dry. In damper areas, it is better to dry the leaves singly on paper or cloth in a dry, airy place. Properly dried leaves are a deep, dark green. They crumble easily and absorb moisture after drying. Therefore, they must be kept in closed containers, or in wooden containers with loosely fitting lids. Nettles can also be dried by hanging them in windows, which has the added advantage that they will repel flies from the room. Dried herb bundles can be stored in a dry, cool place for use in spring as livestock fodder or garden fertilizer. Freshly puréed nettle greens can be frozen for use later in the year.

Seed Saving and Germination

It seems improbable that such a common plant as the stinging nettle should have once been the subject of extensive plant breeding, but this is actually the case. Many different strains and varieties of nettles have been developed for differing fiber content and strength and length of the single fibers, and unfortunately, many varieties have already been lost. These varieties should be propagated solely by root division, or they will cross with each other and with wild plants. If true-to-type seed is nonetheless to be saved, care should be taken to include both male and female (dioecious) plants of the greater nettle, and to use proper isolation techniques.

Gardening Hints

Cloth and paper manufacturers cultivate the greater nettle on a commercial basis. The best plants are tall and sturdy specimens, with long, supple fibers, grown in a damp and sheltered position on rich soil. The greater nettle can be grown from seed, but it is easier to propagate the perennial herb by root division. The Scots once cultivated the lesser nettle as a potherb, but this practice has fallen into disuse.

Nettles are very difficult to eradicate from a field once they have taken hold, which is why so many husbandmen and gardeners consider them a well-rooted nuisance. In their animosity, they forget that even hated weeds can prove helpful in the garden. This is especially true in the case of the nettle: it is second only to comfrey as a compost herb (as long as the plants have not begun to blossom or form seeds!) and as a basis for fertilizing nettle tea. Young nettle plants can be used as mulching material, and growing nettles enrich the soil, help to accelerate the process of decomposition and encourage the formation of humus. Nettles are sometimes planted where no other plants will grow as a guard against erosion, and they are also used to improve the garden microclimate as windbreaks. Nettles attract butterflies and beneficial insects, and are indispensable food plants for many caterpillars. Modern experiments have pointed to their effectiveness in reducing the negative effects of water and earth currents, and even radioactivity (nettles seem to "absorb" radioactivity, cleansing the soil). Companion nettle plants will also stimulate peppermint, valerian, angelica, sage, and marjoram to greater oil production and enhance the keeping qualities of tomatoes. Fresh tomatoes can be stored indoors for a few days on a bed of nettle plants.

A spraying liquid made from nettle leaves soaked in cold water for up to, but not more than, 24 hours contains some of the plants' "sting." If this is sprayed directly onto endangered plants, they will be protected for a short time from harmful insects. Nettle water that has been left for more than 24 hours and has already begun to ferment will probably attract more insects than it will repel, and should only be used as fertilizer.

In Saxony, nettles planted around a cabbage field are thought to discourage cabbage moth caterpillars, and a nettle stalk placed in a field together with a broomstick is believed to protect the crops from birds. According to the Estonians, a nettle stalk should be placed in the ground at planting time and then weighted down with a rock to protect crops against caterpillars.

Culinary Virtues

The stinging nettle is, despite all its stings, a savory vegetable, and can be prepared as a cooked green, soup, or salad. The leaves must be cooked to destroy the prickles, and it is advisable to wear rubber gloves while picking and washing the plant. Nettles are more easily digestible than spinach, and some cooks add nettles to spinach dishes to "dilute" the oxalic acid present in the spinach and make the dish more palatable and nutritious. Nettle salads are prepared from the cooked leaves of very young plants (older plants are gritty), combined with fresh head lettuce, dandelion, or cooked sorrel leaves. Nettles are highly nutritious: they contain many trace minerals, large quantities of protein, and vitamins C and K, and are among the first plants to appear in spring.

Because of these qualities, and also because the leaves taste best when young, nettles are a traditional spring dish in most European countries. Pliny was of the opinion that nettle eating in the spring would keep sickness away all year. Bavarians still believe that a spring nettle meal will help to keep debts away (maybe because it's free food?), and many Germans eat nettles in the spring to better their health and luck for the coming year. Nettles are traditionally served on Maundy Thursday (the Thursday before Good Friday and Easter) in a soup or pancakes prepared from the first green plants of the years: garden chervil, spinach, parsley, sorrel, nettles, daisies, chickweed, cowslip leaves, ground ivy (note: *not* common ivy), dandelion, ground elder (*Aegopodium podagria*, not to be confused with elder leaves, which are poisonous), violet leaves, etc. Although one nettle meal in spring probably has more symbolic than medicinal effect, positive and even amazing effects can be obtained if nettles are served regularly throughout the spring. They are a better source of vitamins and minerals than pills, and have a tonic effect on the entire system. They aid the digestion, help to cleanse the blood of impurities accumulated during the inactive winter months, and are a welcome novel vegetable in the first pale spring days when little high-quality fresh produce is available.

Noteworthy Recipes

Nettle Greens: Only the youngest spring nettles should be used for cooking. If nettles are cut down regularly, they will grow new shoots, which may be used into the summer. In the heat of the year, nettles are gritty, felty, hairy, and generally unpalatable. If the summer plants are cut back, most of them will send up new shoots in fall when the weather cools down. The smallest nettles can be cooked whole, but the stems of larger plants must be removed before cooking. The leaves are washed carefully in plenty of water to remove dirt, and then drained. With kitchen tongs, lift the washed greens into just enough unsalted water to cover the bottom of a saucepan. Nettles, like spinach, will wilt down to almost nothing when cooked. Nettles should not be overcooked, or cooked in too much water, or the nutrients will be leached out. They are simply simmered in the covered pot until the leaves soften. The cooking time will vary according to the amount of greens cooked, but should not exceed 10 minutes. After straining off the excess water, which may be used as a soup base, or even cooled and used as a liquid fertilizer for houseplants, the cooked nettles are seasoned with salt, pepper, nutmeg, and a little butter. Some cooks prefer to purée the cooked vegetable, like spinach, or to chop the leaves and serve them with crumbled bacon. A very tasty soup can be prepared from puréed fresh nettle greens and ramsons *(Allium ursinum)*, thickened with a little cornstarch or mashed potatoes, thinned with stock, and served with a spoonful of mashed potatoes floated in the green soup. Cooked or puréed nettle greens freeze well for use later in the year.

Nettle Pudding: The following is an adaptation of a seventeenth-century Scottish recipe, once recorded by Samuel Pepys in his *Diary:*[105]

Clean one gallon of loosely-packed young nettle tops and shred them finely; slice two large leeks, or a generous handful of ramsons; shred one small head of cabbage; and toss the vegetables to mix well. Place a strong clean muslin (or nettle) dishcloth in a bowl, and alternately layer it with the vegetable mixture and half a pound of rice. Tie the cloth together with a string, leaving enough slack in the bag to allow the rice to swell. Hang the cloth bag in a large saucepan half-filled with strongly salted boiling water, and cook for 25 minutes if a dry rice dish is desired, and 35–40 minutes if a real "pudding" is required. Turn into a pre-warmed bowl, removing the cloth, crown with a pat of butter, and season with nutmeg.

Herb Beer: There are many recipes for herb beer in circulation, and there are many variants of each recipe. Most beer-brewers would agree that the following recipe will give good results the first time, but after that, opinions diverge:

Wash 1 gal. of loosely-packed fresh nettle tops, strain, and bring to a boil in a large enameled pot with 2 gal. of cold water, 2 oz. of crushed fresh ginger root, and the juice and peel of two unsprayed lemons. The leaves of other herbs such as dandelion, goosegrass, cleavers, burdock, meadowsweet, or horehound may be added at this point to vary the flavor, or to enhance the drink's medicinal properties. Boil the herbs and water for 40 minutes, and then strain through cheesecloth. Stir in 2 cups of brown sugar, and let cool to lukewarm. In another bowl, stir 1 oz. of brewer's yeast until liquid with a few drops of water and spread it onto a piece of toasted bread. Float this bread on the surface of the brew, cover, and keep the mixture in a warm place for 6–7 hours. Then skim off the scum and stir in 1 Tbsp. of cream of tartar. Siphon the liquid into sturdy, sterilized bottles without disturbing the yeast sediment with a length of rubber tubing. Cork well with fresh corks that have been softened overnight in cold water. At least ⅓ of the cork should be left outside the bottle, and the corks tied down securely with string. The bottles must be stored in a cool place, or they will explode. They are ready to drink in 2–3 days. It is advisable to chill the bottles before opening. Bottles that have been

---

105.   Pepys, *The Diary of Samuel Pepys*, 2 vol., Ed. Henry B. Wheatley (New York: Random House, undated).

shaken, or stored for too long or in a warm place, may pop their corks or even explode.

If fresh nettle leaves are not available, beer can also be prepared from a quarter as many dried nettle leaves. Nettle beer is a very simple, yeasty beer, and cannot stand comparison with fine ale. People who suffer from flatulence should avoid it, but those with kidney and bladder troubles or kidney stones may profit from it. It is an excellent thirst quencher and has been a traditional drink for farm hands and harvest workers for centuries.

Household Applications

Nettle cloth is often mentioned in fairy tales and legends, and has been a source of wonder and merriment for many readers. But nettle cloth is not a figment of storytellers' imagination: it has been produced commercially over the centuries, and will probably undergo resuscitation in Europe, after the flax and hemp revivals. Various nettle-cloth manufacturing processes are already protected by patent. Large *Urtica dioica* plants have fibers about 1 in. in length that can be worked into rough, sturdy cloth similar to linen and of value as sail cloth.

The first record of nettle cloth manufacture was in 800 AD; the production of *Nesseltuch* (modern muslin is still called by this name in Germany) was widespread in the fifteenth, sixteenth, and seventeenth centuries, and the Scots produced large amounts of household nettle fabric in the sixteenth and seventeenth centuries. In fact, the nettle was also an emergency food for the weavers in industrial Britain, supplementing their starvation wages. Interest in nettle cloth manufacture was revived during World War I. The German government supported attempts to commercially produce nettle cloth as a hemp and cotton substitute, and even issued army uniforms prepared wholly or partially with nettle fibers. At flea markets throughout Europe, it is still possible to find homespun nettle underwear and towels, because the cloth is extremely long-lasting.

Since the Second World War, many attempts have been made to produce nettle cloth on a commercial basis, with varying degrees of success. Nettle fabric can be woven in many thicknesses and textures; its color varies from white to an off-yellow. When new, the fabric is a little scratchy, but it becomes marvelously soft with age.

A green dye can be obtained from nettle leaves, and a yellowish orange color from nettle roots and alum. The green nettle dye is primarily used for woolens, the orange dye for coloring yarn and Easter eggs. The green leaves can also be used to dye woolens, producing tones from gray to yellow to orange-brown, depending on the mordant used.

Nettles are also important dairy plants. Cows fed with carotin-rich nettle roots produce butter of the rich yellow color so desired by dairy clients. Fresh nettle juice can curdle milk and has been used as rennet. Another rennet substitute recipe calls for 3 pints of a strong infusion of the plant, and a quart of salt. Nettle roots have also proved effective in inhibiting the formation of lactic or acetic acid in milk and beer. In 1902, milk women in Berlin placed a carefully scrubbed nettle root in their milk on hot, sultry days to keep it from spoiling. Beer brewers have been known to hang a nettle root on the side of their barrels before a storm to keep a brew from souring.

Other dairy beliefs associated with the nettle are primarily magical in nature. For example, a nettle root is laid in the milk used for the Christmas cheese and then thrown with the whey out onto the dungheap. This is believed to ensure dairy success throughout the year. If milk has been bewitched, or will not turn to butter, the reluctant butter churn is beaten by Bohemians with nettles until the butter comes. The buttermilk is then poured into a hole, a stake is placed in the hole, and the nettles buried next to the stake. In Transylvania, bewitched milk is poured onto a nettle stalk and the stalk is beaten. This will force the witch to appear and undo her spell. In Saxony, nettle plants are addressed with a spell to make the milk turn to butter.

> May God greet you, nettle bush,
> You've got fifty cows, fifty healthy ones,
> Give me the best, let me open the witch's spell,
> Let me take out butter balls,
> If God so wills... [106]

Nettle leaves can be used as non-scratching scouring pads for copper or glass. Nettle juice can also be applied to small leaks in wooden tubs to swell the wood and make the container watertight. Nettle oil can be used as lamp oil. Distilled nettle water is thought to discourage lice, and flies will leave a room if fresh nettle plants are placed in it.

Cosmetic Properties

Nettles, and nettle roots in particular, can help eliminate dandruff problems, stimulate hair growth, and tone the scalp. Nettle roots are the most important ingredient of many hair tonics.

Nettle-leaf tea has blood-staunching, astringent, cleansing, and bracing qualities, and can be used as an aftershave lotion or herbal astringent. Nettle baths and nettle steaming mixtures refresh and help to clear the skin, and nettle tea or nettle vinegar cool skin reddened or burned by the sun. Dirt-darkened hands can be lightened by washing them with the distilled spirits of nettle seeds and then drying them in the sun.

---

106.   Hanns Bächtold-Stäubli, ed., *Handwörterbuch des deutschen Aberglaubens* (1927–42), vol. 1 (Berlin: Walter de Gruyter & Co., 1987), 1554.

Medicinal Merits

Judging from the number of references to nettles in old herbals, they must once have been held in very high esteem. The three major medicinal applications for the herb were as a fever-reducing herb or febrifuge; as a generally purging, cleansing, and diuretic herb; and as an aphrodisiacal herb used for treating female disorders. In the words of northern Italian folk healers,

> Whoever has the little nettle
> Close to the kitchen kettle
> Has a medicine of his own
> To many yet unknown.[107]

According to one Italian herbal, simply holding nettles and yarrow in one's hands is sufficient precaution against illness, fever, and death. A more cautious Pliny recommended the herb as a cure for tertian and quartain fevers. In order to be effective, the roots of *Urtica autumnalis* had to be dug while repeating the names of the patient and his father, and they were then tied to the patient. A widely distributed folk remedy for fevers in general is to strew salt on fresh nettles while repeating a spell against seventy-seven different types of fever. The fever will "dry out" as soon as the leaves begin to wither. Feverish patients were sometimes "whipped" with nettles to bring on a sweat and "break" the fever.

According to Nicholas Culpeper, the nettle "consumes the phlegmatic superfluities in the body of man, that the coldness and moisture of winter has left behind."[108] It was therefore in great demand as a spring tonic and was further used to combat all kinds of growths, swellings, pustules, arthritic complaints, gout, and even cancer. It was eaten to cleanse the stomach; the seeds were taken with honey to open the lungs; it was prescribed against scurvy; the leaves infused in wine were believed to open the brains; and it was administered as an antidote against mushroom, hemlock, quicksilver, henbane or mandrake poisoning, snakebite, scorpion stings, and the venom of mad dogs.

Nettles were also widely used externally. Nettle oil prepared from nettles picked before sunrise was though to protect the skin against frostbite and to ease a hardened stomach; a piece of lint moistened with nettle juice and inserted into the nostril stopped nosebleeds; salt and nettles were strewn on cancerous wounds; smallpox sores were treated with nettle leaves; lumbago was relieved with hot nettle poultices; a plaster of wine and nettles was laid on a swollen spleen; and distilled nettle water, nettle powder, or a decoction of the roots was applied to fresh wounds.

---

107. Giuseppe Delfino and Aidano Schmuckher, *Stregoneria Magia Credenze e Superstizioni a Genova e in Liguria*, vol. 39, Biblioteca Lares (Florence: Leo S. Olschki, 1973), 41.

108. Culpeper, *Culpeper's Complete Herbal* (1653) (London: Foulsham, undated), 250.

As an aphrodisiac, nettle was thought, in Otto Brunfels' words, to "irritate the human body to unchastity."[109] In order to fulfill their marital duties, men and women were advised to eat nettle seeds, onions, egg yolks, and pepper.[110] A decoction of the leaves in wine was believed to "provoke womens courses, and settle the suffocation or strangling of the mother [womb]."[111] Suppositories of myrrh and nettles were introduced into the vagina to induce menstruation. In Bavaria, women with cancer of the womb were told to throw nettle seeds to the four winds before sunrise. Slovakians believed that relief from vaginal problems could be obtained by urinating on fresh nettles. Native American women used the plant to strengthen themselves after a strenuous birth.

> *Tho Nettles stinke, yet make they recompence,*
> *If your belly by the Collicke pain endures,*
> *Against the Collicke Nettle-seed and hony*
> *Is Physick: better none is had for money.*
> *It breedeth sleepe, staies vomits, fleams doth soften,*
> *It helpes him of Gowte that eates it often.*

—THE SCHOOL OF SALERNUM

Modern Medicine

Although many of the older cures are fanciful, if not downright dangerous, the nettle is still called "nature's broom" and is esteemed as a superb tonic and purifying agent. The nettle is one of the most important haematic or sanguinary medicines. It is blood-purifying and cleansing, and a preferred choice for spring cures because of its easy availability. It can aid the formation of new corpuscles, and regenerate blood, and is therefore useful in the treatment of anemia and as a strengthening medicine after hemorrhages, surgery and birth. Nettles can be given to patients with high blood sugar levels with good results. They were once an ingredient of vitamin tonics.

Nettles can help induce menstruation, but can also regulate bleeding because of their high vitamin K content. They are used in combination with rose petals and mullein flowers as a tea for the treatment of bleeding hemorrhoids. Nosebleeds can be stopped with a "plug" of cotton dampened with nettle tea and inserted in the nostril. Nettle tea is a strengthening drink for people with internal wounds and who have been coughing blood, or for women after birth and hemorrhaging, but it goes without saying that further medical help must be obtained in such cases.

---

109. Brunfels, *Contrafayt Kräuterbuch* (1532), facsimile (Munich: Konrad Kölbl, 1964).

110. Ibid.

111. Culpeper, *The English Physician* (London: Peter Cole, 1652).

The nettle works through the kidneys to cleanse the body and rid it of impurities. The most pleasant way to take nettles is in beer form, and this is recommended for those suffering from kidney stones and gravel, or who are under doctor's orders to drink plenty of liquid. Nettle tea is an ideal drink for feverish patients, and can be given to those suffering from rheumatism, gout, or arthritis. A tea made from nettle roots is an even more powerful diuretic than nettle leaf tea, and may be administered in cases of painful water retention. Nettle usually has a laxative effect, but can, under some circumstances, provoke precisely the opposite result. Nettle leaf tea is taken by nursing mothers to increase the flow of milk, and a tea of nettle roots can help to loosen phlegm in the chest or stomach.

New support for the homeopathic principle that like will cure like can be found in the fact that a tea of nettle leaves can help to cure certain kinds of rashes and eczema, in particular the skin ailment known as *Urticaria*. A homeopathic tincture of nettles is used in the treatment of rheumatic gout, asthma, chicken pox, nettle rashes, and swellings of the spleen. *Urtica urens* is employed homeopathically to treat burning pains and burns, bee stings, gout, and rheumatism, as well as problems with the breast glands, and kidney stones. It can be effective as an antidote to allergic shellfish reactions.

- Nettle tea is prepared from 1 Tbsp. of the leaves, or 1 heaping tsp. of the roots for each 2 pints of boiling water. The leaves are brewed with the boiling water and allowed to steep for 10–15 minutes. The roots can be boiled for 1–2 minutes. If a cup of nettle tea produces a feeling of nausea, it is too strong.

Fresh nettle juice is most effective for spring cures. Well-stocked druggists may carry it, or it can be prepared with a juicer and stored in sterilized, sealed bottles for winter use. A nettle-root tea can be used as a gargle for a sore throat, or larger amounts employed to sponge down a sick person. Fresh nettle-leaf tea or nettle tincture may be applied as a soothing lotion for burns.

Special Cures

Spring Tea Cure: A tea mixture for a spring cure can be prepared from the following plants: 3 parts heart's ease, 3 parts walnut leaves, 2 parts each of nettle and dandelion leaves, 2 parts each yarrow and fumitory *(Fumaria officinalis)*, 1 part St. John's wort, 1 part marigold flowers, 1 part each of burdock, parsley, and lovage roots, and, if available, 1 part sassafras *(Sassafras albidum)* roots. The tea is prepared by brewing 2 Tbsp. of the mixed herbs with 1½ pints of boiling water, letting it steep for 10–15 minutes, and then straining into a thermos bottle. This tea should be taken daily for 4–6 weeks.

    The consumption of alcohol and cigarettes must be sharply curtailed, and pork, large amounts of meat, citrus fruits, coffee, tea, and fatty foods avoided for the duration of the cure. If conscientiously followed, such a spring cure can help to purify the blood, cleanse the skin, and combat acne. It can have a curative effect on many skin diseases and give relief to those suffering the first twinges of rheumatism. Last but not least, it can reawaken one's spirits and lead to an enhanced enjoyment of life.

Uses in Husbandry

Nettle fibers are suitable for processing into paper as well as cloth. Twine, ropes, and fish-lines are twisted from nettles. Sugar, starch, and even ethyl alcohol have been produced from nettles in times of scarcity. Chlorophyll was processed from the lesser nettle in Eastern Germany in the 1950s.

Many husbandmen overlook nettles as a possible source of animal fodder because few animals (except asses) will voluntarily eat the fresh plant. But most herbivorous and even some carnivorous animals eat cooked or dried nettles with great enjoyment. Cows, pigs, and household fowl eat dried nettle roots; horses, sheep, geese, chickens, turkeys, goats, and even dogs and cats can be fed cooked or dried nettle leaves as a healthy addition to their diet. According to a Swiss saying, a sick animal is sure to die if he refuses to eat nettles. Horses' and sheep's coats will turn glossy if nettle seeds are mixed with their food; cows, pigs, and horses will retain their good health if fed regularly with nettles; cows will produce more milk on a nettle diet; chickens fed with nettle leaves are said to lay more eggs; and turkeys given meal supplemented with nettles will lay sooner. The manure produced by nettle-fed animals is unusually rich in nitrogen and trace minerals.

In mountainous regions of Java, a local nettle is planted, similarly to hemp in Romania, as a hedge between fields that can be processed into fibers at the end of the growing period.

Another unusual property of nettles is their ability to draw radioactive material out of the soil. Readings after the reactor catastrophe in Chernobyl were much higher for nettles than for most other plants, and these findings were consistent as the years went on: nettles raised on soil with a fairly high radioactive content had consistently higher readings than the soil itself.

Veterinary Values

Nettles are employed in both official and folk veterinary medicine. Nettle fodder keeps animals in good health, and dried nettle leaves can be used as medicinal fodder after bouts of diarrhea, anemia, rheumatism, arthritis, or internal bleeding. Chicks suffering from diarrhea and horses with digestive problems are given dried nettles, and nettle-leaf tea is administered to colicky horses. Cats, dogs, and horses with arthritis can be "whipped" with fresh nettles as a counterirritant, and cooked nettles added to their diet. Dogs troubled with nervousness and eczema can also be treated with cooked nettles. Horses will recover their sheen if their coats are rubbed with a lard and nettle-root salve, prepared like comfrey salve.

In many countries, the entire nettle plant is thought to have antidemonic properties. In Russia, Finland, and Hungary, nettles were hung over stall doors and windows on Midsummer's Day to protect the farm animals from scheming witches. In other areas, nettles were hung over the animal's heads, or they are forced to wear protective nettle amulets. In Czechoslovakia, a nettle was placed on the manure heap on Walpurgis Night (the Eve of May 1st), and beaten with a stick. This was believed to put fear in the hearts of witches wanting to harm the barn animals. In Altenburg, bewitched cows were stroked three times in the name of God from head to tail with three different kinds of pounded nettle roots. The "bewitched" roots were then thrown over the healer's shoulder. According to the Roma (gypsies), the foot diseases of cattle were cured by bending and breaking three nettle stalks through a hedge and repeating the following rhyme,

> This one's for the ox,
> The next one's for the hock,
> And the third one's to make him walk.[112]

Miscellaneous Wisdom

During the Industrial Revolution, food was so scarce in the British Isles that the stinging nettle almost became an endangered species. Many home weavers gathered nettles to supplement their meager diets, and scoured the countryside for anything green and edible.

Because of its burning qualities, the nettle has often been associated with fire, lightning, the sun, and burning lust and love. Midsummer nettles are considered effective against witches, demons, and magic in all of Europe. In Russia, Midsummer celebrants jumped over bonfires, and their cattle were driven through nettle "bonfires" to protect them from witchcraft. This practice was continued until the last century. According to Albertus Magnus, holding fresh yarrow and nettles in one's hand affords protection against all "feare and fantasye." A later writer, Otto Brunfels, believed that holding nettles and chervil could protect against all enemies. In Iceland, sorcerers were beaten with nettles to force them to renounce the magic arts. If nettles grew profusely at a crossroads in Czechoslovakia, it was taken as a sign that witches would soon hold a Sabbath there. Witches supposedly add nettles to their brews so that their sorcery will not be interrupted.

With the exception of the Franconians in Germany, the belief was widespread in Europe that lightning would not strike nettles. In Hungary and northern Italy, nettles were gathered on Maundy Thursday and strewn on the attic floor to keep lightning away. In Germany, nettles were laid on the kitchen fire during a storm to protect the house

---

112. Hanns Bächtold-Stäubli, ed., *Handwörterbuch des deutschen Aberglaubens* (1927–42), vol. 1 (Berlin: Walter de Gruyter & Co., 1987), 1559.

against lightning. A curious extension of this belief came from Prussia: when it thundered, nettles and iron were laid under hatching eggs to keep them from going deaf.

The aphrodisiac, burning qualities of nettles have been recognized for centuries. Ovid wrote of nettle potions believed to lower inhibitions and to increase fertility. Animals, especially prime breeding stock, had their genitals beaten or rubbed with nettles. On the Rhine, a girl is said to be "in the nettles" when she is nubile and willing.[113] According to the Swiss, a girl who has "peed in the nettles"[114] is likely to give birth to an illegitimate child. In Swabia, an old love charm says one must dig a nettle root on Midsummer's Day and then hide it under the altar cloth. The object of one's affections is then rubbed surreptitiously with the root, and forced to listen to three Ave Marias. In northern Germany, the "curly-headed" nettle is invoked by girls to bring them a "curly-headed" lover.

In Roman times, athletes beat themselves with nettles to tone their bodies before contests and races. According to French gypsies, a present of nettles is taken as an encouragement to fight. A century ago in Herefordshire, alder twigs and nettles were nailed to the door of a house of an offensive servant. In southern Ireland, schoolboys still delight in whipping each other with nettles on the first of May, probably a relic of ancient fertility rites. And to round out the list of miscellaneous uses, Albertus Magnus advised fishermen to rub their hands with the juice of nettles and house leeks, and the fish would swim to them.

Oracular Worth

It is said that virgins can touch nettles without burning themselves, and one ancient method of proving a woman's chastity was to have her urinate on the fresh plant. If she was still a maiden, the leaves would retain their virginal freshness, but if she was not, her womanly heat would wilt them. This belief, in somewhat modified form, has survived to this day in Switzerland, where a woman is considered barren if her urine causes nettles to wilt. In Bosnia, young Muslim women use nettles on the Eve of St. George's Day to discover the names of their future husbands.

In the thirteenth and fourteenth centuries, nettles were believed to foretell the fate of sick people. If their urine wilted nettles, or if nettles placed in the chamber pot under the bed wilted, there was little hope. Fresh nettles were taken as a sign of imminent recovery. A white-leaved nettle growing in a garden hedge near the house was taken as a sign of coming misfortune. The Swiss say that a person on his or her deathbed will soon be "in the nettles."

---

113.   Hanns Bächtold-Stäubli, ed., *Handwörterbuch des deutschen Aberglaubens* (1927–42), vol. 1 (Berlin: Walter de Gruyter & Co., 1987), 1556.

114.   Ibid.,1560.

According to Swabian agricultural superstition, nettle leaves punctured with tiny holes forebode hail in summer. If the nettles bloom early, then it is best to sow early; if they grow high in summer, it is taken as a sign that the snow will lie deep in winter.

Herbal Pastimes

Children usually try to avoid nettles, but still manage to get stung, time and time again. Supposedly, nettles will not sting if "picked with mettle" or while holding one's breath. But if one does get stung, wet clay will help to ease the pain, or rosemary, mint or sage leaves can be rubbed into the "sting." The most common remedy is to slowly rub the wounded place with dock leaves (all docks, coltsfoot, and Good King Henry are used indifferently), and repeat a rhyme. Wiltshire children chant,

> Out 'ettle, in Dock,
> Dock zhall ha' a new smock,
> 'ettle zhant ha' narrun [nonc].[115]

In Northumberland, the rhyme goes,

> Nettle in, dock out,
> Dock in, nettle out.
> Nettle in, dock out,
> Dock rub nettle out.[116]

Two other English variations on this theme are "In Dock, out nettle, Don't let the blood settle,"[117] and "Docken in and nettle out, Like an auld wife's dish clout.[118]

In Switzerland, nettle stings are rubbed with Good King Henry (*Chenopodium bonus-henricus*) and the following rhyme chanted:

> In Nomini Patri,
> Rub nettle and nettle petal
> With Good King Henry
> And don't let the nettle settle.[119]

---

115. *Choice Notes from Notes and Queries* (London: The Folk-Lore Society, 1859), 254.

116. Ibid.

117. G. F. Northall, *English Folk-Rhymes* (1892) (Detroit, MI: Singing Tree Press, 1968), 132.

118. William Henderson, *Notes on the Folk-Lore of the Northern Counties of England and the Borders* (London: The Folk-Lore Society, 1897), 26.

119. Hanns Bächtold-Stäubli, ed., *Handwörterbuch des deutschen Aberglaubens* (1927–42), vol. 1 (Berlin: Walter de Gruyter & Co., 1987), 1559.

Literary Flowers

Hoi Marinko, are you going to your mother
to lie down?
Hey nettles green!
I'm not going to my mother:
The covers are short, the night is long,
The North wind blows the whole night through!
Hey nettles green!
Hoi Marinko, are you going to your lover
to lie down?
Hey nettles green!
I am going to my lover:
The covers are short, the night is long,
The South wind blows the whole night through!
Hey nettles green!

—A YUGOSLAVIAN FOLK SONG, INCLUDED IN CESAR BRESGEN'S *LIEBESLIEDER*

One day he saw some peasants busy plucking out Nettles; he looked at the heap of plants uprooted and already withered, and said, "They are dead. Yet it would be well if people knew how to make use of them. When the nettle is young, the leaf forms an excellent vegetable; when it matures, it has filaments and fibres like hemp and flax. Nettle fabric is as good as canvas. Chopped, the nettle is good for poultry; pounded it is good for cattle. The seed of the nettle mingled with fodder imparts a gloss to the coats of animals; its root mixed with salt produces a beautiful yellow color. It is besides excellent hay and can be cut twice. And what does the nettle require? Little as it ripens, and is difficult to gather. That is all. With a little trouble, the nettle would be useful; it is neglected, and becomes harmful."

—FROM VICTOR HUGO, *LES MISERABLES*, QUOTED IN GRIEVE'S *MODERN HERBAL*

The nettle weed is sour and bitter and singes me,
I've lost my fair pretty love, and that's rue to me.

—"A FAMOUS COMPLAINT OF A DISCONSOLATE LOVER,"
LUDWIG UHLAND, QUOTED IN MANNHARDT, *DER BAUMKULTUS DER GERMANEN*

St. John's wort and Dill
Make the storm stay still.

—Swiss folk saying

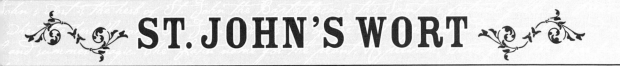

ST. JOHN'S WORT

Name

St. John's wort is the herb of St. John the Baptist, because John the Baptist's festival falls on Midsummer's Day, when the herb blossoms. St. John's wort is one of the most important midsummer herbs used in solstice ritual and summer magic. Known as *Hypericum perforatum*, it is a perennial member of the **Clusiaceae** or **Hypericaceae**, or **St. John's wort**, family. It can be distinguished from other members of this family by its perforated leaves and the reddish juice exuded by the crushed flowers.

The Latin term *Hypericum* stems from the Greek *hyperikon*, which refers to the anti-demonic and anti-spectral nature of the plant. *Perforatum* describes the leaves, which look like they have been perforated by hundreds of tiny needles.

Folk Names

Saynt iohanns gyrs, Saint Johnsgrasse, and Saynt Iohns wurt are all old names for the plant that are no longer in use. The herb is still called hardhay, penny John, rosin rose, tough-and-heal, cammock, amber, and balm of the warrior's wound. Some of the many German names are *Johanniskraut, Hartheu, Tüpfel-Hartheu, Sonnwend-kraut, Mannskraft, Alfblut, Hexenkraut, Teufelsflucht,* and *Liebeskraut*. The ancient Latin term, *fuga daemonum*, pointed to the herb's antidemonic properties, and the ancient Greek name, *dionysias*, to its use in the Dionysian mysteries. The French call it *herbe de Saint Jean, chasse-diable, mille pertuis, herbe à mille trous, herbe aux piqûres,* and *herbe percée*; the Italians, *iperico, scaccia diavoli, erba di San Giovanni, pilatro,* and *mille buchi*; the Welsh, *ysgol grist* and *llysiau ifan*; and the Highland Scots have given it the nickname *ach larson cholumcille*. A Russian name is *zveroboj obyknovennyj*.

Appearance

The St. John's wort of medicinal fame grows to a height of 1–3 ft., its branches spreading out to form a shrub-like plant that is shaped something like an inverted pyramid. The herb is common on waysides and in fields, and takes on a ragged appearance after the first exuberance of its blossom. The herb's two major identifying characteristics are (1) the "blood" that flows when the yellow, flowering tops are rubbed or crushed (other plants that might be confused with the herb will not bleed), and (2) the leaves, which look like they have been struck by miniature lightning bolts or jaggedly punctured with a pin. Culpeper's description of the herb is quite precise:

> Common St. John's Wort shoots forth brownish, upright, hard, round stalks, two feet high, spreading many branches from the sides up to the tops of them, with two small leaves set one against another at every place, which are of a deep green colour, somewhat like the leaves of the lesser centaury, but narrow, and full of small holes in every leaf, which cannot be so well perceived, as when they are held up against the light; at the tops of the stalks and branches stand yellow flowers of five leaves each, with many yellow heads in the middle, which being bruised do yield a reddish juice like blood; after which do come small round heads, which contain small blackish seed, smelling like rosin. The root is hard and woody, with divers strings and fibres, of a brownish colour, which abides in the ground many years, shooting anew every spring.[120]

Place, Season, and Useful Parts

St. John's wort grows throughout Europe and most of Asia to an altitude of 6,000 ft., and has become something of a pest in North America. It is a common meadow plant with a preference for calcareous soil. The most potent plants grow on mountain pastures, but they can also be found on dry, sunny hills and meadows, hedges, waysides, the edges of woods, in light copses and clearings, among underbrush, on moors, sunny heaths, grassy places, riverbanks, cliffs, railroad dams, and on uncultivated ground. The plant flowers from June to August and occasionally in May and September. The flowers alone, or the flowering tops, or the entire flowering plant are gathered when the plants bloom, usually around midsummer. It has been cultivated in Russia, Poland, and East Germany, and is regaining importance as a cash crop because of increased demand.

---

120. Culpeper, *Culpeper's Complete Herbal* (1653) (London: Foulsham, undated), 203.

Gathering, Drying, and Storage

According to modern gathering procedures, the best drug is obtained by cutting off the top 8–12 in. of the plant, before any fruits are formed. Single flowers for St. John's wort oil must be plucked by hand.

Ancient instructions stipulate that you should gather the plant without being seen by anyone and without talking to anyone; you should address the plant before picking it; and you should never, ever cut the plant or touch it with iron. It was considered wise to tell the plant how it was going to be used, and then to repeat an invocation. One sixteenth-century charm was widely used:

> Haile be thou, holie herbe, growing on the ground
> All in the mount Cavalrie first wert thou found.
> Thou art good for manie a sore, and healest many a wound;
> In the name of sweet Jesus, I take thee from the ground![121]

Modern herbalists point out that St. John's wort can cause a hypersensitivity to sunlight. The skin of the sensitive "burns" more readily in the sun, and, in extreme cases, blisters may be raised. People who work with the plant, especially during the harvest, should keep this in mind, and protect themselves with gloves.

The tops of the flowering plant are tied in small bundles and hung up in an airy place to dry. St. John's wort oil keeps best when stored in a cool place in dark glass containers, although its color is so exquisite that a small amount can be kept in a clear glass vial for everyday use and enjoyment. Unless it turns rancid, the oil will retain its potency for two years. Rancid oil must be thrown away.

Seed Saving and Germination

St. John's wort is usually wildcrafted, although it is possible to improve the quality of the herb through selection. Seed should only be taken from the best and healthiest plants. If this selection is kept up over several seasons, and less desirable plants ruthlessly ripped (rogued) out before they blossom, the quality of the plants will steadily improve.

Gardening Hints

St. John's wort is almost always gathered from the wild, for the plants spring up abundantly where they do grow. When the herb does appear in the garden, it is usually treated as a trespassing weed. The rootstock is difficult to remove from the soil, and the plant is aggressive in its search for nutrients, often crippling other plants. If allowed to go to seed, the whole garden may soon be reduced to a forest of St. John's wort. Gardeners should

---

121. Qtd. in Paul Huson, *Mastering Herbalism* (New York: Stein and Day, 1974), 234.

also be careful not to get too much of the plant's juice on their hands while the sun is shining. The unfortunate result may be painful burns, because the juice sensitizes human skin to the sun.

St. John's wort grows best in a sunny position in chalky soil. The larger-blossoming members of this family, such as the Rose of Sharon *(Hypericum calycinum)* are often grown as ornamentals. The seeds are barely covered with soil, and kept moist, but germination is usually erratic, and sowings may have to be repeated.

Culinary Virtues

The plant's Norwegian name, *oelkong*, refers to its employment as a beer flavoring. The practice of aromatizing liqueurs with St. John's wort went out of style several centuries ago, but the custom of laying the herb between cheeses to keep them from spoiling, improve their flavor, and discourage worms has remained alive from Paracelsus' day to the present. The herb should only be used with great caution and moderation as a salad herb because of its strong nature and powerful medicinal properties. The flowers can be used as garnishes, but may "leak" red juice into liquids or oils. At one time, powdered St. John's wort was added to bread to improve its keeping qualities.

Household Applications

Those who place faith in the pendulum will be interested to note that St. John's wort can bring a pendulum to a virtual standstill. Because of this ability, the herb has been used for centuries to counteract the unpleasant and unhealthy effects of earth or water currents running under a house or barn. It is placed in mattresses and pillows to aid fretful sleepers. In the Middle Ages, the herb was hung in bedrooms to prevent nightmares and keep away the nightelf. A modern recipe for a sleeping cushion calls for equal quantities of the dried flowers and leaves of St. John's wort, the leaves and flowers of wild marjoram (organy), chamomile flowers, curled mint leaves *(Mentha spicata)*, rose petals, lavender flowers, and the flowers and leaves of lemon balm, mixed well together, fixed with a few drops of benzoin tincture, and sewn into a pillow covering. The individual herbs in the mixture can be tested for allergic reactions by placing a full bowl of the herb next to the bed overnight. If the herb has an agreeable effect, double the amount in the recipe; if it causes breathing difficulties, omit it from the mixture.

St. John's wort flowers, or the red juice extracted from the flowers, will stain wool and silk a deep yellow, especially if these are fixed with alum. The juice of the entire plant will dye wool a color closer to red. Old seed heads produce a greenish tint. Using stannous chloride as a mordant produces an orange-red; with chrome, the color is yellow-brown. Because of the flowers' sunny color and pleasing aroma, they are often used in herbal sachets and potpourri.

Cosmetic Properties

The rather greasy oil prepared from the flowers of St. John's wort helps to lubricate the skin, and to ease minor aches and pains. It relaxes the muscles, and strengthens ligaments and nerves. It is often used, with the addition of rubbing alcohol, herbal essences, or other oils, as a healing massage oil. St. John's wort oil is applied to fingernails to strengthen and smooth them, to reddened skin to ease the pain of sunburn, and to scars to speed the process of scar formation and to ease itching. It is also used as a liniment or rubbing oil by those suffering from lumbago, rheumatism, backaches, or sore muscles. The oil is applied after bathing to soften dry skin, or a few drops are added directly to the bath water. This will make the bathtub a little slippery, but will ease the task of cleaning it. St. John's wort oil can stain clothes, and should therefore be rubbed in vigorously. A nervine bath mixture is prepared by mixing equal parts of melilot *(Melilotus officinalis)*, St. John's wort, lavender flowers, and rosemary leaves. Four or five generous handfuls of the mixture can be placed in a porous sack hung under the hot water tap, or the herbs are brought just to a boil in a gallon of water and then strained into the bath. The bath bag with its herbs can be dried carefully and reused several times, until it loses its fragrance.

Blossoming St. John's wort is added to steaming mixtures, and applied as a compress to oily or blemished skin. It has a refreshing, invigorating quality that recommends its use as a facial lotion.

Noteworthy Recipes

St. John's Wort Oil: It is wise to go to the trouble of making St. John's wort oil, for the purchased product is expensive and may already have gone rancid on the shelf. In the seventeenth century, John Gerard offered up an interesting recipe (although one that produces a rubbing oil inferior to that obtained by the modern cold extraction method):

> Take white wine 2 pintes, olie olive foure pounds, oile of Turpentine 2 pounds, the leaves, floures, and seeds of St. John's wort of each two great handfuls gently bruised; put them in the Sun eight or ten daies; then boile them in the same glass per Balneum Mariae, that is, in a kettle of water, with some strawe in the bottom, wherein the glasse must stand to boile: which done, strain the liquor from the herbs, and do as you did before, putting in the like quantitie of herbs, floures, and seeds, but not any more wine. Thus you have a great secret for the purposes aforesaid.[122]

---

122.   Gerard, *Gerard's Herball* [1597]: *The essence thereof distilled by Marcus Woodward from the edition of Th. Johnson, 1636.* Ed. Marcus Woodward (London: Gerald How, 1927), 124.

The method approved by modern herbalists uses only the fresh flowers without the stems, gathered shortly before full bloom. Crush a generous handful of these flowers, and place them in a clear glass container and cover with sweet-smelling extra virgin olive oil. Place the closed container in the sun for 7–10 days, and shake it at least once a day. Then strain through cheesecloth or filter paper, squeeze out the excess oil, and repeat the entire procedure. The oil is ready when it attains a handsome blood-red color and smells strongly of St. John's wort. Strain it into a dark glass bottle, stopper well, and store in a cool, dark place. It is a good idea to keep a small bottle of St. John's wort oil within reach of the stove. Any minor cuts or burns treated immediately with this oil will heal easily without leaving a scar.

A word of caution: Some people react strongly to St. John's wort, especially when exposed to sunlight, and may develop light sensitivity. So be sure to test the herb on yourself before using it extensively, and do not go out into the sun after applying the oil. It is not suitable for use as suntan lotion.

Medicinal Merits

Dioscurides, Galen, Pliny, and Paracelsus mentioned St. John's wort in their herbal treatises, and prescribed it for such various diseases as dizziness, epilepsy, shaking limbs, heart attacks, hysteria (also known as a "fit of the mother"), tertian or quartan fever (a fever recurring every 3 or 4 days), asthma, lumbago, insanity, and melancholy. The decoction or tincture of the flowers was accepted throughout Europe until the seventeenth century as a medicine for the treatment of melancholy and insanity. It was also used to cure all diseases caused by witchcraft, black magic, or demons. As Robert Burton wrote in his *Anatomy of Melancholy*,

> Hypericon, or St. Johns Wort, gathered on a Friday in the hour of Jupiter, when it comes to his effectual operation (that is about the Full Moon in July): so gathered, and borne or hung about the neck, it mightily helps this affection, and drives away all phantastical spirits.[123]

The plant's "blood" was believed, according to the doctrine of signatures, to point to its efficacy to treat wounds, cuts, and burns. It was administered to those who spat blood (tuberculosis), and used to treat anemia as well as other "female" complaints. The "blood" of the herb was even believed to keep mad dogs at bay. Because of its yellow flowers, St. John's wort was also considered a diuretic herb. In Austria, twigs of the herb were laid under a child's bed to stop him or her from bed-wetting, and it was famous in Germany as a treatment for jaundice.

---

123.   Burton, *The Anatomy of Melancholy* (1621) (London: Tudor, 1977), 596.

Modern Medicine

Most of the ancient cures based on the doctrine of signatures have been recognized by present-day medicine. The herb is still used to treat all "disbalanced" diseases such as epilepsy, problems caused by adolescence and menopause, anemia, sexual disorders, winter depressions, and painfully cramped conditions. It is also employed in the treatment of insomnia, somnambulism, nervous heart conditions, and to help relieve mental exhaustion. Taken regularly for several weeks alone or in combination with circulatory herbs such as rosemary, horse chestnut flowers, or yarrow, it can have a curative affect on chronic depression and some types of headaches. Winter depressions due to lack of sunlight have been treated with surprising success with St. John's wort. This may be due to the plant's ability to sensitize people to sunlight, and therefore to render the few rays of winter sunlight more effective. A bitter tea prepared from St. John's wort, chicory leaves, and dandelion leaves can help to stabilize cholesterol imbalances if taken regularly for 4–8 weeks before meals and supported by appropriate dietary measures.

St. John's wort is a prime remedy for disorders of the organic nervous system, and has been called the "arnica of the nervous system." Any disorders that are hard to localize, but are supposedly of a nervous nature, respond well to treatment with St. John's wort, or a stronger mixture of St. John's wort, valerian roots, and lemon balm leaves, either in tea or tincture form. St. John's wort is also an ideal tea for children. It helps to calm their fears and ease those symptoms that some generalist once descriptively dumped together under the term "growing pains." It is interesting to note the hormonal imbalances and subsequent complaints of adolescence were almost unknown in the past, but seem to have graduated to one of the most widespread "childhood diseases" today. Even some cases of bed-wetting can be stopped by the consequent use of St. John's wort tea. A cup of St. John's wort, sweetened with honey, has a soothing effect on students before an examination, and can help to ease school pressure.

The reddish juice of fresh St. John's wort is applied to staunch wounds; the tea, juice, or tincture can help regulate menstruation and lessen bleeding and cramps, and St. John's wort is considered a soothing tea for patients with bleeding ulcers. The yellow, bile-like color of the flowers points to the herb's use as a digestive medicine to strengthen the liver, gall bladder, spleen, intestines, and stomach, soothe an acid stomach, and help prevent ulcers. The tea prepared from the flowers also helps to expel urine from the body.

St. John's wort oil is not only a cosmetic preparation. It can be taken internally, 6–10 drops on a lump of sugar or piece of dried bread, to relieve stomach complaints and colics. It is applied externally to cuts, burns, scratches, sores, swellings, boils, fresh scars, and scrapes. It is rubbed on to relieve the pains of gout, rheumatism, arthritis, backaches, stiff joints, shooting pains, lumbago, neuralgia, torn or damaged sinews, nerves, ligaments, and muscles. St. John's wort oil can be applied to damaged nerves and even to painful tumorous growths. As Culpeper once stated, "the ointment opens obstructions, dissolves swellings, and closes up the lips of wounds."[124]

Homeopaths prescribe an essence of the plant after nerve operations and operations where nerves were damaged, and also after concussions. It is an amazing remedy for those who have just suffered a fall on the coccyx, and can be taken hourly until the pain subsides. It is also an excellent palliative for those suffering from tooth pain, or from pain after a trip to the dentist. It can be alternated with arnica to help treat tooth trauma.

Special Cures

Teas for Children: St. John's wort is especially valuable in the treatment of children's diseases because it is a bitter, but not unpleasantly bitter-tasting, herb. The tea, unsweetened or sweetened with a little honey, has a soothing, strengthening effect on the digestive tract. Its soothing qualities help to dispel stomachaches and childhood terrors and to lessen the effects of those hidden disorders that adults often only discover when it is too late. The adult dose of St. John's wort tea is ½ oz. of the dried drug for each quart of boiling water. The tea is strained into a thermos bottle, and can be taken ½ hour before meals, 2–3 times a day. This dosage should be reduced by at least half for children.

One of the most unpleasant, and embarrassing, childhood disorders is that of chronic bed-wetting. It is obvious that herbal teas can have little effect if the complaint is of a psychological nature, but may be of great use if the condition is due to minor anxiety on the part of the child, or is due to bladder weakness. 3 parts of yarrow flowers should be mixed with 2 parts of agrimony leaves and 2 parts of St. John's wort, and spiced with 1 part of masterwort *(Peucedanum ostruthium)* or pellitory *(Anacyclus officinarum)* roots. One cup of the tea (1 tsp. for every ½ pint of boiling water) should be given 1 or 2 hours before the child goes to bed so that he or she will have time to go to the bathroom before falling asleep. If the case is stubborn, a second cup of tea should be given in the morning, and the child woken up a few hours after going to bed to empty his or her bladder.

For the treatment of childhood anemia, a tea of equal parts of St. John's wort, linden flowers (also called lime flowers or lime tree flowers, *Tilia europea*), and hawkweed *(Hieracium pilosella)* may be given in the same dosage as above. A stronger tea, for children as well as adults, can be prepared from 3 parts each of St. John's wort, agrimony, heart's ease, and linden flowers, 2 parts of the entire flowering chicory plant with roots, 2 parts elecampane *(Inula helenium)* roots, ½ part juniper berries, and 1 part gentian roots *(Gentiana lutea)*. Mix well, and prepare and serve a tea of 1 tsp. of the mixture before meals. Special care should be taken

---

124.   Culpeper, *Culpeper's Complete Herbal* (1653) (London: Foulsham, undated), 203.

with fair-skinned or sensitive children, in case they become sensitized to sunlight through continued use of the herb. St. John's wort cures should be limited to at most 6 weeks of continual use.

Uses in Husbandry

St. John's wort is sometimes called hard hay for the obvious reason that the plant, when cut and dried, produces unusually hard hay. In the northern Palatine (Germany), this hay is thought to have aphrodisiacal powers. It is called Stierkraut, or Bull's herb, and is fed to breeding stock. St. John's wort hay, and especially Midsummer's Day St. John's wort, is given to cows before calving to ease delivery; and cattle that are believed to be bewitched are set on a St. John's wort diet. In Silesia (Germany), Midsummer's Day St. John's wort is placed in the four corners of the barn to drive away mice and rats.

Veterinary Values

St. John's wort oil can be applied to the wounds, cuts, sores, scrapes, strained muscles, and burns of cats, chicken, dogs, swine, cattle, and horses. It is also given internally on a piece of bread to relieve stomach cramps, diarrhea, and nervous intestinal disorders. Albino or white-skinned animals may become sensitized to the sun if they have eaten St. John's wort regularly or in large amounts. If the condition persists, they may even develop sunburns and blisters.

Miscellaneous Wisdom

In European folk belief, the series of days from June 21st to June 24th (Midsummer's Day) is a time of magical power. June 21st technically marks the summer solstice, when the sun (*sol*) is thought to stand still (*stasis*), pausing at the point furthest from the equator before returning, but June 24th is the feast day of St. John the Baptist and widely considered to be the "real" Midsummer's Day. In heathen Europe, an attempt was made to encourage and persuade the sun to return to the northern countries at midsummer by means of festivals, celebrations, sacrifices, and the lighting of fires on the hilltops. These rituals gradually became a direct celebration of the return of the sun.

The midsummer fires were lit to symbolize the rekindling of the sun's warmth. The celebrants rejoiced, thinking of the months to come in which the crops would ripen, the trees would grow, the animals fatten, and humans could live a life of ease, forgetting all about hunger. The celebrants knew that the cold winds would soon blow again after the September equinox, hail and snow would fall again, the fields would whiten with frost and grow barren, and the animals huddle together for warmth. They knew that they, the summer worshipers, would soon sink into winter melancholy. Therefore, they leapt over the midsummer fires while the going was still good, hoping to experience the full bounty of nature's fertility in the short summer months. It was considered self-evident that herbs found blossoming or growing on this day of days would be more potent than everyday herbs, balanced in their action, not too fiery, nor too cold and damp. They had in them all the memories of the chilly months and the budding promise of the summer months, and the strengthening medicine of solar influences. The herb with the fiery sun-colored flowers, St. John's wort, was considered especially valuable and was gathered under lunar influence at midnight on St. John's Eve, or under solar influence at noon on St. John's Day.

This midsummer herb was famous, from Sweden to Wales, from France to Bosnia and Russia to Sicily, as an antidemonic plant. It was thought to drive away witches, evil spirits, and demons, ban enchantment, and counteract poison. It was *the* most popular herb among Italian folk healers, and the French idiomatic saying, *"employer toutes les herbes de Saint-Jean,"* means "to try all in one's power." In Somerset, a twentieth-century saying praises the herb:

> Blessed, blessed in the ditch,
> Cures the itch and the stitch
> And drives away the witch.[125]

In the northern counties, the saying goes,

> Trefoil, vervain, St. John's wort, dill
> Hinder witches of their will.[126]

Crosses made of St. John's wort are laid on the windowsills, over the threshold, or in the windows to dispel even a suggestion of evil influence. Fresh plants are stuck in the four corners of the house and fields to protect farm animals and crops, and houses are fumigated with the burning herb to drive away all evil beings. The herb is eaten or worn as a spell against enchantment, the Evil Eye, and poison, and is carried to church to be blessed on August 15th (the Day of Mary's Ascension) in Germany. St. John's wort stalks are bound to the first sheaf of a harvest to protect the crop against mice. A wreath is made by children on St. John's Eve and hung over the door to protect the house against witches and misfortune. Tyrolean women cross themselves with the bloody juice of the plant to free themselves from witchcraft for one day, and girls throw St. John's wort wreaths into the midsummer fire and then bite into them. According to belief, they will then be freed from toothache for an entire year.

On the Isle of Man, whoever steps on St. John's wort after sunset will be carried off by faery horses. Fumigating new mothers and their babies as well as anyone at danger

---

125. Ruth L. Tongue, *Somerset Folklore* (London: The Folk-Lore Society, 1965), 32.

126. William Henderson, *Notes on the Folk-Lore of the Northern Counties of England and the Borders* (London: The Folk-Lore Society, 1897), 227.

of being "taken away" or "exchanged" by the faeries with St. John's wort is a standard precautionary procedure. In the Palatine, St. John's wort is added to a child's first bath to protect against heathen influence until the child can be christened. St. John's wort hung in a bedroom is supposed to have a discouraging effect on night elves, and to protect sleepers against nightmares. Young couples hang St. John's wort up in the bridal chamber to prevent any interruptions of marital confidences and intercourse.

St. John's wort is also considered to be an excellent aphrodisiac. As the German saying goes,

> Many have the mad notion
> To dig St. John's wort before day,
> Which makes people knowledgeable about each other
> Even before they have met.[127]

In the Slavic countries, barren women drink tea prepared from blessed St. John's wort in order to receive the blessing of a child. In the Middle Ages, St. John's wort was included in love philters and was an important remedy for those who suspected bewitchment in affairs of the heart.

Because of its association with the sun and midsummer fires, St. John's wort is also linked with fire and lightning. St. John's wort that is gathered in the midnight darkness of St. John's Eve and then hung up in all four corners of the house, or burned during a storm, is considered effective in preventing fires and keeping lightning from a house. The plants worn by midsummer celebrants are also formed into wreaths and tossed onto the roof. In Thurgau, in Switzerland, wreaths are thrown onto the roof during particularly violent storms and the rhyme is repeated, "St. John's wort and Dill / Make the storm stay still."[128]

According to a Belgian legend, a voice once called out from a cloud in the middle of a storm, "Does here no lass / Know about St. John's grass?"[129]

Oracular Worth

In Franconia, if St. John's wort blossoms early in April, then storms will surely follow. According to classical writers, women count the holes on a St. John's wort leaf to discover how many children they will have. This oracle seems outdated today, since the number of children any one woman bears has gone down dramatically. In Denmark,

---

127. Hans Vintler, qtd. in Hanns Bächtold-Stäubli, ed., *Handwörterbuch des deutschen Aberglaubens* (1927–42), vol. 3 (Berlin: Walter de Gruyter & Co., 1987), 1489.

128. Hanns Bächtold-Stäubli, ed., *Handwörterbuch des deutschen Aberglaubens* (1927–42), vol. 3 (Berlin: Walter de Gruyter & Co., 1987), 1488.

129. Ibid.

girls dig up two plants and plant them under the roof beams on Midsummer Day. If they grow toward each other or even begin to twine around each other, then the "girl" and the "boy" will soon marry. This same oracle can be consulted to learn the fate of relatives: if the "mother" plant grows upwards, then the real mother will be blessed with a long life. If the plant droops downward, the mother's health will deteriorate.

St. John's wort, and particularly midsummer's St. John's wort, is commonly consulted as a love oracle. In Wales, where it is called *llysiau Ifan*, women go look for it at midnight on St. John's Eve, each carrying a glow worm in her hand. Only those plants growing among ferns are gathered. They are then hung on the bedroom wall. If the leaves are still fresh in the morning, the woman will marry within the year; if wilted, then she will spend her days as an old maid, or die soon. Germans consult St. John's wort by rubbing the herb between two fingers, and repeating the rhyme,

> If our love is right,
> Then the blood is red;
> If our love is dead,
> Then the water's white.[130]

Needless to say, this is an oracle that can't go wrong.

Legends

St. John's wort is, by legend, a virtuous plant. The saints, Mary, and Jesus were supposedly witnesses of the plant's power, and the devil nurses hate against it to this day. The highland name for the plant, *ach larson cholumcille*, or "little armpit of Columba," originated because Saint Columba once came to a child herding cows. The little herder was crying because he was afraid that his cows would stray during the night. Columba comforted the weeping boy, plucked some St. John's wort flowers, and tucked them under the child's arm. "Now you can sleep in peace," said the saint. "Your cattle won't stray any more, but will stay safe and close to you the whole night long."

St. John's wort is often associated with St. John the Baptist, and the "blood" that flows from the flowers is said to be his blood. In the Austrian Inn Valley, the legend goes that St. John's enemies hung a plant on the window of his house to point it out to his pursuers. The next morning, every house in the town was miraculously adorned with St. John's wort.

The Virgin Mary is also associated with the herb. The "blood" from the flowers is thought to be a reminder of her bloody tears or of her menstrual blood. The bloody juice exuded by the plant is also associated with the labor pains she suffered to bring forth

---

130. Hanns Bächtold-Stäubli, ed., *Handwörterbuch des deutschen Aberglaubens*, vol. 3 (Berlin: Walter de Gruyter & Co., 1987), 1490.

Jesus. Another Mary, Mary Magdalene, is believed by northern Italians to have anointed Jesus' feet with a St. John's wort salve while he was on the cross, hence the folk name *il balsamo de la Madalena*. In other areas, the belief is that the herb sprung from drops of Christ's blood as they fell from the cross.

Belief in the devil's antagonism toward the plant is just as tenacious as the belief in its saintly origins. Some say that the devil went to the plant at night and tried to kill it by brutally puncturing the leaves with a needle. He considered the "saintly" plant an affront to his powers. But the herb was protected by St. John, and survived this harsh treatment. The plant's leaves still bear Satan's marks, and are as potent as ever for combating evil and supporting the powers of light.

Tarragon, Draco Herba, of Spanish Extraction; hot and spicy:
'Tis highly cordial and friendly to the Head, Heart, Liver, &c.

—John Evelyn, *Acetaria*

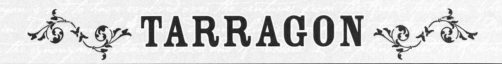

TARRAGON

Name

The word "tarragon" is said to have evolved over the centuries from the Arabic *tarkhun*. The Arabic word is of uncertain origin. Known botanically as *Artemisia dracunculus*, tarragon is a perennial member of the **Asteraceae** (**Daisy**) family and is also known under the synonyms *Artemisia glauca* and *A. inodora*. It is a plant sacred to Artemis, and was called *dracunculus* (a little dragon or worm) because of the form of its roots. In antiquity, the plant was used to treat snakebites and the wounds of dragons.

Folk Names

Old English names for tarragon were *sallade herbe* and *draco*; modern English names are little dragon, little dragon mugwort, dragon sagewort, and dragon wormwood. Germans call the herb *Estragon, Dragun, Dragon, Ragu, Kaisersalat,* and *Dragunwermut*. French names are *estragon, esdragon,* and *dragon*. Italians call it *dragone, dragoncello,* and *serpentaria*; the Spanish, *taragona*; the Danish, *drageurt* or *kongenssalat*; the Russians, *polyn estragon* or *tarchun*; and the Irish, *dragan*.

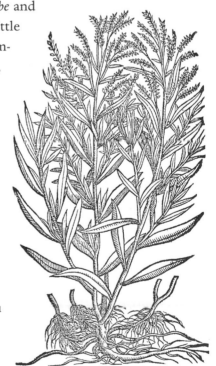

Appearance

Tarragon has an unkempt, bushy appearance, with many green, woody stalks that appear late in spring. The small, elongated leaves have a penetrating, aromatic odor. The plant can grow to a height of 4 ft., depending on the variety. Russian tarragon is usually taller and weedier, and French tarragon is bushier and compacter. Tarragon resembles hyssop, but the leaves are much longer than hyssop leaves, and are unique in their form, resembling an elongated fleur-de-lys. Their color is an unusual light green, and they are shiny, and not hairy. Tarragon seldom flowers, and many people overlook the flowers when they do appear: they look like yellow miniature balls, and never open fully. The herb's roots are long and fibrous, and produce many underground shoots that resemble tiny snakes.

Place, Season, and Useful Parts

Tarragon originally came to Europe from the East, and can still be found growing wild in Siberia, Hungary, the Himalayas, and Afghanistan. It also grows wild in some parts of the American West. It is cultivated in the temperate zones to an altitude of 4,500 ft. It is grown as far afield as Indonesia, but does best at a lower altitude, in a warm and dry climate. It sometimes escapes from cultivated areas. Tarragon blossoms, when it does flower, from May on into September.

Gathering, Drying, and Storage

Tarragon leaves can are gathered in June, and then cut again as needed, until as late as September. The leaves should be used while still fresh, stripped from the stems and dried. Tarragon oil is distilled from the freshly gathered plant, or from the leaves.

Fresh tarragon has a much more delicate flavor than the dried herb. Dried tarragon must be stored in dark, airtight containers, and does not keep long. After several months, it is almost worthless, and resembles straw. It can be dried in bunches hung from the rafters in an airy attic, or the leaves stripped from the stalks and dried quickly in a heated room on cloths or screens. The leaves must retain their pale green color on drying.

Tarragon may be frozen with better results, or pressed down in wide-mouth bottles, sealed, and then processed under pressure. Another method of preservation is to press the leaves in wide-mouthed bottles, cover them with good strong vinegar, and then cork the bottles securely. Tarragon vinegar is prepared with a sprig of fresh tarragon placed in wine vinegar.

Seed Saving and Germination

Tarragon varieties will vary widely in oil content and aroma. Various varieties are maintained vegetatively, through plant and root division. Russian tarragon can be propagated by seed, but it is generally inferior in quality. The fastidious cook will do well to ask around for a particularly aromatic variety, and then propagate it.

Gardening Hints

There are two major kinds of garden tarragon: Russian and French tarragon. Russian tarragon can be grown from seed and is often listed in seed catalogs, but is by far inferior in taste to French tarragon. French tarragon must be propagated by root division or cuttings, since it does not set seed in colder climates. Because of this, it is much harder to find. Specialty herb growers often offer several varieties, but the buyer should only trust his or her nose—growers may try to get rid of inferior tarragon varieties by selling them to novices.

Tarragon needs well-fertilized, loose soil, and a sheltered, sunny position. It prefers well-drained soil, and will not prosper in heavy, waterlogged soil. All tarragons withstand frost well, although they die back each year and only come up late in the season.

French tarragon is usually barren. This caused ancient herbalists and agriculturalists to believe that the plant could be raised from a flax seed planted in a hollowed onion. Much better results can be obtained by buying young plants, by dividing existing plants in spring, or by rooting stem cuttings in July or August. The herb spreads quickly, and should be given at least 2 ft. of room in each direction. If the plant is not divided, it will spread quickly through subterranean shoots, which root easily. The spent stalks should be cut down after the first frost and dressed with mulch or straw as a protection against frost heaves, which can damage the plant. Tarragon only sends out shoots late in the following year, and can easily be dug out. It needs to be fed well at the beginning of summer, and should be transplanted or divided every few years to keep it from depleting the soil, and robbing nutrients from other plants.

Russian tarragon sprouts best in very warm weather, and should only be sown after all danger of frost is past.

Culinary Virtues

As John Evelyn stated in his *Acetaria: A Discourse of Sallets*, "Tarragon is one of the perfuming or Spicy Furnitures of our Sallets." Because of its fine and distinctive taste, tarragon vinegar is justly the most famous of all herbal vinegars. A fresh green salad flavored with tarragon vinegar can become the highpoint of a meal, instead of just another insipid side dish. According to John Gerard, tarragon also tempers the cold, and therefore noxious temperament of salad greens. Chervil, chives, and tarragon are often used in combination as salad herbs. Tarragon is also added to mustards and various pickles. Olive oil can be perfumed by the addition of a few tarragon stalks.

Russian tarragon tends to taste insipid, or too intensive. Good cooks prefer French tarragon with its high oil content, and always employ it sparingly in the kitchen. As Ogden Nash is reported to have said,

> There are certain people
> Whom certain herbs
> The good digestion disturbs,
> Henry VIII
> Divorced Catharine of Aragon
> Because of her reckless use of Tarragon.

Tarragon clashes with some herbs, and the uncertain cook does well to use it alone when in doubt. It is said to increase the appetite, and to aid digestion. French chefs employ the herb widely and wisely in their recipes. Tarragon chicken is world-famous; Bearnaise, Hollandaise, and Mousseline sauces are often flavored with tarragon, and many herbal butters owe their delicate taste to it. Tarragon can also be used to enhance the natural taste of game, fish, seafood, lamb, pork chops, sausages, omelets, Yorkshire pudding, and chicken livers. Its taste can improve consommé, chowders, and vegetable juices as well as chicken, mushroom, and tomato soups. Tarragon jelly is sometimes served with fowl or game. Adding tarragon can aromatize artichokes, asparagus, avocado, bean salads, salsify, spinach, and zucchini.

Tarragon purée, made by heating the herb in white wine and incorporating the liquid into a Béchamel sauce, can be served with pastries and vegetables. A thinner tarragon sauce complements boiled chicken, fish, grain, and meat dishes. Slovenian cooks prepare herb strudels made with tarragon (see parsley chapter). Tartar sauce usually contains tarragon, and other fish sauces are prepared with tarragon, horseradish, and vinegar. The herb is a common ingredient of pickles, ketchup, and pickled vegetables. Tarragon is occasionally used to flavor liqueurs and date wines.

Noteworthy Recipes

Tarragon Vinegar: William Kitchiner offered this receipe in the nineteenth century:

> This is a very agreeable addition to Soups, Salad Sauce and to mix Mustard. Fill a wide-mouthd bottle with fresh-gathered Tarragon-leaves, i.e. between Midsummer and Michaelmas (which should be gathered on a dry day, just before it flowers), and pick the leaves off the stalks, and dry them a little before the fire; cover them with the best Vinegar, let them steep fourteen days, then strain through a flannel Jelly Bag [or cheesecloth] till it is fine, then pour into half-pint bottles: cork them carefully, and keep them in a dry place. Obs. You may prepare Elder-flowers and Herbs in same manner; Elder and Tarragon are those in most general use in this country.[131]

---

131. Kitchiner, *The Cook's Oracle* (1817) (London: Samuel Bagster, 1860), 262.

Spicy Herbal Vinegar: Those who desire a spicier vinegar for seasoning hot sauces may want to use this recipe. Stuff 3 handfuls of tarragon, 1 diced white onion, 7 diced shallots, a few scrapings of lemon peel and nutmeg, 2 laurel leaves, 5 sprigs of thyme, 15 peppercorns, 7 cloves, 1 clove of garlic, and a pinch of dill seeds into a wide-mouthed bottle, and pour 2 qt. of the best white wine or cider vinegar over the herbs. Stopper the bottle, and let stand for 3 months in a warm place before straining and re-bottling. Those who like it hot can add a tiny chili pepper to the vinegar mixture.

Tarragon Sauce: This is a rather unusual tarragon sauce served with cold meat. Add the following herbs and spices to 1 pint of tarragon vinegar and 5 oz. of olive oil in a wide-mouthed jar: a small handful each of finely-chopped fresh tarragon, parsley, chives, chervil, garden cress, sorrel leaves, and salad burnet; 2 handfuls of chopped shallots; 1 oz. of chopped capers; 4 oz. of minced salted anchovies; ½ pint of French mustard; 1 oz. of sugar; and a pinch of pepper. Mix the ingredients, pour into jars, seal well, and store in a cool place, or freeze. Before serving, blend the mixture with the yolks of hard-boiled eggs in the blender.

Household Applications

Because of its penetrating odor, tarragon is added in minute amounts to potpourri and herbal cushion mixtures. Pretty bottles filled with good vinegar and a sprig or two of tarragon make good, inexpensive gifts.

Cosmetic Properties

Tarragon oil is combined with other oils by perfumers to produce fantasy odors. Tarragon leaves can be used in combination with chamomile flowers in facial masks.

Medicinal Merits

Tarragon, the little dragon, was used in ancient times as an aphrodisiac. It was prescribed for women before and after birth, as well as during menopause for its sedative effect. It was also used to treat gout and alleviate toothache.

Modern Medicine

Tarragon is not now generally considered to be a healing herb, aside from its warming effect on the digestive system and its stomachic properties. It can help to expel worms, and can be taken by those afflicted with gout, rheumatism, or heartburn. A poultice of fresh tarragon leaves is still thought to ease toothache.

Good morrow, good yarrow, good morrow to thee,
I hope by the morrow my lover to see.

—AN ENGLISH SAYING

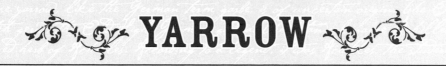

YARROW

Name

The English name "yarrow," like the German term *Garbe*, is of uncertain origin. The Old English form was *gearwe*; the Dutch, *gerw*; the Old High German, *Garwa*. The botanical name, *Achillea millefolium*, means "the thousand-leaved herb of Achilles." According to legend, it was Achilles, the student of Cheiron, who discovered the healing properties of the plant.

The yarrows are perennial members of the **Daisy** or *Asteraceae* family. *Achillea millefolium* is the name of common yarrow. Among the many yarrow species, several subspecies are also of medicinal interest. Many decorative forms have been developed in recent years for garden use, but these do not possess the same medicinal value as the wild forms.

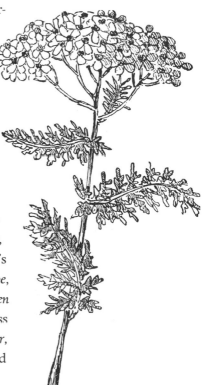

Folk Names

Yarrow is known under many local names: common yarrow, bloodwort, sanguinary, nosebleed, arrowroot, sneezings, stanchweed, stanch grass, squirrel tail, thousand-seal, carpenter's grass, soldier's woundwort, knight's milfoil, milfoil, thousand-leaf, thousand weed, thousand-leaf clover, hundred-leaved grass, yarroway, field hops, traveller's ease, yellow, yarra grass, seven-year's-love, old man's pepper, old man's mustard, bad man's plaything, snake's grass, devil's plaything, and devil's nettle. Germans call the plant *Schafgarbe, Schafrippe, Garbe, Tausendblatt, Herrgotts Ruckenkraut, Jungfrauen Augbraune, Grundheil,* and *Heil aller Schaden.* The French address the herb as *millefeuille, Achillée, saigne-nez, herbe à charpentier, herbe à la coupure, herbe de Saint Joseph, herbe à la taille,* and *sourcils de Vénus*. Italians have named it *millefoglio, erba dai millefiori, erba per i cento tagli, tagiola*, and *erba militare*; the Spaniards, *plumajillo*. The Dutch call it *yerw*; the Irish, *athair thalún*; the Portuguese, *millfohlas*; the Russians, *tysjačelistnik obyknovennyj*.

Another important member of the **Daisy** family, *Achillea ptarmica*, is called sneeze-wort, sneezeweed, white weed, hard head, bastard pellitory, European pellitory, adder's tongue, goose tongue, goosewort, angel's breath yarrow, old man's pepper-box, wild fire, shirt buttons, pearl yarrow, and fair maid of France. Germans call it *Dorant, Orant, weißer Dost, weißer Dorant, Wild-Fräulein-Kraut, Sumpf-Schafgarbe, Hemdknöpchen, deutscher Bertram, Wiesenbertram, Bertramskraut*, and *Schneeballen*. It is called *erbe à ètenuer, bouton d'argent, pyrethre sauvage*, and *Achillée sternutatoire* in France; *tysjačelistnik ptarmika* in Russia; yerba *estornutatoria* in Spain; and *bottone d'argento* or *tarmica* in Italy.

Another yarrow, *Achillea erba-rotta ssp. moschata* (musk milfoil), is known as *Moschus-schafgarbe, Wildmännlikraut*, or *Wildfräulikraut* in Germany because of its association with the mountain "little people."

Achillea ageratifolia is called sweet yarrow or Greek yarrow, and *Leberbalsam-Schaf-garbe* in German. It grows wild in Portugal and the western Mediterranean, and was once used as a medicinal and a perfumer's herb.

In North America, Native Americans have used *Achillea lanulosa*, also known as plumajillo or wooly yarrow, for centuries. Its medicinal action is stronger than that of its European cousin.

Appearance

The most striking feature of the yarrow plant ("an upright and not unhandsome plant ... [that] grows two feet high"[132]) is its flowers. These can be off-white or pink, and are gathered together in umbel-like clusters resembling miniature clouds. Yarrow flowers grow on stiff, angular, and hairy stalks that rise in clumps from a strong system of light brown, crawling, wiry roots, rootlets and stolons. Finely segmented, feathery, dark green leaves grow outward from the stems. The leaves resemble the backbone of a fish, and are covered with fine hairs. They end in a sharp point. Yarrow florets are tiny, and are gathered together into flower heads that have a smell reminiscent of honey. The leaves and stems have a strongly aromatic fragrance and a bitter and spicy taste. The plant produces a leaf rosette in its first year, and flower stalks in its second and following years.

Sneezewort is a perennial plant that grows to a maximum height of 4 ft. Its leaves are not as feathery as those of the common yarrow, and are serrated but undivided. The single flower heads are 3–4 times as large as yarrow, and very numerous. They are usually white.

---

132.   Nicholas Culpeper, *Culpeper's Complete Herbal* (1653) (London: Foulsham, undated), 397.

Place, Season, and Useful Parts

Yarrow blossoms from June until the first frosts. It grows in most of the northern regions to the polar cap, and can also be found in Australia and the Americas, but only rarely in the Mediterranean countries. It will grow wherever grain grows, on poor or sandy, but not too moist, soil. It thrives in dry, grassy places, and can be found at the edges of fields, in meadows, pastures and gardens, and on paths, roadsides, and rubble heaps to an altitude of 9,000 ft.

Sneezewort prefers damp soil, moors, and meadows, and is fairly common next to ponds, lakes, or woods, or in ditches and damp fields in most of Europe and northern Asia as well as North America. It grows to an altitude of 13,500 ft., and blooms from July through September. Musk milfoil grows where common yarrow will not grow, and at higher altitudes.

Gathering, Drying, and Storage

The ancient Romans believed that the best medicinal yarrow must be picked between eleven and one o'clock. Modern herb-gathering manuals only stipulate that the herb should be gathered on a sunny day, as soon as the dew has dried. They usually go on to warn harvesters that they may develop an allergic reaction to the plant. The flowers should be picked or cut just after they open, and care must be taken to avoid including stalks and discolored flowers. Since the stems are wiry, gloves are helpful while stripping the blossoms from the stems. The top 8 in. of the plant can also be cut in July or August when the plant is flowering.

Yarrow should only be dried in the shade, spread out in layers, or hung up in bundles. It keeps well for one year if properly dried.

Seed Saving and Germination

Yarrow self-seeds readily, and can also easily be propagated by root division. Where it is a prevalent weed, garden strains can easily become crossed or confused with wild plants, and must be isolated. The best way to save seed is to cut the flowering stalks before the blossoms become overblown, and dry them on cloth in a dry, shady place. The seeds will fall out and can easily be sifted out from leaf debris. But it is even easier to divide clumps of existing plants. The plants respond well to transplantation if the stem is cut back and they are kept moist until established. Because of the ease of root division propagation, there is little need to keep the seed stored for longer periods.

Gardening Hints

Despite the fact that wild yarrow is often considered a bothersome weed, it can be used to excellent advantage by the unorthodox gardener. Yarrow is one of the best compost herbs, and can be combined with stinging nettles, dandelions, oak bark, comfrey, chamomile, valerian, and elder leaves to speed decomposition and to add valuable nutrients and minerals to the compost pile. Many so-called compost starters are nothing but these dried herbs mixed with lactose. The freshly layered compost pile should be "inoculated" by poking holes with a stick and pouring a teaspoon of the powdered herbs into the holes, covering them, and then watering the pile thoroughly. Another method is to powder the herbs finely, mix them with water in a watering can, and then water the compost pile with the mixture. Yarrow is especially beneficial for soils deficient in copper.

Yarrow increases the aromatic properties of the herbs grown in its vicinity, and has a similar effect on vegetables when grown in a border, or along a garden path. Care should be taken, though, to keep yarrow from spreading its wiry runners too far, and subsequently leaching the soil of nutrients. Its roots are difficult to eradicate once they have taken hold. Decorative yarrow varieties possess many of the same beneficial properties as the wild plant. They are available in a wide array of colors, from yellow to red, and are not as invasive as the wild plant.

Yarrow can be grown on the poorest and even on alkaline soils. It is the pasture plant of last resort on very poor ground, on peat, or in meadows dotted with molehills. The plant is self-propagating through runners and has very tough roots. Yarrow is winter-hardy, and will stand extremes of heat and cold, but not dampness. It grows best in a sunny, dry position, and needs little watering. Existing stands propagate themselves by seeds or runners; new plots can be planted with divided plants in the fall or spring, or sown with yarrow seeds in the spring. Yarrow seeds germinate best if they are not covered, but simply pressed into the soil. The seedlings usually emerge in 10–14 days. Once established, the plants should be divided every other year to prevent crowding. Fertilizing with manure is advantageous to prevent the plants from leaching the soil. The stems of decorative varieties should be cut back just after the blossoms begin to fade. This will prevent them from seeding all over the garden.

Culinary Virtues

Small amounts of young yarrow leaves add a spicy and distinctive taste to greens or salads. Chopped fresh yarrow can also be eaten on bread and butter. Yarrow is valued for its fresh taste and high vitamin content, and for the fact that it is one of the first herbs to appear in spring. The feathery leaves are recognizable as yarrow leaves even when very small, and can be picked as soon as the snow melts. Because of this, yarrow leaves are often included in traditional Maundy Thursday soups. The fresh young leaves combine well with nettles, with sorrel, and with plantain. Young yarrow leaves should be carefully washed to remove all grit, and then cooked quickly or steamed to retain nutrients. Older leaves must be boiled in one or two waters to remove their bitter taste. Sneezewort can also be added to salads in small amounts as a spicy seasoning. Musk milfoil is used, especially in Switzerland, in the manufacture of liqueurs. In England and Sweden, a powerful beer is brewed with yarrow.

Household Applications

Yarrow flowers, especially the pink and yellow varieties, can be dried and added to sachet and to potpourri mixtures. The entire flowering yarrow plant (without roots) can also be gathered and hung upside down to dry. These dried yarrow flowers make unusual winter ornaments. Dried or fresh yarrow can, like so many members of the **Daisy** family, be boiled to produce a yellow dye for woolens. With copper as a mordant, dark bronze tones can be obtained, with iron, a dark olive green, and a deep moss green with oxalic acid. The addition of ammonia to the rinse water will produce vibrant green shades.

Cosmetic Properties

One of yarrow's greatest medicinal merits is its ability to stimulate the circulation. This is of great cosmetic interest, for a rosy appearance and clear skin are often due to proper circulation. Yarrow can be given in tea form, or used externally in yarrow-tea compresses or in facial steaming mixtures. Yarrow-leaf powder may also be added to facial masks. Yarrow exerts a drying and astringent action on the skin, and can be used by those with oily skin or thread veins to good advantage. Thread veins are best treated by substituting caffeine and alcoholic beverages with yarrow tea. The skin is washed with yarrow infusion, but never steamed. Yarrow compresses can also ease the pain of sore nipples. Milk in which yarrow has been macerated for several hours can be applied as an astringent blackhead-removing lotion. Oily hair is treated with yarrow, both inwardly in tea form, and outwardly as a rinse. Baths prepared with the herb are stimulating for the entire body, and yarrow and sea salt foot baths soften corns and calluses.

A note of caution: allergic reactions to yarrow are fairly common, especially in combination with sunlight. Yarrow, like St. John's wort, can cause excessive sensibility to sunlight and result in sunburn, or rashes. If these symptoms develop, use of the herb should be discontinued.

- A tea that can be given to young people suffering from acne and poor complexions is prepared from 1 part each of linden or elder flowers, peppermint, yarrow, and thyme, with a pinch of chamomile and sage. This tea should be taken 2 hours before going to bed every evening for 1–2 months. Drinking the tea every once in a while will not lead to success—it needs to be taken every day in order for the cure to be successful.

Medicinal Merits

Yarrow was a healing herb familiar to Hippocrates, Dioscurides, and Pliny. Hildegard von Bingen wrote of its ability to clear clouded eyes, and treat rabies and tertian fever. Nicholas Culpeper praised it for staunching violent bleeding and staying the running of the reins (kidneys) and the whites (*fluor albus*). In Central Europe, white-blossoming yarrow plants were thought effective against women's whites and uterus infections as well as stomach disorders. The pink or red-blossoming plants were used to induce and control menstruation.

In Orkney, yarrow was given to those suffering from melancholy. In Lincolnshire, the traditional folk remedy for depression was yarrow tea seasoned with a little gin. An Irish cure for incipient blindness and pains in the head was concocted from yarrow, honey, and fish gall. In Austria, menopausal women laid sacks of yarrow on their feet and hearts to ease the symptoms of their condition. In other areas, yarrow wreaths were hung up to drive away the plague; and a nine-day-fever was treated by giving the patient a soup prepared from 9 yarrow leaves on the first day, 8 on the second, 7 on the third, and so on, until the fever had run its course. Yarrow was also used to treat backaches, malevolent growths, menstrual problems, intestinal catarrh, tuberculosis, anemia, coughs, and headaches.

In North America, both yarrow and *Achillea lanulosa* have been used for centuries as healing herbs, especially in the treatment (breaking) of agues and fevers, to alleviate diarrhea, and to strengthen a weakened stomach. It has also been applied externally as a wound herb. The Ojibways used *Achillea lanulosa* in poultice form to treat spider bites, and it was burned to fumigate patients with headaches, and to drive out evil spirits.

I will pick the smooth yarrow that my figure will be more elegant, that my lips may be warmer, that my voice may be more cheerful; may my voice be like a sunbeam, may my lips be like the juice of the strawberries.

May I be an island in the sea, may I be a hill on the land, may I be a star when the moon wanes, may I be a staff to the weak one: I shall wound every man, no man shall wound me.

—a traditional Gaelic folk charm, from *A Celtic Miscellany*

Modern Medicine

Today, yarrow is considered to be one of the most important healing herbs, and is ranked next to chamomile by some herbalists because of its unusual versatility. Yarrow exerts a positive effect on the circulation and the blood vessels, and all the problems caused by poor functioning of these vessels. If only for this, it deserves more attention in a world plagued with "civilized" diseases such as heart disease and cancer. Yarrow flowers help to regenerate red corpuscles and marrow, and therefore to improve the circulation, but also to slow and stop bleeding. It is especially effective in increasing circulation in the pelvic area. Yarrow is a gentle tonic and stimulant, and may be given with good effect to menopausal women, women with fibroid tumors, and those troubled with anemia. It is a useful addition to blood-purifying herbal mixtures.

Yarrow flower tea not only regulates blood circulation, but also helps to regulate excessive or irregular bleeding: it is therefore prescribed to normalize menstruation and heavy bleeding. Pregnant women should be cautious in their use of the herb, especially if they have a history of miscarriages. It is further employed as a wound herb, and to treat hemorrhoids and chronic diarrhea. Some children know that sticking a yarrow leaf up one's nose will cause a nose bleed (a good trick to make adults feel sorry!), but often do not know that squeezing a drop of the plant's juice into the nostril will stop the bleeding just as quickly. Chewing fresh yarrow or sneezewort leaves can also lessen the bleeding and ease the pain caused by a trip to the dentist.

The list of yarrow's medicinal virtues does not end here. Yarrow flower tea gently stimulates the kidneys and counteracts weakness of the bladder by virtue of its astringent qualities. The herb is an invaluable aid to those suffering from water retention. The liver, stomach, and gall bladder are gently stimulated by the bitter principle present in the herb. Loss of appetite, flatulence, a sluggish stomach, and mild cases of intestinal catarrh can all be treated with yarrow. Children with poor appetites should be given a tea prepared with yarrow blossoms and St. John's wort. Yarrow can help to cleanse the lungs, and is added to many cough mixtures and to teas for patients with laryngitis, bronchitis, influenza, measles, chills, and fever. The powdered roots and flowers of the sneezewort plant are taken as snuff to clear stuffy heads (hence the name). Yarrow may be administered in tea form, as a juice extracted from the fresh plant and taken regularly during the summer months, or as a tincture prepared for winter use. Pregnant women, and people who develop an allergic reaction to yarrow, should avoid any internal use of the plant.

In homeopathy, yarrow is widely employed as a wound herb, staunching blood and strengthening the capillaries of the lungs, nose, and uterus. Painful varicose veins are treated with the remedy, as well as bruises and after-effects of a bloody fall. The blossoming plant is prescribed for women with circulatory disorders and female complaints.

The folk names Carpenter's grass, Stanch weed, Knight's milfoil, and Soldier's woundwort all point to the fact that fresh yarrow leaves (like clean, freshly spun cobwebs) can be applied directly to cuts and wounds as emergency bandages. These "bandages" help to stop bleeding, speed healing, and avoid excessive scar formation. A wound salve can be prepared from the herb, or the fresh juice may be applied directly. Chilblains and hemorrhoids are often treated with yarrow juice or yarrow salve, which is made in the same manner as marigold salve (see that chapter). Large yarrow plasters can be applied to poorly healing wounds or to the liver area. Yarrow baths strengthen children with the rickets, and ease the pains of gout and rheumatism.

Special Cures

Tea for the Circulation: Yarrow is one of the most important circulatory herbs and is often included in mixed teas. A good circulatory tea can be prepared from yarrow or from a combination of yarrow with other herbs such as goosegrass *(Potentilla anserina)*, melilot *(Melilotus officinalis)*, and club moss *(Lycopodium clavatum)*. This tea can be taken for a long time to improve the circulation. Patients suffering from hemorrhoids may find relief by drinking a tea 2–3 times daily made from equal measure of yarrow flowers, rose petals, dandelion leaves, and mullein flowers. If bleeding is present, then the tea mixture should consist of equal parts of rose petals, stinging nettle leaves, and mullein flowers.

Yarrow Tincture: Yarrow tincture can be made by pounding or blending the flowers, covering with high-proof alcohol and expressing the juice through cheesecloth. Add an equal amount of alcohol and allow to stand one week in a dark, cool place. Filter through filter paper and store in dark bottles.

Uses in Husbandry

Lincolnshire farmers insist that cattle pastured in yarrow fields are more docile than animals fed with ordinary hay. The herb responds well to manure fertilizers, and even fresh manure, although it will also grow if not fertilized. It will tolerate peat, and is not sensitive to drought, excessive heat, or excessive cold. These properties make it an annoying weed in gardens and lawns, but recommend it to husbandmen growing fodder crops on poor soil. Some, however, warn against feeding yarrow to dairy cows, since it will interfere with the curdling process for cheesemaking. Sheep and turkeys thrive on yarrow. Native Americans used it as a stimulant, applying it externally to horses. In the Palatine, yarrow is hung in stalls as magical protection against lightning. Yarrow leaves can be dried and used to add body and spice to herbal tobacco mixtures, or powdered as snuff.

Veterinary Values

Many centuries ago, Pliny described a yarrow salve used to heal the wounds and sores of plowhorses. Modern farmers rub their horses down with bunches of the fresh herb before turning them out to pasture, in order to discourage flies. Horses, sheep, and cattle suffering from cramps and flatulence are given yarrow tea to ease their pains. Piglets with intestinal disorders are also subjected to a yarrow cure. Animals suffering from recurrent internal bleeding should have yarrow added to their diet as a supplement.

Miscellaneous Wisdom

Yarrow was depicted as a symbol of sleep on Roman sarcophagi, and was mentioned in Hildegard von Bingen's works as a sleep-inducing plant with antidemonic properties. In France, some old wives still lay yarrow leaves on children's eyes to help them fall asleep, have sweet dreams, and not be startled out of their slumbers. In Lincolnshire, it is said that a witch will lose all her powers if she inadvertently sits on yarrow. Yarrow is therefore strewn on doorsteps and laid in the cradle to keep witches away from the house and the babe happy and healthy. In England, yarrow is carried for good luck by farmers going courting or on their way to market. Bridesmaids wear it to church in the hopes that they, too, will marry within seven years. Some northern Italians believe that yarrow worn next to the skin has the power to drive away ghosts. It is generally considered to be a magical herb in the Germanic countries. Germans include it in the Kräuterbusch blessed on Assumption Day (August 15th), and then hang it up in the house and stall to protect animals and humans from harm. Sneezewort is strewn on the stove during storms in the Rhine area as a protection against lightning.

Yarrow is not only believed to avert evil, but also to impart magical powers. The prosecutor at one English witch trial based a large part of his case on the fact that the supposed witch used yarrow to cure distemper, and to make predictions. In Hesse, Germany, a man wishing for good luck at cards and dice should go and dig up the "Margaret herb" yarrow during the eight days preceding and following St. Margaret's Day, while the moon is waxing. He must find three red worms among the roots, should place them carefully in a clean cloth, tuck the cloth into a pouch, and wear it on his right side. The Swiss believe it possible to find treasures with the help of the mountain yarrow.

In England, boastful men are sometimes called "yarrows." This is because men working near yarrow fields often become a little woozy from the smell and have been known to say things, in their state of temporary insanity, which they later regretted.

Oracular Worth

The Chinese *I Ching* oracle is consulted with yarrow stalks allowed to fall at random. In the West, lovers often consult yarrow oracles. Lincolnshire girls tuck a sprig of yarrow into their dresses and then try to attract the attention of young men. If they are ignored, then they must wait until the next full moon to consult the yarrow. If the man shows interest, the girl walks barefoot with closed eyes through a yarrow patch at the stroke of midnight, picking flowers at random. The flowers must then be placed in a drawer or laid under the bed. If the flowers are still fresh in the morning, the girl can take it as a sign that the young man is willing. If the flowers wilt overnight, she will have to face her disappointment, and repeat the whole process one month later when the moon is full. In other areas of the shire, lovers hoping for happy dreams gather the flowers on St.

Swithin's Day (June 15th) and then place them under their pillows. Before going to sleep at night, they repeat the rhyme,

> Good morrow, good yarrow, good morrow to thee,
> I hope by the morrow my lover to see;
> And that he may be married to me.
> The colour of his hair and the clothes he does wear,
> And if he be for me may his face be turned to me,
> And if he be not, dark and surly may be he,
> And his back turned to me.[133]

In England, it is traditional to gather yarrow on All Hallow's Eve (Halloween), and sew an ounce of it into a piece of flannel. Before going to sleep, repeat the spell,

> Thou pretty herb of Venus' tree,
> Thy true name it is yarrow,
> Now who my bosom friend must be,
> Pray tell me thou to-morrow.[134]

In Cornwall, yarrow is placed under the pillow during the full moon:

> Goodnight, fair yarrow,
> Thrice good night to thee;
> I hope before tomorrow's dawn
> My true love I shall see.[135]

In Sussex and Devonshire, a girl should pick yarrow from the grave of a young man, and then repeat the rhyme before placing it under her pillow.

> Yarrow, sweet yarrow, the first that I have found,
> In the name of Jesus Christ I pluck it from the ground.
> As Joseph loved sweet Mary, and took her for his dear,
> So in a dream this night, I hope, my true love will appear.[136]

One other method of love divination is to stick a leaf of yarrow up one's nostril and then to say the words,

---

133. *Relics of Popular Antiquities*, Publication of the Folk-Lore Society (London: Nichols & Sons, 1878), 156.

134. Ibid, 157.

135. *The Folk-Lore Journal*, vol. 5 (London: The Folk-Lore Society, 1883–89), 215.

136. William Henderson, *Notes on the Folk-Lore of the Northern Counties of England and the Borders* (London: The Folk-Lore Society, 1897), 101.

Green 'arrow, green 'arrow, you bears a white blow,
If my love love me, my nose will bleed now;
If my love don't love, it 'ont bleed a drop;
If my love love me, twill bleed every drop.[137]

Legends

Achilles is believed in some places to have been the first healer to use yarrow medicinally, or to have learned about it from Chiron the Centaur. He bound it on the wounds of his soldiers, and was able to cure them of their pain. He is also reported to have healed King Telephos with yarrow.

In Austria, mountain elves hold the herb in high esteem. A mountain mannikin once came to an old woman and told her that she would be cured of all her ills if she would eat the herb with the skin and hair, the one humans call yarrow.

Literary Flowers

Here finds he on an Oake Rheume-purging Polipode;
And in some open place that to the Sunne doth lye,
He Fumitorie gets, and Eye-bright for the eye:
The Yarrow, where-with-all he stops the wound-made gore.

—MICHAEL DRAYTON, *POLY-OLBION*, SONG XIII

---

137. *Relics of Popular Antiquities*, Publication of the Folk-Lore Society (London: Nichols & Sons, 1878), 156.

LUNAR
HERBS

I bring angelica for the lucky child. It protects Mankind from lechery.

—CHARLES DE COSTER, *TYLL ULENSPIEGEL*

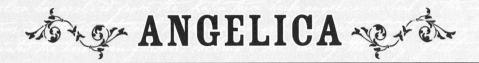

ANGELICA

Name

The name "angelica" evolved from the Latin term *herba angelica*, or "herb of the angels." The sixteenth-century herbalist Tabernaemontanus was the first to call the herb "archangelus," associating it with the highest of angels. Otto Brunfels elevated the herb even further, calling it the "root of the Holy Ghost."

Angelica archangelica (also known as *Archangelica officinalis* or *Archangelica angelica*) is a biennial, and often perennial, member of the **Carrot** or **Apiaceae** family. *Angelica archangelica var. archangelica* is widely cultivated for the large, fleshy roots so prized by herbalists. *Angelica sylvestris* grows wild in Europe, and there are many angelicas that can be encountered in the New World, including a poisonous variety called *Angelica lineariloba*. Several Oriental angelicas are used in the cosmetic industry, as well as for medicine and food. True masterwort *(Peucedanum ostruthium)*, although a completely different species, belongs to the same botanical family as angelica and has similar healing powers.

Folk Names

Angelica is also called archangel, garden archangelica, garden angelica, angelic herb, Holy Ghost, Jack-jump-about, ground ash, ghost-kex, smooth-kesh, water kesh, water squirt, kedlock, jeelico, skytes, and, misleadingly, ground elder, wild parsnip, and masterwort. German names are *Angelica, Engelwurz, Erzengelwurz, Heiliggeistwurz, Heilingenbitter, Theriakwurzel, Zahnwurzel,* and *Brustwurz.* The French call the herb *angélique, archangélique,* and *herbe du Saint Esprit;* the Italians, *angelica, angelica domestica, angelica di Boemia,* and *archangelica.* In Holland, the plant is known as *engelwortel*; in Flanders, as *engelkruid*; in Greenland, as *quaunor* or *kuanek*; in Iceland, as *hvönn*, *aetihvönn*, or *spisekvan*; in Sweden, as *strätta* or *ädel kvanne*, in Ireland, as *ainglice*, and in Russia, as *djagil lekarstvennzj*.

Appearance

Angelica can grow to a height of 6 ft., and spreads outwards to overpower other plants. The entire plant is imbued with a fragrant, aromatic odor. Cultivated and wild varieties are difficult to differentiate, and special care should be taken when gathering wild angelica because of its poisonous look-alikes such as hemlock. As a rule, poison hemlock is a much smaller plant and does not have angelica's characteristically pleasant fragrance. It is also not visited by as many insects.

Angelica has thick, brownish-gray roots filled with honey-colored sap. Their odor is strongly aromatic, even musky, with a resinous, sweetly bitter taste. Angelica stalks are thick and upright, hollow inside, and smoothly ribbed outside, seeming smooth at first glance. They are green, occasionally tinged with purple or red. Angelica leaves grow on long, sheathed, hollow footstalks, and are divided three times, and then again three or more times. They vary in size and shape, becoming smaller at the top of the stalk, a brilliant green above, and a blue green below. Angelica flowers are greenish or yellowish white, sometimes tinged with purple, and are gathered together in umbels. They smell as sweet as honey, and are visited by a great number of insects. Angelica fruits are ribbed and straw-colored.

Place, Season, and Useful Parts

Garden angelica is cultivated in Europe, China, Japan, Korea, India, and North America. It prefers the colder and temperate regions of the Northern Hemisphere, and can even be grown with success in Siberia, Greenland, and Iceland. It often escapes from cultivated areas and crosses with wild varieties in Europe, Siberia, Alaska, the Pyreneans, the Alps, and the Himalayas. It can be found in gardens, graveyards, on riverbanks and lakesides, on beaches, dams and moors, or in damp pastures. It occasionally grows near hedges and copses. According to tradition, angelica is said to blossom on the day appointed to the Archangel Michael, the 8th of May. On closer examination, this only holds true in southern regions. In the north, the herb only begins to blossom in summer.

Gathering, Drying, and Storage

The stems and stalks of angelica plants can be cut for candying from May through July. Angelica leaves should be gathered before the plant blossoms. The seeds are harvested as they ripen, usually in August, September, or October. The rhizomes of two-year-old plants can be gathered in the late fall or early spring. They are washed and then hung up to dry in an airy, dry room. Tiny roots can be braided together to form a large root "rope." Skin is often irritated by many plants of the **Carrot** family, causing swelling, especially in combination with sunlight. Angelica is no exception to this rule, and allergic reactions can be severe. Just to be certain, it is best to wear gloves when handling the plant.

Angelica leaves should be dried in a shady, airy place, or with the help of artificial heat. They must retain their light green color when dry. Angelica roots should be washed quickly under running water, split, and then hung up on a string to dry, without the aid of artificial heat. Well-dried roots are gray and wrinkled on the outside, and spongy white inside. They may be stored for several years in airtight containers. Angelica seed umbels are cut and spread out on cloths in an airy place. They dry, under normal conditions, in 7–10 days, and are then threshed and sifted, and stored in airtight containers.

Seed Saving and Germination

The most important thing to remember when trying to reproduce angelica is that the seeds are notoriously poor germinators, and will only retain their viability for a few weeks. They should be sown *immediately* after harvest to ensure a good crop of seedlings. Ideally, the seeds are sown in damp ground similar to the moist places in which the plant occurs naturally. In the case of angelica, it is often easier to keep it in its natural habitat, such as a damp meadow, instead of transferring it to the garden. Small plants can be transplanted in spring into damp garden soil.

Angelica seeds shatter easily, which means that they fall to the ground before all the seeds ripen. As with most umbels, the best seed is in the central umbel, and not in the secondary ones. This means that the central umbel should be harvested from as many plants as possible instead of trying to harvest all the seed from one plant. Because the seeds do not stay viable in storage, no special precautions are necessary, as long as they are kept cool and dry.

Gardening Hints

According to the ancient sagas, angelicas were grown in the very first Scandinavian gardens at the turn of the last millennium. Wild angelica was fenced in to protect it from browsing reindeer and other animals, and the roots were sold as a market commodity. Angelica was introduced to Central Europe in the fifteenth and sixteenth centuries, and soon became a favorite confectionery herb.

Wild angelica can easily be transplanted in the spring, and brought into the garden. The seeds can also be collected when ripe, sown immediately outdoors, only lightly covered with damp soil. Otherwise, they may refuse to sprout altogether, even if subjected to the cold vernalization period they require. It is also possible to start the seeds indoors and then to transplant them to their final position. The seeds germinate so slowly that it is advisable to cover the seedbed loosely with mulch or pine boughs throughout the winter months. Seedlings can be transplanted to allow 3 ft. between plants, but older plants should not be disturbed. Seedlings will spring up under older angelica plants allowed to go to seed, and should be removed or transplanted. Angelica is such a stately ornamental plant that it can be placed against a wall, or given a place near a small garden pool, or in a far corner of the yard or back border. New plants may also be obtained by dividing angelica roots in the fall. The divided plants and seedlings are set in deeply worked, humus-rich, moist soil in a sunny spot, preferably next to running water. Angelica responds well to regular feeding, but will not tolerate fresh manure. Garden angelica is usually biennial, dying back each year, but can be kept for 3 years if prevented from going to seed. Another alternative is to allow the seeds to fall out, producing a new crop of seedlings the following year. Some inventive organic gardeners use dry angelica stalks as nest material for beneficial insects, or as hiding places for earwigs.

Culinary Virtues

Angelica is highly prized as a vegetable herb in the extreme north because it grows to great size in the coldest climates. Oriental angelicas are also widely used in the kitchen. All parts of the European angelica can be used at the proper time of year for culinary purposes. The young leaflets are boiled in one or two waters, and served together with milder greens as a tonic spring vegetable. These tender leaves impart a fine flavor to fruit salads, cream cheese, and fruit drinks. Angelica leaves, and especially the stems, are so sweet that they can be used as a mild sweetening agent, especially in combination with mint and sweet cicely. The leaves make a pretty garnish for fish, meat, or canapés.

Angelica stalks are cut, peeled, and eaten like celery in the fall, when they are juiciest. Some like to slice the peeled stems onto buttered bread, or even to add them to rye dough before baking. The stems can also be baked in hot ashes, or the blanched stems and leaf-ribs boiled as a vegetable. The peeled stems are cooked with rhubarb, and used to flavor and sweeten jellies.

Angelica roots can be eaten raw, or baked in bread. They can even be grated, and then fermented like sauerkraut.

Angelica flowers are employed in Lapland as rennet: reindeer milk is boiled and then poured over the flowers. The resulting liquid is emptied into scrupulously cleaned reindeer intestines, like a sausage, and hung up to dry. This angelica cheese is reputed to have excellent qualities as a digestive food.

Angelica seeds are added as a flavoring to pastries and sweetened breads. Digestive angelica comfits are prepared in the same manner as coriander and caraway.

Although most people have not had the opportunity to taste fresh reindeer cheese or angelica root sauerkraut, most Europeans have eaten candied angelica at one time or another. It is added to fruit puddings and cakes, to jams, and even to ice cream. Young stems and leaf stalks are cut in May, peeled, cut into finger-long pieces, and then candied. The candied stems are also used to decorate pastries, confectioners' goods, and Christmas sweets. Angelica essence can impart a delicate flavor to custards, crèmes, and soufflés. Candied angelica roots are added to sweet beverages, and angelica roots and seeds flavor stomach bitters and such assorted alcoholic beverages as Chartreuse, Vespestro, Eau de Mélisse, gin, vermouth, angelica brennivin, melissa cordial, ratafia, and Benediktiner. The roots of wild angelica are distilled into clear spirits in Iceland and Norway, as well as in Alaska and northern Asia. Hop bitters are sometimes flavored with dried angelica leaves. A tasty angelica wine is prepared by simply infusing the seeds in a light white wine for twenty-four hours.

Noteworthy Recipes

Candied Angelica: There are many different recipes for candied angelica. According to one old and complicated recipe, the stems are harvested in May or June, and then cut into 4-inch-long pieces. Steep them for 12 hours in salted water. Then place a layer of cabbage or cauliflower leaves (or vine leaves) in a clean copper pan, arrange the angelica stems on the leaves, and cover with a second layer of cabbage leaves. Add fresh water and a little vinegar until the leaves are submerged. Boil the mixture slowly until the angelica turns green, and then strain the angelica and discard the cabbage leaves.

Make a heavy syrup with water and 1 lb. of sugar for every pound of strained angelica stems. Boil the syrup for 10 minutes, and then pour it over the angelica. Let the mixture stand for 12 hours, and then pour off the syrup into a saucepan. Boil it for 5 minutes, and pour it back onto the angelica. Let the mixture stand again for another 12 hours, and then it bring to a boil. The angelica can now be frozen or canned in syrup, or the stems can be taken out and strained, laid on a baking sheet, sprinkled with sugar, and dried in a slow oven. In dry climates, the angelica can be dried on a baking sheet in a warm, dry place. The remaining syrup can be used fresh, or bottled separately.

Modern cooks will usually want to omit the cabbage leaves, and use stainless steel or enameled cookware. The cut stalks are first plunged into boiling water until soft. Drain and peel, and then soak in a mixture of half sugar and half water for 24 hours. Strain off the liquid, and boil it until it reaches a temperature of 225° F. Add the angelica stems, and bring to a boil again. Freeze or can the mixture. If the candied stems are to be used for decoration, they should be dried in a slow oven before storing.

Angelica Liqueur: A pleasing angelica liqueur can be prepared by placing 2 lb. of finely cut angelica stalks in a clear glass container (such as a canning jar) with 1 qt. of good brandy or clear wine spirits. Close carefully, and place the container in direct sunlight or a warm spot for several weeks. Then dissolve 1 lb. of sugar in a little water over a low flame. Add the cooled syrup to the strained angelica liqueur, close the jar, and let the mixture settle for several days before straining through filter paper and funneling into bottles. Cork the bottles securely.

Household Applications

Angelica leaves and flowers, or finely ground angelica roots, are added to potpourri, to herbal cushions, and to sleeping-pillow mixtures. Wild angelica can be processed to produce a yellow dye for woolens. The stems of most angelicas can also be cut, dried, and used as large straws. A relatively pleasant way to suck the air out of plastic bags before freezing is through a sweet-smelling angelica "straw." The seed heads of all the angelicas can be cut, hung upside down to dry, sprayed with a fixative, and included in winter flower arrangements. Large dried angelica stems and seed umbels make striking arrangements when placed in vases or large bottles on the floor.

Cosmetic Properties

Angelica is highly valued as a perfumer's herb. If the stem of the plant is cut near the crown in spring, it will exude a resin with an aroma similar to musk benzoin. This resin, and the ethereal oil extracted from angelica roots and seeds, is added in small amounts (singly or in mixture) to bath and toilet waters and perfumes. During the eighteenth century, angelica water was sold as "angel-water … a curious wash to beautify the skin."[138] Angelica leaves can also be applied to the skin as a compress to relieve itching and irritation. *Angelica sinensis (A. polymorpha)* is employed in China as a cosmetic preparation against freckles. Rinsing one's teeth regularly with a decoction of angelica roots or stems in addition to regular brushing can help to prevent tooth and gum decay.

Medicinal Merits

The Oriental angelicas have been employed medicinally in China for at least four thousand years as painkillers, and as yin and immune system tonics. Our Western angelica was used as medicine against the Black Death (plague) during the Middle Ages. In fact, one large medical treatise of this time devoted itself exclusively to a discussion of the

---

138.   From *The Accomplished Female Instructor* (1719), qtd. in Robert Nares, James O. Halliwell, and Thomas Wright, *A Glossary: Or, Collection of Words, Phrases, Names, and Allusions to Customs, Proverbs, Etc.,* vol. I (London: Gibbings, 1901; digitized), 25.

relative merits of angelica and holy thistle to treat and prevent the plague. Angelica was also used extensively to treat the victims of the Spanish influenza epidemic of 1918–19. It was once included in the ancient panacea theriak, and is now added to the "Swedish herb mixture" that has come into vogue. Ancient physicians considered angelica capable of comforting and defending the heart, blood, and spirits; of easing intestinal disorders; of cleansing the womb of poison and obstructions; and of ridding the body of poison, worms, harmful humors, and excess water.

Modern Medicine

Angelica roots and angelica seeds are now recognized as strengthening and tonic medicines for the glandular and circulatory systems, with a beneficial effect on the nerves, the respiratory and reproductive organs, the skin and the digestion. Angelica products are used externally as counterirritants, often in the form of a salve. Angelica roots can be administered like masterwort and burnet saxifrage *(Pimpinella saxifraga)* as tonic and strengthening medicines. Of the three roots, angelica is the mildest, followed by burnet saxifrage, and then masterwort. The mountain forms of these herbs are appreciably more potent than lowland plants.

Angelica seeds are used to fortify the body against infection, aiding the circulation, and strengthening weakened nerves and a weakened constitution. Chronic illness and general debility can also be treated with angelica seed tea.

The roots of the plant are given to cleanse the lungs, stomach, and intestines of mucus, to counteract the effects of excessive alcohol and tobacco consumption, as well as the aftereffects of such poisons as hemlock. It is interesting to note that angelica and hemlock often grow in close proximity to each other in their natural habitat. The roots are also prescribed as preventive medicines against contagious diseases such as influenza, and can be used to induce perspiration and to "break" a fever. Angelica has a warming and comforting effect on the digestive organs, and can relieve flatulence, expel worms, and soothe an overacid stomach. Angelica should not be given to diabetics, and pregnant women should also avoid using the herb. Oriental angelica has been widely marketed under the name Dong quai in the West as a tonic and regulatory yin medicine for the female system that can be taken over an extended period. Dong quai contains phytoestrogens, helps to heal vaginal yeast infections, and helps to enhance the immune system. It should not be taken when diarrhea is present, and should be administered carefully if the patient is bleeding.

The juice of the fresh angelica plant is applied externally to help ripen boils and abscesses. Angelica salve and angelica spirits are used in the treatment of rheumatism, gout, and neuralgia. Angelica baths, prepared from 5–8 oz. of coarsely ground angelica roots, are helpful for those weakened by nervous disorders, a weak immune system, or distressed by rheumatism.

Angelica sinensis is used homeopathically for pre-menstrual syndrome, weight changes, leucorrhea, and thyroid problems. It is prescribed as a tonic medicine for asthmatics, the sleepless, and those with digestive disorders.

Angelica sinensis is called honeywort or mountain celery in China, and is often added to herbal mixtures as a flavoring agent, and also as a blood tonic to treat menstrual complaints, tonify the body, improve the muscle tone, moisten the intestines, relieve pain, reduce swelling, and strengthen the immune system. It contains phytoestrogens, and is used to treat yeast infections. The plant root is divided into three parts—the head, the body, and the tail—each of which is used to treat different complaints. Another angelica, *Angelica dahurica*, known as Chinese angelica root, is used to expel dampness, to treat sinus congestion and head colds, and to reduce swelling and carbuncles.

Special Cures

Angelica Honey: This thickened syrup is prepared from 1 part finely ground angelica root powder, 3 parts (European) juniper berries, water, and sugar. Boil the juniper berries with water and sugar until the mixture attains a syrupy consistency. Then add the angelica powder, stir the mixture several times, strain, and pour into sterilized jars. Seal carefully, and store in a cool place. If desired, the sugar can be omitted. This angelica "honey" is spread on bread and butter, or taken a teaspoonful at a time to relieve respiratory problems or to loosen a cough. Pregnant women and diabetics should avoid its use altogether, and patients with kidney or bladder infections should use it conservatively.

Angelica Wine: Angelica wine is prepared from 1 oz. of the powdered roots or 1 oz. of the seeds infused in 1 pint of white wine for 24 hours. Then strain the mixture through filter paper, adding a few kernels of cardamom as flavoring. Bottle and seal. This wine can be taken a teaspoonful at a time for digestive purposes and as a preventive measure against infectious diseases.

Swedish Herb Mixture: This consists of a mixture of 30 grams of granulated aloe, 15 gr. pure camphor, 7.5 gr. carline thistle roots, 7.4 gr. gentian *(Gentiana lutea)* roots, 30 gr. manna (the sugary sap of the manna ash, *Fraxinus ornus*), 7.5 gr. granulated myrrh, 15 gr. China rhubarb *(Rheum officinale)* roots, 15 gr. senna *(Cassia senna)* leaves, 15 gr. zeodary roots *(Curcuma zedoaria)*, 15 gr. Venetian theriak, and 2 gr. pure saffron. These herbs and resins are infused in 1 qt. of clear spirits, and placed in a stoppered bottle in a sunny place for 2 weeks. Shake daily. Strain and filter the mixture at the end of 2 weeks, and fill into small bottles, corking them securely.

The resulting tincture can be taken a few drops at a time for a great number of disorders, and also applied externally.

Uses in Husbandry

Lice are said to dislike the smell of angelica seeds: a few drops of the oil are added to lice-deterring mixtures. Angelica leaves are sometimes dried for use as herbal snuff, or as a tobacco substitute. Bohemian angelica is considered to be the best commercial angelica.

Veterinary Values

Wild angelica leaves can be fed to cattle, with the exception of recently-bred cows. Angelica roots are added in miniscule amounts to the food of animals troubled with digestive or nervous disorders or cramps. *Angelica keiskei* is used in Japan as a fodder plant.

Miscellaneous Wisdom

Angelica's healing abilities are often attributed to angelic beings or to the Holy Spirit, and it is worn as an antidemonic amulet, just like the related osha *(Ligusticum porteri)* in the North American southwest. When the plague was still a dreaded disease, so much angelica was harvested for its roots that the herb was close to extinction, like ginseng and coneflower *(Echinacea sp.)* in our day and age. Herbalists once recommended that their patients hold the roots under their tongue to deter plague, witches, poison, sorcery, and evil vapors, as well as impotence. The roots were said to relieve that queasy feeling occasioned by swallowing a spider, and were included in love potions.

Children love to dry angelica stalks and use them as peashooters, whistles, and straws.

Legends

The story goes than an angel was concerned with the suffering of men. He then told one of them in a dream of the healing properties of an angelic herb and its power against all diseases and the plague in particular. Since then, angelica has been a staple medicinal remedy in Europe.

And the house of Israel called the name thereof Manna:
and it was like coriander seed, white;
and the taste of it was like wafers made with honey.

—EXODUS 16:31

ANISE & CORIANDER

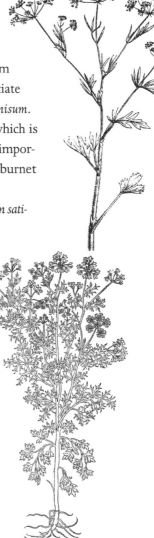

Name

Anise and coriander are both annual members of the ***Apiaceae***
or ***Umbelliferae*** (**Carrot**) family. The word "anise" has developed from the Latin *anisum*, a Roman and originally a Greek term
for both dill and anise. Later, an attempt was made to differentiate
between dill and anise, and anise became known as *Pimpinella anisum*.
The term *pimpinella* developed from the Latin word *bipinella*, which is
a botanical designation for a plant with bipinnate leaves. Other important healing herbs also carry the name *Pimpinella*—for example, burnet
saxifrage.

"Coriander" and the first part of its botanical name, *Coriandrum sativum,* are derived from the Greek and may originally have
been Eastern words. *Koros* means "bug": the name was
probably used to describe the penetrating "buggy" odor of
the plant's leaves, which in turn repelled insect pests such as
bedbugs and lice. *Sativum* means that the plant is, despite its
strong smell, edible.

In addition to *Pimpinella anisum*, anise is known by the
synonyms *Carum anisum, Apium anisum, Anisum officinarum,*
Selinum anisum, and *Anisum vulgare.*

Several varieties of garden anise have been developed over
the years, of which green anise is the most famous. Star or Chinese anise *(Illicium verum)* has an odor and taste similar to anise,
but it belongs to a completely different family as well as species.

Folk Names

Anise was known in Old English as *anyse*, and in one old
herbal was termed *anacetum*. Modern folk names are sweet alice,

sweet cumin, Chinese parsley, and heal-bite. German names are *Anis, süsser Kümmel*, and *römischer Fenchel*. Some French terms are *anis, anis vert*, and *boucage*; some Italian terms are *anice, anica verde*, and *anaci*. In Spanish, the herb is known as *anis*; in Irish, *ainís*; in Sanskrit, *shetapusapa*; in Turkish, *anason* or *anasur*; in Russian, *anis obyknovennyj*; in Chinese, *ou hiu hsiang* or *huai hsiang*; and in Japanese, *anasu*.

Coriander is also known as bug-herb, cilantro, and (incorrectly) Chinese parsley. Earlier names were collendre, coliander, and corriandir. Between 1730 and 1800, the name coriander was used as slang term for money or coins. Old High German names were *Chullentar* and *Collander*. Germans now call the plant *Koriander, Schwindelkorn, Wanzendill*, or *Galander*; the French have given it the names of *coriandre* and *persil arabe*. Italians address it as *coriandolo, coriandro, coriandolo selvatico, erba cimicina*, and *erba puzza*. Spaniards know it as *cilentro, culentro, culantrico*, and *cilantro*; Turks as *kisnis*; Russians as *kišnec* or *koriandr*; and Japanese as *koendoro*. In China, it goes by the name *xe hu yn, yuan sui*, or *hsiang sui*. The Sanskrit name was *dhanyaka*.

Appearance

Anise has a single, spindly, annual root. The plant's stem is round and ribbed. It grows to a maximum height of 3 ft. but is usually only half that tall. Anise leaves vary from the bottom to the top of the same plant. The lower leaves are heart-shaped, and the upper leaves resemble those of dill. The whole herb, especially the fruits, is imbued with a characteristic aroma that is its most important identifying characteristic. Because it is a member of the **Carrot** family, there is danger of confusing anise with other less wholesome herbs. The anise stalk branches out to produce flat-topped double umbels of small white or pinkish flowers. These flowers later produce hairy fruits that open to reveal two grayish-brown seeds decorated with 10 ribs apiece.

Coriander grows to a maximum height of 3 ft., and is recognizable by the usually unpleasant odor of its leaves, similar to that of crushed lice or bedbugs. Coriander aficionados will certainly protest, because they have gotten used to the plant's smell, and find it exhilarating. It is nonetheless possible to confuse coriander with other umbels, since the first leaves differ in form from the later. The only certain method of identification is to compare fruits. Coriander fruits have an almost perfect spherical shape that is unusual for members of this family. The plant has a thin, spindly root. Its erect stems are slender, ribbed and strongly branched, looking a little like inverted pyramids. Unlike anise, they are not covered with hairs. Coriander leaves, like anise, vary from the bottom to the top of the plant. They are shiny and bright green, and very finely cut. Coriander flowers are mauve or white, and produce symmetrical clusters of fruits shaped like tiny balls. These fruits have a mildly buggy smell that turns pleasant once they are dried. The taste is sweet and at the same time spicy and a little bitter.

Place, Season, and Useful Parts

Anise originally came to Europe from the Orient or the Middle East and is now culti-vated in gardens in temperate climates the world over. It sometimes escapes from culti-vated areas, but only survives for a short time as a wild plant. It often begins to blossom in May, and then continues on into September. Anise usually produces fruits in August and September. It may not produce seeds in northern countries.

Coriander originally came from the area east of the Mediterranean, and is now widely cultivated in Europe, Asia, North and South America, and Northern Africa. Euro-peans usually turn up their noses at the herb, but it is an essential part of the cuisines of most southern and eastern areas. It often escapes from cultivated areas, and can now be found on all these continents as a wild plant. It may appear in grain and pea fields, in gardens, potato patches and vineyards, on rubble and riverbanks, or in open meadows to an altitude of 4,500 ft. It flowers from June through August. Both the leaves and the seeds are harvested.

Gathering, Drying, and Storage

Anise fruits are harvested in August and September, when they ripen, on a sunny, dry day, as soon as the dew has dried. The first ripe central umbels are cut first, with a second harvest a little later. The fruits will not fall off the stems like coriander, and can easily be dried on cloths in the shade, or, if a spell of bad weather is predicted, in the midday sun. For the second harvest, the plants are cut as soon as most of the fruits begin to darken and the stalks lighten in color. Anise plants can be dried outdoors on sheets or trays, weather permitting, or they are bundled, brought indoors and hung up in a dry, airy place over sheets to dry. The plants are threshed to remove the fruits as soon as the stalks are dry. Properly dried anise fruits are gray or light brown in color.

Coriander plants lose their fruits easily. To prevent shattering, they should therefore be harvested carefully in the morning, as soon as the dew has dried. The harvest takes place just before the fruits fully ripen, as soon as they begin to lose their penetrating odor in July, August, or September. They are then laid out to dry on cloths in the sun or in a dry and airy place. Unlike most herbs, the aromatic qualities of coriander fruits improve with age, and they can be stored for as long as 5 years. The fresh herb is cut like parsley before blossoming, and should be used immediately, because it will not keep long.

Seed Saving and Germination

Fewer anise forms exist than coriander. Over the centuries, a surprising diversity of coriander varieties has been developed. The major selective criterion is either for fruit or leaf production. Local varieties have been developed the world over by farmers to adapt the plants to local growing conditions, and the oil content can also vary greatly from one variety to another. Coriander varieties will cross readily with one another, so single varieties should be isolated to maintain genetic purity.

The best seeds are formed in the first umbels the plants produce. It is therefore better not to wait until the secondary umbels ripen, but to concentrate on the first ripe fruits for seed harvesting. This selection will also, over a number of years, help to produce an earlier variety. Fruits saved for seed should be dried slowly but evenly indoors, and stored in as cool, dry, and dark a place as possible. Anise seeds retain a high germination rate for 2–3 years, but coriander seeds very quickly lose their viability. They can still be used for cooking if they do not germinate.

Gardening Hints

The cultivation of anise was recommended by Charlemagne for European cloister gardens, and it has been a common garden plant ever since. Anise grows best next to coriander, and vice versa. Both plants require light, well-aerated soil enriched with humus and limestone. They prefer a warm position and damp, yet warm weather, and are usually very sensitive to drought, baking sun, or cold northern winds. They should be protected from wind and the beds kept well weeded and well watered. Anise should be rotated with other crops, and only grown once every three years on the same plot.

Anise seeds, like those of many other members of this family, take their time about germinating. It may take up to four weeks until the first seedlings show their heads. The soil should be neutral or slightly alkaline. The seeds can be sown in peat pots under glass in February to May to lessen transplantation problems in cooler climates. In warm climates with a long growing season, they are sown outdoors after the last frost. Plant out the peat pots after all danger of frost is past, or thin the seedlings to allow 4–5 in. between plants. Anise succumbs easily to the first cold snap.

Coriander may occasionally winter over, although it is an annual herb, and readily re-seeds itself. In milder areas, special varieties can be grown as a winter crop. Coriander seeds germinate relatively quickly, usually in less than a week. Unlike anise, which requires a long growing season, coriander can be sown in its final position outdoors in April. It usually begins to flower 2 months later. A distance of 8–10 in. should be allowed between rows, but the distance between plants varies greatly according to variety. Coriander should be freed regularly from weed competition, and may be subject to insect infestation, especially aphids. It is therefore often used as a decoy plant by organic gardeners to keep aphids away from more important or endangered crops. Fennel should not be planted in the vicinity of coriander, or it will produce fewer seeds.

Culinary Virtues

Anise is one of the oldest culinary herbs. A spice with a similar taste, star anise, has been used for millennia to flavor foods in the Far East, but it is not related botanically to our garden anise. Anise was employed in the kitchens of the ancient Egyptians and Greeks, as well as the Cretans, Cypriots, and Syrians. In ancient times, Greeks sprinkled anise fruits on their bread, and added them to sauces and wines. In Rome, an anise cake called *mustacca* was served at the end of a meal to relieve the digestive problems caused by over-indulgence. In present-day India, a dish of anise fruits is sometimes placed on the table after a meal for the same reason.

Anise, like its relatives fennel, caraway, and coriander, can be added to "windy" dishes to prevent and counteract flatulence. It is a good seasoning for convalescents, and is often used to flavor bread, cakes, biscuits, pastries, and pancakes. Anise fruits and anise oil can help to prevent mold from forming on confectioners' paste. The fruits are also employed to season marmalades, jellies, jams, candies, stewed apples, pears, and quinces, and to preserve pickles and cheese. Ground anise can be added in small amounts to shrimp cocktails, sweet-and-sour dishes, as well as to lobster, cod, crab, or shellfish. Cabbage and cauliflower soups, as well as spinach and cream cheese dips can be seasoned with anise. Freshly chopped anise leaves taste good in salads, and are added in small amounts to baby carrots or fresh cottage cheese or ricotta. Anise fruits should always be bought from a reliable source or grown at home, since they are occasionally adulterated with the seeds of poisonous *Apiaceae*.

Coriander is also an ancient seasoning herb. The Chinese and Romans made use of it at an early date, and it has been discovered in prehistoric sites in Britain. The ancient Egyptians flavored wine with it, and it was mentioned in the Talmud. Coriander was widely used as a seasoning in both North and South America before Europeans discovered these continents, and Saxons were familiar with its culinary properties well before the Roman Conquest. According to Varro, Romans preserved meat during hot summers by rubbing it with wine vinegar and crushed coriander fruits before curing. The coriander also helped to keep away flies. Pickling mixtures always included coriander.

Coriander fruits are excellent for seasoning and preserving smoked and pickled meat, lamb, sausages, roasts, stews, and meat loaves, as well as grain stews and soups. Boiled wheat, spelt, barley, millet, rice and oats, cheese, cabbage, red beets, spinach, carrots, pickles, savory puddings, and lentils can all be flavored with coriander fruits or coriander leaves. The aroma of the fruits is enhanced by roasting and then crushing them before use. Some cooks are very partial to the spicy taste of coriander vinegar, and the crushed leaves and fruits are an important addition to curry powders, piccalillis, and chutneys.

Fresh coriander leaves (cilantro) are rarely used by Europeans, Americans, and Canadians, but are an essential ingredient in Central and South American, Thai, Indian, and Caribbean cuisine. Cilantro is as important to many cuisines as the "fines herbes" of French cooking are to the Western world. Coriander is used in American cooking primarily in combination with chili, but also together with turmeric and cumin seeds. Coriander flowers can also be used for seasoning purposes. Southwestern American and Mexican cooking makes extensive use of the herb as a parsley substitute and as a distinctive seasoning. In Thai cooking, even the roots of the coriander plant are employed.

Coriander fruits are in great demand by bakers and confectioners. Unscrupulous practitioners have been known to use the musky taste of the seeds to overpower the flavor of stale flour. In Germany, fresh rolls are seasoned with coriander fruits, and *Lebkuchen* (gingerbread) spice mixtures usually include crushed coriander fruits. Whole coriander fruits can also be roasted and then dipped in sugar and fashioned into candy balls and "comfits" for children. These coriander comfits not only taste good, but also help to comfort the stomach and expel wind. They were once so popular that the Italian name *coriandolo* came to be synonymous with comfit, and is still used to designate the traditional white candies prepared from seeds or single almonds, and distributed at Mediterranean weddings and christenings.

Distillers as well as home brewers employ both anise and coriander. Anise wines and anise beers were very popular drinks in the Middle Ages. Anisette, Pastis, Mistrá, Ouzo, Allasch, Raki, and Mannheimerwasser, to name just a few alcoholic drinks, are now prepared with anise. Beers brewed from wheat (Weissbier) are sometimes flavored with anise. Eau de Carmes and Melissengeist are usually flavored with coriander fruits, and gin often owes its unique flavor to juniper berries and coriander. In ancient Egypt, wine enhanced with coriander was considered highly intoxicating.

Noteworthy Recipes

Anise Liqueur: To prepare anise liqueur, place 1 oz. of bruised green anise fruits in a clear glass quart bottle, and fill with clear spirits such as wine spirits or plum brandy (Slivovitz), leaving some head room. A spicier liqueur can be created by adding 1 small stick of cinnamon and ½ oz. of coriander fruits. Cork well and place in a warm spot. Infuse for 4 weeks, and then strain the mixture through filter paper. Dilute the spirits with cooled syrup made from a small amount of sugar dissolved in boiling water. Anise liqueur is taken after a meal to prevent flatulence.

Aqua Composita: Very adventurous cooks may want to distill their own Aqua Composita from a recipe given by Sir Hugh Platt in 1594:

> Take a gallo[n] of Gascoigne wine, of ginger, galingale, cinnamon, nutmegs & graines [he probably meant cloves], Annis seeds, Fennell seeds, and carroway seeds, of each a dram; of Sage, mints, red Roses, thyme, Pellitory, Rosemary, wild thyme, camomil, lavender, of each a handfull, bray

the spices small, and bruise the herbs, letting them macerate 12. houres, stirring it now & then, then distill by a limbecke of pewter keeping the first clear water that commeth, by it selfe, and so likewise the second. You shall draw about a pinte of the better sort from euerie gallon of wine.[139]

Springerle: The following is a traditional northern German recipe for Christmas cookies:

Beat 2 eggs and 1 cup of very finely sifted powdered sugar in a copper bowl (if available) with a whisk for at least half an hour. Add the grated rind of one lemon, 1–2 tsp. of whole or freshly crushed anise fruits, and 2 cups of fine cake flour sifted with ½ tsp. of baking powder and ⅛ tsp. of salt. Continue to beat the mixture for another quarter of an hour. Roll the dough out on a floured board to a thickness of ¼ of an inch. Press a lightly floured wooden Springerle board onto the lightly floured dough, and cut out the squares. If you do not have a board, cut the dough into 1½ x 1 in. rectangles. Let these rise for 10 hours on greased and floured baking sheets. Bake in a moderate oven for 10–20 minutes, until dry, but not brown.

Some cooks prefer to dispense with the baking powder, and use carbonate of ammonia dissolved in spirits, or simply increase the number of eggs. The carved Springerle board produces very pretty cookies, but may be omitted if unavailable.

Cold Cucumber Soup: In a blender, combine 1 large, peeled cucumber with 1 cup of chicken or vegetable broth, ½ cup cilantro leaves, and ¼ cup sour cream. Season to taste with salt, freshly ground black pepper, and a little lemon juice. Serve at room temperature, or chill in refrigerator for 2–3 hours.

South of the Border Cole Slaw with Cilantro: Mix 2 cups of finely shredded white cabbage and 2 cups of finely shredded red cabbage in a salad bowl. Add ½ cup of finely chopped cilantro leaves, the juice of 1 large lime, 1 Tbsp. of water sweetened with honey or sugar, ½ Tbsp. of crushed cumin seeds, and salt to taste. Coleslaw should be prepared 1–2 hours ahead of time, and served at room temperature.

Fresh Salsa: There are innumerable recipes for salsa, but most of them include coriander leaves as one of the main ingredients. Salsa is often served with tortilla chips, but it also mixes well with other Mexican dishes, beans and rice, or even with bread and cheese.

Take 4 juicy tomatoes, and peel and dice them. Add, according to taste, either mild or sharp chilis that have been roasted over a flame, the seeds and dividing walls removed, and then chopped small. Mix in 2 cloves of chopped garlic, and 4 finely chopped green onions. Stir the mixture in a ceramic bowl, and add 2 Tbsp.

---

139.   Platt, *Delightes for Ladies* (1594) (London: Penguin, 1948), 59.

of fresh lime juice, ⅛ cup of finely chopped cilantro, 1 Tbsp. of finely chopped oregano, a pinch of sugar, and salt and pepper to taste. Some may want to add a pinch of crushed cumin seed *(Cuminum cyminum)* to accentuate the taste of the cilantro. Let stand, covered, at room temperature for 2 hours before serving to intensify the flavor.

Household Applications

The pleasing and refreshing scent of anise seeds recommends them to sachet and pot-pourri-makers, who often combine powdered orris root *(Iris germanica var. florentina)* with crushed anise seeds. Anise and coriander seeds can help to freshen a room, and drive insects away. Anise seeds are also used as bait for mice, and are often included in moth-repelling mixtures.

Small amounts of crushed coriander fruits can be added to potpourri, or to incense mixtures. Ethereal oil of coriander combines well with other oils if used sparingly. A sweet-smelling incense was once prepared from coriander and was enjoyed for its mild narcotic properties. Coriander is valued for its ability to drive away flies, fleas, and even bedbugs. This is probably why it was originally so widely grown in southern countries.

One of the most handsome products prepared from anise and coriander are spice balls or wreaths. They impart a spicy, holiday aroma to a room, and make excellent gifts. Take a small wreath or ball form made of styrofoam or a natural product such as straw, and cover it with pretty single-toned paper before fastening the whole spices to it with glue or wire. Cloves, cinnamon sticks, star anise fruits, dried ginger roots, white or brown nutmegs and laurel leaves are obvious decorative choices. Smaller balls can be covered with fennel, anise, caraway, coriander, mustard, or poppy seeds, or even peppercorns, and then fastened to the larger form. Vanilla pods and tonka beans, as well as orris, licorice, and galingale roots, are unusual additions, and a touch of color can be added with red hawthorns, rose hips, and rowan berries, or white unhulled pumpkin seeds. With a bit of imagination, pleasing patterns and color/scent combinations can be invented.

Cosmetic Properties

Anise and coriander oils are employed today by perfumers and soap makers to titillate the nostrils of their customers. Commercial mouthwashes made from anise freshen the breath and strengthen the gums, and some toothpastes contain oil of anise.

In the seventeenth century, it was fashionable among the upper classes to wear golden "apples" as neck ornaments. These apples opened up into segments, and each segment contained a costly perfume: musk, ambergris, and civet, as well as essence of anise. This was not a purely ornamental practice, but served a very practical need. Bathing was not as popular then as it is today, even among the monied classes, and great quantities of perfume were necessary to overpower unpleasant body odors and drive away parasites.

When baths *were* taken, John Shirley's book gave an expensive and complicated recipe for a coriander herbal bath:

> To make a sweet Bath
>
> Take the flowers or peels of Citrons, the flowers of Oranges and Gessamine, Lavender, Hysop, Bay-Leaves, the flowers of Rosemary, Comfry, and the seeds of Coriander, Endive and sweet Marjorum; the berries of Myrtle and Juniper; boil them in Spring-Water, after they are bruised, till a third part of the liquid matter is consumed, and enter it in a Bathing-tub, or wash yourself with it as you see occasion, and it will indifferently serve for Beauty and Health.[140]

For the modern bather, citron and orange blossoms are fabulous bath additions if you happen to live in the south. For the rest of us, lavender, hyssop, rosemary leaves, and marjoram are excellent aromatic bath herbs, and can be used alone, or flavored with a little anise or coriander.

- The easiest way to use these herbs is in the form of ethereal oils. Just 1–2 drops of anise oil can be mixed with a natural body oil such as avocado, almond, or jojoba. Add a little liquid soap, and shake the mixture before bathing to distribute the anise. The mixture is added to the hot water before the bath is filled—otherwise, the sharp oil may burn the skin. If fresh herbs are available, barely cover the herb mixture with water and boil it in a closed pot for no more than 10 minutes. Then strain the mixture into the bath water. Those who are in a hurry may simply want to fill the herbs into a coarse "bath bag," and hang it under the hot water tap.

Herbs should never be added directly to the bath water without straining: unpleasant messes, clogged drains, and stained enamel may result. Most experts recommend increasing the temperature of the herbal bath by several degrees after the first few minutes, and then continuing to increase it until the water is pleasantly warm, but not hot. Adding a few drops of high-quality oil such as jojoba or olive oil to the bath water helps to avoid stains and simplifies cleaning. Herbal baths should be enjoyed for 15–20 minutes, followed by 15–20 minutes of complete relaxation in a warm bed. Those with circulatory or heart problems should be careful about using stimulant herbs such as rosemary, especially in the evening.

---

140.   Shirley, *The Accomplished Ladies Rich Closet of Rarities* (London: N. Bodington, 1688), 66.

Medicinal Merits

Ancient writers considered anise to be a warming herb, capable of drying out scrofula and phlegma, easing epileptic fits, strengthening women after the ordeals of childbirth, and helping runners to catch their "second wind." As the saying goes, "With Pimpinel! Sweet Pimpinel! Mother and Babe are doing well!" It was also prescribed to stop "yeoxing or hicket" (the hiccups), increase the appetite of the lazy, and heal "broken" ears. It was said to provoke venery, and was placed under pillows to prevent bad dreams. Dioscurides summed it up: "Anisum hath generally a warming, drying, sweet breathmaking, paine easing, dissolving, ureticall, discussing faculty."[141]

Coriander was thought to be a much more powerful, and subsequently more dangerous, herb. Dioscurides warned against it in his Herball: "It is engendering of seed. But being taken too much it disturbs ye understanding dangerously, whence men ought to avoid the overmuch, & too often use of it." Otto Brunfels seconded this opinion, and wrote that overuse would "anesthetize and enebriate the brain." It was generally considered to be an effective aphrodisiac, which may explain why it is so assiduously avoided, even today, in most of the Protestant world. The Chinese even credited the plant with the ability to render human beings immortal. Women who were having trouble giving birth were advised in the herbal of Pseudo-Apuleius to find a chaste person, and to tie 11 or 13 coriander seeds to his or her thigh. Coriander seeds were also thought to stimulate the liver and the intestines, and were administered to counteract poison and to treat recurrent three-day fevers. European herbalists did not use coriander leaves medicinally.

Modern Medicine

Modern practitioners consider anise to be a mild herb capable of soothing and strengthening mothers and their young children, of warming and comforting the digestive organs, and of expelling mucus from the body. Pregnant woman may drink anise tea in moderate amounts to cleanse the mucous membranes before birth, and then after birth to increase the milk flow. The milk of mothers who drink anise seed tea is also beneficial for the newborn child: it comforts the child, cleanses its lungs of mucus, and eases digestive disorders. Anise baths also help to increase the milk of nursing mothers. Teething children calm down somewhat if anise tea is used to dilute their milk. Anise can relieve flatulence in both children and adults, ease digestion and intestinal cramps, and strengthen the stomach. In the words of *The School of Salernum*,

> The stomach it doth cleanse, and comfort well:
> And fourthly, it doth keep and cleanse the sight.

---

141.   Robert T. Gunther, ed., *The Greek Herbal of Dioscurides* (New York: Hafner, 1959), 299.

And thus the seed and hearbe doth both excell.
Yet for the two last told, if any seed
With Fennel many compare, 'tis Annis-seed:
Some Annis-seed be sweete, and some more bitter,
For pleasure these, for medicine those are fitter.[142]

Anise may be administered either in wine or water, or it can be laid on the stomach in warm sacks. It helps to expel phlegm from the body and also eases coughs, congestion of the lungs or uterus, and earaches or headaches. Anise seeds may be combined with sage and then infused as a gargle for sore throats, or the smoke of the burned fruits inhaled to clear the head. Some modern herbalists believe that anise stimulates the nerves, and that it can even help to strengthen the spinal nerves. Anise is further applied as a salve to ease skin irritations, as an eye-water to cleanse the eyes, and as a tea to combat sleeplessness. In aromatherapy, anise oil is used primarily to calm nervous digestive troubles, flatulence, and nausea. Overuse of the herb over an inordinately long time can lead to the same symptoms as alcohol poisoning. Star anise is the homeopathic treatment of choice for patients with pain around the third rib.

Coriander seeds are carminative, which means that they counteract flatulence, and can be used as strengthening agents for the digestive organs. They are included in many digestive spirits (*Aqua carminativa, Karmelitergeist, Spiritus aromaticus, Spiritus melissae compositus*), and are added as a flavoring agent to many others. They help to relieve stomach troubles, ease intestinal cramps, colics and flatulence, stomach catarrhs, indigestion, and diarrhea. Coriander seeds should not be used excessively, for large amounts have been known to cause headaches and dizziness. Some patients swear by a sleeping draught of coriander seeds in mulled wine. In aromatherapy, the oil is used internally for intestinal and digestive troubles, cramps and nervous states of exhaustion. It is employed in rubbing mixtures for the treatment of rheumatism. The intake of excessive amounts of coriander oil can cause drunkenness and consequent states of depression. Coriander leaves, cilantro, can aid detoxification when fasting or undergoing a cleanse.

Anise is used in Chinese medicine to treat constipation and difficult urination, as well as low back pain. Coriander is considered good for provoking perspiration, and resolving feelings of fullness and abdominal discomfort. It can cause measles to break more quickly into the rash stage. In China, coriander leaf is cooked with fish to increase the warm energy of these colder foods, and to imbue them with fragrance.

---

142.   Sir John Harrington, trans., *The School of Salernum* (Salerno, Italy: Ente Provinciale per il Turismo, 1953), 47.

Special Cures

Anise Tea for Children: A child or infant with a cold can be given a teaspoon of warm anise seed tea every hour. Boil ½ tsp. of the fruits (or a little more for older children) in 1 pint of water for several minutes and let stand, covered, for 15 minutes before straining. For adult use, prepare the tea from ⅙ oz. of the dried fruits in 1 pint of water. If children will not drink the tea, try sweetening it with a little honey, but do not let this become a habit. In Europe, the alarming state of pre-school children's teeth is caused to a large degree by the instant commercial herb tea widely used to calm infants.

Anise to Induce Menstruation: A tea mixture to induce menstruation can be prepared from equal parts of anise, caraway, and fennel fruits, together with a mixture of half that amount of peppermint leaves, marigold flower petals, and English chamomile flowers. Best results can be obtained by boiling ½ tsp. of the fruit mixture in 1 pint of water for 10 minutes before removing from the heat. Then add a weak tablespoon of the looser herb mixture before steeping, covered, for 15 minutes. This tea should be taken 2–3 times a day in small quantities for 1 week before the expected date of the period.

Anise for Nursing Mothers: Nursing mothers who do not have enough milk to feed their babies may want to drink a tea prepared from equal parts of fennel, dill, anise fruits, and lady's mantle leaves. This tea can be prepared in larger amounts and stored for up to a day in a thermos bottle. The mother should religiously drink a small cup before and after each nursing session. An added bonus is the calming effect exerted on the child through the mother's milk.

Uses in Husbandry

Both anise and coriander plants are visited by bees. Although large amounts of anise oil are harmful for birds, a few drops can be rubbed onto pigeon roosts, and a few fruits mixed with their food when they are brought to a new home. Some breeders recommend giving the birds cooked peas and thyme, or barley flavored with anise, to accustom them to a new roost. Others suggest giving pigeons a piece of anise bread on Candlemas (February 2nd, the day birds begin to sing again after the dark months of the European winter) and on every day for the next 4 weeks to improve their health.

Horses are partial to the taste and odor of anise, and many horses have been lured against their will by grooms who keep some crushed anise, fennel, and hemp seeds in their pockets along with a few lumps of sugar, or by owners who perfume themselves with lavender oil.

Dairy cattle can be given a maximum of 3 oz. anise fruits mixed with their fodder to increase milk production. Goats should not be given more than 1 oz. Mice and moles can occasionally be forced into abandoning their homes if their tunnels are stopped up with freshly blossoming coriander plants.

Coriander has been used to impart a spicy flavor to tobaccos, and the bark of star anise is incorporated into some Japanese incenses.

Veterinary Values

Anise is used by veterinarians for animals in many of the same ways it is administered to humans. Animals' fur is rubbed down with oil of anise to drive away fleas and lice. Anise and coriander fruits are added to fodder in small doses to relieve cramps and flatulence. Pneumonia can also be treated with larger doses of anise. Horses and cattle may be given as much as 2–3 oz. of the crushed fruits, while pigs only tolerate ⅙ as much, and dogs only a fraction as much as pigs.

Miscellaneous Wisdom

Because of their strong aromatic odor, both anise and coriander are thought to possess strong antidemonic properties. Anise is reputed to avert the Evil Eye, as well as to prevent stomachaches and colics. The fruits are worked into tiny lockets and amulets hung around infants' necks. In Prussia, coriander stalks were once hung up in stalls on Midsummer's Day to protect the cattle from the machinations of witches, and any woman suspected of being a witch was tested with coriander or caraway bread. If she ate the bread, then she was not dangerous, but if she refused it, it was taken as a sign of her association with Satan. Anise and coriander were combined with camphor and other herbs to produce a scrying incense capable of producing visions and aiding the work of conjuration.

Anise was once held in great repute as an aphrodisiac. Anise in wine or anise spirits were favorite drinks of young people when they met at traditional spinning parties to work, drink, tell stories, and meet new friends. On November 30th, otherwise known as *Anischtag*, or Anise Day, Bohemians believed that anise exerted extraordinary powers. In Malaysia, an aphrodisiac potion is still prepared from coriander seeds, peppercorns, cloves, nutmeg, and the brain of a goat. Pregnant English women were once told to eat great quantities of coriander and quinces in order to impart geniality to their unborn children, and to prevent vaporous afflictions.

...It makes a man merry and joyfull: which thing also the old verse concerning Borage doth testifie: Ego Borago gaudia semper ago. I Borage bring alwaies courage.

—JOHN GERARD, THE *HERBAL*

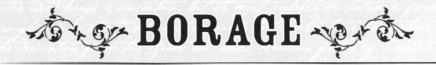

BORAGE

Name

The etymology of the word "borage" is uncertain, but its most probable derivation is from the Latin word *borra* or *burra*, meaning "rough hair" or "short wool" and referring to the plant's hairy stems and leaves, which are similar to those of a burro. The theory that it is derived from the Arabic *abu arak*, meaning "father of sweat," is hypothetical, and the attempt to seek its origins in the Celtic language seems fanciful.

The annual, and occasionally biennial, *Borago officinalis* is a member of the **Boraginaceae** or **Borage** family, also known as the **Forget-me-not** family.

Folk Names

Other names for the plant are burrage, burridge, herb of gladness, star-flower, bee bread, alkanet (the herb is often confused with true alkanet), talewort, cool tankard, virgin's robe, and common bugloss. Germans call it *Borretsch, Gurkenkraut, Borgelkraut, Gurkenkönigskraut, Liebäuglein,* and *Blauhimmelstern*; the French, *bourrache* or *bourrouche*; the Italians, *borragine, buglosa* (it is also confused with bugloss), *lingua bovina,* and *borandella*; the Spaniards, *borraja*; the Brazilians, *borragem*; the Turks, *hodan*; and the Russians, *ogurečnik*.

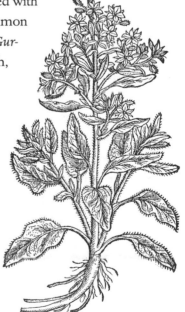

Appearance

The most noticeable feature of the borage plant is its hairy calyx, with a five-petaled, star-shaped flower with a black point in its center. The flowers are occasionally pink or white instead of blue. They grow on short flower stalks and droop downward. Borage flowers are small in comparison with the herb's thick, wide, rough, hairy, veined, and somewhat prickly leaves. The mature plant attains a height of 2 ft., and its stalk is thick, juicy, sometimes woody, and always covered with furry hairs. When bruised, borage leaves smell like cucumber seasoned with a hint of onion. The plant's taste is most pronounced after a sunny spell. Borage roots are branched, white, and relatively small for the weight of the plant. They have a juicy, slimy consistency and a sweet taste.

Place, Season, and Useful Parts

Borage is primarily a garden plant, but is hardy enough to survive as a garden escape in many parts of the world. It can be found growing wild on compost and rubbish heaps, near houses and abandoned places, in brackish fields or shady places, in vineyards or on the edges of lakes, to an altitude of 4,500 ft. Borage's original homeland is thought to have been Spain or Northern Africa. It blossoms during the months of June, July, and August into September, and occasionally in May or October.

Gathering, Drying, and Storage

Young borage leaves and flowers can be plucked singly as needed during the growing period, or the entire plant is harvested as soon as it begins to flower. Plants that have become unsightly should be cut back regularly. Borage can easily be confused with other members of the **Borage** family, such as viper's bugloss (*Echium vulgare*) or alkanet (*Anchusa officinalis*). This is not a cause for panic, since both the plants are healing herbs in their own right, and not poisonous.

It is almost always best to use fresh borage, for it loses many of its beneficial properties during the drying process and does not keep well. It may be frozen for kitchen use.

Seed Saving and Germination

There are slight variations between borage strains, including both white and blue-flowered varieties. These different varieties will cross with each other, and should be isolated for varietal purity. Borage flowers produce seeds very quickly, and these often fall to the ground before they can be harvested. The best method of seed harvesting is to cut the seed-bearing stalks singly, after most of the flowers have blossomed. The hanging seed receptacles contain two long black, pointed seeds. These will fall out if the cut branches are placed in a dry, airy place in the shade on white paper. Seeds that are not yet ripe will ripen quickly, even after picking, as long as the leaves and stalks do not begin to mildew, which is a problem in damp climates. Many of the seeds will hide within the receptacles, and have to be pressed or rubbed out. Borage seeds remain fertile for 2–3 years if stored well, but can also be dried with silica gel and then frozen.

Gardening Hints

Because of the plant's lush growth and delicate blue or white flowers, borage is considered an ornamental plant as well as a culinary and medicinal herb. Planting borage in the vicinity of strawberries, squash, or tomatoes will increase the strawberries' resistance to disease, discourage tomato and squash worms, and improve the growth of all of these plants. The seeds are usually sown in their final position outdoors in April. Loose, airy, yet not too dry soil and a sunny position are ideal. It is theoretically possible to transplant borage, but only a small fraction of the plants will survive transplantation. The plants should reach maturity in June or early July, and continue blooming until the first frost if the plants are cut back to harvest the seeds. If necessary, small amounts of borage seeds can be re-sown at regular intervals to ensure a continual crop of fresh borage leaves and flowers. Borage is an easy herb to grow, and makes few demands on the gardener. In fact, most gardeners only buy a packet of borage seed once, and then continue to harvest the plant for years afterwards, for it seeds itself. Surplus plants (without seeds) can be fermented in rainwater together with comfrey leaves as a liquid garden fertilizer. The fermented mixture is diluted 10:1 or 20:1 with water, and then distributed with a watering can in the early morning or evening.

Culinary Virtues

Borage loses its seasoning and flavoring strength when dried, and is therefore usually used fresh or preserved by freezing. Borage leaves have a mild, unobtrusive, but distinctly cucumber-like taste and are an excellent seasoning for salads and cucumbers, if harvested when young and tender. Borage flowers can also be included in salads for their unusual color. Fresh young borage leaves (older leaves turn felty, tough, or even prickly) are chopped and used as sandwich fillings, or cooked whole as potherbs, or dipped in batter and deep-fat fried. They are also chopped and added to dips, cream or cottage cheese, or used as a seasoning for soups and egg dishes. The fresh juice is extracted and added to vegetables juices. Borage-leaf jelly is served with meat, and the fresh leaves are used to season sweet-sour foods.

Several centuries ago, Robert Burton recommended a seasoning mixture of borage, fennel, parsley, bugloss, dill, lemon balm, and chicory for those suffering from melancholy. This has been seconded by modern scientists, who prescribe borage oil for those suffering from a lack of essential gamma linoleic (Omega 6) oils in their diet. Some modern diets are deficient in these oils, and the consequent use of borage oil can help to cure or relieve stubborn cases of depression and generally support well-being. Borage oil should not be heated, but used fresh.

Borage flowers are used in the same manner as the leaves: as a seasoning herb, in salads, fried in batter, or baked into apple pies. They are a tasty garnish for fruit salads and grapefruit dishes. The flowers can also be frozen inside ice cubes as a very decorative addition to chilled drinks, or floated in claret cups, cider, chilled wine drinks, lemonade, or even beer. They are occasionally added to vinegar to give it a blue tinge. The leaves and the juice of the fresh plant are also used to flavor drinks. A beautiful blue syrup can be prepared from the flowers, or they are added to jams and jellies, or candied. Borage and nasturtium flowers, along with marigold flower petals, are very decorative as garnishes, and can also be tossed in a fresh salad.

Noteworthy Recipes

Candied Borage Flowers: This sixteenth-century recipe for candying borage flowers is relatively difficult for modern cooks to follow (more modern recipes are given in the violet chapter):

> To candie Marigolds, Roses, Borage, or Rosemary Flowers. Boile Sugar, and Rosewater a little uppon a chafingdish with coales, then put the flowers (being throughly dried, either by the sunne or on the fire) into the sugar, & boile them a little, then strewe the powder of double refined sugar vpon them, and turne them, and let them boile a little longer, taking the dish from the fire, then strewe more powdred sugar on the contrary side of the flower. These will die of themselves in two or three hours in a hot sunne days, though they lie not in the sunne.[143]

Sommer Borage Salad: The prettiest summer salad is one of the easiest to prepare: green lettuce, halved red cherry tomatoes, and, if available, fresh rocket leaves (also called arugula or rucola), tossed with a vinaigrette dressing. Just before serving, add whole blue borage flowers without the calyx, and the flower petals of marigolds.

John Shirley employed the same herbal combination in his unusual recipe,

> To boil a Pullet, Capon or Chicken, the best way. Truss them, and put them into Mutton-broth, with Mice (mace), Spinnage and Endive, marigold-flowers, bugloss, Borage, Sorrel and Parsley: and when they are enough, garnish the dish with Borage and Marigold flowers, and serve them up in sippits.[144]

Cucumber Salad with Borage: This traditional borage recipe is easy to prepare, and may help to drive away the blues. Take 3 large cucumbers, and slice very thinly with a slicer (the vegetable absorbs the flavor of the dressing better this way). Salt lightly and let stand for a few minutes, until water begins to exude from the cucumbers. If you don't like a watery salad, pour off this liquid. Then place the cucumbers

---

143. Sir Hugh Platt, *Delightes for Ladies* (1594) (London: Penguin, 1948), 24.

144. Shirley, *The Accomplished Ladies Rich Closet of Rarities* (London: N. Bodington, 1688), 110.

in a salad bowl, and add ½ cup of sour cream and 2 cups of plain yogurt. Season with cider or rice vinegar, add several tablespoons of freshly-chopped green chives or multiplier onions, and ¼ cup of very finely-chopped tender young borage leaves, as well as 1–2 Tbsp. of good olive, flax, or borage oil. Season with salt and pepper to taste, and chill before serving. Serve with garnishes of fresh borage flowers and marigold flower petals.

Household Applications

The blue flowers of the borage plant are dried for potpourri and sachets for their unusual color. Dry borage leaves contain so much nitre that they spark when burned, and flame up easily, like match paper.

Cosmetic Properties

An effective eyewash for eyes irritated by wind or dust can be prepared from infused borage leaves. Add a little salt before bathing the eye.

Medicinal Merits

Ancient herbalists were unrestrained in their praise of borage as a sovereign remedy for melancholy and mental disease. The blue color of its flowers was interpreted as a sign that it should be prescribed as a vein, heart, and brain herb capable of driving away melancholy. Pliny's adage "Ego Borago gaudia semper ago" ("I, borage, always bring joy") has been quoted in herbal after herbal over the centuries. In his colossal work *The Anatomy of Melancholy*, Robert Burton spends many pages dealing with the excellent properties of this plant:

> Borage and Hellebore fill two scenes,
> Sovereign plants to purge the veins
> Of melancholy, and cheer the heart
> Of those black fumes which make it smart;
> To clear the brain of misty fogs,
> Which dull our senses, and soul clogs.
> The best medicine that e'er God made
> For this malady, if well assay'd.[145]

According to John Evelyn, the seventeenth-century gardener,

> Borrage, Borrago, hot and kindly moist, purifying the Blood, is an exhilirating Cordial, of a pleasant Flavor: The tender Leaves, and Flowers especially, may

---

145.   Burton, *The Anatomy of Melancholy* (1621), vol. 1 (London: Tudor, 1977), 8.

be eaten in Composition; but above all, the Sprigs in Wine, like those of Baum (lemon balm), are of known Vertue to revive the Hypochondriac, and chear the hard Student.[146]

Francis Bacon believed that borage "hath an excellent spirit to repress the fuliginous vapour of dusky melancholie."[147] One further expert, the thirteenth-century physician Arnoldus Villanovanus, reports that borage

> drives away leprosy, scabs, clears the blood, recreates the spirits, exhilirates the mind, purgeth the brain of those anxious black melancholy fumes, and cleanseth the whole body of that black humour by urine. To which I add, that it will bring madmen, and such raging bedlams as are tied in chains, to the use of their reason again. My conscience bears me witness that I do not lie, I saw a grave matron helped by this means; she was so choleric, and so furious sometimes, that she was almost mad and beside herself; she said and did she knew not what, scolded, beat her maids, and was ready to be bound, till she drank of this borage wine, and by this excellent remedy was cured, which a poor foreigner, a silly beggar, taught her by chance, that came to crave an alms from door to door.[148]

However strange and extravagant these claims may seem, borage has been prescribed again and again, down to the present day, for those ailments that can be loosely classified under the antiquated term "melancholy": heart weakness, loss of memory, hypochondria, epilepsy, excessive sorrow, a tendency to faintness or to feverish dreams, ringing in the ears, hangovers, depression, tiredness, mental disease, and general debility. It was also considered one of the four best cordial, or heart-strengthening, herbs. Modern medicine has attempted to explain and corroborate these claims by pointing out that borage is unusually rich in mineral salts, acids, and nitrate of potash, and that it may exert direct influence on the adrenal gland. Recent research has proved that borage oil is unusually rich in gamma linoleic oils, and doctors often prescribe it, together with black currant and evening primrose oil, to treat deficiencies of these essential fatty acids. One of the common results of a deficiency of essential fatty acids is depression.

Modern Medicine

Borage is obviously not a wonder drug with immediate and astounding medicinal action, but is a gradually effective herb that can be taken over an extended period. It exerts a positive influence on patients with minor heart irregularities, psychological dis-

---

146. Evelyn, *Acetaria: A Discourse of Sallets* (London: B. Tooke, 1699), 13.

147. Qtd. in Mrs. Maude Grieve, *A Modern Herbal* (1931) (London: Penguin, 1976), 120.

148. Qtd. in Robert Burton, *The Anatomy of Melancholy* (1621), vol. 2 (London: Tudor, 1977), 224.

orders, or circulatory complaints, and has a good track record in the supplementary treatment of depression. In view of the steadily growing ranks of patients with depressive disorders, it is only reasonable to look more closely at a plant with such a reputation. A few years ago, little attention was paid to the role that St. John's wort plays in the treatment of this disease, and the herb can now be found on supermarket shelves.

Borage can cleanse the body of wastes, poisons, and fevers by inducing perspiration, lowering body temperature, dispelling urine, and purifying the blood. A warm tea of the fresh herb, or the juice of the fresh plant, is capable of "breaking" a minor fever, of lessening the effects of a chest cold, and of easing some of the symptoms caused by a hardened liver or malfunctioning kidneys. The juice can be used alone, or combined with the juice of other plants as a blood-purifying spring cure, taken daily for 4 weeks. Used externally, borage has a softening effect and is applied as a compress for painful varicose veins, bruises, and inflamed eyes. Homeopathic medicine uses borage to treat high blood pressure, joint problems, and tension headaches. Borage is also included among the Bach flower essences discovered by Edward Bach at the beginning of the last century, and is used to raise the spirits and instill courage, much in the manner of earlier herbalists.

Uses in Husbandry

Borage is considered one of the very best plants to have in the vicinity of the bee hive, second only to its close cousin, viper's bugloss *(Echium vulgare)*. Cattle and poultry also profit by being fed small amounts of the herb after an especially long winter. Feeding finely chopped borage leaves in milk can increase the milk production of bitches with a large litter. Dogs will of their own accord search out borage leaves to induce vomiting or to ease a cough. A blue varnish has been produced at various times on a commercial scale from borage flowers.

Miscellaneous Wisdom

Legends

The ancient Greeks believed that borage could turn cowards into lions; this belief is mirrored in a Lincolnshire legend. Cromwell's soldiers, given borage leaves to chew, became so courageous that they were able to fight for a day and night without resting.

According to legend, borage was one of the healing herbs held up on the point of a spear to Jesus on the Cross. Victorians believed borage to be the symbol of bluntness.

For though Chamomile, the more it is trodden on the faster it grows,
yet youth, the more it is wasted the sooner it wears.

—WILLIAM SHAKESPEARE, *HENRY IV*

CHAMOMILE

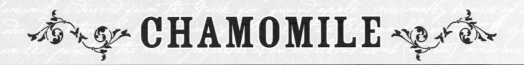

Name

The term "chamomile" is derived from the Greek for "ground apple," presumably because of the herb's sweet, apple-like odor. The botanical Latin name for the plant is *Chamomilla recutita*. A synonym, *Matricaria chamomilla,* points to the herb's properties as an excellent womb (or *matrix*) medicine.

Both *Chamomilla recutita* (an annual) and *Chamaemelum nobile* (English chamomile, a perennial) are members of the **Asteraceae** or **Daisy** family. *Chamaemelum nobile,* according to its etymology, is a noble flower. These two chamomiles are often confused with each another and with other similar plants, especially the wild chamomiles.

True chamomile (*Chamomilla recutita,* formerly known as *Chamomilla officinalis, Matricaria chamomilla, Matricaria suaveolens, Leucanthemum chamaemelum,* or *Chamomilla vulgaris*) has small, yellow-centered blossoms with white outer petals. Chamomile tea is made from these sweet-smelling flowers. English chamomile *(Chamaemelum nobile)* has larger, white flowers that taste bitter.

Other herbs, such as mayweed, feverfew, or stinking chamomile, resemble these plants but do not have the same medicinal properties. Feverfew is a healing plant in its own right, but with different medicinal merits. English chamomile is not as widely used medicinally as its more common chamomile cousin.

Folk Names

Chamomile, camomile, common chamomile, true chamomile, German chamomile, Germain chamomile, camel, camomine, single chamomile, pinheads, and matricary are common names for the herb. Antiquated names are maythen and horse gowan. In Germany, the plant is known as *Kamille, echte Kamille, deutsche Kamille, Matronenkraut, Hermännchen,* and *Aepfelchrut.* Italians call it *camomilla* and *capomilla*; the French, *camomille* and *camomille vraie*; the Spaniards, *manzanilla* and *manzanilla dulce*; the Irish, *fiogadán*; and the Russians, *romaška aptečnaja* and *romaška obodrannaja.*

To confuse matters, English chamomile is also called common chamomile, noble chamomile, Roman chamomile, sweet chamomile, perennial chamomile, ground apple, garden-scotch, lawn chamomile, and double chamomile. German names are *römische Kamille, welsch Kamille, Römerei,* or *Handknöpf.* In Italian, it is *camomilla romana*; in Spanish, *manzanilla romana*; in French, *camomille romaine*; and in Russian, *rimskaja romaška.*

Appearance

It is very easy to confuse true chamomile with a host of similar plants such as mayweed, feverfew, dog herb, corn chamomile, pineapple-scented chamomile, unscented or stinking chamomile, etc. Because it is easy to confuse the herb, many people prefer to grow chamomile instead of gathering it from the wild. The "other" chamomiles are not poisonous, but they do not have the same medicinal properties as true chamomile, nor do they have the same pleasant taste. Their flowerheads are usually flat, and do not contain a hollow space.

True chamomile can be distinguished by its pleasing, apple-like, fresh odor. The flower has a petite and wholesome appearance. Its hollow flower heads are characteristic and unique. The yellow flower center of mature flowers is raised, the white petals bend downwards, and a hollow space can be seen when the stem is broken off. Young chamomile flowers have a less clearly defined hollow space, and the white flower petals do not bend as much. The roots are short and spindly, and the plant's round upright stem grows to a maximum height of 2 ft. The plant is often dwarfed if water is scarce. The leaves are light green, divided and feathery, and their taste is bitter and aromatic.

English chamomile attains a height of 1 ft. and sometimes even 1½ ft. Its leaves are gray-green, small, divided, and threadlike, and the entire plant is covered with down. It has a well-developed rootstock and often propagates itself through runners. The flowers of wild growing English chamomile plants are single while the cultivated forms have double and filled flowers. The flower petals of English chamomile are much broader than those of true chamomile, are not hollow, and only turn downward at night or before rainfall. The yellow flower center is small and unobtrusive, giving the plant the appearance of a white daisy. Cultivated forms often look like frilled white buttons. English chamomile flowers exude a pleasant, vanilla-like odor.

Place, Season, and Useful Parts

True chamomile was originally a native of the Near East, as well as eastern and southern Europe. It has now established itself in most of Europe, and is at home in Asia, Australia, and North America, to an altitude of 5,000 ft. A large part of commercially sold wild chamomile comes from eastern Europe, India, and Egypt.

Chamomile is often cultivated in gardens, but also grows wild and escapes from cultivated areas. It can be found in grain, turnip, potato, clover, or alfalfa fields, or in village waste places, on rubble, on open gravelly fields or walls, near construction sites, and in vineyards. The chamomile with the highest oil content is rumored to grow in grain fields. The plant flowers from May through September, and should be gathered then.

English chamomile blossoms from June to September. It grows wild on dry, sandy soil with a high limestone content, on cliffs, sand dunes, or near streams and lakes. It does not grow wild in the southernmost part of Europe, but is cultivated widely in Central and eastern Europe and in parts of the United States.

Gathering, Drying, and Storage

Chamomile flowers must be picked as they appear, which makes gathering a tedious process. Ideally, they are harvested every 2–3 days in dry, sunny weather, just after the heads have opened in the morning. They must be dried immediately. Chamomile flowers can be picked by hand, or they are harvested with special combs. Care should be taken to include as little stem as possible with the harvested flowers, and to avoid collecting chamomile from fields that have been sprayed with herbicides or pesticides. Most chamomile is gathered from the wild, although cultivation is becoming more widespread. Since its harvest is so labor-intensive, commercial chamomile is often adulterated with other herbs.

It is easy to keep fresh chamomile available in the garden: sow it in an unused corner, water it well until established, and then forget about it. The flower heads can usually be harvested in the middle of the summer. If it is too much trouble to harvest the flowers singly, then pull out the plants, and cut off the heads over a large bowl, taking care that no dirt gets in the bowl, and that a few flower heads are left to go to seed outdoors for next year's crop. Dry the flowers and store.

It is difficult to dry chamomile flower heads well. Older flowers tend to fall apart, and large amounts of flowers will ferment if dried in thick layers, or too slowly. Chamomile flowers should be dried quickly in very thin layers on cloth, paper, or thin mesh in a shady, airy place. They should be handled as little as possible and not turned while drying.

Storage in a very dry environment, or in airtight containers, is essential. The dried flowers should be inspected regularly for mold, and if necessary, kept dry with a desiccant material such as silica gel.

If chamomile flowers do fall apart during the drying process, the resulting drug can be sifted. The entire flower heads are used for tea, and the yellow chamomile dust stored separately for poultices or chamomile baths.

Pure essential chamomile oil can be stored for a long time in closed dark containers or bottles. It will change color after contact with air, first from blue to green, and then from green to brown or yellow.

Seed Saving and Germination

Miniscule chamomile seeds develop from the yellow flower centers, and fall out easily, which can lead to patches of chamomile spread throughout the garden. When saving seeds, cut the stems with the blossoms shortly after full bloom, when they begin to look scraggly. Spread the flower heads on cloths in a dry and shady place to ripen, taking care not to include any soil. The ripe seeds fall out as the flowers dry, and can be easily removed by rubbing the flower heads through a sieve. Pass through various sieves to remove debris. Chamomile seeds mold easily in wet conditions, and should therefore be dried carefully and stored in airtight containers. Silica gel can be used to extract moisture from the seeds before storage in a glass jar or aluminum packet. Properly dried and stored chamomile seeds will keep their vitality for several years, and even longer if stored in airtight containers in the freezer.

There are many different chamomile varieties, since they have developed differently in their wild habitat. These varieties vary in azulen content, as well as in botanical characteristics. Single varieties can be maintained in isolation, or a genetically diverse mixture of different varieties, well adapted to local conditions, can be developed.

Gardening Hints

True chamomile once grew abundantly in grain, turnip, potato, or clover fields, but has now been decimated by herbicides. It does best in a dry, warm climate suitable for growing wine, and especially likes sandy soil. But chamomile will also thrive in most garden soils if they are not too acidic or alkaline. If sown between the months of April and August, chamomile will flower two months later and reappear the following year if allowed to go to seed. In some climates, it may even develop into something of a pest.

English chamomile is best sown indoors in trays and then transplanted to its final place in the garden. Germination is not always good. English chamomile, as John Lyly noted in "Euphues and His England," grows well in pathways or other thoroughfares: "The chamomile, the more it is trodden and pressed down, the more it spreadeth." It requires a sunny yet damp spot, and prefers light sandy soil to clay. English chamomile can be sown from seed in the spring or again in the fall, and should be trodden in well after sowing. Runners can also be set, or the roots divided in the fall. The plant is perennial, as opposed to normal chamomile, and will soon form a thick carpet if allowed to spread.

Both chamomiles are excellent compost plants, since they help to stimulate yeast growth and contain calcium. The presence of chamomile plants will usually aid the growth of young plants. The chamomile must be removed, though, before it begins to flower, or it will compete with the neighboring plant for nutrients. Setting a few chamomile plants in the mint bed for a short time, and then removing them can increase the oil content of the mint. Chamomile will also aid the growth of onions if planted 3 ft. away, and cabbage plants seem to profit from the presence of some chamomile. Potatoes are an exception to the rule: they will not grow well if there are any chamomile plants in the vicinity.

Culinary Virtues

Chamomile flowers are seldom used in cookery except as a flavoring for meat stock or as a garnish. One very useful, but little-known culinary property of chamomile is its deodorizing effect on strong-smelling pieces of meat, game, or fish. Simply dipping the offending piece in cold chamomile tea before cooking will remove most of the unpleasant odor. Cutting boards and utensils can also be washed with chamomile tea to sweeten them and to keep bacteria from spreading.

Chamomile tea (tisane) is often given to people with a weak stomach, but is also soothing after a large meal or too much wine.

Chamomile flowers and the bitterer English chamomile flowers can be used to flavor beers, wines, and liqueurs. Chamomile beer was often served in the Middle Ages, and English chamomile was sometimes combined with wormwood as a hop substitute for bitter beers. English chamomile can also be brewed with ginger root as a mildly bitter herbal beer. Digestive aperitifs are prepared from English chamomile, a little wormwood, and a mixture of other bitter herbs steeped in wine. Manzanilla sherry is flavored with *manzanilla* (Spanish chamomile).

Household Applications

Dried chamomile flowers are often added to sachet, potpourri, and moth-repelling mixtures. Strongly diluted chamomile extract, or a weak infusion of chamomile flowers, is an excellent deodorant and mild disinfectant that deserves a better reputation among housekeepers. Refrigerators can be rinsed out with chamomile infusion, "sour" kitchen sponges can be soaked in it and then dried in the sun, and dishcloths can be rinsed or deodorized with it. It can be added to dish water or used to scrub down shelves and cupboards to make them smell sweeter. Wooden utensils or boards are also rinsed in chamomile tea to remove unpleasant odors.

English chamomile was planted in Tudor times in scented lawns and pathways. Both chamomiles can be used as dye plants (light yellows). Another member of this family, dyer's chamomile, *Anthemis tinctoria*, has yellow flowers that have been used for centuries as a reliable yellow dye. Chrome mordant will produce an orange hue, and iron a brownish color.

Cosmetic Properties

Chamomile is one of the best cosmetic herbs. Azulen has a mildly cleansing, deodorizing, disinfecting, softening, pain-killing, and astringent effect on the skin, and only rarely causes allergic reactions. It can be used on even the most sensitive, young, or aged skin, and is often added as a healing agent to baby oil. Chamomile tea is a very mild astringent. Yarrow has stronger astringent properties, and is often combined with chamomile to strengthen facial tonics. Chamomile tea can be patted on the face and allowed to dry, or added to steaming mixtures to remove blackheads. Steaming with chamomile is recommended for dry skin, and chamomile boiled in milk has a healing effect on broken and chapped skin. A beaten egg white, thinned with chamomile tea, is applied as a face mask to reduce puffiness or to remove dark circles under eyes after a particularly long night. Chamomile is also recommended as a healing drink for those with dilated or broken facial veins. English chamomile is occasionally used in perfumery.

Chamomile baths have a soothing and at the same time stimulating effect. Nicholas Culpeper was a great supporter of chamomile baths:

> The bathing with a decoction of chamomile taketh away weariness, easeth pains to what part of the body soever they be applied. It comforteth the sinews that be over-strained, mollifieth all swellings: it moderately comforteth all parts that have need of warmth, digesteth and dissolveth whatsoever hath need thereof by a wonderful speedy property … [149]

Besides disinfecting and deodorizing, chamomile baths help to keep insects away. Strongly diluted chamomile extract may be added to douche water, or to hand and footbaths. Mixing in some powdered chamomile can also enhance the deodorizing properties of ordinary talcum powder.

Both chamomiles are important hair care herbs, and true chamomile is an essential ingredient of many hair tonics. Well-strained infusions of chamomile flowers can be used as a hair wash or added to mild shampoos. English chamomile will also lighten

---

149.   Culpeper, *Culpeper's Complete Herbal* (1653) (London: Foulsham, undated), 74.

blonde highlights. A mild hair lightener can be prepared from powdered English chamomile flowers and a thickening agent such as egg yolk or Irish moss. This paste is applied generously to damp hair, and left for at least one hour before rinsing. A strong infusion of English chamomile flowers and blue cornflower petals *(Centaurea cyanus)* is a good rinse for brightening ashen blonde or white hair.

Work-toughened hands can be bathed in chamomile infusions or softened with chamomile compresses. Inflamed eyelids are treated with warm chamomile tea bags, or pads moistened with strongly diluted chamomile extract. Rinsing the mouth with chamomile tea after a visit to the dentist will help to relieve pain, remove unpleasant odors, and prevent infection.

Noteworthy Recipes

A Deodorant Bath: An excellent disinfectant and deodorizing bath can be prepared from equal parts of sage, rosemary, and thyme, and three times that amount of chamomile flowers. Ten handfuls of this mixture are covered with water and brought to a boil in a large pot. Allow to steep for 10–15 minutes, and then strain into the bath, adding a little oil to the water to facilitate cleaning (sage tends to stain enamel). The dried herb mixture can also be filled into a cloth bath bag if this procedure is too time-consuming. The bag is tied to the hot water tap, and allowed to steep in the hot tub for at least 10 minutes before removing. The bath herbs can be dried after the bath, and reused 2–3 times.

A Bath for Weak Nerves: A bath with a soothing and strengthening effect on the nerves can be mixed as above from equal parts of chamomile, lavender, rosemary, marjoram, and wild thyme. Herbal baths are most effective if they are followed by at least half an hour's complete rest in a pre-warmed bed.

A Facial Herbal Tonic: A good facial tonic can be prepared from 1 handful of chamomile flowers, and half a handful each of lavender, sage, rosemary, and coltsfoot leaves. Place the herbs in a bowl, and add 2 oz. of high-proof spirits and enough distilled water to completely cover the herbs. Let the bowl stand, closely covered, in a warm place. Add more distilled water if necessary. After one week at cool temperatures, strain the mixture, pour it through filter paper to remove all residue, and add a few tablespoons of mild cider vinegar, or the strained juice of 3 fresh lemons as preservatives. Rose or lavender water can be added as a perfuming agent if desired. Store the tonic in airtight containers or bottles in the refrigerator, for it will not keep indefinitely. If necessary, it can be frozen for later use. This tonic is ideal for tightening and toning the skin.

Medicinal Merits

Chamomile has been a recognized healing herb for centuries, although it has never been as highly thought of as it is today. Ancient Egyptians anointed patients from head to toe with chamomile oil, and then wrapped them in blankets to induce perspiration. Galen mentioned chamomile, and Dioscurides ordered tubercular patients to sit next to a bed of chamomile and inhale deeply. Pseudo Apuleius listed it as an eye herb. Otto Brunfels considered it to be warming and drying, and recommended it for a host of minor complaints and illnesses. German botanist Hieronymus Bock (sixteenth century) was the first to lavish praise on the plant:

> The very common Chamill
> is the Doctor's Prescription Number One
> for they cannot cure much
> without the help of this flower.[150]

Modern Medicine

It is almost impossible to misuse chamomile. Its medicinal action is of a very mild, yet gently effective nature if taken regularly in small doses for a long time. It helps to soothe the gastrointestinal tract and the mucous membranes, and can relieve cramps. It has a softening, weakly antiseptic, and soothing effect on the kidneys and uterus, and can be used to treat infection, either internally or externally. It combines well with other herbs, and can be added to both tonic and bitter herbal mixtures.

Chamomile is such a mild and soothing herb that it can be given in small doses to newborn babies, or to nursing mothers. It helps to ease the nervous tension of mother and child, and to ease minor uterine cramps and strengthen the womb. Chamomile will help relax a teething, cranky, sleepless, or irritable child, and calm colics. Despite its mild nature, some people do have pronounced allergic reactions to the herb, and should avoid its use.

Chamomile baths, compresses, douches, enemas, bandages, and hot pillows can be used on any part of the body. They have a mildly cleansing, healing, soothing, antiseptic and fungicidal effect, and help to soften and strengthen the skin and the mucous membranes. Wounds or infected eyes can be washed out with chamomile tea. Chamomile steam baths help to relieve the pains of colds, flu, headaches, sinus troubles, and toothaches, and chamomile oil can be applied directly to soothe the pains of colic, rheumatism, arthritis, and gout. The homeopathic remedy *Chamomilla* is prepared from German chamomile, and is the primary treatment for fretful, teething babies who want to be carried all the time. Colds, conjunctivitis, and colics are also treated with it. Adults who overuse cof-

---

150. Bock, *Kreütterbuch* (1565), facsimile (Munich: Konrad Kölbl, 1964).

fee can benefit from *Chamomilla*, and it is a constitutional remedy for oversensitive, overly nervous, or elderly people who tend to suffer from pains, cramps, spasms, and asthma.

English chamomile is not as mild a medicinal herb as true chamomile, and should be used sparingly. It can be taken as a bitter tea before meals to help relieve congestion of the liver, gastrointestinal disorders, or colics due to gallbladder insufficiency. It is often prepared as a cold infusion. It is a vermifuge, and has a curative effect on some kinds of diarrhea and coughs. It helps to promote menstruation, relieve obstructions of the womb, and soothe cramps. English chamomile should not be prescribed when strong bleeding is occurring.

Special Cures

Teething Aids: John Shirley gives this unusual recipe for the "hard Breeding of Teeth" in his *Rich Closet*:

> Give the Child Candle made of Virgins-wax to nabble on, and foment the cheeks with the Decoction of Althea (marshmallow); Cammomoil-flowers, and the Seed of Dill.[151]

Today, we would probably omit the beeswax, rub chamomile and marshmallow onto the gums and cheeks, and give homeopathic preparations of chamomile hourly to the fretful, teething child. A warm chamomile tea bag or hot chamomile pillow can be applied if the child will allow it.

Hot Chamomile Pillows: Fill a linen or cotton sack half-full with chamomile flowers, tie or sew it shut, and then place it on a rack above a pot of boiling water. The chamomile in the sack will swell as it absorbs the steam. When the pillow is warm but not too damp, remove it and let it cool a few minutes before applying to the body. A chamomile pillow can be kept at a constant temperature for a long time by placing a hot water bottle on top of the pillow. After removing the pillow, dry the skin area carefully with a clean towel and cover well to prevent loss of heat. The contents of chamomile pillows can be reused two or three times if they are dried carefully and stored in a dry place between applications.

Uses in Husbandry

The leaves of English chamomile are sometimes dried and employed as tobacco and as snuff. In some parts of Germany, chamomile and St. John's wort were once tied into the first sheaves of the grain harvest to protect it from insect infestation.

---

151. Shirley, *The Accomplished Ladies Rich Closet of Rarities* (London: N. Bodington, 1688), 89.

Veterinary Values

Chamomile flowers have such a gentle healing effect that they can be given to most animals as a universal remedy under the motto that if it doesn't help it can't hurt. Wounds and cuts are washed with chamomile tea or strongly diluted chamomile extract, and infected eyes swabbed with chamomile tea. Kittens with crusted eyes can be effectively treated with a chamomile tea bag moistened with boiling hot water, cooled and then pressed out, and applied directly. Chamomile tea is especially useful in the treatment of calves' diarrhea, and beginning hoof rot can be alleviated with compresses of chamomile, chervil, and lemon balm, applied for 20 minutes. Afterwards, the hooves must be dried carefully and the animals bedded down on clean straw. Chamomile can be added to the diet of a whelping bitch, and chamomile tea can also be used to dilute the flakes given to puppies or to sick dogs and cats. Chamomile tea is given as first aid if the dog or cat is suffering from diarrhea or stomach upsets, and as a strengthening and soothing drink after bouts with poison, usually in combination with charcoal tablets.

Miscellaneous Wisdom

In ancient Egypt, chamomile was consecrated to the sun. In northern Germany, the plant was considered powerful enough to secure any person against enchantment if carried on the body. Chamomile hung from the rafters in bundles will supposedly begin to swing to and fro the minute a witch enters the room. One unexplained and uniquely German superstition is that chamomile should be treated with respect, for chamomile plants are actually enchanted soldiers (*Hermännchen*). English chamomile was once invoked as a magically healing herb in the famous Anglo-Saxon Nine Herb Charm.

According to folk belief, the best chamomile is gathered on Midsummer's Day. Supposedly, this chamomile has not been attacked by worms or touched by witches. After midsummer, it is believed that witches foul the plants, evil insects attack it, or the plant changes magically into stinking chamomile. According to northern Italian folk belief, the best chamomile is gathered with the left hand under the influence of the new moon.

Oracular Worth

The popular belief is widespread that anyone who takes a whiff of stinking chamomile (*Anthemis cotula*) will subsequently lose all sense of smell.

CHERVIL & SWEET CICELY

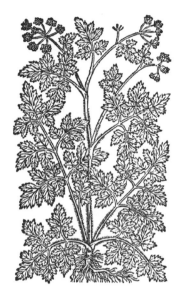

Name

The Greek name for chervil was *chaerophyllon*, which is composed of two words: the verb "to rejoice" and the noun "leaf." "Chervil" is therefore just another name for a joy leaf. In Latin, the name became *chaerophyllum*.

Now called *Anthriscus cerefolium,* chervil is an annual (and occasionally biennial) member of the **Carrot** family *(Apiaceae)*. It used to be called *Chaerophyllum sativum*, *Chaerophyllum cerefolium*, or *Scandix cerefolium* (*cerefolium* means "waxy leaf"). Caution should be exercised when gathering the plant, since it can be confused with other poisonous members of the **Carrot** family.

The name "sweet cicely" is derived from the Greek word *seselis*, which is also used for other members of the **Carrot** family. Sweet cicely's botanical name, *Myrrhis odorata*, literally means "an odoriferous perfume."

Sweet cicely is also, confusingly, called "wild chervil." It is a perennial member of the same family as chervil, and therefore closely related, not only by name. American sweet cicely does not differ appreciably from the European herb.

Another related plant, *Chaerophyllum bulbosum* (turnip-rooted chervil or parsnip chervil), has for centuries been cultivated for its edible roots, especially in eastern Europe and northern Europe, Turkey, and Siberia.

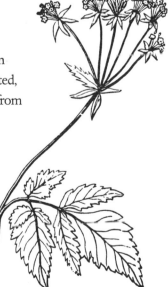

Folk Names

Chervil, chervill, salad chervil, or garden chervil is known in Germany as *Kerbel*, *Kerbelkraut*, or *Suppenkraut*;

in France as *cerfeuil*; and in Italy as *cerfoglio* or *mescolanza*. Its Anglo-Saxon name was *cer-fille hynne leac*.

Sweet cicely is also known under the names of sweet chervil, great chervil, cow chervil, wild chervil, sweet fern, British myrrh, garden myrrh, holy grass, anise, sweet bracken, sweet-cus, sweet humlock, sweets, the Roman plant, sheperd's needle, smooth cicely, and smoother cicely. German names are *Myrrhenkerbel*, *Süßdolde*, and *Anis-Kerbel*. In French, it is *cerfeuil musqué*; in Italian, *finochiella*; in Spanish, *perifolio*; and in Dutch, *roomse kervel*.

Appearance

Chervil, when small, resembles carrot, parsley, hemlock, and other members of the **Carrot** family. It can best be distinguished from these plants by its sweet-spicy smell when bruised, by its feathery leaves, and long, thin, black seeds. The fragrance of the growing plant is unobtrusive, yet somewhat sweet and aromatic. Chervil has a feathery appearance, like hemlock, and seems to be covered with a blue sheen when viewed in direct sunlight. The roots are thin, hard, spindly and white, and smell a little like anise. The round, rilled, hollow, reddish, or bluish stalks rise to a maximum height of 2 ft. (usually less) and are covered with hair at each joint. The leaves are of a light green color, and strongly divided. Chervil flowers are small, green or white in color, and grouped together in umbels. Ripe chervil seed is black, shiny, and long, resembling tiny stems.

Sweet cicely has somewhat darker, fleshier, and much broader leaves, and a sweeter, but also bitterer, flavor than chervil. It grows to a height of 3 ft., and its hollow, large, furrowed stem ends in large downy, fern-like leaves and cloudy white flower umbels. The roots are large, fleshy, and white, similar to stubby parsnips.

Place, Season, and Useful Parts

Chervil originally came from southeastern Europe or western Asia, but is now cultivated in most parts of the world to an altitude of 3,750 ft. It flowers from May to August, and may occasionally be encountered wild as a garden escape on rubble or compost heaps, at roadsides, and in vineyards, light woods, or hedges.

Sweet cicely grows wild in northern and mountainous Europe, as well as in Chile, and is widely cultivated in cottage gardens the world over. It can be encountered on mountain pastures, grassy places, abandoned gardens, and in hedges and woods. It blossoms from April to June, depending on the climate.

Turnip-rooted chervil grows as far north as Scandinavia and Siberia, and as far south as Turkey and Iran.

Gathering, Drying, and Storage

Chervil and sweet cicely plants mature shortly before they blossom, about six weeks after sowing. The leaves are then gathered for culinary purposes, and for medicinal purposes when they flower. The fruits are gathered as they ripen, from July to September.

Chervil does not dry well, but can be frozen with good results. Small portions of the chopped herb are frozen without water in an ice cube tray, and the cubes are then placed in the freezer in plastic bags for individual use. Sweet cicely is also used fresh, but can be dried as a sweet addition to herbal teas. It must be stored in airtight glass jars.

Seed Saving and Germination

Chervil seeds remain fertile for at most three years, although it is easy to maintain a variety by letting it self-seed. There is some variation between different strains, especially in the size and tenderness of the leaves. Single varieties must be isolated to maintain purity, since the seeds fall out easily.

Sweet cicely seeds are large, and ripen in large amounts. They need a period of cold weather to germinate, but once established can become invasive through self-seeding.

Turnip-rooted chervil is a notoriously poor germinator, and must be sown as soon as possible after harvest to maintain its vitality. It may also be propagated by root division. Because it does not germinate well, it is becoming increasingly endangered, and can be included among the neglected food crops or underutilized plant species.

Gardening Hints

Chervil was unknown to the ancient Greeks, and is neglected even today in Greece. The ancient Romans, on the other hand, were so enthusiastic about the herb that they considered it an insult to Mercury to omit chervil from any garden.

Chervil does not make great demands either on the gardener or the garden, and can be sown generously in regular intervals. The seeds germinate in less than 2 weeks. Chervil thrives in warm, well-fertilized, moist, humus-rich soil, and prefers partial shade in the summertime and little wind. It likes well-mulched soils, and germinates easily under the shade of trees. If the garden is to its liking, it will self-seed readily. Chervil should be sown during the last days of summer or fall, well before winter frosts, to ensure an early spring crop. It can be re-sown and covered lightly against frost in February or March, and then re-sown again in regular intervals until August. This will guarantee a continual supply of the fresh herb. Chervil cannot easily be transplanted, and should be sown in its final position. It will go to seed quickly and die back if placed in too sunny a spot in the garden, as it prefers a shady and moist situation.

Radishes grown next to chervil have a more biting taste than other radishes. The herb re-seeds so easily that it can be used as a green manure crop for unused beds in the garden. Chervil can be tilled or dug into the soil quickly, providing nourishment and building humus. It is also suitable for planting in window boxes, provided that they are protected from too much sun.

Sweet cicely prefers partial shade and moist soil. Many gardeners have trouble with germination, since the seeds require a few months of winter weather (vernalization) to sprout. Seed sown in the spring will simply refuse to come up. Seeds sown in the fall may sprout the following spring, but may also pause and only appear the year after that. The herb can best be propagated if some seeds are allowed to fall out from an existing stand. They fall on moist soil under the plant, are covered with the frond-like leaves that decompose into rich humus, are subjected to frost in winter, and spring up massively in the spring. Although larger plants usually do not like to be transplanted, the tiny seedlings can be dug out and redistributed. Once established, the roots of sweet cicely are bulky and difficult to remove. The stands of sweet cicely still found in many abandoned gardens are witnesses to the tenacity of the herb. This is why the plant should be divided in regular intervals, or it will try to take over the garden. It flowers early with frothy white blossoms, which makes it a valuable ornamental in the herb and flower garden. In a dry year, the plants will be stunted: the plants are starved for the sake of the roots, which will spring up with renewed vigor the following spring.

Culinary Virtues

In his nineteenth-century cookbook, William Kitchiner describes chervil's flavor as "a strong concentration of the combined taste of Parsley and Fennel, but more aromatic and agreeable than either.[152] Other cooks have described it as "finer parsley," while still others include it among the "fines herbes" of French culinary fame. It is somewhat sweeter and softer than parsley, and may be used as a parsley substitute in many recipes. It is best used alone or in combination with chives, tarragon, and basil because of its sweet, penetrating taste. Chervil should always be used fresh to retain its delicate flavor, and added at the last minute before serving. It may be finely chopped and frozen in ice cube trays for winter use.

Chervil is often eaten in Germany as a Lenten herb, or added to Maundy Thursday soups because of its blood-purifying and cleansing properties. It is one of the very first herbs to appear in spring, and should be more widely grown than it is. In recent years, it has become increasingly neglected, even in traditional growing areas.

Chervil leaves are added to bouillon, soups, salads, egg dishes, dips, cottage or cream cheese, remoulades, white sauces, fish or herb sauces, broccoli, spinach, peas, asparagus, or sorrel. It may be baked in bread, or eaten with bread and butter. The feathery leaves make a useful garnish. The roots of ordinary chervil can be eaten if desired, and the roots of bulbous chervil *(Chaerophyllum bulbosum)* are cultivated for culinary pur-

---

152.   Kitchiner, *The Cook's Oracle* (1817) (London: Samuel Bagster, 1860), 272.

poses. Both are prepared like Chinese artichokes *(Stachys sieboldii)*, and can also be used in bread-baking and distilling. Herbalist John Gerard recommended boiled chervil roots sliced in salads as a medicinal food for the elderly. These roots are capable of comforting the heart, strengthening the body, and imparting courage. He also suggested adding the fruits of the chervil plant to salads to make them more agreeable to the stomach.

Skirret *(Sium sisarum)*, turnip-rooted chervil, and earthnut *(Bunium bulbocastanum)* were once widely used as winter root vegetables in Europe, but have become neglected since other vegetables are more widely available all year round.

Sweet cicely has a sweet, anise-like flavor and is often used as a seasoning for beverages or fruit dishes. The leaves, fruits, and the roots of the plant are so sweet that they can be used to replace sugar in many recipes, or to flavor foods for diabetics. Like chervil, sweet cicely mixes well with other herbs and can increase the appetite and aid digestion. Fresh or dried sweet cicely leaves may be added to rhubarb (less sugar is needed), to tart fruits, to fruit salads, to salads or lemon salad dressings, and to vegetable juices and summer drinks. The seeds can be cooked in chutneys or in apple jellies, added to avocado dishes, or used as a substitute for anise seeds. They are also added to *aquavit*. The roots and leaves are boiled and eaten as a vegetable. Sweet cicely roots are sometimes boiled and eaten with white sauce, or they are candied. The leaves are occasionally dipped in batter and deep fat fried.

Noteworthy Recipes

Chervil Soup: Chervil soup can be prepared quickly. The flavor can easily be varied with the addition of various garden herbs and vegetables. Melt 2–3 Tbsp. of butter in a saucepan, and make a roux by adding 4 Tbsp. of flour or cornstarch. Stir quickly until the mixture just begins to brown, and then stir in 3 cups of meat or vegetable stock slowly. Add 4 Tbsp. of finely chopped chervil, stirring all the time, and season with salt and pepper to taste. Cover and let simmer for 10 minutes. Serve piping hot with a dollop of sour cream or yogurt in every dish, and sprinkle with fresh, finely chopped chervil.

If you are not partial to the floury taste of this soup, substitute 1–2 lb. of peeled potatoes for the roux. Brown the potatoes in the butter lightly, add ½ an onion, chopped fine, and the stock. Cook at moderate heat until soft, and then blend in a mixer or food processor. Season, add chervil, let simmer, and serve.

Household Applications

Fresh chervil is said to drive away ants when set out in open bowls. Sweet cicely is often added to sachets and potpourri because of the sweet fragrance of its leaves, or placed in sacks in the linen closet. Sweet cicely fruits are also pressed to produce oil, which is added to furniture waxes to improve their aroma. A cheap, homemade furniture wax can be prepared by thinning liquefied white wax or beeswax with a little turpentine, adding powdered sweet cicely fruits, setting the mixture in the sun, and then beating it until smooth.

Cosmetic Properties

Chervil is not widely used as a cosmetic herb, although it is rumored to smooth wrinkles while bracing the skin. Russian women once added a mixture of chervil leaves and chamomile flowers to beauty baths. Sweet cicely was more widely used in the past than it is today. Its sweet scent is occasionally added to aromatic mixtures by perfumers.

Medicinal Merits

Although chervil has gone out of official usage, it was once thought to possess fiery and sanguine powers, and the Chinese considered it to be one of the few herbs capable of prolonging human life. Pliny recommended it as a stomachic herb, and other herbalists praised it for its water-provoking, cleansing properties. They prescribed it for such various ailments as tuberculosis, plague, worms, scrofula, dropsy, gout, and clotted blood in the veins.

Modern Medicine

Chervil is recognized as a blood-purifying herb rich in vitamin C, and is considered helpful in the treatment of colds, catarrh, or asthma. It has a stimulating effect on the glandular and lymph systems, and can be a dietary supplement for liver or digestive troubles, gallstones, or female disorders. It is taken internally, applied externally, or used in salve form to disperse milk. Fresh chervil poultices are applied to chilblains and bruised or stiff joints. An infusion of the herb can be employed as eyewash.

Sweet cicely is only rarely used medicinally, except as a tea with a strengthening effect on a weak stomach or as a sweetner for herbal teas and pharmaceutical products. The roots can be mashed and applied as an antiseptic and healing wound poultice.

Uses in Husbandry

Chervil leaves are occasionally added to herbal tobacco mixtures. Sweet cicely is favored by bees and other insects, providing them with valuable nectar early in the year. In the north, the herb is often one of the very first garden plants to flower profusely.

Literary Flowers

Now she stands out among Lydian women like the rosy-fingered moon after sunset, surpassing all the stars, and its light spreads alike over the salt sea and the flowery fields; the dew is shed in beauty, and roses bloom and tender chervil and flowery melilot.

—SAPPHO, *GREEK LYRIC*, VOL. I

People who are always sick and anemics should treasure ramsons like gold.
The young people would then flower like a climbing rose.

—Johann Künzle, *Chrut und Uchrut*

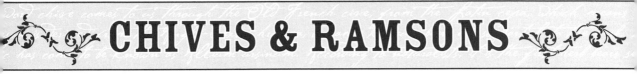

CHIVES & RAMSONS

Name

The word "chive" comes to us through the Old French *cive*, from the Latin *cepa*, meaning "onion." Chives are among the smallest members a vast botanical tribe called the Alliums. The botanical name for chives is *Allium schoenoprasum*, and they are perennial members of the **Alliaceae** family.

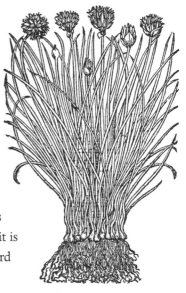

Most of the Alliums are edible, and vary botanically according to local habitat. Ramsons are one example of the many wild garlics to be found within this botanical group. Bears are quite partial to ramsons, and consequently "bear's garlic" has come to be known as *Allium ursinum*. According to naturalists, it is the first herb bears seek out after their long hibernation. The word "ramson" is derived from the Anglo-Saxon *hramsa*, or ram.

Among the many different types of onions, the top-setting onions *(Allium x proliferum)* and the Welsh or bunching onions *(Allium fistulosum)* can be used like chives. Chinese chives *(Allium tuberosum)* combine the taste of onions and garlic.

Folk Names

Other English names for chives are cive, cive garlic, civet, rashleek, and sedgeleek. One ancient term is *sweth*. In Germany, the plant is called *Schnittlauch*, *Schmallauch*, and *Suppenkraut*; in France, *vivette*, *ciboulette*, *petit pourreau*, and *civette*; in Italy, *cipoletta* and *cipollina*; in Spain, *cebollino*; in Holland, *bieslook*; in Russia, *šnittluk* and *rezanec*; and in Ireland, *síobhas*.

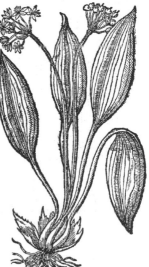

Ramsons, or bear's garlic, is blessed with a whole list of descriptive folk names: wild garlic, ramps, ramshorns, ramsey, rommy, hog's garlic, gipsy's gibbles, gipsy's onions, devil's posy, badger's flower, onion stinkers, snake's food, stinking jenny, water leek, brandy bottles, iron flower, moly, stink plant, wild leek, and broad-leaved wild garlic. Germans call the plant *Bärlauch*, *Wald-Lauch*, *Rämschelen*, *Teufelsknoblauch*, *Zigeunerlauch*, and *Hexenzwiebel*. A Russian name is *luk medvežij*.

Appearance

Chives grow close together in tufts up to 1 ft. high. The plant's "leaves" are hollow, thin shafts growing upward from tiny bulbs and enclosed in white sheaths at the bottom. Chive flowers are clustered into a ball, and are usually white with a purplish or bluish tinge. Ripe chive seeds are flat, wrinkled, and black. They are either carried by the wind or fall to the ground, and sprout easily.

Ramsons also grow in groups, although the plants are spaced a little further apart than chives. The plants can always be recognized by their penetrating garlicky smell that can carry for several hundred yards, and perfume a whole forest. Some poisonous plants resemble ramsons in appearance, but not in smell. Ramsons grow to a height of 1 ft., and produce 2 or 3 large, lance-shaped green leaves in early spring. Flower stalks and clusters of star-shaped white flowers follow somewhat later. Young ramson leaves roll in at the edges when young, but flatten as they grow older.

Chinese chives are somewhat larger than normal chives, and the leaves are almost flat. The flowers are white, and so decorative that they can be grown in the flower garden.

Top-setting onions look like smaller onions, but grow bulblets at the end of the shafts. These can be rounded, elongated, red, white, or green. The plant then grows upward until the shafts become too heavy and break off. The bulblets root in the soil, and produce new plants. Top-setting onions are perennial, and easy to grow.

Place, Season, and Useful Parts

Chives and similar wild onions grow wild in the northern temperate zones and are cultivated in gardens the world over. Wild onions and wild chives can be found in mountain meadows and moors, in swampy places, and on riverbanks and in damp meadows. Chives appear early in the spring. They can be harvested repeatedly, if the plant is kept from flowering, from then until the winter frosts. They usually blossom in July, July, and August, and quickly set seed.

Ramsons are found under deciduous trees, especially beeches, or in the moist soil of valleys and riverbanks. In some areas, the plants does not appear at all, but in others, they forms deep green carpets in spring. Ramsons can be gathered very early, from March until they die back in June.

Gathering, Drying, and Storage

Chives should be cut with sharp scissors, shears, or a knife on dry days about 1 in. above ground. They seem to thrive on repeated cuttings. If chives are cut on rainy days, water will run down into the stalks and they may turn yellow and wither. Chive blossoms can be gathered singly for use in the kitchen, or cut back to force the plant to produce more greenery. Chinese chives and top-setting onions can also be cut back repeatedly. Ramson leaves are plucked before the plant flowers, and the bulbs are dug in late fall. Ramson bulbs can be used as onion substitutes in times of scarcity. Chives and ramsons can be frozen or freeze-dried with good results. They do not dry well.

Seed Saving and Germination

Different chive varieties will cross with each other, so isolation techniques are necessary if more than one variety is to be maintained in a garden. Chive seeds do not keep well for more than 1–2 years. Chinese chives do not cross with regular chives, and can be grown at the same time in the garden. The seeds are also short-lived, and must be dried and frozen if they are to be kept for a longer period in storage. Stratification may be helpful in germinating ramson seeds. As a general rule, it is best to sow the seed immediately after harvest. The plants do not produce much seed, and are usually propagated vegetatively. Top-setting onions can only be propagated vegetatively, by placing the bulblets in the soil or in a flowerpot and lightly covering with soil. Because they do not flower, they will not cross with each other or other onions, and several varieties can be maintained in one garden, as long as the bulblets do not root near another variety. There are several very striking varieties that can be planted as attention-getters in vegetable and ornamental gardens.

Gardening Hints

One of the most persistent gardening superstitions is that begged or stolen herbs grow better than bought herbs. Stolen chives are, according to this maxim, better than honest chives. Bavarians believed that chives should never be set during the waning moon, or they would crawl underground. Chives are usually planted in Bavaria on the eve of St. George's Day (April 23rd). In most parts of Germany, a garden in which chives flourish is said to be the garden of a mean and stingy woman.

Chives do not grow equally well in all soils, but once established need little attention beyond weeding, fertilizing, and occasional transplanting. Chives are thankful for an occasional side dressing of compost and coffee grounds (onions and earthworms both seem to like coffee grounds). The plants can be propagated by division in late fall or in spring. Many gardeners suggest replanting chives each and every year to keep the soil from becoming depleted. This will also discourage the proliferation of disease. The seeds are sown in March or April, and must be kept moist until the first shoots appear. Chives can also be transplanted to flower pots and brought indoors for winter use. If these become spindly and produce few shoots, place the entire pot in a cool place and do not water it for a while. Then transplant the divided rootstock into fresh soil (preferably a compost/garden soil mix), bring it back into the room, and begin regular watering. Potted chives can also be sent "on vacation" into the garden in summer. They are then divided and repotted before the winter months. Chives spring up promptly every spring before most of the larger onions have managed to push their way up out of the cold soil, which makes them especially valuable as a fresh source of vitamins after the long winter months.

Chives, like garlic, can be planted next to roses to repel aphids. This companion planting helps to improve the growth and fragrance of the roses, as well as the pungency of the chives. Chives are also planted next to celery, lettuce, and peas as a protection against aphids. A chive infusion is used to spray apple trees for scab, and gooseberries against mildew. Tomatoes, cucumbers, and carrots will all grow better in the vicinity of chives.

Ramsons are seldom cultivated, although Czech horticulturalists have worked on breeding better ramson varieties. Seeds gathered from wild plants are sown under glass, and must be planted in a moist, shady place, if possible under beech trees.

Culinary Virtues

Chives have been employed by cooks for at least 5,000 years, but were, strangely enough, often overlooked by ancient Greeks and Romans. Charlemagne recommended their use in cloister gardens. Nicholas Culpeper once warned his readers that raw chives could harm the brain and the eyesight, and make sleep fretful, but these objections have not been verified by modern herbalists and researchers. Chives are rich in iron and vitamin C, stimulate the digestive organs, and are so mild that they can be given to convalescents and to people with sensitive stomachs. They have the additional virtue of being one of the first plants to peek through the snow in spring. Therefore, they are often included in the soups and pastries traditionally served on Maundy Thursday. These herb dishes are supposed to protect the family from disease for the rest of the year. In Russia, chive pastries are traditionally served on May 20th.

Chives should always be eaten fresh to avoid vitamin loss. Finely chopped chives can be eaten directly on bread and butter, or they are added to salad dressings and to cream cheese, dip, and cottage cheese mixtures. Chives, or single chive blossoms, are a handsome garnish for soups, vichyssoise, hors d'oeuvres, pancakes, boiled or baked potatoes, squash and rice dishes, sauces, boiled beef, and omelets. Chive butter is served with grilled meat and fish. Chive bulbs can be pickled like pearl onions, although they are somewhat small. Incidentally, the diversity of true pearl onions has, in the last few years, become endangered, because they are only grown by commercial producers and have lost their place in small gardens.

Chive blossom vinegar makes a pretty gift from the kitchen garden if prepared in decorative bottles. The freshly chopped herb can be frozen in small portions in ice cube trays for winter use.

Ramsons are much, much stronger in flavor than chives. Fresh ramson leaves can be boiled or steamed, and they combine well with the taste of nettles or spinach. They are prepared just like these greens. Cooked ramsons can be gathered in large amounts in the spring, and frozen with good results in small portions or preserved in pesto form for later use. Ramsons are often considered to be a better medicinal than culinary herb, because of their strongly cleansing and laxative action, but this is no reason to forego their strong taste in moderation. In any case, it is advisable to first try a small portion before going on a ramson orgy. Those who like strong foods may even want to eat ramsons raw in soups and salads, or with cream or cottage cheese. According to the old adage that the best accompaniment to meat is the vegetable the animal likes to eat, wild onions and wild garlic are the perfect accompaniment to game, especially bear meat.

Noteworthy Recipes

A Cold Chive Sauce: Hard-boil 2 eggs, and mix the hard-boiled yolks with an uncooked yolk. Add several tablespoons of freshly pressed sunflower or flax oil and half the amount of wine (not balsamic) vinegar until a thick sauce is formed. Add a pinch of salt, and a handful of finely chopped fresh chives. This sauce can be stretched by adding a few teaspoons of breadcrumbs or the chopped hard-boiled egg whites. If a spicier sauce is desired, add some French mustard. Other herbs such as tarragon, chervil, sorrel, or salad burnet are complementary to the taste of chives. This sauce can be served with fish, but also with cold meat.

Chive Blossom Omelet: Beat 3 eggs together with salt, freshly ground black pepper, and 2 tsp. of chopped fresh parsley. Heat 1 tsp. of olive oil in an omelet pan or iron skillet, and then pour in egg mixture so that it thinly covers the bottom of the pan. Shake the pan. Sprinkle the single flowers of 3 chive blossoms and 2 Tbsp. of grated cheese (Swiss, cheddar, or Monterey Jack, according to taste) into the middle of the omelet until the cheese begins to melt. Fold the omelet, and serve with single chive or borage blossom garnishes.

Herb Strudel: The following is a traditional Alpine recipe for herbal pastry. The dough is prepared from approximately ½ lb. of white flour and a pinch of salt mounded onto a board, and 1 egg, 2 oz. of melted butter, and a few tablespoons of lukewarm water poured into the hole in the mound. Work this until a stiff yet workable dough is formed (adding a little water if it is too stiff, and some more flour if it is too soft). Chill, and roll the dough out on a large floured cloth with a floured rolling pin as thin as possible. Then, leaving the stretched dough on the cloth, brush the top with melted butter. Beat ¼ pint of thin cream and 5 or 6 eggs together in a bowl, and spread the mixture onto the dough. Season with salt and pepper, and cover the cream mixture with mixed chopped herbs such as chives, parsley, chervil, sorrel, salad burnet, dill, and/or sweet basil.

Roll the filled dough by loosening it from one end of the cloth, folding it over, and then rolling it off the cloth until a long "log" is formed. Transfer the roll carefully to a buttered baking form, bending it as needed. Bake in a moderately hot oven until the top begins to take on color, then remove and brush with melted butter. Return to the oven, and bake until the strudel turns a rich golden brown. Serve as a hot meal or a side dish.

Ramson Soup: Pick several handfuls of fresh ramsons in spring, and, if available, the first fresh tips of nettles, or dead nettles (pick the nettles with rubber gloves and tongs). Wash carefully to remove all grit, using gloves to wash the nettles, and then strain in a colander. Put a pot half full of salted water on the stove, and add peeled and diced potatoes until almost full. Cook until almost done, and then add the ramsons and/or nettles. Let simmer until the greens are cooked, and then put though a blender (or food processor) until puréed, or use a handheld blender. Serve warm with a spoonful of mashed potatoes floated in the green soup. Cooked ramsons and nettle greens freeze well for use later in the year.

Medicinal Merits

Chives have never been considered important medicinal herbs, but ramsons are still held in high regard as excellent tonic and depurative herbs. Ancient naturalists observed that hungry bears would waddle over to the next ramson patch after their long winter's sleep, and eat their fill there. Soon, the bears' shaggy coats were sleek and glossy, and they were ready to turn to the serious business of spring hunting. Following the example of their ursine relatives, humans tried eating the leaves in spring, with excellent results. Since then, most herbalists have prescribed the plant as a blood-cleansing and tonic herb. Nicholas Culpeper wrote that it can "work miracles in phlegmatic habits of body," and recommended it to open the lungs and intestines, to combat asthma, and to ease windy colics.

Modern Medicine

Wild ramsons are praised by modern herbalists as expectorant, vermifugal, laxative and depurative. They can be helpful in the prevention of arterial and circulatory disorders, especially high blood pressure. Ramsons cause the uterus to contract, and also have a healing and antiseptic effect when applied externally to cuts and wounds. People with poor facial color, acne, or the first twinges of rheumatism, can profit by eating wild ramsons, or drinking ramson tea in spring.

Those who take offence at ramsons' strong odor can turn to chives, their milder cousins. Chives, like ramsons, are harmful if consumed in inordinately large quantities, but can be beneficial if eaten regularly and with moderation. Chives, like ramsons, help to cleanse the intestines, lungs, and blood, and they are useful in the treatment of anemia. Carrot and chive juice can be taken regularly for several weeks to discourage intestinal parasites. Glandular swellings are treated with poultices of chopped chives, and poultices of bruised ramson leaves also have antiseptic properties. Chives are used in Chinese medicine to warm cold conditions, and to move blood, as well as counteracting nausea and lack of appetite.

Uses in Husbandry
Animals, especially cattle but also dogs and cats, can be given a small amount of chives mixed with their fodder. The herbs will help to prevent worm infestation and act as a general tonic and blood-purifying medicine.

Miscellaneous Wisdom
The city of Chicago owes its name to the Native American word *sikaakwa*, meaning "a place that smells of wild onions and garlic."

In Germany, if the chives in the garden start to "grow wrong," then superstition says that the head of the house will die.

He need neither Physition nor Surgeon,
that hath Bugle and Sanicle.

—A FRENCH PROVERB

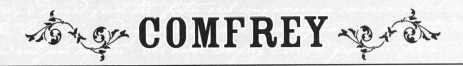

COMFREY

Name

The name "comfrey" is derived from the Latin verb *confirmare* or *conserva*, which describes the plant's healing properties. Comfrey's modern botanical name, *Symphytum*, which is probably derived from the Greek *symphyo* ("to make whole") and *phyton* ("plant"), also points to the plant's ability to make bones "grow" or "join together."

A perennial member of the ***Boraginaceae*** (**Borage**) family, *Symphytum officinale* has also been known as *Symphytum consolida, S. patens, S. bohemicum, S. tanaicense, S. uglinosum, S. stenophyllum, S. ambiguum,* and *S. majus*. There is a good deal of confusion about the various comfreys. The larger forms, such as *Symphytum asperum* and *Symphytum x uplandicum*, are usually used as fodder plants. *Symphytum peregrinum* has been the subject of a large amount of gardening and media interest in the last few years; the plants that are sold under this name, unfortunately, are often nothing other than common comfrey, or the comfrey hybrid *Symphytum x uplandicum*.

Folk Names

Common comfrey is also known as consound, boneset, bugle, middle comfrey, knitback, knitbone, boneheal, healing herb, slippery root, wallwort, blackwort, church bells, gooseberry pie, pigweed, snake, coffee flowers, suckers, bruisewort, gum plant, and ass ear. It was known as *ban vyrt* to the Anglo-Saxons, and *Beinwella* in Old High German. Modern German names for the plant are also numerous: *Beinwell, Beinwurz, Wallwurz, Schmierwurz, Hasenbrot, Milchwurzel,* and *Schwarzwurzel*. French names are *consoude, herbe à la coupure, langue de vache, oreille d'âne, oreilles de vache;* Italian, *consolida maggiore* or *consolida*; Russian, *opopnik lekarstvennyj*; Spanish, *consuelda major* and *bourrache*; Irish, *meacan*; and Russian, *okopnik lekarstvennyi*.

Appearance

Comfrey can, under favorable conditions, grow to a height of 3 ft., although it is usually only half that tall. Its hairy, hollow, and thick stem is graced with large, pointed, prickly, dark green leaves that droop downward. The leaves are hairy, and sandpapery to the touch. Comfrey's bell-shaped flowers are found in drooping clusters on one side of the stem. The flowers of common comfrey are purple or dirty red, and occasionally white. A wild relative, *Symphytum tuberosum*, which does not have the same healing properties, sports yellowish-white blossoms, and the garden plant *Symphytum caucasicum* has brilliant blue flowers. The plant's roots are spindle-shaped and up to 1 ft. long, or even more in light soil. They are extremely brittle, and ½–1 in. thick. They branch easily, are black outside and whitish inside, and are of an unusually slimy and fleshy consistency.

Ancient herbalists divided the comfreys into male and female plants, each used for different healing purposes. The white-blossoming forms were considered to be female, and the purple-flowering common comfrey was believed to be the male comfrey.

Place, Season, and Useful Parts

Common comfrey grows wild in most of Europe and as far east as western Siberia, as well as in North America in damp places and in meadows. It also can be found on salty, moist, or shady ground, on rubble heaps, near fences, ditches, streams, brooks, or ponds, and in copses and lightly wooded areas to an altitude of 3,250 ft. It is widely cultivated in gardens, and occasionally raised commercially as a medicinal herb. Common comfrey is also grown in Brazil as a fodder plant. In temperate areas, where grass does not grow well, various comfreys are used as important fodder plants with high protein contents.

Comfrey blooms from April or May to September and occasionally even into October. The roots and leaves are widely used in medicine. Some herbalists gather the flowers separately.

Gathering, Drying, and Storage

The comfrey plant is often confused with similar **Borage** family members, and can be gathered in their place, or vice versa, without danger. Most members of this family are healing herbs in their own right, and none are dangerously poisonous. Comfrey leaves are gathered either before or during flowering, from May to October. The thick stems should be removed from the leaves, which must then be dried with great caution to avoid spoilage and mildew. Commercially produced comfrey leaves are often exorbitantly expensive or only available in specialty stores, because of the difficulties involved in drying them without alkaloid loss. Keeping a plant or two in the garden does not take up much room, and will bring forth fresh leaves for most of the year. It will also produce valuable plant material for the compost pile or mulching.

Comfrey roots are gathered after the plant has flowered from October to November, or when the ground thaws, before the plant blossoms, in the spring. Comfrey roots are best dried near a source of constant low heat. They should not be parched or overheated. They can be dried on a clothesline hung over a warm radiator or stove, on a rack over the pilot light in an oven, or in a dehydrator set on low heat. Mildewed roots should be discarded immediately. Comfrey roots must be completely dry before storage, or they will mildew. They keep best in airtight containers.

Seed Saving and Germination

Comfrey plants are best propagated by plant division or root cuttings, and not from seed. There are several forms with ornamental properties, such as white flowers and variegated leaves, as well as the hybrids (such as Bocking 14, developed by Lawrence Hills of the Henry Doubleday Research Association in England) and many local forms. The plants are fertilized by bees and bumblebees (this herb is one of their favorites). They self-seed readily, as well as propagate themselves through root division. Each piece of root can easily grow into a new plant. Because of this, they can become something of a nuisance in a garden. If you are interested in saving the seeds of non-hybrids, gather the whole stalk while the upper flowers are still flowering, but the bottom blooms have faded. Shake the seeds out onto a cloth, and remove them. Leave the plants to dry on a cloth in the sun. Shake out the seeds again, and remove them. If the weather allows, dry the stalks outdoors for another day, shaking out the seeds at the end of the day or removing the seeds with a sieve. The stems will mildew quickly, even in a dry climate, and ruin the seeds, if the stems are not turned and removed regularly. Comfrey seeds germinate best if sown immediately, but can also be dried and frozen for future use.

Gardening Hints

Henry Doubleday, the nineteenth–century horticulturist, saw great commercial potential in the comfrey plant as a substitute for rubber and spent a fortune researching the possibilities. The organization that grew out of his endeavors, the Henry Doubleday Research Association (HDRA), is still active, promoting organic gardening and the maintenance of plant genetic resources. Unfortunately, Henry Doubleday was not able to find lucrative commercial applications for the comfrey plant, but did develop several hybrids with better growth habits. The sisters of the Abbey Fulda in Germany have also adopted the plant, and written a monograph on the varied uses to which comfrey can be put, especially as a compost and mulch plant.

A stand of comfrey, once established in a fairly damp position, will spread so rapidly that it may endanger other garden plants. It is extremely difficult to get rid of comfrey because of the brittleness of the plant's roots: each root section is capable of producing a new plant. To make matters worse, comfrey is extremely hardy, and is only attacked by one major disease, rust. The only effective method of discouraging the plant is to drain the soil, or let it dry out repeatedly, and then sow a thick green manure crop of hemp or mustard in the comfrey patch 2 years in a row, cutting back any plants that manage to make it through the greenery. Nonetheless, comfrey is a valuable plant to have in the garden.

It is best to plant comfrey in an unused, shady or damp corner of the garden or yard, and let it spread at will. The informed gardener knows that comfrey is one of the best compost plants, especially when used together with stinging nettle leaves, because it decomposes very quickly and is an excellent source of potassium. The leaves and stems can be spread as exceptionally good mulch under tomato and celeriac plants or bush fruits such as raspberries and gooseberries, and they can also be strewn in potato trenches. If the garden soil is potassium-rich, gardeners should ease off on comfrey, and only use it as a fertilizer for tomatoes and potatoes. Some organic gardeners prepare a fermented liquid fertilizer made from comfrey leaves and water. An even easier method is to stuff comfrey leaves into a container, pack them down, and close it tightly. The comfrey leaves contain so much fluid that they will quickly decompose into a thick black liquid. This comfrey "tea" should be diluted with 10–20 parts of water and used as a liquid fertilizer for tomatoes or potatoes.

Comfrey seeds are sown in the fall, or root cuttings taken throughout the year, or existing plants divided in fall or spring. If planting commercially, a distance of 2½ ft. should be maintained between rows. The plants grow especially quickly if watered and fertilized well. They usually suppress most weeds. Compost or old manure can be spread around the plants or between the rows in winter to ensure a more luxuriant crop.

Caucasian comfrey is an attractive garden perennial that requires little attention, and can even become invasive on damp or shady soil. Its brilliant blue flowers are especially effective in mass plantings under trees.

Culinary Virtues

Comfrey is similar in appearance, if not in family relationship, to black salsify (*Scorzonera hispanica*), a garden vegetable cultivated for its fleshy, delicate black roots. Comfrey roots can also be eaten as a vegetable in times of scarcity, although they cannot be considered a delicacy. Children sometimes eat them as "survival food" when playing "desert island." If roasted and parched over a slow fire, comfrey roots make a passable coffee substitute. Very young comfrey leaves may be boiled as a vegetable, added to soups, dipped in batter, fried in butter or oil, and added to salads. Young comfrey leaves can also be used to flavor vegetable juices and vegetable cocktails, or passed through a juicer when making carrot or apple juice. Only add a few leaves at a time, alternating with apples or carrots, because comfrey has so much mucilage that it will block the juicer and strain the motor. This method of preparation maintains the many nutrients and high protein content of the leaves. Comfrey is unusual because it has such a high vitamin B12 content, a nutrient that is usually lacking in the diets of vegetarians. Older leaves are not palatable because they are so felty and prickly. Young comfrey shoots can be blanched like sea kale by covering them with a mound of earth. They are then eaten like asparagus. Young comfrey flowers can be used as garnishes, but they wilt quickly, like borage flowers.

Wine can be produced from comfrey roots in the same manner as parsnip wine, but the flavor is not very satisfactory, and probably does not justify the work involved.

Household Applications

A bright yellow dye can be prepared from the flowering comfrey plant, harvested without roots, using tin as a mordant. Chrome as a mordant will produce a darker color, tinged with green.

Cosmetic Properties

Comfrey leaves and roots have healing, soothing, and astringent cosmetic qualities. They are used in much the same manner as marshmallow roots or aloe vera:

- A comfrey hand or body cream will help to soften and cure rough, chapped skin.
- Comfrey sunburn lotion can ease the pains of sunburn and prevent excessive peeling of the skin.
- Steaming with comfrey leaves has a healing effect on acne.
- Comfrey baths (the fresh leaves should be enclosed in a linen bath bag or pochette and hung under the hot water tap) are healing and help tone the skin.
- Comfrey compresses can be applied to swollen or roughened skin on feet, elbows, and hands.
- Some users report that the regular use of comfrey leaf poultices and comfrey baths helps to heal and prevent fungal skin diseases.

Young, tender leaves are used if possible. Older, tougher leaves are acceptable as bath additions, or if the comfrey is heated. Comfrey salve is prepared in the same manner as marigold salve, and can be often be employed in the same manner. Some people develop an unexpected allergic reaction to the herb. In this case, its use should immediately be stopped.

Noteworthy Recipes

Comfrey Water: In the seventeenth century, John Shirley gave a recipe for a distilled cleansing water that he claimed would make "a young Face exceeding Beautiful, and an old Face very Tolerable":

> Take of Benjamine [Benzoin] two handfuls, Scabeous [Devil's bit, *Succisa pratensis*] the like quantity, the Roots of Comfry a handful, Penny-royal and Rosemary, of each a handful: wash and pick them clean, then steep them a day and a night in White-wine, sprinkling them afterwards with a Powder of Myrrh; and so put them into a cold Still, and the Water so drawn off will exceed any wash in use, and not at all prejudice the party when she leaves it off, as those which are Chymically prepared do, by rendering those old and withered even in the prime of their youth, who accustome themselves thereto.[153]

Comfrey Steaming Mixture: Those who do not happen to have a still or a handful of benzoin in their apartment can still make effective use of comfrey as a cleansing herb. If the skin is blemished or damaged (but not sensitive or marked with broken veins), a steam bath with fresh comfrey leaves can work wonders. Place a warmed bowl on the kitchen table, add a handful of fresh comfrey leaves or combine with other mild herbs such as chamomile flowers or lady's mantle leaves, and pour boiling water over the leaves. Cover the bowl with a tightly fitting lid and let steep for 5–10 minutes. Prepare a tent out of a bath towel and place your face over the steaming bowl, taking care to avoid overheating the skin. Enjoy the steam for at least 10 minutes, and then dry off your face carefully. Do not go out into the cold for at least an hour after a steam bath, but close the pores with witch-hazel lotion or herbal vinegar. The treatment should be topped off with a nourishing moisturizing cream and a good night's sleep.

Medicinal Merits

Comfrey has in recent years become quite a fashionable medicinal herb, and battles have raged over the extent of the plant's medicinal virtues or its harmful qualities. Comfrey is certainly not the panacea enthusiasts would make it out to be, nor is it a noxiously harmful drug that necessarily causes liver cancer in humans, as its detractors claim. It is, very simply, a medicinal herb used externally to speed the healing process of broken bones or damaged tissues, and internally as a mild astringent with cleansing properties. It should not be taken for an extended period as a "totally harmless" herb,

---

153.   Shirley, *The Accomplished Ladies Rich Closet of Rarities* (London: N. Bodington, 1688), 154.

as some devotees would suggest, or eaten in inordinately large amounts, but should only be used regularly over several weeks for specific ailments, or added occasionally to foods. It may cause allergic reactions in some patients.

Comfrey has always seemed to attract controversy and superlatives. Otto Brunfels claimed that the plant could heal meat in a pot, and another German herbalist, Zwinger, was of the opinion that

> if one boils this herb together with the roots in water for a bath, and lets young widows bathe in it every once in a while, then they will be like unto virgins again.[154]

In his herbal, John Gerard quoted a French saying about the herb: "He need neither Physition nor Surgeon, that hath Bugle (Comfrey) and Sanicle."[155]

It is doubtful if any of these statements were believed literally, even by contemporaries. Instead, they were meant as metaphorical and hyperbolical praise of the plant. In actual practice, comfrey was prescribed as a vulnerary herb for the treatment of wounds, broken bones, open boils, bruises, and hernias, or as a poultice herb for gouty limbs or breasts sore with milk fever. Local Shropshire healers thought the purple comfrey effective for men's wounds, and the white comfrey better for women's complaints. Comfrey was also used to still bloody fluxes or vomitings, and to cleanse the breast of "damp vapors" and phlegm.

In Somerset, one folk cure for a broken limb was to tie a comfrey plant around the arm or leg and then repeat three times:

> Our Lord rade
> The foal slade
> Sinew to sinew and bone to bone
> In the Name of the Father, Son and Holy Spirit.[156]

In northern Germany, hernia patients were treated during the waning moon. The healer made three crosses over the patient with comfrey roots just before dawn and then buried the roots with a spell, but without saying another word to a living soul, just before the sun rose.

---

154. Qtd. in Gustav Hegi, *Illustrierte Flora von Mittel-Europa*, vol. V, part 3 (Munich: Lehmanns, 1913–1918), 2226.

155. Gerard, *Gerard's Herball* [1597]: *The essence thereof distilled by Marcus Woodward from the edition of Th. Johnson, 1636.* Ed. Marcus Woodward (London: Gerald How, 1927), 144.

156. Ruth L. Tongue, *Somerset Folklore* (London: The Folk-Lore Society, 1965), 37.

Modern Medicine

Comfrey poultices and salves are still widely used to aid the healing of broken bones and operation scars, to soften and heal growths, bruises, joints swollen with gout, rheumatism, and arthritis, hardened milk knots and varicose veins as well as skin diseases, and to ease the pains and scars of freshly-operated hernias, burns, and amputated limbs. Wounds heal better after the application of comfrey leaf or root poultices, leaving less scar tissue. Comfrey salve is particularly helpful after joint replacement surgery, rubbed in alternately with arnica salve, first on the surrounding tissue, and then on the scar, as soon as the stitches or staples are removed. Some forms of eczema can be treated with comfrey, although allergic reactions may occur, and an experienced herbalist should supervise the treatment. Homeopathic tinctures are prescribed internally and externally to aid the cell growth of bone as well as nerve and connective tissue, and to treat bleeding gums. Either fresh or dried comfrey leaves are used as healing compresses, but poultices of powdered roots are more effective.

Comfrey roots are further used internally in the treatment of respiratory problems, pneumonia, tuberculosis, and angina, and as an astringent medicine for stomach ulcers, diarrhea, and hemorrhoids, or for some cases of internal hemorrhage, under expert supervision. A strong electuary for those suffering from persistent coughs and catarrh can be prepared from comfrey roots and honey. The healing properties of comfrey roots are thought to be due to the alkaloid allantoin, and to the unusually high levels of calcium, phosphorus, and potassium the leaves and roots contain.

Special Cures

Comfrey Tea: Comfrey root tea should never be prepared in an iron pot, or it will turn black. One teaspoon of the roots can be boiled in ½ pint of water for several minutes, and then allowed to steep, covered, for 15 minutes. A better method is to let the roots soak overnight in cold water, and then to heat the mixture gently in the morning before drinking. This way, fewer of the ingredients are harmed by high temperatures.

Comfrey Poultices: Comfrey poultices are prepared from a strong decoction of the chopped or powdered roots. If using chopped roots, boil them with twice the amount of water until a slimy, very thick consistency is obtained, and let cool to body temperature. Strain out the remaining root particles, place the thickened mass on a piece or gauze or clean cloth, and apply as a plaster. Comfrey root powder is much more practical to use: it is simply stirred to a paste-like consistency with hot water, and applied directly. The patient with a comfrey poultice should remain quiet, with cloths wrapped around the hurt area, until the roots begin to dry and crumble. Then the poultice is removed, and the skin rubbed down carefully to remove dampness and remaining powder. Wrap warmed cloths around the limb or damaged area to prevent it from becoming chilled. A comfrey root poultice can be applied in place of a plaster cast in emergency situations, before medical help can be obtained. Comfrey leaf poultices are prepared from the fresh leaves or from dried leaves reconstituted with hot water. They are generally used for treating broken bones, sprains, and beneficial growths or knots. Comfrey leaf poultices are applied to open wounds or minor bruises and lacerations.

Comfrey Salve: Comfrey salve can be prepared with wax and lanolin, but this requires good equipment and some experience with salve preparation. The simplest comfrey salve, which has been used by farmers for centuries, is made with lard. Heat the lard slowly until liquid in an enameled or stainless steel pot, and then add a generous handful of the fresh leaves, and half as much of the powdered roots. Cook over a very low flame for 10–15 minutes, and then cover and set aside overnight. In the morning, reheat the mixture, and then strain the liquid lard through a fine sieve or a piece of cheesecloth. Press out the remaining residue. Pour into ceramic, enameled, or glass pots and store in a cool pantry or refrigerator. If the mixture begins to smell rancid, throw it out, and prepare a fresh batch.

Comfrey salve, applied several times every day for a period of several weeks, can encourage the hasty mending of broken bones. Many hospitals are not willing to accept self-treatment with comfrey, but a discreet tin of good comfrey salve can certainly be rubbed into traumatized muscles and tendons after surgery. It is especially good for use on animals. Because of the lard, many animals will accept a comfrey salve more readily than other medicines. Cats and dogs will of course lick most of it off, but that can also help to speed the healing process.

Comfrey Gel: Another method of preparing comfrey is to heat 2–3 Tbsp. of the chopped roots with 1–1½ cups of cold water. Simmer for a few minutes, and then let the roots cool in the water. Reheat, let cool again, and reheat. Carefully strain out the roots with cheesecloth, pressing out the residue. Pour into a ceramic pot or squirt bottle, and refrigerate. The result should be a jelly-like liquid that can easily be applied to hurt limbs and joints. If the mixture does not jell sufficiently, heat again and repeat the process. Apply cold. The cold comfrey applications are especially effective in treating bones and limbs after major surgery, such as knee or hip replacements, but also simple sprains or fractures. They act similarly to ice to cool inflamed areas, and also aid tissue formation and repair.

Uses in Husbandry

Beekeepers appreciate comfrey's virtues as a bee herb, and plant it in the vicinity of their hives. Farmers consider it a pasture weed because it spreads easily and robs nutrients from the soil, but does not make good hay because of its tendency to mildew. On the other hand, fresh or cooked comfrey leaves and stems, mixed with crushed grain, make excellent fodder for pigs, horses, cows, rabbits, and poultry, and are often used as a supplement to mixtures given to young animals. If a pig has an unusually large litter, the piglets can be given comfrey leaves. Even animals in zoos such as elephants, rhinoceroses, and giraffes, or house pets such as parakeets, eat comfrey and profit from the high protein and nutrient content. Dogs and cats prone to arthritis, rheumatism, or hip problems should be given comfrey in their food as preventive medicine. Comfrey leaves are added to the fodder of racehorses and poultry as a general tonic. Foresters also use comfrey as a decoy plant to lure deer away from freshly planted tree seedlings. Young comfrey leaves can be added to mixed herbal tobaccos.

Veterinary Values

Comfrey salve is widely used in the treatment of both animal and human complaints, primarily to help healing processes after breaks, sprains, or swellings, and for the first-aid treatment of cuts, sores, lacerations, or bites. Comfrey salve should be standard in any veterinary medicine cabinet, since it can be used on so many animals. A lard salve is preferable to a wax salve.

Living short but merry lives, / Going where the devil drives,
Having sweethearts, but no wives, / Live the Rakes of Mallow

—IRISH BALLAD FROM 1753

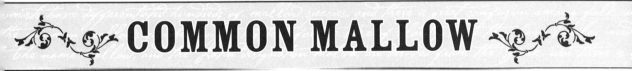

COMMON MALLOW

Name

Taxonomists have differentiated hundreds of mallow species, and there is great confusion among folk names. But the common mallows can be grouped together for the sake of clarity, since they have similar medicinal merits.

The name "mallow," and the Latin designation *malva*, are derived from the Greek word *malakos*, meaning "soft" and "pliable." The **Mallow *(Malvaceae)*** family includes a large number of useful and healing plants, from garden hibiscus to okra, cotton, jute, the common mallows, hollyhocks, musk mallows, marshmallows, and vegetable mallows. Since none of the mallows are particularly harmful, confusing the species is not dangerous. The annual *Malva neglecta*, or dwarf mallow, has also been known as *Malva vulgaris*, *Malva rotundifolia*, and *Malva parvifolia*. The annual or biennial *Malva sylvestris* has also been called *Malva grandifolia* and *Malva mauritiana*, and a common subspecies is now known as *Malva sylvestris ssp. mauritiana*. The annual *Malva verticillata* was once called *Malva crispa* and includes several subspecies.

Folk Names

Folk names for the mallows are even more numerous than botanical names and are often used indiscriminately, since most of the members of this family have similar uses. *Malva neglecta* is known as dwarf mallow, cheeseplant, cheeses, and common mallow in English; *Wegmalve, kleine Malve,* and *kleinblütige Käspappel* in German; *petite mauve, mauve des chemins, herbe à fromage, fromageon,* and *guimauve* in French; *malvetta* in Italian; and *katost* in Danish.

Malva sylvestris was known as *hoc leaf* in Anglo-Saxon, and now goes under the English names of common mallow, high mallow, blue mallow, mallow, cheeses, cheese-log, fairy cheeses, doll cheeses, and round dock. A few of the innumerable German names are *Käsepappel, Käspappel, Rosspappel, Hasenpappel, Saupappel, Ganspappel, Waldmalve, wilde Malve, Twieback, Pannkoken, Zuckerplätzchenkraut, Katzenkäse, blaue Malve, Algiermalve,* and *mauretanische Malve*. Italians call the herb *malva, malve,* and *riondela*; the French, *grande mauve, mauve sauvage, mauve, fausse guimauve, fromage,* and *petit fromage*; the Russians, *mal'va lesnaja* and *prosvirnik lesnoj*. One Thai appellation for the plant is "mother blossom," because of its widespread use by midwives.

Malva verticillata is one of the oldest healing herbs, and has been used as a vegetable in China for many centuries. English names are curled mallow, curled-leaved mallow, farmers' tobacco, and large whorl mallow. Germans call it *krause Malve, Gemüsemalve, chinesische Malve,* or *krausblättrige Malve*; the French, *mauve frisée*; and the Italians, *malva crispa*.

Appearance

Dwarf mallow *(Malva neglecta)* grows to a maximum length of 3 ft. but is usually much shorter, forming a small, rounded bush. It is a crawling plant and can easily be overlooked in other greenery, for its flowers are pale and small and it has a tendency to hide under tall grasses. The leaves are heart-shaped or rounded, and the plant is ever-bearing, producing flowers, fruits, and seeds at the same time on the same stalk. The fruits are the typical tiny mallow "cheeses."

Blue mallow *(Malva sylvestris)* is a robust plant that grows to a height of 4 ft. The plant's fleshy tap root gives off an odor vaguely reminiscent of cloves when crushed. Its rounded hairy stem is woody at the base, and filled with dry pith. The stem either crawls or climbs, and exudes no particular smell. The grass-green, hand-shaped mallow leaves are similar to lady's mantle or to some geranium leaves. Flowers of the blue mallow have 5 petals and are showy and fairly large, of a pink, violet, or even white color. Each petal has 3 dark purple stripes, which guide bees visiting the plant to the nectar and pollen. Mallow fruits have the form and color of tiny cheeses or, to draw another parallel, they look like rolled-up, smooth-skinned caterpillars. They separate into sections when ripe to reveal the plants' seeds.

Curled mallow *(Malva verticillata)* is as vertical in its growth habit as the dwarf mallow is horizontal, up to 6 ft. high, and leafy to the top. The leaves vary according to variety, but are usually large and tender, and often curled or puckered on the outside, resembling a large geranium leaf in a frilly petticoat. The flowers are small, white, and nondescript, and the seed is brown.

Place, Season, and Useful Parts

Many mallow species are native to the tropics, and only a few are indigenous to the northern latitudes. The dwarf mallow tends to spring up in soil that has been disturbed on the edges of fields, and is so widespread as to be almost cosmopolitan. The entire plant should be gathered when it blossoms for the first time, before the fruits have a chance to ripen. The first leaf crop can be harvested in June or July, when the plants are quite small. If the plants are cut back rigorously and watered well, a second crop can be gathered in September. It is also possible to simply cut off the tops of the plants as needed.

Blue mallow grows in most of the world to an altitude of 3,000 ft. It is often cultivated in gardens, but can also be found growing wild on uncultivated ground. It flowers from summer to early autumn. Mallow leaves are picked singly before they blossom. The flowers can be plucked as they appear, or the entire blossoming plant harvested from June to September, and the roots dug in March or April, and then again in October.

Curled mallow is a cultivated plant, although it sometimes escapes from cultivated areas. The large leaves are picked singly.

Gathering, Drying, and Storage

Mallow leaves and shoots are usually gathered before they blossom, and the flowers are gathered just before they open fully, in several harvests. The roots are dug in fall or the early spring.

The flowers and leaves are dried quickly in shady, airy rooms. The flowers must be stored in dark, moisture-proof containers or they will turn pale and begin to decompose. They cannot be stored for longer than 1 year. The roots should not be washed, but simply brushed or scrubbed to remove dirt and then split or cut into slices, and dried.

Seed Saving and Germination

The mallows retain their germinating vitality for up to 5 years in good conditions. The easiest way to reproduce mallows is to allow the plants to self-seed. If plants with larger leaves or flowers are desired, then weaker plants should be rigorously ripped out. Over the years, this constant selection for plants with the desired characteristics will result in a new strain, which can be reproduced by isolating the plants, collecting seeds, and sowing them the following year. Wild plants will have to be removed in order to keep them from combining with the improved plants.

Vegetable mallows must be kept isolated to keep different vegetable mallow varieties pure. They will cross with each other, but not with other mallows. The tall plants produce masses of seeds that can be harvested more easily than those of the marshmallow.

Gardening Hints

The common mallows are cultivated for their flowers as border plants, as greens in the vegetable garden, or as healing herbs in the herb garden. The fruits of the wild plants are sown in April and then again in late summer, on rich but not freshly fertilized soil. Blue mallows will usually only blossom in the second year, and should be sown in summer. The fruits are said to germinate more rapidly under the influence of light, which is why they do so well when they self-seed. At this point it is only fair to point out that mallows may cause more mischief than anything else in a garden, although the purple blossoms are pretty and are much appreciated by bees. The plants tend to spread rapidly, and their roots are difficult to eradicate once they have taken hold. The best place to grow mallows is in an unused corner of the yard at some distance from the main garden. Here the mallows can spread as much as they want, and thrive with little attention, little trouble, little water, and little or no hoeing. Even the showy blue mallow can compete very well with grass, and may spring up uninvited in the lawn. Enthusiasts of wild greens may want to plant mallows next to an existing nettle patch to ensure their supply of fresh wild greens through the spring and summer months.

The blue mallow *(Malva sylvestris)* is biennial, and is sown in summer and can then be transplanted to its final position. It needs 16 in. between plants, and will grow to over 3 ft. high. The curled mallow *(Malva verticillata)* is an annual, and is sown in spring. It will grow to 6 ft., but does not branch as much as the blue mallow. The curled mallow is a garden plant in its own right, and is used as a vegetable, as a backdrop for more showy flowers, or as a decorative element in the vegetable or herb garden. It is easy to grow the plants from seed by direct-seeding them in April, or they can be transplanted when still small to fill in gaps. Once a stand is established, it will usually reproduce itself by self-sowing and require little further attention besides watering. The cultivated mallows will self-seed as readily as the wild representatives of the family.

Culinary Virtues

Various mallows have been used as vegetable plants for centuries, if not millennia. The practice began in China, then developed in Southeast Asia and on into Europe and North America. Hesiod was one of the first classical authors to mention the use of mallows as food. Otto Brunfels recommended a salad prepared from the tips of young mallow plants and mallow flowers, olive oil, vinegar, and salt. It was once medicinal practice to prepare a conserve of blue mallow flowers as cough medicine. Aside from its healing action, this conserve had a pretty purple color and an agreeable taste.

The young shoots, leaves, and flowering tops of *Malva verticillata*, *Malva sylvestris*, and *Malva neglecta* are still used today as vegetable and salad herbs. The use of mallows in cookery was once especially prevalent in China, but is now popular in France and Italy.

The best mallow leaves for cookery are those of *Malva verticillata*, because of their large size and soft texture. They can be used in much the same way as spinach in most recipes, and also make excellent garnishes, especially for desserts. Blue mallow flowers are often overlooked as edible garnishes for a variety of foods, from spicy salads to puddings.

Mallow "cheeses," as the plants' fruits are called, are eaten greedily by children, and are sometimes added to salads or boiled as an unusual, if somewhat insipid, vegetable for adults. A strong decoction of mallow cheeses contains so much albumin that one American herbalist suggests it be used as an egg-white substitute by strict vegetarians, and whipped like egg white.

Noteworthy Recipes

Spring Mallow Soup: A tasty soup that also has blood-cleansing properties can be prepared from a mixture of garden vegetables and mallow leaves. Gather a handful each of spinach, kale, chard, endive, and young salad leaves (or any combination of the fresh leaves available in your garden), a handful of wild or cultivated sorrel leaves, and two generous handfuls of mallow shoots, leaves, or flowers, without stems. Melt a dab of butter in a saucepan, and then add the washed, drained, and chopped greens. Cook very gently over a low flame until the vegetables begin to change color, and then add water or stock to barely cover the greens. Season with salt, pepper, and maybe a little freshly grated nutmeg, and let simmer until all the leaves are soft. The texture can be improved by mixing everything in a blender before serving, and enriching it by adding a little sour cream or plain yogurt before serving.

Household Applications

Blue mallow blossoms are added to potpourri because of their brilliant color. *Malva sylvestris*, *Malva verticillata*, and *Malva neglecta* all contain fibers that can be processed in much the same manner as Chinese Jute *(Abutilon theophrasti)*, another member of the widespread mallow family.

Cosmetic Properties

A compress or poultice of mallow leaves can soften, cleanse, and gently disinfect the skin. A mallow-leaf facial is therefore of great value to those with dry, chapped skin, or dry skin combined with acne. Work-roughened or weather-chapped hands, or even diaper rash can be softened with mallow-leaf compresses, or mallow-leaf hand baths. A softening hand lotion or cold cream can be prepared from a strong infusion of mallow leaves and thickening agents such as quince seeds, Irish moss, honey, lanolin, or beeswax, and preserved with alcohol, borax, or benzoin tincture. Toothpaste can also be prepared from powdered mallow root, or a piece of the root chewed to cleanse the teeth.

Medicinal Merits

The common mallow is an ancient medicinal herb. The Chinese were already using it 5,000 years ago to help relieve digestive and respiratory problems. In the Bible, Moses treated the feverish with mallow tea. Dioscurides recommended it as an antidote for all deadly poisons, and Pliny wrote that one cup of mallow tea, taken daily, could guarantee freedom from ill health. Pliny also considered the herb to be so cooling that it could lessen the heat of scorpion and wasp stings. According to him, scorpions will deep-freeze if placed on mallow leaves.

Otto Brunfels was a great supporter of the herb. He prescribed mallows for a variety of ills, in particular for female disorders. He recommended laying childbearing women on beds of mallow leaves to aid delivery, and prescribed a mallow bath or douche to ease a hardened uterus. A mallow-leaf and fennel-seed potion was used to draw out a woman's milk, and a poultice of the boiled roots and black wool was used to soften any hardenings of the breast. He administered mallow tea as a universal remedy for bladder pains, and men who suffered from premature ejaculation were told by Brunfels to tie mallow plants around their arms. He prescribed the plant for feverish people, melancholiacs, epileptics, and those with a cough, and used it to treat eye sores, and obstructed stomachs. Mallow leaves were employed to draw out splinters. A supposedly sovereign remedy was a concoction of barley meal, chicken broth, two egg yolks, violet oil, and mallows, applied externally to ripen an abscess or to soften a hardened liver or spleen. Brunfels applied mallows and spit to extended thyroid glands, and rubbed in mallows steeped in urine as a dandruff remedy.

Rural folk medicine has adopted some of these remedies. Birthing women are still placed on mallow beds in secluded mountain areas, or given mallow tea to drink before delivery. A mallow footbath is believed to bring on menstruation and ease labor pains. Soothing vaginal douches are prepared with mallow-leaf tea. Mallows cooked in milk and sweetened with sugar are administered for a cough. The distilled water of mallows is used for toothaches and earaches, suppurations, and inflammations. In the words of an Italian folk saying, "the mallow can save you from every ill."[157] In other words, it is a versatile herb with a wide range of healing properties.

Modern Medicine

Modern herbalists are more cautious in their praise and use of mallows and usually consider them a harmless and gentle home remedy. Mallow leaves can soften swollen, infected tissue or mucous membranes. They can aid healing, and calm the patient.

---

157. Hanns Bächtold-Stäubli, ed., *Handwörterbuch des deutschen Aberglaubens* (1927–42), vol. V (Berlin: Walter de Gruyter & Co., 1987), 1559.

They also soothe and gently combat infections and free the body of poison. They are especially helpful in the treatment of infections in the respiratory, digestive, and urinary tracts. Mallow tea is one of the best medicines for those who have to contend with a nervous or sensitive stomach. European doctors who pooh-pooh all alternative medicines still recommend that their patients drink mallow tea for chronic stomach problems or after an operation. Mallow tea, like chamomile, is easily available and can be given to anyone suffering from mild infectious diseases, and it can also be used in steaming mixtures to relieve the symptoms of a cold. Mallows can be taken for extended periods without harmful side effects. An enema of mallow-leaf tea has a soothing and cleansing effect, and can relieve intestinal colics.

Because fresh mallow leaves also contain some astringent qualities, they are often used externally as compresses and poultices to soften swellings and draw out infections. An abscess or boil can be ripened with a warm mallow-leaf compress, and then opened with another compress of warm mallow leaves mixed with St. John's wort oil. Compresses of mallow leaves can also be used to soften swollen or hardened glands, hemorrhoids, or benevolent growths. Mallow leaves brought to a boil in olive oil and allowed to cool are applied to frostbitten hands and feet.

Purple mallow flowers are gathered separately and used specifically to treat colds, coughs, sore throats, and chest or lung complaints, and are administered to children with measles, tonsil infections, and colds. The fresh flowers crushed in olive oil and applied immediately to bee or wasp stings help relieve pain and swelling. A crushed fresh leaf will also give some relief. Chewing the fresh flowers is said to lessen toothache, and chewing fresh mallow roots is a recognized method of strengthening the teeth and gums and preventing trips to the dentist.

Special Cures

Tea for a Nervous Stomach: A simple tea mixture for a nervous, acid stomach can be mixed from 2 parts each of mallow leaves and chamomile flowers, 1 part each of hops, St. John's wort, and marigold petals, and ½ part of freshly crushed linseed. It is important that the flax seeds are fresh, for they quickly turn rancid, and are then worthless or even harmful. The tea is brewed with fresh boiling water, allowed to steep for 10–15 minutes, and drunk ½ hour before main meals for a period of 2–3 months. The linseed can be omitted if it causes internal griping, and a tablespoon of fresh flax oil taken instead.

Gargle for Sore Throats: A softening gargling infusion for infected tonsils and sore throats can be prepared by mixing equal amounts of mallow leaves, marshmallow roots, mullein flowers, colt's foot leaves, and cooked or canned elderberries (*Sambucus nigra*, also *Sambucus racemosa*). Add 1 Tbsp. of the herb mixture to ½ pint of cold water, let stand for 6 hours, and then heat until just warm before straining. The best method is to strain it into a thermos bottle and to take sips of the brew as soon as the throat starts getting scratchy.

Uses in Husbandry

A tincture of blue mallow flowers *(Malva silvestris)* is employed as a delicate chemical test to determine the presence of alkalis. Chickens are fond of mallow seeds, and bees are strongly attracted to most mallow flowers, especially the blue mallow. Curled mallow is occasionally grown as a fodder plant.

Veterinary Values

The leaves of the common mallow (or the roots of the marshmallow) are used as poultices to cleanse and soften the wounds of household and barnyard animals. Cats suffering from colds can be given milk thinned with mallow-leaf tea, and freshly chopped green leaves are added to their diet as vitamin and nutrient-rich supplements.

Miscellaneous Wisdom

Greeks offered mallows (representing humankind's first source of nourishment) to Apollo at his temple. Mallows were also planted on graves: the ring-formed "cheeses" of the plant's fruits were considered suitable food for the dead. The Pythagoreans classed the mallow as sacred and refused to eat it because of its association with the death cult. *Malva alcea* is still planted on graves in Austria.

In Germany, mallows were buried under the threshold to prevent witches and milk thieves from entering the house or barn. In England, mallow flowers are woven into garlands or strewn in front of the door in traditional May Day ceremonies.

A sympathetic parallel, between the seeds of the mallow plant and lice, was once drawn in Bavaria: a person who eats too many mallow cheeses will consequently be plagued with lice. In Posen (Poland), the belief is that anyone who gorges himself on mallow cheeses will certainly go crazy.

Herbs closely linked with death are also often associated with birth and marriage as well, and this is true of the mallow. In the East, brides and grooms were showered with mallow leaves after the ceremony. Marriage beds adorned with mallow flowers were believed to bring many children. The Greeks also thought that mallow seeds were imbued with aphrodisiacal properties.

Oracular Worth

In the fifteenth century, mallows were used as a primitive pregnancy test. The woman's urine was poured on fresh mallow leaves. If the plants were still green three days later, then it was taken as a sign that she was expecting a child. Two centuries later, the same test was used to determine a girl's virginity: dried leaves denoted chastity, while green leaves were an indication of the girl's experience in the mysteries of love. In very isolated regions, these oracles are still consulted today.

Herbal Pastimes

Mallow cheeses were favorite playthings of children. They were picked, peeled, eaten, stored away, and used as wheels or cheeses in dollhouses and doll shops. John Clare, the nineteenth-century English poet, considered playing with mallow fruits one of the "joys that came wi spring," and observed,

> The sitting down when school was oer
> Upon the threshold by his door
> Picking from mallows sport to please
> Each crumpld seed he called a cheese
> And hunting from the stackyard sod
> The stinking hen banes belted pod
> By youths vain fancy sweetly fed
> Christning them his loaves of bread ... [158]

We can only hope that not too many children tried to eat the poisonous "bread" made of henbane.

Legends

In Malta, a legend is told of the time when there was no bread. Jesus was still a child, but when he realized that he and his mother had no bread to eat, he told her to go to the front of the hut and to break off the mallow plant growing there. Mary did as she was told, and carried the plant to the baker. At first the baker wanted to have nothing to do with the weed. But then he saw the tiny golden seed rolls growing on the plant, and his annoyance turned to wonder. The plant was given the name *Hobbeiza*, or "flower rolls," and was eaten for centuries whenever there was a shortage of bread.

Literary Flowers

> *Exhausted by the journey and his grief,*
> *The old man plucked some grain from patches wild,*
> *And mallows from around the courtyard well,*
> *As in the days when but a little child.*
> —HAN POEM FROM CHARLES BUDD, *CHINESE POEMS*

---

158. John Clare, *The Shepherd's Calendar* (1827) (London: Oxford Univ. Press, 1964), 56.

The flow'ry May, who from her green lap throws / The yellow cowslip, and the pale primrose.
Hail, bounteous May, that dost inspire / Mirth, and youth, and warm desire!

—JOHN MILTON, "SONG ON MAY MORNING"

COWSLIP & PRIMROSE

Name

The term "cowslip," despite all attempts to give it a more appetizing etymology, is derived from the Old English term *cū* and *slyppe*, or "cowpat." Anyone who has seen the plants growing in cow pastures, peeking through old cow dung, can reconstruct the reasoning behind this name.

The English word "primrose," along with the Latin name *Primula*, point to the seasonal properties of this plant: it is the *prima rosa*, the first "rose" to appear in spring. Cowslips and primroses are both members of the **Primrose (*Primulaceae*)** family.

In North America, however, the term "cowslip" is also used to designate a totally different and somewhat poisonous plant: *Caltha palustris*, otherwise known as marsh marigold. One ancient folk name for cowslips and primroses, "paigle," is derived from the old verb "to paggle" (meaning "to shake and hang downward").

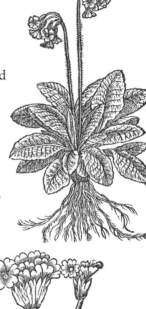

The members of the **Primrose** family are very numerous and varied, with many species and subspecies. Some of them are so closely related that they hybridize readily, confusing botanical classification. So, for the purposes described in this chapter and the sake of simplicity, keep in mind that all European yellow-blossoming primroses and cowslips (*Primula veris*, *Primula elatior*, and *Primula vulgaris*) can be employed medicinally (although the common meadow cowslip, *Primula veris*, is preferred). Colorful garden hybrid varieties do not have the same qualities. *Primula auricula*

(mountain or alpine cowslip) and *Primula farinosa* (bird's eye primrose) have also been part of the primrose healing tradition.

Folk Names

In old herbals, the cowslip had many names: *herba paralysis*, *verbascum odoratum*, *arthritica*, and *betonica alba*. Modern English names for the herb also abound. The names primrose, cowslip, and oxlip are often used indiscriminately and interchangeably, although the the plants are botanically distinct. Other names are paigles, peagles, peggle, plumrocks, palsy wort, petty mulleins, herb peter, key flower, key of heaven, Our Lady's keys, artetyke, cowslop, spring cowslip, butterrose, buckles, crewel, fairy cups, password, drelip, and May flower. German names for the cowslip are just as numerous: *Schlüsselblümchen*, *Primel*, *Himmelsschlüssel*, *Frauenschlüssel*, *St. Petersschlüssel*, *Wiesenschlüsselblume*, *Fastenblume*, *Schmalzschlüsseli*, *Pluderhose*, *Eierblume*, *Pankooksblume*, *gelber Scharnigl*, and *weiße Petonie*.

The oxlip *(Primula elatior)* is known as *hohe Primel* or *wald Primel* in Germany. The French call it *primevère*, *primerolle*, *coucou*, *printanière*, and *primevère à grande fleurs*; the Italians, *primavera*, *pestalache*, and *occhio di civetta*. The Welsh call the herb *briallu mair*.

Primula auricula is known as the mountain cowslip, dusty miller, auricula, and bear's ear in English; and *Aurikel*, *Platenigl*, *gelbes Gamsveigerl*, *gelber Speik*, and *Gamsbleamerl* in German.

Appearance

The cowslip is one of the first flowers to poke its head out of the ground in spring, often through the snow. Cowslip leaves are easily recognizable: they are relatively large, egg-shaped, ridged, and strongly wrinkled, and of a pale vivid green color. They are felty on the underside, with rolled edges. The leaves have no particular smell, but taste slightly bitter. The cowslip produces leaves in the fall, 2 tiny leaves in February, and then a full leaf rosette in late February or early March. A long stem shoots forth from the rosette in April, which in turn produces a bunch of small, yolk-colored, sweet-smelling, bell-shaped flowers. The blossoms usually have 5 petals, and each petal has a gold-colored spot on it. The flowers' fragrance is sweet and smells like honey.

Garden primrose flowers appear on single flower stalks. Other primulas have short flower stems, and pink, yellowish, or even brown-colored flowers in a wide array of shapes, usually with dark yellow or orange honey guides for bees. Cowslips and primroses rarely grow taller than 10 in.

Cowslip roots are perennial, short, grayish-brown on the outside, and yellowish-whitish on the inside. The plant has many secondary rootlets. The roots taste extremely bitter, but have a pleasant anise-like fragrance that becomes more intense when the root is dried.

Place, Season, and Useful Parts

Cultivated cowslips and primroses can be found in most parts of the world with moist climates. Cowslips, oxlips, and primroses grow wild in Asia Minor and most parts of Europe, with the exception of arid areas or the extreme North. The alpine cowslip, *Primula auricula*, grows to an altitude of 5,000 ft. but also flourishes in gardens at sea level.

The cowslip has a definite liking for sunny, open places and low altitudes. It can usually be found in dry pastures and meadows, on sunny slopes, in open fields or under hedges and light underbrush. The first *Primula* to appear in spring, the oxlip, *Primula elatior*, prefers a damp position on shady slopes or damp meadows, in woods and field borders, or under thick underbrush. It thrives up to alpine regions. The mountain primrose does best in drier soil, in hedgerows, pastures, or along railway embankments.

Gathering, Drying, and Storage

Cowslip roots should be dug before the plant begins to blossom in the spring. Since the species are often endangered in the wild, they should only be gathered where allowed by law, or from garden plots. Even picking the plants is prohibited in some areas. Cowslip flowers can be picked when fully opened with or without the green flower receptacle, or calyx. Cowslip leaves can be gathered shortly before or while the plant is flowering. Wilted, yellowish, or diseased leaves must be discarded. They should be packed loosely in baskets to avoid bruising the leaves or flowers as much as possible. It is advisable to wear cotton gloves when harvesting cowslips and primroses, or a painful rash may develop.

Cowslip leaves and flowers must be dried quickly if they are to retain their color. They should be laid out in very thin layers on paper or cloth, and the cloth changed often to remove the tiny insects that are usually gathered with the herb. Cowslip roots should be brushed clean, or washed quickly under running water to remove all dirt particles, and then split lengthwise and hung up on a string to dry in a shady, airy room.

Seed Saving and Germination

There are numerous garden primroses, and these can be best propagated by plant division. For medicinal use, the wild varieties are employed, and these can be propagated by plant division, or by sowing the seed as soon as it ripens in leaf mold or loose, damp soil.

Gardening Hints

Since so many of the wild-growing primroses and cowslips are now protected, it makes sense to grow primroses in the lawn or back yard for private enjoyment and use. An astounding array of ornamental primroses has been bred for garden use, or as winter houseplants. These hybrids have little or no medicinal value, but great attractive worth.

The mountain cowslip, *Primula auricula*, is often grown in gardens, and the simple primrose is also of value in wild areas of the garden, in lawns, under fruits trees, and even in the perennial border.

Cowslips need a combination of sun and shade as well as moisture to flourish. They should be protected from the glare of the midday sun, and planted in rich soil. Layers of mulch or leaf mold will help protect the plants' delicate crowns and short roots, and retain moisture. Compost or mulch should be worked in around the plant as soon as it stops flowering. The wrinkled leaves funnel all rain and moisture directly down to the roots, but it is nonetheless almost impossible to overwater the plants. They wilt if exposed to the direct midday sun, or if not watered enough.

The mountain cowslip, or dusty miller, should be placed in a sunny, open position. It requires less moisture than its thirsty cousin. Birds are often a problem, because they peck at the young leaves and blossoms, but planting the herb underneath lavender or other larger bushes can solve that problem.

Garden varieties of primroses can be propagated by plant division, or, in some cases, by seed. Wild primroses and mountain cowslips do best if propagated by plant division in fall. Seeds can be thinly sown in leaf mold in a cold frame, as soon as the weather permits in spring. Germination is erratic, and older seeds should be stratified. Seedlings are then transplanted into boxes, or a weed-free area, allowing at least 2 in. between plants. The resulting large plants should be transplanted into their permanent positions in November or the following spring. After two years of growth, the plants may be divided. If desired, primroses can also be raised indoors in shaded window boxes.

Some Swiss gardeners believe that the mountain cowslip is the daughter of the true cowslip because it only appears after the former has stopped blossoming. In northern Germany, primroses transplanted on Maundy Thursday are thought to produce more, and more colorful, flowers than those transplanted on any other day.

Gardeners who work with primroses may develop allergic reactions, especially if the skin is exposed to sunlight. It is advisable to wear garden gloves when touching the plants.

Culinary Virtues

Fresh cowslip leaves can be added to mixed green salads, or included in potherb mixtures. A few chopped cowslip leaves also combine well with mixed herbs used for seasoning. Cowslip flowers make excellent garnishes, and they can be tossed into a salad, cooked with greens, or used, together with day lily buds, to make an appetizing flower broth.

Cowslip preserves or cowslip flower powder can be added to cakes, pies, and tarts to give them a distinct flowery flavor. One famous English rice dish was prepared with honey and almonds, saffron, and ground primroses. Cowslip flowers are often candied and used as garnishes, or added fresh to green salads. A decorative vinegar can be made by adding cowslip flowers to white wine vinegar.

But the cowslip is best known in culinary circles for the wine prepared from the flowers. This drink contains the medicinal virtues of cowslip tea, as well as its sleep-inducing properties. It keeps well and is refreshing, with an aroma slightly reminiscent of honey. Alexander Pope once praised cowslip wine in one of his letters: "For the future I'll drown all high thoughts in the Lethe of cowslip-wine."[159]

Noteworthy Recipes

Cowslip Wine: Mrs. Isabella Beeton provided this recipe in the nineteenth century:

> Ingredients. To every gallon of water allow 3 lb. of lump sugar, the rind of 2 lemons, the juice or the rind and juice of 1 Seville orange, 1 gallon of cowslip pips (cowslip pips, or peeps, are the yellow flowers gathered without the flower receptacle or calyx). To every 4½ gallons of wine allow 1 bottle of brandy.
>
> Mode. Boil the sugar and water together for ½ hour, carefully removing all the scum as it rises. Pour this boiling liquor on the orange and lemon-rinds, and the juice, which should be strained; when milk-warm, add the cowslip pips or flowers, picked from the stalks and seeds; and to the 9 gallons of wine 3 tablespoonfuls of good fresh brewer's yeast. Let it ferment 3 or 4 days (stoppered with a thistle tube to let fermenting gases escape); then put all together in a cask with the brandy, and let it remain for 2 months, when bottle it for use.
>
> Time. To be boiled ½ hour; to ferment 3 or 4 days; to remain in the cask 2 months.
>
> Seasonable. Make this in April or May.[160]

Candied Cowslips: In the seventeenth century, John Shirley offered this recipe "to Conserve or Keep any sort of Flowers, as Roses, Violets, Cowslips, Gilliflowers, & c":

> Take your Flowers well blown and clean picked, bruise very small in a Mortar, with three times the weight of sugar; after which take them out, and put them in a Pipkin; and having thorowly heated them over the fire, put the Conserve up in Gally-pots for your use.[161]

Cowslip Paste: And almost a century earlier, Sir Hugh Platt suggested the following:

159. Pope, *The Poetical Works of Alexander Pope*, vol. 1, Ed. Robert Carruthers (London: Ingram, Cooke, and Co., 1853), 34.

160. Beeton, *The Book of Household Management* (1861) (New York: Farrar, Straus & Giroux, 1977), 881.

161. Shirley, *The Accomplished Ladies Rich Closet of Rarities* (London: N. Bodington, 1688), 36.

To make paste of Violets, Roses, Marigolds, Cowslips, or licorice. Shred, or rather powder the dry leaves of your flower, putting thereunto some fine powder of Ginger, Cinnamon, and a little muske if you please, mixe them all confusedly together, then dissolue some sugar in Rosewater, and being boiled a little, put some saffron therein, if you worke vpon Marigolds, or else you may leaue out your saffron, boile it on the fire vnto a sufficient height, you must also mixe therewith the pappe of a roasted apple being first well dried in a dishe over a chafing-dish of coales, then pour it vpon a trencher, being first sprinkled ouer with Rosewater, and with a knife worke the paste together. Then breake some sugar candy smal, but not to powder, and with some gumme Dragagant, fasten it heere and there to make it seeme as if it were roche candied, cut the paste into peeces of what fashio(n) you list with a knife first wet in Rosewater.[162]

A simplified version of this very complicated historical recipe calls for 2 lb. of finely crushed flower petals. At least 4 lb. of white sugar are boiled in a little water until the thread stage is reached on a candy thermometer. Let it cool, and add the crushed cowslip flowers and an equal amount of tart apple jelly. Cook over a minimal flame just long enough to thoroughly combine all the ingredients. Skim the mixture to prevent crystallization, and pour into sterilized glasses or jars. Seal and store in a cool, dry place.

Household Applications

Cowslip flowers are sometimes substituted for black tea or added to it to make the taste more "flowery," like the jasmine tea served in oriental restaurants. A decoction of the flowers will dye Easter eggs a pretty yellow. Because of their sweet smell and cheery color, the flowers are also added to sachets and potpourri. Cowslip root has been employed as an additive to commercial powdered detergent, for it is rich in saponines that cleanse fabric without harming it. Because of its high saponine content, the cowslip has also been used in the production of effervescent drinks.

Cosmetic Properties

In the sixteenth, seventeenth, and eighteenth centuries, cowslip water and cowslip wine were famous facial cleansing lotions. The sixteenth-century herbalist William Turner commented on these cosmetic aids:

---

162.   Platt, *Delightes for Ladies* (1594) (London: Penguin, 1948), 36.

Some weomen we find, sprinkle ye floures of cowslip wt whyte wine and after still (distill) it and wash their faces wt that water to drive wrinkles away and to make them fayre in the eyes of the worlde rather than in the eyes of God, Whom they are not afrayd to offend.[163]

The fresh juice of the cowslip or an ointment made from cowslip flowers was also used to remove wrinkles, freckles, or blotches, and to soften and bleach facial skin. Since a milk-white face is no longer considered a necessary attribute to beauty, the use of the cowslip in cosmetics has suffered a setback. The flowers are now occasionally added to floral facial waters, to facial steaming mixtures, and to fragrant bath pochettes.

Like St. John's wort, cowslips can cause skin problems in some people if they use the plant on their skin and then expose it to sunlight. Those with sensitive skin should avoid all cosmetic use of cowslips.

Modern Medicine

The cowslip is a soothing, calming, and pain-easing plant that works mildly in different areas. It can be taken alone as a sleep-inducing and painkilling herb, or it may be combined with more specific medicinal herbs in order to strengthen their action. Alexander Pope even advised in his *Satires*, "If your point be rest / Lettuce and cowslip wine: Probatum est."

The cowslip has three major areas of gentle medicinal influence beyond its soothing properties:

- It can help relieve and regulate the symptoms of poor circulation and low blood pressure such as dizziness, headaches, and migraines, and also can ease some of the unpleasant effects of menopause. It can aid those suffering from arteriosclerosis, paralysis, and the after-effects of a stroke. For these reasons alone, it cannot be recommended enough as a medicinal tea for the elderly.

- The second area of action is as a mild diuretic, laxative, and vermifuge. The entire plant possesses these qualitites to some degree, and the roots to a larger extent. The cowslip can therefore be of value in the treatment of gout and rheumatism, and is used as a blood-purifying spring tonic herb.

- Above and beyond this, the cowslip has expectorant and sudorific qualitites that render it an effective medicine for the treatment of colds, coughs, and mild bouts of influenza.

---

163. Qtd. in Mrs. Maud Grieve, *A Modern Herbal* (1931) (London: Penguin, 1976), 231.

Cowslip tea is usually prepared from cowslip flowers, or from a combination of leaves and flowers. Root tea can be substituted if stronger medicinal action is required. A homeopathic cowslip tincture is used in the treatment of neuralgia, dizziness, kidney complaints, threatened strokes, eczema, and severe headaches such as migraines.

Many people are extremely sensitive to primrose pollen, so sensitive that they receive a rash from simply touching the plant. It goes without saying that these people should avoid the primrose as a medicinal herb, and that a primrose cure should be immediately interrupted if an allergic reaction occurs.

Cowslip leaves are applied as warm anesthetic poultices to rheumatic or arthritic joints, or to bruises and sprains, and the entire plant can be added to baths, relieving stiffness in the joints. Cowslip tea is mixed with linseed oil and applied as first aid to alleviate the pains of minor burns.

Special Cures

Prevention Tea for the Elderly: A simple tea made from a combination of 2 parts of cowslip flowers, 1 part lavender flowers, 1 part vervain *(Verbena officinalis)*, and ¼ part masterwort *(Peucedanum ostruthium)* roots can be warmly recommended to the elderly and those who suffer from loss of memory. This is a good preventive tea, used either alone or in combination with a tea for blood pressure regulation against arteriosclerosis. It can help to lower the risks of arterial clogging, and in some cases, even improve mental confusion and loss of memory.

Uses in Husbandry

Like mulberry leaves, *Primula vulgaris* leaves are fed to silkworms. The flowers have orange honey guides for bees, and are avidly visited by these insects. In the thirteenth century, Albertus Magnus recommended a powder—made from cowslip flowers gathered before sunrise on May Day—as magical medicine for sick animals, and his advice has been followed in some areas until the present day. Primrose leaves are used in combination with other herbs as herbal snuff.

Miscellaneous Wisdom

The cowslip is one of the very first flowers to appear in spring, and therefore the very first cowslips are believed to have extraordinary powers. In Denmark, anyone who swallows the first three cowslips of the year is believed to be immune against thyroid complaints for the entire year.

According to widespread agricultural superstition, it is extremely unlucky to bring too few primroses or cowslips into a house in spring. The French believe that this will cause the goslings to suffocate in the egg. In the northern English counties, it is thought that all the poultry will die. In Norfolk, bringing less than 13 primroses into the house will cause most of the chicks to remain in the egg. In Shropshire, the poultry is endangered if someone brings a single primrose into the house. In Somerset, less than 13 primroses placed under a child's cradle are believed to harm the child, more than 13 to protect it. But on the northern German island of Rügen, householders believe that cowslips, no matter how many, will bring luck to a house. Cowslips are often carried on treasure hunts and visits to Faerieland. Many people believe that the golden flower "keys" are a magical combination lock to open hidden doors if they are carried in the right number. The Swiss believe that cowslips can also magically transform themselves into hidden treasure.

Primroses are believed to either harm humans, or to protect them from harm. In Somerset, it is considered wise to always carry violets together with the traditional catkins and primroses to church at Easter. This way, the violets will counteract any harm caused by picking the wrong number of primroses. According to German folk belief, one should pick a primrose and eight other flowers on May Eve, and then lock the flowers in a chest. If strange noises are heard coming from the chest, it is a certain sign that a witch has been captured. In Ireland, primroses are hung over the threshold on May Day to protect the house against witches and faeries. In Somerset, a primrose ball is hung over threshold on May Day. Primroses are also hung in the stalls, and tied to horses' and cows' tails to keep them from harm. In Somerset, one is only allowed to wear green on May Day if protected against pixies by late primroses and forget-me-nots. Primroses are also believed to offer general protection against all magic on Midsummer's Eve.

Oracular Worth

Some Germans believe that the barley and hemp will grow to a good height if the cowslips grow tall in the spring. According to Italian superstition, if a cowslip flowers every month throughout the winter, it can be taken as a bad omen for the coming harvest. The Welsh have their own saying, "Untimely fruit, untimely news." They consider it extremely unlucky if primroses bloom again in June. The English take a blooming primrose plant at Christmastime as a certain sign of coming illness or disaster.

Cowslips and primroses are consulted as love oracles in many countries. German girls who find cowslips blooming during the Easter week believe that they will marry within the year. In the northern English counties, young people cut off primrose stamens with sharp scissors and then hide the tops away in a secret place. If the stamens grow back to their original size within 24 hours, and the young person has thought of his or her sweetheart the entire time, then their love will also flourish.

Herbal Pastimes

In Lincolnshire, children often wear peagles on May Day. In other parts of England, the custom of making primrose balls is widespread. They are affectionately called tosties, cucking balls, or tissty-tossties. To make a tissty-tossty, several dozen flowers with short stalks are joined together to form a yellow ball with a piece of sturdy thread.

Legends

Before the cowslip came to be associated with the Virgin Mary and St. Peter, northern Europeans believed it to be a flower of Freya or Hulda. Its blossoms were considered to be the keys to open the treasure palaces of these goddesses.

According to Tyrolean legend, cowslips first grew on earth when pagans copied the keys to the Heavenly gates. When St. Peter heard of the sacrilege, he let his own keys fall in fright. He immediately sent an angel to pick up the keys, but by the time the heavenly messenger had reached the earth, tiny flowers, later known as St. Peter's keys, had sprung up around the real keys.

Literary Flowers

And I serve the fairy queen,
To dew her orbs upon the green.
The cowslips tall her pensioners be:
In their gold coats spots you see;
Those be rubies, fairy favours,
In those freckles live their savours:
I must go seek some dewdrops here,
And hang a pearl in every cowslip's ear.

—WILLIAM SHAKESPEARE, *A MIDSUMMER NIGHT'S DREAM*, II.1

Pale primroses,
That die unmarried, ere they can behold
Bright Phoebus in his strength,—a malady
Most incident to maids; bold oxlips and
The crown-imperial; lilies of all kinds,
The flower-de-luce being one! O, these I lack,
To make you garlands of; and my sweet friend,
To strew him o'er and o'er!

—WILLIAM SHAKESPEARE, *THE WINTER'S TALE*, IV.III

Blind nettle, dumb nettle, deaf nettle, dead nettle,
how can the Archangel have chosen thee?

—Author Unknown

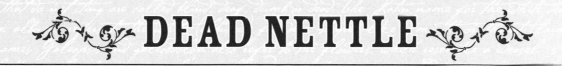

DEAD NETTLE

Name

Nettles that do not sting are called "blind," "deaf," "dumb," or "dead." Dead nettles are members of the **Lamiaceae** or **Mint** family.

The Latin name for the white dead nettle, *Lamium album*, refers to its white (*album*) flowers, which are shaped like a mouth or throat (*laimos*). A perennial, the white dead nettle is also known as *Lamium capitatum* and *Lamium vulgatum*.

The yellow dead nettle, also a perennial, goes by the botanical name *Lamiastrum galeobdolon (Lamium galeobdolon* or *Galeopsis galeobdolon). Galeopsis* and *galeobdolon* also refer to the flowers, which resemble a weasel's face and have all the peculiarities of a weasel's smell.

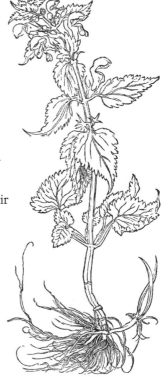

The spotted dead nettle (a perennial) is known as *Lamium maculatum*. Yet another purple dead nettle is called *Lamium purpureum*. *Maculatum* means spotted and *purpureum* means purple. *Amplexicaule* is a term referring to a botanical detail: the leaves clasp the stem.

Unless otherwise stated, the dead nettle referred to in this chapter is the common white dead nettle. Because dead nettles are difficult to tell apart until they have blossomed, it is easy to confuse them with each other—and also with stinging nettles.

Folk botany only differentiates the plants by the color of their blossoms.

Folk Names

The dead nettle is also known as blind nettle, dumb nettle, deaf nettle, archangel, and bee nettle. German names are *Taubnessel, tote Nessel, zahme Nessel, milde Nessel, Lugnessel, Bienesaug,* and *Zauberkraut*. A Spanish term is *ortiga muerta*; Italian, *ortica bianca* and *ortica che non punge*; French, *lamier*; and Danish, *tvetand*. The Chinese call it the "herb of the smiling mother."

Dead nettles with yellow flowers are called weasel's snout, yellow archangel, and dummy nettle; *ortie haune* in French; and *ortica gialla* in Italian. The spotted dead nettle goes by the name of *ortie rouge* in France, and *dolci mele* or *milzadella* in Italy. Purple dead nettle is called *pied de poulet* in France, and *erba ruota* or *ortica fetida* in Italy.

Appearance

White dead nettles tend to grow in the vicinity of stinging nettles, and it is often difficult to tell the plants apart until they flower. Dead nettles have lighter green, downier, and softer leaves than stinging nettles. The hollow stalks are four-cornered and hairy. The leaves are situated in opposite pairs on the stalk, and the entire plant gives off a somewhat unpleasant odor when crushed. Flowers are clustered together in whorls of 6 to 12, and are of a creamy-white or an off-white color. White dead nettle flowers suggest an open mouth, vulva, or maw, an impression strengthened by the flower's long neck. Some herbalists see a weasel's face in the plant's blossom. The seeds are tiny, and are expelled from the plant when ripe. White dead nettle grows to a height of 20 in., and the top-heavy flowering stalks often bend under their own weight. The roots are stringy and of a whitish color, and lie close to the surface.

Yellow dead nettle roots do not creep as much as the roots of the white dead nettle. This plant is somewhat shorter and the flowers are yellow, occasionally blotched with red and similarly shaped, except that they are broader.

The stalks of the purple dead nettle are square and somewhat hairy, like the white dead nettle. The leaves are small, tinged with purple, dented about the edges, and grow out of the joints. The smell of the plant is extremely unpleasant, and the smallish flowers are of a reddish or brownish-purple color.

Place, Season, and Useful Parts

Dead nettles grow in the vicinity of human habitations. As Culpeper says, "they grow almost every where, unless it be in the middle of the street; the yellow most usually in the wet grounds of woods."[164] Dead nettles normally appear in large numbers, but may be missing altogether from some areas. The plant has traveled westward and northward with humans, and the seed is often carried into improbable places by ants and magpies. Dead nettles can be found in most of Europe and the Orient, and grow sparsely in North America to an altitude of almost 7,000 ft. They grow in large groups next to fences, hedges, walls, buildings; on village paths, rubbish heaps, field borders, and railroad banks; in graveyards and overgrown gardens, fields, and meadows; on untilled

---

164. Nicholas Culpeper, *Culpeper's Complete Herbal* (1653) (London: Foulsham,undated), 29.

ground and on the edges of woods. The yellow dead nettle prefers damp, shady woods, and is partial to heights.

The white dead nettle flowers, with or without the calyx, or the entire blooming plant is gathered from May until the end of August, and again in the fall and into winter. The yellow dead nettle flowers, or the entire flowering herb, can only be gathered from April to July; the purple dead nettle can be gathered from April to September.

Gathering, Drying, and Storage

According to one estimate, 90 gathering hours are necessary to pick 2 lb. of dried white dead nettles flowers, hence the exorbitant prices often demanded for the drug. Many people prefer to gather the entire plant, or the flowers with the calyxes. The herb should only be harvested on very dry, sunny days, and packed loosely in baskets to avoid crushing. It is wise to wear rubber gloves while picking dead nettles because of the stinging nettles that often grow between the plants.

Dead nettles should be dried in dark, airy rooms or attics, spread out thinly on cloth or paper. Artificial heat often has to be used to avoid spoilage. The distinctive and unpleasant dead nettle odor lessens with drying. Properly dried white dead nettle flowers should retain their ivory color.

Seed Saving and Germination

Dead nettles are almost always gathered from the wild, since the plants tend to grow in great numbers where they do occur. The easiest way to propagate them is to encourage them to spread by weeding competing plants, and mulching with leaf mold.

Gardening Hints

White dead nettles often grow around the edges of vegetable gardens or on the border of wooded areas, and should be encouraged to do so, for they aid the growth of vegetables near them. Some organic gardeners even plant them in borders for this purpose. Purple dead nettles are, however, not welcomed in the garden. They are among the first plants to appear in spring, and if left undisturbed will soon seed massively and literally take over the garden. But, as weeds go, they are fairly easy to control. These annuals, once weeded, will not return unless allowed to go to seed, or if the flowering plants are added to the compost heap.

Dead nettles are rarely cultivated, but existing stands can be encouraged by collecting the seeds and then sowing them, or by dividing the plants, or even taking cuttings.

Folk wisdom says that the inhabitants of a house will find cures for their ailments in the plants growing in the vicinity of the house. For example, if white dead nettles are profuse, the mistress of the house will probably have problems with uterine infections, and should make use of the herb. If this belief at first seems fanciful, there is a grain of truth in it. Many herbs are signal plants, only growing in masses when certain soil conditions and minerals are present in certain microclimates. These conditions can, in turn, aid the development of certain diseases.

Culinary Virtues

All dead nettles can be eaten as greens while they are still young and tender, although purple dead nettles are less felty and hairy than other dead nettles. They are prepared in the same manner as stinging nettles. In times of scarcity, dead nettle roots have been boiled and served with salt, oil, and vinegar as a salad. Dried and pulverized dead nettle flowers can be used as a medicinal additive to foods. John Gerard suggests conserving or preserving the flowers in sugar, similar to violets (see violet chapter). The distilled water of white dead nettles was once administered to lighten the heart, bring fresh color to faded cheeks, and invigorate the spirits.

Household Applications

Dead nettle roots, like those of the stinging nettle, can be boiled in water to produce a yellow dye. The Slavic Wends once rinsed their milk containers with a boiling dead nettle and sneezewort (*Achillea ptarmica*) decoction to drive away witches and protect the milk from spoilage. This may seem to be pure superstition, but nettles (both dead and stinging nettles) can help to inhibit the formation of lactic acid, and thereby prevent the milk from spoiling.

Medicinal Merits

Folk medicine has a simple approach to the medicinal merits of the dead nettles: in consonance with the ancient doctrine of signatures, white dead nettles are thought to counteract colds and infections in the genital/urinary tract. They are also used to stay the "whites" of women. Yellow-blossoming dead nettles are used to combat serious or insistent infections; the purple dead nettle is administered to stop bleeding and, as Culpeper so carefully phrases it, women's "reds." Modern science has reaffirmed the validity of these applications, as well as the efficacy of treating paleness and anemia with white dead nettle.

Modern Medicine

The white dead nettle is among the most important "women's herbs." It can help to contract the uterus and tone and strengthen the female organs, as well as relieve uterine cramps. It can also, under certain conditions, act to regulate the blood flow and to regularize menstruation. Due to its disinfectant and diuretic action, the white dead nettle can help to dispel mucus and the "whites," ease painful urination, and replenish the blood supply after a difficult period. Women would be much less predisposed to genealogical complaints if they would make a habit of drinking a tea composed of equal parts of white dead nettle flowers, lady's mantle, and alpine lady's mantle. Men, particularly older men suffering from mild prostate troubles, can also find relief from the white dead nettle. Drinking a tea consisting of a strong diuretic herb such as horsetail or goldenrod *(Solidago virgaurea)* and the blossoming white dead nettle for 4 weeks at a time is a superb prophylactic measure against kidney and bladder troubles in both men and women.

The secondary properties of the white dead nettle are antibacterial, cleansing, and softening. Any internal infections can profit from treatment with the white, or in more stubborn cases, with the yellow dead nettle. White dead nettle flowers are blood-purifying, and have been used with success to treat eczema, rashes, and skin problems. Because of its gelatinous quality, the herb is sometimes boiled with water until a thick consistency is reached, and then cooled. The resulting jelly-like mass can be applied as a disinfectant and healing plaster to wounds or to fresh burns, or applied outwardly to hardened or swollen body parts to soften them.

The yellow dead nettle is used alone or together with the white dead nettle if the complaint is of an infectious or chronic nature.

The purple dead nettle has blood-staunching and also blood-building qualities. The flowers are used as a tea to help stop bleeding, or to lessen the menstrual flow. The bruised leaves can be applied directly to fresh wounds. Cotton wool moistened with purple dead nettle tincture is also valuable in the first-aid treatment of cuts and wounds. The crushed fresh herb is applied to the nape of the neck to stop nosebleeds. The herbal mixture of 1 part shepherd's purse, ½ part tormentil roots *(Potentilla erecta)*, and 2 parts purple dead nettles, infused as a tea and drunk in small sips over a period of several days, can work minor wonders as a blood-stilling medicine. If tormentil is not available, substitute 1 part of periwinkle *(Vinca minor)* leaves. The purple dead nettle has one negative side effect common to most blood-staunching herbs: it can cause constipation.

Lamium album homeopathic preparations treat headaches, especially those moving backward and forward on the head. *Lamium purpureum* is used to quiet bleeding.

Uses in Husbandry

The dead nettles are favorites with bees. Smaller bees gather nectar of the purple dead nettles, but the white and yellow dead nettles have such long and narrow flower throats that bees often have difficulty visiting the plants, and may just bite their way through the blossom's "jugular."

Cattle turn up their noses at dead nettles and their peculiar smell. They refuse to eat them while fresh, and will only occasionally condescend to do so when the plants are dried as hay.

Veterinary Values

Crushed purple dead nettles are applied to the wounds of cattle and other barnyard and household animals as poultices and emergency bandages to stop bleeding.

Miscellaneous Wisdom

In the thirteenth century, Albertus Magnus wrote that thieves could be forced to return pilfered goods with the help of a complicated ritual involving running water and the white dead nettle. In southern Germany, roots of the white dead nettle are dug on the day the cows are led to pasture, washed first in running water and then in wine, and used as amulets to protect the wearer against theft, envy, and enmity. In the eighteenth century in Eberfeld, the white dead nettle was used to cure a cold, rheumy fever. The patient had to urinate on the plant and repeat the following rhyme:

> I let my water on this plant's seed
> In the name of every fever
> Fever go away and leave me
> Till I come and try to cut off the sun.
> In the Name of the Holy Ghost, God the Father, and the Son, Amen.[165]

Children love to pick the long-necked flowers and to suck out the honey. They sometimes fashion large stems into whistles.

---

165. Hanns Bächtold-Stäubli, ed., *Handwörterbuch des deutschen Aberglaubens*, vol. VIII (Berlin: Walter de Gruyter & Co., 1987), 706.

As the Sun enters into Leo, an eye awakens in the fields.

—Sister Clarissa

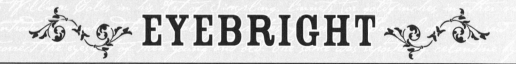

EYEBRIGHT

Name

According to William Coles in his *Art of Simpling*, linnets (or goldfinches, in other versions of the story) first introduced mankind to the healing properties of eyebright.[166] Careful observers saw that the birds used eyebright to correct the eyesight of their young and old. The same has been reported of celandine, by various authors from Pliny on.

The botanical name for eyebright, *Euphrasia*, was once thought to have evolved from the Greek word for linnet. But more likely origins for the word can be found in the Greek word for happiness, and consequently, the name of one of the three graces—*Euphrosyne*. Eyebright may have been named *Euphrasia* because it was supposed to promote gladness, or because of its pleasing daintiness, or because of its efficacy in healing eye troubles.

The English name "eyebright" has obvious origins. The herb has, since the beginnings of recorded herbalism, been known for its ability to help heal eye diseases and to clear the eyesight. The term "eyebright" was already common in the fifteenth century.

Eyebright belongs to the **Orobanchaceae** family, and is an annual hemiparasite. Local eyebrights vary widely, especially in the color of their flowers, and there are disputes in learned circles as to the proper classification of the variants. The species of greatest medicinal importance is *Euphrasia rostkoviana* (once known as *Euphrasia officinalis*).

---

166.   Coles, *The Art of Simpling* (London: J. Streater, 1656).

Folk Names

Medieval Latin names were *herba luminellas*, *ocularis*, and *ophthalmica*. The herb is known in English as eyebright, eufrasy, euphrasine, and euphrasia; in German, as *Augentrost*, *Augendank*, *Milchdieb*, *Grummetblume*, *Augustinuskraut*, and *Nitnützle* (good-for-nothing). French names are *casse-lunettes* and *luminet*; Italian, *eufragia* and *eufragia*; and, in the Italian canton of Switzerland, *erba agostina*. In Spain, the herb goes under the name of *eufrasia*, and in Turkey, *gozlukotu*.

Appearance

Eyebright is a small herb, only growing to a height of 2–18 inches. It therefore often goes unnoticed, getting lost underfoot. But when meadows have been cut and the grass is not too tall, eyebright's flowers sprinkle the fields with white, a preview of the coming winter snows. The plant looks like a miniature shrub with ridiculously short roots. The root base and the stalk are sometimes too weak to support the herb, which has to lean on other plants for support. Eyebright's flowers are white, shaped like miniature holy water fonts, and marked with yellow or orange and purple honey guides to attract bees to the plant. These honey guides also give the plant its "signature," for they resemble the pupil of an eye. The herb's odor is weak but pleasant, and its taste is spicy and grassy.

Place, Season, and Useful Parts

Eyebright grows in both dry and wet pastures and meadows; in moors, heaths, light woods, in the lowlands and the mountains. It requires a fair amount of sun and the presence of host plants, but is nonetheless very common where it does occur, primarily in Europe, the Balkans, and in Russia. In some areas, it is highly endangered and should not be harvested. In others, it grows in extremely large populations. It is an annual, and blossoms from July until the first frosts. The entire blossoming plant without roots is gathered when the plant is at its healthiest, in July and August.

Gathering, Drying, and Storage

The entire plant may be cut, taking care that the roots are not included in the final drug. Eyebright is dried in an airy spot in the shade, laid out on paper. The blossoms will fall out onto the paper during the drying process. The best storage containers allow some air to circulate, and should be kept in a dry place.

Seed Saving and Germination

Eyebright germinates best if the seed is allowed to ripen on the plant, and falls out onto cut grass. If a place is to its liking, it germinates massively. It can often be found in hayfields or in moors, and can be encouraged through timely cutting of competing plants. No cultivated varieties are known, although local variants exist.

Gardening Hints

Eyebright is a semi-parasite, drawing mineral nourishment from other plants, and is therefore not often welcomed in the garden. It grows in abundance in the wild, and is easy to harvest. But if desired, it can be transplanted to a grassy space, for it is dependent on grass to furnish nutrients and protect it from the weather. Eyebright does not usually damage its host plant because its root-suckers die off each fall, giving the plant time to recuperate before spring.

In order to keep eyebright proliferating in a meadow, it is necessary to avoid overgrazing, although most animals are not partial to it. Mowing schedules should be timed so that the grass is cut before the plants start blossoming, and again when the seeds are ripe. The seeds will fall out of the plants as they dry, allowing the plants to reproduce themselves.

Culinary Virtues

Eyebright may be powdered and added to soups, although it probably has more medicinal than culinary worth. It was cultivated in England during the Middle Ages for this purpose. Both Gerard and Culpeper swore by a mixture of the powdered herb, sugar, mace, and ground fennel seeds as a medicinal food additive.

Cosmetic Properties

Eyebright deserves more attention as a cosmetic eye herb. It works from within to make eyes shinier, to clean and clear them, and to help with wrinkles, red eyes, and puffiness. Well-strained eyebright tea with a pinch of salt dissolved in it can be used as eyewash, or the herb applied as a warm compress. Eyebright tea can be kept for a limited time in the refrigerator, but should be heated to body temperature before use. Eyes washed out with eyebright start to water, rinsing out any impurities. Therefore, eye make-up should always be applied after using eyebright, and not before.

- Eyebright tea is not brewed as strongly as other herbal teas. At most, 1 tsp. of the fresh herb is taken for every ½ pint of water, and the infusion should only be allowed to steep for 1–5 minutes. This tea can be taken internally, applied as a compress, or used as an eyewash.

Medicinal Merits

Old herbals speak of many different healing properties of eyebright, but these have now been neglected. Hildegard von Bingen, one the most important herbalists of the twelfth century, recommended eyebright as a wound herb. Italian and English healers praised its ability to provide relief for melancholy, hysteria, sleeplessness, headaches, stomach troubles, and colds. It was also supposed to improve memory by increasing circulation in the brain (is this an indication that it may be helpful in the treatment of Alzheimer's disease?). Very little scientific work has been done to prove or disprove these beliefs. In fact, even the nature of eyebright's main chemical constituent, *acubin*, remains something of a mystery to modern science. Until more proof is forthcoming, it is best to suspend judgement on eyebright's secondary medicinal merits.

> *If the herb was but half as much used as it is neglected, it would half spoil the spectacle maker's trade and a man would think that reason should teach people to prefer the preservation of their natural before artificial spectacles ...*
>
> —NICHOLAS CULPEPER, QUOTED IN GRIEVE'S *MODERN HERBAL*

Modern Medicine

Eyebright is an eye herb, first and foremost. It can be employed both internally and externally to clear and lighten the eyes and to ease eyes strained with overwork, too much time spent in front of the computer, or too much reading. Eyebright poultices are applied to soften sties. Eyebright can help to alleviate eye infections and diseases in their initial phases, and also help to prevent glaucoma and relieve the sore, red, or runny eyes associated with colds, allergies, or hay fever. It is furthermore prescribed as a specific medicine for conjunctivitis, especially by homeopaths. Its action is astringent and tonic, and it has proved useful in the general treatment of hay fever. Patients with damaged liver function should avoid using the herb, and it should only be taken for 3–4 weeks at one time. Commercial eyebright extract, diluted with rose water, fennel-seed tea, or distilled water, can be also used as eye drops. Eyebright is known homeopathically as *Euphrasia*, and prescribed for hay fever and allergies, as well as eye disorders.

Special Cures

An Eye Cure: Bitter aloe powder and eyebright can bring about almost miraculous cures for eye troubles such as minor eye and sinus infections. A tiny pinch of aloe powder is stirred well in an eye bath or small glass with boiling water and cooled to body temperature. Wash the eye with the mixture, being careful to dry the eye area thoroughly after each application. The treatment should then be continued with a lightly salted eyebright infusion for at least 1 week. This will ensure a complete cure, and strengthen the eyes against subsequent infection.

Eyebright Wine: Eyebright ale was drunk as a medicinal draught during the reign of Queen Elizabeth I, and eyebright wine has been prescribed since at least the sixteenth century. Eyebright is gathered in the late summer and fall, when newly fermented wine is plentiful.

Infuse a small handful of the herb (without roots) in 1 qt. of white wine or sweet must for 1 week, and then strain, filter, and bottle it. This wine can be taken internally, a small glass at a time, every day for a period of several weeks.

Uses in Husbandry

Eyebright has been included in herbal tobacco mixtures all over the world. It is an ingredient of British herbal tobacco, a mixture smoked to relieve colds. The mixure consists of 16 parts coltsfoot leaves, 8 parts each eyebright and buckbean *(Menyanthes trifoliata)* leaves, 4 parts wood betony *(Betonica officinalis)*, 2 parts rosemary, 1½ parts wild thyme, and 1 part each lavender and chamomile flowers mixed well together and rubbed through a sieve. The resulting "tobacco" can be enjoyed in a pipe or rolled in cigarette papers. In the Middle Ages, smoking eyebright was believed to impart clairvoyance.

Veterinary Values

Animals are treated with smaller doses of eyebright than their human counterparts to strengthen strained, runny eyes and to cure infected tear ducts and conjunctivitis. Eyebright should not be given internally to cattle, as it may poison them. Cows that have pastured too heavily on eyebright often give bloody milk. They should be forced to drink warm chamomile tea and eat eyebright-free hay until cured. The reddish milk is not fit for human consumption and must be discarded.

Miscellaneous Wisdom

The healing properties of eyebright were once so highly valued in Bavaria that simply hanging a sack with the herb around a patient's neck was believed to effect a perfect cure.

Because eyebright blossoms when cows begin to give less milk, the herb was thought to be the cause of the milk loss. Witches were accused of using the herb in their incantations to draw milk from healthy cows, or to poison them and make them give bloody milk. One German name, *Grummetblume*, points to the fact that eyebright becomes visible after the second hay cutting, and can easily be gathered then.

Oracular Worth

In Swabian rural belief (Germany), a field covered with eyebright blossoms is taken as a sure sign of a hard winter. The Czechs believe that winter will come early if the plant blossoms heavily. Fall crops must be sown earlier than usual if eyebright flowers are clustered at the top of the stalk.

Literary Flowers

> *To nobler sights*
> *Michael from Adam's eyes the film removed*
> *Which that false fruit which promised clearer sight*
> *Had bred; then purged with euphrasine and rue*
> *His visual orbs, for he had much to see.*

> —JOHN MILTON, *PARADISE LOST*

"Oh, Lord! My eyes have grown weary with weeping, and my breast heavy with sighing. Oh, Lord, I cannot see but to cry!"

At first, man received no answer to his prayer. God wasn't listening, or didn't care.

But the linnet listened, and listened again, and, finally, swooping down from the birch tree, spoke to him in a sweet, ringing voice, "I shouldn't tell you this, for God gave me the keeping of the secret, but I can't bear to hear you suffering. Use eyebright, and it will bring gladness to your heart, ease to your breast, and light to your eyes. Stop your moaning, and make the herb serve you. Stop your crying, and sing with me today."

Man followed the bird's advice and did, indeed, enjoy happiness for a day.

> —A MODERN PARAPHRASE OF THE OLD LEGEND,
> WILLIAM FLETCHER, *SUPERSTITION IN REVIEW*

As the Sun enters into Leo, an eye awakens in the fields. The sun is radiant before autumn, the fields in their last glory before winter, and the cows, suffering in the heat and the changing seasons, begin to give less milk. Eyebright, gathering dew in its miniature font, draws its strength from underground rivers of stolen milk. A tiny, milk-colored flower with orange and purple markings springs to life. The longer it grows in the meadow and the longer it looks at us, the more we come to realize that it is the eye of the sun in its autumn clarity. It is balm for eyes wearied with looking and poison for the unwary cow who attempts to eat back her milk.

Eyebright knows the ways of summer as well as those of fall, presenting humans and animals with the gift of clearer sight, and cleansing their eyes like the autumn rain.

> —SISTER CLARISSA'S *UNPUBLISHED BOOK OF NATURAL OBSERVATIONS*

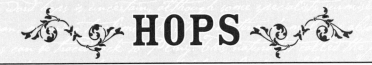

HOPS

Name

The final origin of the word "hops" is uncertain, although some specialists surmise that the term developed from the Anglo-Saxon *hoppan*, meaning "to climb." The European hop is known in botanical circles as *Humulus lupulus*. *Humulus* is also of uncertain origin, but the secondary name, *lupulus*, can be traced back to Pliny. This naturalist called the plant *lupus salictarius*, or "a wolf among the willows," because of its aggressive habit of climbing or "leaping" onto trees and willows.

Hops is an annual plant with a perennial rootstock. It is classed among the **Cannabaceae** or **Hemp** family. In slang, "hop" is another name for heroin. (Of course, hopheads are not addicted to hops, but to the big H.)

Folk Names

Hops are also known as common hops, hop vine, and bine. The German name is *Hopfen*, and female plants are called *Läufer* while male plants are referred to as *Femmelhopfen*. French names are *houblon*, *houblon vulgaire*, *houblon à la bière*, and *vigne du nord*; and in Russian, it is *chmel obyknovennyj*. Italians call hops *luppulo* and *cervoglia*; Spaniards, *lupulo*; Dutch, *hop*; Japanese, *hoppu*; and, in Ireland, the plant is simply known as *lus*.

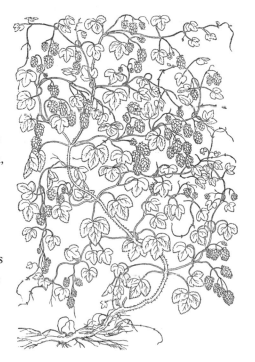

Appearance

The hop is a crawling, climbing plant, and has vines that may grow to be as long as 3–6 yards. Hops are a botanical curiosity because the vines and tendrils wind to the right, in a clockwise direction (most vines wind toward the left). As Nicholas Culpeper notes in his herbal,

> The Hop runs to a great height, climbing up, and twisting round the poles which are placed for its support, the branches are rough and hairy, being large, rough, vine-like leaves, divided into three parts, serrated about the edges. On the tops of the stalks, grow clusters of large, loose, scaly heads, of a pale greenish yellow colour when ripe, and a pretty strong smell.[167]

The plant has a stout, firm root that John Gerard describes as "folded one within another."[168] The stems are square and sturdy and flexible, and are covered with white down. Hop leaves resemble vine or maple leaves, but they are not as smooth. They are hand-shaped, divided into 3 or 5 segments, and dark green in color. The edges of the leaves are finely toothed, and the entire plant is rough and bristly. Hop plants may be either male or female. The male plants produce loose bunches of flowers, and the females the aromatic fruits called catkins. Hop fruits are shaped like pine cones, and are covered with brownish scales that rustle in the wind. They contain yellowish glands and occasional seeds. Hops can easily be confused with the poisonous white bryony (*Bryonia dioica*).

Place, Season, and Useful Parts

Hops grow wild in northern temperate Europe, and in Asia and Australia as well as North America, and are cultivated in Europe, India, China, and North America. They do not grow in the extreme north, and are completely missing in Norway, Iceland, Ireland, and Finland. A related species, *Humulus scadens* or Japanese hops, can be found in the Far East and in northeastern North America.

The hop is a climbing plant, and thrives in hedgerows, among underbrush, and next to streams and ponds. It will climb over trees (especially willows) as well as walls, fences, hedges, and briars. Because of this, it is often overlooked. The plant flowers in the summer, and usually produces fruits in the fall. Herbalists employ hop catkins and the glands that fall out from the catkins in powder form, and there is occasional demand for the roots. The young shoots are gathered in spring for culinary purposes.

Gathering, Drying, and Storage

The fruits are harvested from August through October, when they turn amber and while still firm, are papery to the touch. The best catkins contain few seeds and a large

---

167. *Culpeper's Complete Herbal* (1653) (London: Foulsham, undated), 191.

168. Gerard, *Gerard's Herball* [1597]: *The essence thereof distilled by Marcus Woodward from the edition of Th. Johnson, 1636.* Ed. Marcus Woodward (London: Gerald How, 1927).

amount of yellowish gland powder. They can be picked singly, or the entire plant is harvested, and then hung up to dry. Commercially harvested hops are pressed into cakes. The herb must be dried completely within a few hours of picking to preserve all the active principles. The hop glands are sifted from the catkins as soon as possible in order to exclude all leaf and stem particles from the cleaned drug. Hop glands must be stored in airtight containers to avoid spoilage. Those who work with hops for a long time may develop allergic reactions to the drug.

Hop fruits should be dried as quickly as possible after picking, and should also be used as quickly as possible after drying. Fresh hops are of a bright greenish-yellow color, and feel clammy to the touch. Older hops are golden or even brown, and contain yellowish gland powder. Very old hops develop an unpleasant, cheese-like odor. Some unscrupulous dealers treat their hops with sulphur to freshen the color of their wares.

Hop roots are dug in fall or spring, and hand-long shoots that have not yet developed true leaves, or the very tips of the young hop plants, are gathered in April or May.

Seed Saving and Germination

European hops have been improved by crossing in North American wild material, in much the same manner as the development of the grapevine. There has been a lot of breeding in Europe and in New Zealand of an amazing number of different varieties and lines for beer production. Different hop varieties can best be maintained vegetatively through plant and root division, or stem cuttings.

Gardening Hints

The best areas for hop cultivation are said to be Bohemia and Bavaria (hence the superior quality and reputation of the beer produced in these areas). Hops were cultivated in Germany as early as 700 AD. They were introduced into England in the sixteenth century (the saying goes that they traveled on the same ship that brought peacocks and heresy to the northern isles), and into the United States in the 1620s. Because of the amount of care they require and the amount of space they appropriate, their cultivation is only profitable on a commercial scale.

The gardener who wants to grow a few specimens can buy one-year-old plants from a nursery, or may grow them from cuttings from root crowns of old plants or pieces of stem 12–18 in. long with at least 45 eyes. These pieces should be placed at a slant in the earth in the fall, allowing 6 ft. of distance between plants. Hop plants can also be found growing wild, and can be transplanted and placed in garden soil next to a wall or in an unused corner of the yard next to trees or shrubs. The germination of hop seed is difficult and erratic. If hops are to be harvested, it is necessary to have both male and female plants for fertilization. Hops are also used to hide walls or unsightly corners of the house with greenery.

Hops will not grow on poor soil, nor will they thrive in freshly manured ground. They require a southern position, and humus-rich, warm soil. Hops like to be fertilized with composted manure and ashes or with blood meal and lime in fall. Rows between plants should be mulched heavily with bracken or other organic matter to retain moisture. Hop plants cannot be over-watered, and often spring up wild on riverbanks. Air must be allowed to circulate freely around the plants if they are to produce disease-free catkins, and this is why the plants are trained onto poles or wires in their third year of growth. In the house garden, they look particularly attractive if allowed to climb up into trees.

Hop plants grow little in the first year of their life, using these months to establish their extensive root systems. They die back in fall, and shoot up the next spring with renewed vigor. They produce catkins the following year, and care should be taken to prevent these flowers from going to seed so that the plants will keep on producing. Hop fields must be fertilized generously each year, and the plants trimmed and trained onto poles with at least a slope of 45 percent before they blossom. Bavarian hop farmers believe that hops should not be pruned when the influence of Cancer is at its strongest, or their growth will suffer.

Culinary Virtues

At one time, beer-brewing and bread-baking were considered women's work. The word "lady" originally meant a woman who kneaded dough. Bread-baking and beer-brewing were tasks reserved for the mistress of the house or the highest-raking female servant, and hops were often used to leaven both bread and beer, and make them keep better. The production of beer was thought to be a magical process, which was aided and abetted, or harmed, by household elves. When beer-brewing came to be a commercial venture, men started brewing, and hops came to be used in beer to the exclusion of other herbs such as yarrow and horehound. Hops flavored Dutch beer as early as the fourteenth century, but only came to be generally accepted as a beer flavoring toward the middle of the eighteenth century. Henry VIII opposed the use of hops in beer, since it was considered by some to be a cause of melancholy. Supporters of hops countered these arguments by saying that it made the beer keep longer and imparted a pleasantly bitter taste as well as tranquilizing properties to the liquid. In the words of John Gerard, "The Hops rather make it a Physicall drinke to keep the body in health, then an ordinary drinke for the quenching of our thirst."[169]

---

169.   Gerard, *Gerard's Herball* [1597]: *The essence thereof distilled by Marcus Woodward from the edition of Th. Johnson, 1636.* Ed. Marcus Woodward (London: Gerald How, 1927).

Young shoots of the hop plant can be blanched like asparagus and eaten as a vegetable, or added to vegetable soups and rice dishes, or boiled and served in salad form. Bread dough is said to rise more evenly if moistened with hop water.

Noteworthy Recipes

Hop Shoots: The young shoots of hop plants are gathered as they begin to unfold, before they develop true leaves. Some recipes also call for the flowers of the male hop plants, but these are more difficult to digest and stronger in flavor than the young shoots. Gardeners mound hop plants with earth in the spring to blanch the shoots, and then harvest them like asparagus. Very fresh hop shoots are cooked in boiling salted water, with a few drops of vinegar or lemon juice added to the cooking liquid. When properly cooked, their texture should be a little firmer than that of asparagus. As soon as they are cooked, they are plunged into cold water and then drained. If they are bitter or older, they are plunged into boiling water and then drained. They can be reheated with butter or cream, or gravy, or are served cold as a salad with oil and vinegar. Soups, omelets, and risotti can all be flavored with hop shoots. In Belgium, the vegetable is traditionally served as a side dish, garnished with poached eggs and croutons cut into the shape of cock's combs.

Hop Drink: Place 2 handfuls of dried hops and several unsprayed orange leaves (or 2 oz. of bruised ginger root) in a 5 gallon crock. Add 2 lb. of sugar dissolved in water, stir well, and then add 1 glass of mild cider vinegar. Add enough water to fill the crock, and stir well. Allow to stand, covered, in a warm place for 2 days, stirring often. Strain the mixture, and siphon into sterilized bottles made of strong glass. Cork securely, and tie the corks down. Store in a cool place in an upright position for no longer than a few months (otherwise, the bottles may explode!).

Hop Beer: Commercial beers are prepared from barley that has been allowed to sprout and is dried or roasted before being mashed, heated with hops, and fermented. The average home brewer does not have the knowledge or equipment to reproduce and correctly control these procedures. As a result, many home brews often turn out depressingly different from those obtained by commercial brewers.

For those who nonetheless want to try their hand at brewing, take 1 gal. of water together with 3½ oz. of hulled barley, a generous handful of dried hop catkins, and 1 lb. of unrefined sugar, and simmer for 1 hour. A copper vat is ideal for brewing, but any other large pot (not iron or aluminum) will do. Strain the mixture, cool, and then add 10 qt. of clear spring water and ½ oz. of baker's yeast. Some color can be given to the brew by adding a few cleaned dandelion or chicory roots before heating, or some caramel to the liquid before fermentation. Cover the tub well, and let ferment for 4 days. Then draw the liquid carefully off the sediment into bottles, and cork securely, tying down the corks as a precautionary measure.

Hop Ale: This bitter drink calls for 4 oz. of dried hops mixed with 3 oz. of fresh dandelion roots and 1 oz. of gentian root *(Gentiana lutea)*. Simmer the herbs in 6 gal. of water for several hours. Strain the mixture and then cool to lukewarm before adding 3 lb. of unrefined sugar and 3 Tbsp. of brewer's yeast. Stir and cover. On the following day, draw the liquid off the sediment, strain, and place in a small cask. Cork it, and let stand several days before serving. The ale must be drunk quickly after opening the cask, or it will spoil.

Household Applications

Hop stalks are occasionally used to make baskets, and for wickerwork. A reddish-brown dye can be produced from the leaves and flower heads, and a vegetable wax extracted from the tendrils. Dried hops, softened with a little alcohol mixed with a few drops of glycerine to prevent rustling, are used to fill sleeping pillows. The addition of sweet-scented herbs such as orange blossoms, lemon balm, rose petals, and chamomile will make them smell sweeter and enhance their tranquilizing effect.

Cosmetic Properties

Cosmeticians add hops to relaxant herbal baths, and oil of hops is occasionally employed by perfumers. In the seventeenth century, women believed that their hair would grow especially thick and lustrous if they buried a lock next to hop creepers.

Medicinal Merits

Hops were once supposed to cause as well as to cure melancholy, and were used to cleanse and open the liver and spleen and to treat jaundice. Hop tea was also said to lighten the breast and provoke the expulsion of water. The tips of hop plants were administered to those plagued with venereal diseases, and the seeds given to those afflicted with worms. Oil of hops was also sprayed to stop tuberculosis from spreading.

> *Hop is a sovereign remedy; Fuchsius much extols it; it purgeth all choler and purifies the blood. Matthiolus wonders the Physicians of his time made no more use of it, because it rarifies and cleanseth: we use it to some purpose in our ordinary beer, which before was thick and fulsome.*
>
> —ROBERT BURTON, *THE ANATOMY OF MELANCHOLY*

Modern Medicine

Modern herbalists consider the hop glands to be the most potent part of the plant. The glands are located inside the catkins and the powder is released when the plant is dried. Yellow lupulin powder is a very strong relaxant that can be dangerous if taken in large amounts. The powder is recommended for the treatment of extreme sexual excitability, for weakness of the bladder, for kidney and bladder infections, gonorrhea, menstrual or gastrointestinal cramps, and for some kinds of migraines and neuralgia, especially if they are a result of hormonal imbalance.

The female catkins, the hops themselves, are sedative to a lesser degree. Hop tea is prescribed to ease nervous intestinal disorders and heart ailments, to relieve sleeplessness, to soothe excitable and nervous natures, to strengthen the stomach and liver, and to relieve gastric inflammation. It also helps to expel excess water, urine, and perspiration. Delirious and hysterical patients can often be calmed with hops. Fresh hop tea has a strong effect on the hormonal household, with estrogen-like effects. Because of this, hop tea should only be taken for at most 4–6 weeks at a time, and then replaced with other calming herbs such as valerian, passion flower, or lemon balm. Lying on a hop pillow is said to lessen the pains of an ear infection and to aid sleep, and hop compresses can be applied to inflammations, swellings, neuralgia, boils, and rheumatic pains. Steaming the genital area with hops is occasionally used to treat stones in the bladder.

Homeopathic hops can be used to treat a hangover, especially if it is combined with nausea, dizziness, and headache. It is also effective as a specific treatment for the *delirium tremens* of alcoholics, and has been administered for infantile jaundice and various nervous complaints.

Special Cures

Stomachic Teas: A strengthening tea for a weak stomach can be prepared from a mixture of the following herbs: 1 part hop catkins, 2 parts bogbean (*Menyanthes trifoliata*) leaves, 2 parts centaury (*Centaurium erythraea*), 2 parts lemon balm, and 2 parts horehound. One cup of this bitter tea should be taken half an hour before every meal.

Another stomachic tea, used to soothe an inflamed or ulcerous stomach, can be prepared from 1 part each of crushed fennel seeds and crushed fresh flax seed; 2 parts each of marigold flowers, St. John's wort, chamomile flowers, and hop catkins, as well as 3 measures of mallow leaves. Take the tea before meals 2–3 times a day for several weeks.

Uses in Husbandry

Like other members of the **Hemp** family, hops are also fiber plants. They can be cultivated for the manufacture of hop paper, cardboard, string, and coarse cloth. Long hop fibers can be spun, and a rough cloth can be woven from the fibers after they have been soaked and softened in water for one winter's time. Vegetable sacks and rough household linen were once produced in Sweden exclusively from hops. Hop ashes are one of the craft secrets of the world-famous Bohemian glassworks. In northern Italy, casks were cleaned with hop water. Spent hops and hop leaves can be fed with good results to cattle and to sheep, and hops are occasionally included in herbal tobacco mixtures.

Veterinary Values

Hops are given to dogs, as well as humans, to ease hysterical or nervous disorders. If no other herbs are available, hops can be applied to wounds as emergency dressings.

Miscellaneous Wisdom

In the Slavic countries and in Finland, it is customary to throw hops instead of rice at the newly married couple. In Germany, it is believed that hop plants produce shoots and flowers every year during mass on Christmas Eve.

Because hops grow so quickly, the English terms "as fast as hops" and as "thick as hops" have come into common parlance. Someone who is as "mad as hops" is also known to be "hopping mad."

Oracular Worth

In Swabia, Prussia, and Bavaria (Germany), a snowfall on Christmas Eve is taken as a sign that the hops will be plentiful the following year. The pupae of the hop moth also supposedly foretell the hop harvest: gold-ornamented pupae mean that the catkins will sell well, but silver-spotted pupae presage a bad year. If the pupae are covered with gold spots, and ladybirds with black dots, then the price will be high.

Legends

According to an East Prussian legend, when God was creating the world, he sent his angel Satan into the depth of the ocean to find some soil. Satan dutifully carried the earth back to God, but placed a little bit in his mouth, thinking that he could use it to his own advantage a little later. But God saw what Satan had done. As soon as he had finished molding the fields and the forests and the mountain ranges, God caused the earth to swell, and to grow, and to multiply itself. The soil in Satan's mouth began to grow as well. Satan screamed, and spit out the earth in disgust. On this soil, tobacco and hops began to grow, and they still grow to this day.[170]

---

170. From Oskar Dähnhardt, *Natursagen*, vol. I (Leipzig, Germany: Teubner, 1909), 55.

Sweet candied horehound cakes and pepper mint
Or streaking sticks of lusious lolipop …

—JOHN CLARE, *THE SHEPHERD'S CALENDER*, "AUGUST"

HOREHOUND

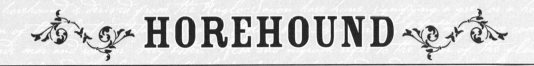

Name

The name "horehound" is derived from the Anglo-Saxon *hare hune*, signifying a gray or a hoary plant. The final origin of the plant's botanical name, *Marrubium*, is uncertain, but it may have come from the old Hebrew words *mar* and *rob* for "very bitter." Horehound flowers are white, and the flowers of the black stinking horehound are dark purple, almost black. *Alba* and *nigrum* refer to the color of the flowers.

White horehound *(Marrubium vulgare* or *Marrubium album)* is a perennial member of the **Mint** family *(Lamiaceae)*. Black or stinking horehound *(Ballota nigra* or *Marrubium nigrum)* belongs to the same botanical family.

Folk Names

English names for white horehound are houndsbene, marvel, and hoarhound. Paradoxically, the herb is often called European horehound, although it is probably better known in the Americas as a healing herb than in Europe. Other names are water horehound, American horehound, common horehound, and hoarhound. Some German names are *Andorn, Gottvergess, Gotteshilf, weißer Dorant, weißer Andorn, Berghopfen, Dauerrang, Marobel,* and *Lungendank.* The French call the herb *marrube* or *marrube blanc*; the Italians, *marrobio, mentastro,* or *erba apiola*; the Spaniards, *marrubio*; the Danes, *kransburre*; the Russians, *šandra obyknovennaja*; and the Irish, *grafán*.

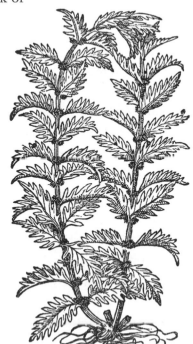

Appearance

The primary identifying feature of the horehound plant is the rounded, small, silvery-olive green color and wrinkled look of the unique leaves, coupled with their bitter taste. The plant resembles a small dead nettle with rounded leaves, and is completely covered, on the underside of the leaves and on the stems, with a white woolly fur that gives it a hoary appearance. The leaves are thick, oval, extremely wrinkled, woolly, more or less pointed at the ends, and as large as the first joint of an index finger. They are marked with a whitish net. The flowers only appear after the second year, in clusters of 6–8 long whitish tubes, in tight whorls on the stems next to the leaves. Nicholas Culpeper wrote,

> Common horehound grows up with square hairy stalks, half a yard or 2 feet high, set in the joints with two crumpled rough leaves of a sullen hoary green color, of a good scent but a bitter taste. The flowers are small, white, and gaping, set in a rough hard prickly husk about the joints, wherein afterward is found a small round blackish seed. The root is blackish, hard and woody, with many strings; and abides many years.[171]

Black stinking horehound has a distinctly weedy appearance. It not only tastes bad, but also smells bad. It is somewhat taller than the white horehound and has darker leaves. The flowers are red or a dull, dark purple.

Place, Season, and Useful Parts

Horehound can be found growing wild in Asia, Australia, South Africa, the Americas, and Europe, including the Azores and the Canary Islands. White horehound was originally a native of Central Asia, but has been carried by sheep and goats, as well as by human cultivation, to most parts of the globe, with the exception of the tropics and some deserts. It usually grows in dry soil near human habitations, on village paths, waysides, and rubble, on rocky soil, in waste places and lean pastures, in hedges, and near fences and the resting places of cattle. The black stinking horehound prefers a shady situation behind houses, fences, and hedges, or near graveyards. The horehounds are found to an altitude of 3,500 ft., or even higher. They blossom from June to September.

Gathering, Drying, and Storage

The entire horehound plant, without roots, is gathered when it begins to flower in June and August. The leaves alone can also be gathered from May on. Many herb gatherers believe midsummer horehound to be the best for medicinal purposes, because the herb is at its peak at this time of year.

---

171. Culpeper, *Culpeper's Complete Herbal* (1653) (London: Foulsham, undated), 192.

Horehound leaves are dried in an airy, shady place. The plant's pleasant aroma is lost during the drying process, but the leaves only seldom mildew.

Seed Saving and Germination

The major drawback with saving seeds of the white horehound is that it is very difficult to determine the proper time to harvest the seed-bearing stalks: the seed receptacles may already be empty before the harvest. A magnifying glass can help to show when the seeds are ripe. They are very insignificant and brownish, and often have to be rubbed out of the bristly seed receptacles. The seeds remain fertile for 2–3 years if stored in a cool, dry place, and much longer if dried with silica gel and then frozen. Silica crystals are now cheaply available as kitty litter.

Gardening Hints

Although white horehound is often cultivated for medicinal purposes, many gardeners consider it to be a weed. It is easy to raise, spreads rapidly, and is only rarely attacked by insects. It requires well-drained, dry, poor, limestone-containing soil, and may fail if the ground is too wet. It will do well in years of drought, and tolerates heat as well as frost. Horehound usually stays gray-green throughout the winter, especially under snow cover. The seeds can be sown in April, and will germinate in 2–3 weeks, although often erratically. They should be pricked out or thinned to allow 9 in. between plants. The roots can be divided in October or March, and cuttings can also be taken. If the plants are allowed to self-seed, new plants may spring up in all corners of the garden, for ants are very industrious in carrying the seeds around. Fruit growers have noticed that canker worms and other insects can be discouraged if horehound is planted under fruit trees. A fermented horehound brew can be sprayed directly on other plants to drive away insects.

Culinary Virtues

Horehound is much too bitter to be cooked as a vegetable, but is sometimes used to give a bitter touch to beers and liqueurs. In the United States, horehound candy is still prepared to this day, although it is unknown in other countries.

Noteworthy Recipes

Horehound Beer: Horehound beer is brewed from fresh horehound leaves, ginger, lemon juice, and brown sugar. It can be given a brown color by adding a little molasses. It has an unusual taste, and is bitterer than beer made with hops. The beer-making procedure is the same as that followed for nettle beer (see the nettle chapter).

Horehound Candy: Horehound's bitter taste combines well with sugar. Horehound candy or cough drops are made by brewing 2 handfuls of fresh horehound leaves in 2 cups of water in a covered saucepan over a low heat for 10 minutes. Strain the herb mixture, and add 2 cups of sugar and a few tablespoons of corn syrup. Boil until the hard-crack stage on a candy thermometer is reached (300° F), and then pour into a well-buttered pan or mold. Cut into small squares before the mixture hardens, roll the candies in powdered sugar or slippery elm powder, and store in airtight containers.

Household Applications

According to folk belief, horehound, like fly agaric, is supposed to keep flies out of a room when placed in a bowl of milk. This has not been corroborated, but the herb does have a deterring effect on many insects. Butter will keep better if the butter containers are carefully scrubbed with horehound. It is thought to keep even better if the horehound is gathered between eleven o'clock and midnight from a cemetery. Flower bouquets can be "framed" around the edges with silvery horehound leaves.

Cosmetic Properties

Black stinking horehound was once employed as a skin and hair rinse, presumably to discourage lice and other parasites. Because of the plant's unpleasant fragrance, it is not employed in cosmetics anymore.

Medicinal Merits

Dioscurides recommended horehound for "ye venemous beast-bitten, & to such as have drank some deadly thing."[172] It was once administered as an antidote to poison, and ancient Romans treated malaria and malaria-like illnesses with it. Later herbalists confirmed its use as a bitter herb capable of strengthening the liver and therefore counteracting poison. It was also supposed to clear the body of phlegm, impurities, and worms. Women were given horehound to hasten delivery and to induce menstruation. The juice was applied externally to sores and ulcers, or dropped into eyes and ears.

Herbalist Otto Brunfels considered the black stinking horehound to be better medicinally because it was less biting, hot, and dry in nature than white horehound. He also believed black horehound to be the male version of the plant, and the white the female.

Modern Medicine

Modern medicinal practitioners and herbalists only use white horehound as a bitter digestive and liver herb, and as an expectorant. Fresh horehound juice with honey, horehound syrup, horehound candy, horehound tea, or horehound powder can help to cleanse the

---

172.   Robert T. Gunther, ed., *The Greek Herbal of Dioscurides* (New York: Hafner, 1959), 349.

lungs, stomach, and intestines of mucus, and to relieve coughs, asthma, allergic reactions, bronchitis, beginning tuberculosis, and some forms of diarrhea. For excessive morning sickness or nervous indigestion with vomiting, it has been used together with chamomile as a tea, although some practitioners do not recommend it under any circumstances for pregnant women. The tea should be taken in small amounts spread over the day, preferably from a thermos bottle. Horehound taken ½ hour before a meal can help to relieve digestive disorders, and ease a hardened spleen, liver, or treat jaundice. The herb further acts as a general stimulant for the weak and anemic, but should never be used over an extended period. It is applied externally to fresh wounds, hardened glandular knots, chilblains, frostbite, skin diseases, and rashes.

Horehound is not widely used homeopathically, but can be employed to help dispel an afterbirth, as a bitter digestive tonic, and for chronic intestinal or pulmonary catarrhs.

Uses in Husbandry

Bees kept in the vicinity of horehound plants will produce a uniquely bitter honey known as horehound honey. According to German beekeeping tradition, bees will reproduce better if horehound is placed under the hive. Cattle generally avoid both horehounds. But, according to folk medicine, hanging black horehound around their necks is said to increase their appetite.

Veterinary Values

Dogs with ear problems not due to ear mites can benefit from having their ears cleaned with a horehound infusion.

Miscellaneous Wisdom

Horehound was familiar to ancient Egyptians under the name Seed of Horus, Bull's Blood, and the Eye of the Star. It is one of the five bitter Passover herbs.

In the Lincolnshire Fens, it was once thought extremely unlucky for a woman to give birth on May 1st. In order to induce the birth on April 30th, she was given a strong tea of horehound and rue and then forced to jump up and down. (It goes without saying that this procedure cannot be recommended because of the possible toxic effect of the herbs.)

The Holly and the Ivy, Now they are both full grown
Of all the trees that are in the wood, The ivy tree wears the crown.

—Traditional English carol

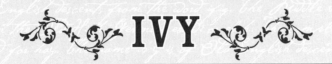

IVY

Name

Ivy is a perennial, evergreen member of the ***Araliaceae*** family. This family only contains a few species, including our common *Hedera helix*. *Hedera* is of Latin origin, and the term *helix* is of Greek ancestry, referring to the plant's winding, spiraling tendency. Other ancient terms for the herb were *Kissos* and *Dionysias,* after the god (or maybe the god was named for the plant?).

The name "ivy" is of Old English descent, from the word *ifig*. The Middle High German forms were *Ep-höu* and *Ebewe*, originating from the Old High German *Ebawi* or *Ebah*. The complete meaning of the word is not clear, but *Höu* was the word for "hay."

The English expression "go pipe in an ivy leaf" means to occupy oneself with useless or idle tasks. The modern equivalent would be to "go take a flying leap at the moon."

Folk Names

Alternate English names for ivy are bindwood, bentwood, woodbind, ivens, ivery, hibbin, love-stone, and English ivy. Ancient names were *poetica, dionysia,* and *silvae mater*. Germans call the herb *Ffeu, Ewigheu, Wintergrün,* and *Baumtod;* Italians, *edera, elare,* and *ellera.* French names are *lierre commun, lierre grimpant,* and *lierre des poetes;* Dutch, *klimop;* Spanish, *cistero* or *hiedra;* Welsh, *eiddew, eiddiorwg,* or *ióreg;* Irish, *eidhneán;* and Russian, *pljusč obyknovennyj.*

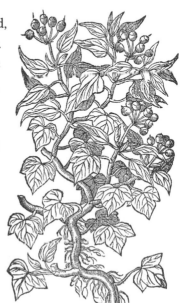

Appearance

Ivy is a creeping, climbing vine that may grow to be 400 or even 1,000 years old. Such ancient specimens have thick, woody stems as thick as 3 ft. in diameter. These Methuselahs may creep to a length of 30 yards.

Ivy often grows in oak, nut, fruit, and beech trees, in chestnuts, pines, poplars, whitethorns, acacias, and bays. It does not grow in holly trees and is never troubled with mistletoe, which may explain why these plants are considered separate magical beings and brought into the house at Christmastime. Ivy may grow on the ground in woods as a creeping plant, but these specimens do not blossom and gradually lose their ability to climb. Unlike the sunflower, ivy turns its leaves *away* from the sun to protect them from sun-scald.

The supporting roots of the ivy plant are amazingly strong, making it extremely difficult to remove the plant from a tree or wall. Ivy's creeping branches are like arms, and can find a hold on even the smoothest surface with the help of small suction disks. The leaves, which are very numerous and showy, are dark green and shiny on the upper side, peculiar in shape, and leathery in texture. They remain green throughout the winter. The leaf is divided 3 to 7 times, and sometimes has white veins. At the top of the plant, the leaves are almost ovular. Ivy flowers late in the year, from September into November, and in some places a little earlier. The flowers are small and inconspicuous, yellow in color, and appear in groups of 3 to 7. They are self-pollinating, and have little scent but some nectar. In good years the fruits hang in heavy clusters, bending the branches with their weight. They are round, and the size of a pea. Their color varies from violet to dark brown to a deep black. The fruits are filled with pitch, and are aromatic in smell but nauseously bitter to taste.

Place, Season, and Useful Parts

Ivy grows in most of Europe, and in Asia, Africa, and North America to an altitude of 5,400 ft. It is not particular as to its position, but does prefer limestone soil. It attaches itself to underbrush, trees, cliffs, walls, ruins, grottoes, and castle walls, and can also be found in graveyards, gardens, and stony woods. It blossoms in the late summer, fall, and even winter, and produces berries in the late fall and winter. These usually ripen around the time of the winter solstice, and stay on the plants until spring.

Gathering, Drying, and Storage

Green ivy leaves are especially valuable in the winter, when few other green leaves are available. The leaves should be dried quickly in an airy place, if necessary with the help of artificial heat. They can be stored for 1 year. Fresh berries are gathered when ripe for external use. The berries and the resin are harvested commercially and processed into pitch. Ivy wood has occasionally been used medicinally.

Seed Saving and Germination

There are various ornamental ivy varieties available. These are usually propagated by cuttings (with or without a heel), which must be kept consistently damp until they root. No further isolation is necessary in order to maintain various varieties beyond removing seedlings. If several varieties are being kept next to each other, care must be taken that seedlings do not take root and grow up between varieties. Ivy seeds can also be planted, but the plants take time to establish themselves. The seeds will sprout after 10–15 days, if kept evenly moist and well covered with earth.

Gardening Hints

Ivy is the only European plant with *three* different kinds of roots: clinging roots, nourishing roots, and aerial roots. It is not a true parasite, but can harm trees to the point of killing them. Fruit trees, especially pear trees, bear poorly if they are burdened with ivy, and other trees can be strangled if ivy stems are allowed to wrap themselves tightly around the supporting trunk. Oak trees, on the other hand, seem to grow better with ivy.

Ivy is one of the very few climbers that will not normally damage walls and stonework unless these are in poor shape, and is therefore encouraged on the outside of houses. The effect of an ivy-covered wall is picturesque, and there are also practical advantages: the wall does not have to be painted or decorated as carefully, it is protected from the elements, and the ivy will draw excess moisture up from the ground and away from the stonework.

Generally, ivy plants only blossom after 8–10 years' growth and are then visited by thousands of honey-seeking insects. They also serve as food for butterflies and moths. Ivy prefers a mild sea climate and grows best in areas warmed by ocean winds. The plants will usually survive, but not thrive, in areas where the winters are long and bitterly cold. Ivy can be grown as a covering plant for walls, trees, shady places, or graveyards, and decorative varieties can even be raised indoors by gardeners who are not superstitious. The leaves are impervious to smoke, exhaust fumes, air pollution, and light frosts, making ivy a valuable plant for city gardeners. The young shoots are planted in the spring, and kept damp until they are established. Ivy usually does not like extremely hot weather, and should be kept far away from sources of direct heat if planted indoors. The plants put up with too much shade much better than with too much sun or heat. A striking effect can be produced by planting ivy beside a room divider, or in planters and baskets hanging from the ceiling.

Culinary Virtues

The wood of thick ivy stems is extremely porous, and has occasionally been used as a filter for wine. The belief was once prevalent that water could be separated from wine by passing it through ivy wood, and that cups made from ivy wood would keep drinkers from feeling their wine. According to Grimmelshausen, red wine poured into an ivy cup would cause it to fall to pieces by the time the drinker counted to 3,000.

It was once customary to advertise taverns with bundles of ivy, or with signs decorated with ivy and hung outdoors. It was also customary to steep ivy leaves in wine cups. The sign depicting an owl inside an ivy wreath was taken as an injunction to "be merry and wise," a fitting motto for the wine-loving philosopher or the thoughtful tavern-keeper.

But as Publilius Syrus once put it, "You need not hang up the ivy-branch over the wine that will sell."[173] The English writer John Lyly observed, "Things of greatest profit are set forth with least price. Where the wine is neat, there needeth no ivy-bush."[174] In Shakespeare's words, "Good wine needs no bush."[175]

Household Applications

Because of their porous texture, slices of very large ivy stems are sometimes used as filters. The wood of peeled ivy stalks is decorative, and often used in flower arrangements. An orange-brown dye can be produced from very young ivy shoots, and ivy pitch is sometimes added to incense mixtures.

- An infusion of ivy leaves can be satisfactorily used as a substitute for soap. Two handfuls of fresh ivy leaves should be brewed with ½ gal. of boiling water, and then allowed to steep for 2 days before straining. The resulting liquid is an excellent detergent for wool. Those who desire a stronger solution for linen should add some washing soda to the ivy liquid.

Ivy is an excellent garland plant. In ancient Greece and Rome, poets and musicians were often wreathed with its flexible stems and fresh green leaves. The plant was also employed at banquets to cool the brow of revelers, and to lessen the effects of intoxicating wine fumes. Other authors report that an infusion of ivy leaves in wine was used as an antidote for wine poisoning. Rubbing ivy berries on one's temples was also said to draw off vapors and harmful influences.

Yet other sources warn against bringing ivy into the house. Ivy is generally accepted as a green climber for adorning the outside of houses, but is believed to exert unwholesome influence and to even cause death if allowed indoors. In northern countries, ivy is welcomed into the house only during the twelve days of Christmas. Then it is used,

---

173. Syrus, Maxim 968.

174. Lyly, "Eupheus and His England," *The Complete Works*, 3 vol. (Oxford: Oxford Univ. Press, 1973).

175. William Shakespeare, *As You Like It*, Epilogue.

together with fir, pine, holly, mistletoe, and rosemary, to decorate kitchen windows, mantels, and wainscoting, and to impart a festive air to a holiday table. Christmas greens should, however, be burned on the morning of January 6th. If not, then bad luck will cling, like ivy, to the house that year.

Cosmetic Properties

The soapy liquid obtained by brewing ivy leaves is as thorough and mild a cleansing solution for sensitive skin as it is for soft woolens. Ancient herbalists recommended a decoction of ivy leaves in wine for cleaning infected or diseased skin. Modern herbalists add ivy to soap and massage liquids to help tone and strengthen the skin. The pitch obtained from ripe ivy berries was once prized as a depilatory before the invention of the razor and chemical depilatories, and was even used as a filling for cavities. A decoction of ivy pitch and water was considered a good deterrent for lice and other unwanted insect guests. The juice obtained from fresh ivy berries was applied directly to hair to darken it, and to color gray strands. Since sunburn and suntan were not considered suitable for a lady's skin, women once smeared their faces with ivy leaves dipped in honey and rose oil, or with a sunburn butter prepared from fresh cream butter and ivy stems.

> *"Womens beauty ... is like vnto an Iuy bush, that cals man ti the tauern, but hangs itselfe withoute to winde and wether."*
>
> —JOHN FLORIO, 2ND FRUITES

Medicinal Merits

According to Otto Brunfels, the sixteenth-century German botanist, ivy is a plant of contradictory nature. It is allied with the earth and cold tempers, but it is also a warm plant that draws much of its nourishment from the air. The cooling properties of the plant were once used to ease the pain of burns, the biting fire of a swollen spleen and jaundice, red smarting eyes, headaches, and sharp ear pains or toothaches. The plant's warming properties were thought capable of dissolving corns, drawing out impurities and cleansing the face, speeding the birth process, countering uterine bleeding, and exciting the female organs as well as easing chronic coughs and catarrhs. In France and England, drinking wine out of an ivy cup was supposed to be an infallible cure for whooping cough. One folk remedy for burns from the Modena (Italy) area called for layers of ivy, virgin wax, and slices of hog lard dropped alternately into a hollowed-out juniper branch. The branch was heated slowly over a fire and the resulting warmed liquid dropped onto the burns. Dioscurides recommended that the berries be used as a pessary to hinder conception. Large amounts of ivy tea were believed to cause sterility in women.

Iuy ys good and glad to se;
Iuy is fair in hys degre.
Iuy is both faur and gren,
In wynter and in somer also,
And it is medicinable, I wen,
Who knew the certus that long therto;

—AN OLD ENGLISH CAROL, FROM RICHARD L. GREENE'S *THE EARLY ENGLISH CAROLS*

Modern Medicine

Because of its relative unreliability, ivy has fallen out of favor as a medicinal herb. The pitch obtained from the fresh plant and the berries is still official in some southern countries, but even that drug varies widely according to locality. There have been some cases of poisoning from ivy pitch, ivy juice, and berries. The most widespread internal use of the herb is as a weak tea, prepared from the berries, for the treatment of whooping cough or an insistent, spasmodic cough. The leaves are occasionally taken as a stomachic, sudorific, and circulatory medicine with a positive effect on the female organs, and have proved useful in the treatment of rheumatism and podagra.

A homeopathic preparation is prescribed for sinus disorders, asthma, and exhaustion, as well as for hemorrhoids, cough, thyroid gland swellings, rickets, and cataracts.

Ivy can be used externally without danger of unpleasant side effects. The Swiss herbal priest Johann Künzle recommended elevating the legs and then placing ivy leaves in one's shoes as a remedy for a sudden rush of blood to the head. Modern herbalists prescribe plasters of fresh ivy leaves on the neck and shoulders as a cure for sleeplessness due to nervous disorders. The fresh, bruised leaves can also be laid onto burns, wounds, rashes, or infected skin, and are applied as poultices to relieve earaches, headaches, and toothaches, as well as the twinges of rheumatism. The plant is especially valuable in the winter months, when few other fresh herbs are available.

Uses in Husbandry

Birds like to nest in ivy branches, for the evergreen leaves provide shelter against rain and snow in winter and the sun in summer. The berries, ripening at a time when little other nourishment is available, are an added attraction. Wood pigeons, thrushes, starlings, and blackbirds descend upon the plants in winter and early spring and greedily devour the berries. In warm climates, bees gather nectar from these late-blossoming plants to produce a dark, pleasant, and spicy honey.

Goats are very fond of ivy leaves, and will produce more milk if a few leaves are regularly added to their diet. Sheep and deer also eat the leaves on occasion. Dogs, rabbits, and cattle generally avoid the plant, and canaries can be poisoned if they eat too many berries.

Highland farmers believe that milk, butter, pigs, and cattle can be all be protected from witches with ivy wreaths. The wreaths should be hung on the animals or tucked under milk containers, or, as a general precaution, hung over the threshold on the Eve of May Day (otherwise known as Walpurgis Night).

The hard wood of thick ivy stems can be used as a substitute for other woods such as boxwood, and it is employed by English leather dressers to sharpen their knives.

Veterinary Values

Goats are given a handful of ivy leaves after birth to ease the passage of the afterbirth, or to help expel retained kids. Calving cows are occasionally given ivy tea. According to folk medicine, animal miscarriage can be prevented by hanging ivy on the door before noon on Christmas Day. Some Herefordshire farmers believe that ewes will bear twins if they are fed ivy blessed at Christmas Mass. Navel hernias or the cut foot pads of dogs can also be massaged with a strong ivy brew laced with witch hazel. Bears eat ivy leaves as medicine when they are wounded, according to Pliny.

Miscellaneous Wisdom

Ivy is thought to be a symbol of immortality, of love, friendship, company, and delight. Ivy roots grasp the soil, and the stems twine like the embrace of lovers. Priests in ancient Greece presented newlywed couples with the green leaves. Participants in the Elysian mysteries carried ivy, myrtle, and silver poplar, and the herb was also liberally used during religious festivities in March. The plant was associated with Osiris in ancient Egypt, Dionysus in Greece, and Bacchus in Rome. Dionysus is often represented wearing an ivy wreath. His thyrsus was topped with pinecones, and wound with ivy and grape leaves. One of Dionysus' nicknames was Kissophoros, or "the ivy-carrying one." His companions—the Bacchae, the Satyrs, and the Silenes—often decorated themselves with ivy leaves. Musicians and poets, as well as revelers, were garlanded with the herb.

Ivy is not only associated with godlike immortality, but also with human mortality. Ivy was once thought to be parasitical, and to owe its unusual vigor and fresh green color in winter to vampire-like traits. Its reputation suffered because it grows especially well on cemetery walls and graves, and provides shelter for sleeping snakes. In southern France, virgins' graves were traditionally decorated with ivy leaves.

Therefore, according to folk logic, ivy is one of the unluckiest plants to bring into the house. Because ivy likes to grow on ruins and in cemeteries, ruin and death are often associated with it. Eastern and northern Germans say that it will destroy marital harmony if brought into a house, and some Thuringians, in central Germany, insist that girls brought up in a house with indoor ivy will never find a husband. The Swiss say that bringing ivy into a house will cause a family member to be carried out, and ivy growing next to a house will demand a death every seventh year. If the ivy falls down from a house, the owners will suffer a financial setback, or be forced to sell the house.

During the twelve days of Christmas, rosemary, holly, mistletoe, laurel, ivy, and evergreens are welcomed into the house, and allowed to spread themselves out on the mantelpiece, join in the jollity and merriness, and partake of abundant food and drink. The mistress of the house must, however, take care to discreetly burn all her green and merry guests before the morning of Epiphany, January 6th. Otherwise the ivy would turn into pixies and other sprites and haunt her the whole year through. Despite all attempts to discontinue these "heathen" practices, the green wood spirits still continue to be taken into houses and even churches during the Christmas holidays.

Two plants, the holly and the ivy, were believed to represent the opposing male and female principles. They are thought to be incompatible in everyday life, but are brought together with great ceremony in fertility rites throughout the year. In the words of the scholar Sir Thomas Browne, ivy

> seldom ariseth about holly or not to great bignesse, the perpetual leafing prevent the arise, or hindring the growth or twisting of [the ivy]. Whether there be not also a dissimilitude in their natures, not one enduring the approximation of the other.[176]

The Irish saying goes, "One should always have a mouth of ivy, and a heart of holly."

At Christmas, when holly and ivy are brought indoors, they immediately begin to contend for mastery of the house. This amorous battle was once acted out by human actors in singing games. Many old rhymes and carols tell of the battle of the holly and the ivy. In Somerset, this song was still sung in 1906:

> O the ivy O, she is Queen of old
> And the holly he is red
> Hang'n high on the farm and he wont come to no harm
> Till the Christmas Days be told.
> O the ivy O, she is Queen of old
> And the holly he is red.[177]

In the seventeenth century, merrymakers used to sing,

> Now kindly for my pritty Song,
> Good Butler draw some beer,
> You know what Duties do belong

---

176. Browne, *The Works of Sir Thomas Browne*, vol. 3 (London: Faber & Faber, 1965), 386.

177. Ruth Tongue, *Somerset Folklore* (London: The Folk-Lore Society, 1965).

To him that sings so clear:
Holly and Ivy, drink will drive me,
To the brown bowl of Perry,
Apples and Ale, with a Christmas tale,
Will make this threshold merry.[178]

In Kentish villages, holly and ivy effigies were burned on Shrove Tuesday, the day before Lent. The girls banded together to steal the holly doll from the unmarried men, and the boys made off with the girls' ivy effigy and burned it. Bunches of ivy were sometimes used as "palms" on Palm Sunday. In England, street sweepers celebrated the coming of spring by designating one of their mates as "Jack the Green." He was dressed up, and a green pyramid crowned with ivy and holly was set on his head. Jack the Green and the street sweepers then swept through the streets in jubilant procession.

Children should not be allowed to play with ivy plants unattended, for the berries have been known to cause poisoning. Nonetheless, the plant figures in many children's rhymes, such as the following nineteenth-century "begging" song:

Holly and ivy
Mistletoe bough,
Give me an apple
And I'll go now.
Give me another
For my little brother,
And I'll go home,
And tell father and mother.[179]

Oracular Worth

The ancient Greeks and Romans associated grapevines and ivy with each other. Even today, French, Swiss, and Germans believe the grapes will be plentiful and the wine good if the ivy flowers profusely. But farmers are not happy when ivy plants set great quantities of fruit, for that means that the winter will be hard on animals and humans.

On New Year's Eve, at the beginning of the twelvemonth, English answer-seekers once consulted an ivy-leaf oracle. They laid an ivy leaf in a dish (ivy was a cheap substitute for the expensive Rose of Jericho), covered it, and placed it in a safe place. On January 5th, on the eve of the feast of the Epiphany, they uncovered it, and looked at it carefully. Fresh green leaves denoted health in the coming year; spotted leaves foretold disease. The position of the blackened spots could also give information about the organ

178.   Richard Leighton Greene, *The Early English Carols* (Oxford: Clarendon Press, 1977), cxxiii.
179.   Ibid., cxxii.

or body part likely to cause trouble. Thanks to this oracle, preventive measures could be taken to ward off illness.

On the eve of St. Matthew's Day, February 24th, it was once customary in Germany for girls to gather together at a spring. Candles were lit and, one by one, each girl threw one wreath made from ivy and other wintergreen plants, and one wreath made of straw, into the water. She then danced and sang and, walking backward, tried to fish one of her wreaths out of the spring. If she came up with the straw wreath it was taken as an ill omen, but the ivy wreath was a sure sign that she would soon marry. Another method of divination was to float three ivy leaves in a bowl filled with water from three springs on the eve of St. Matthew's Day. If the leaves came together, then the girl would marry within that year.

On the eve of All Hallows Day, Halloween, Irish boys go to the ivy plant and, without speaking, pluck off ten leaves. One of the leaves is then thrown away, and the remaining nine placed under the boy's pillow. That night, he will dream of his future wife. Similarly, Scottish girls pin three ivy leaves to their nightshifts on quarter days in the hopes that they will dream of their future husbands. In Cornwall, whoever pins four ivy leaves to the four corners of his or her pillow will dream of the Devil.

According to Swiss sources, the ivy plant also knows if a girl is a virgin. Virgins fumigated with the plant will not be affected, but other girls will be unable to hold their urine.

Legends

Ivy was sacred to Osiris, Dionysus, and Bacchus, and was used at times by Apollo, Heracles, Aphrodite, Artemis, Ganymede, and the Muses, as well as Pan, Priapus, Cheiron, and the Satyrs. Celtic priests also revered the plant.

Ivy was said to grow abundantly at Nyssa, Dionysus' childhood home, and the herb therefore came to be closely associated with that god. One of Dionysus' attendants was named Kissos, a rambunctious youth who never came to rest. Dionysus transformed him into the leaping, jumping, and hardy ivy. Ivy was so closely linked with Dionysus that the mere presence of great quantities of the plant in India led Alexander the Great to believe that Dionysus had already visited the place.

According to tradition, Dionysus' life was saved by ivy when he was still a child. Hera, jealous as usual, convinced Dionysus' mother Semele to demand that her lover Zeus appear to her in his godly form. Bound by his oath, he was forced to fulfil her wish. The shining fire of his presence burnt her, and set the house aflame. According to one version, Zeus was able to rescue his son from his mother's womb and carried him for three months in his hip, but the other version insists that nymphs rescued the baby and bathed him in ivy baths to heal his wounds. Consequently, Hera hated ivy more than any other plant. While still a child, Dionysus was captured by Tyrrhenian pirates. When he awoke, Dionysus demanded the sailors take him to Naxos. They jeered at him, and refused to follow the orders of a slave child. Dionysus then let ivy and grapevines grow from the depths of the ocean, and trap the ship in their tendrils. He changed himself into a lion, and threw all the sailors except one into the ocean. The one remaining sailor sailed with him to Naxos, and the other sailors turned into dolphins.

Literary Flowers

You have seen how ivy twines
Its leaves round a lofty elm, from the earth's bosom
Lapping its supple arms around the whole tree till it finds
A way to the very top, and hides all the wrinkled bark
With a mantle of green…

—WAHLAFRIDUS STRABO, *HORTULUS*

Hung wi the ivys veining bough
The ash trees round the cottage farm
Are often stripped of branches now
The cotter Christmases hearth to warm
He swings and twists his hazel brand
And lops them off wi sharpened hook
And oft brings ivy in his hand
To decorate the chimney nook.

—JOHN CLARE, *THE SHEPHERD'S CALENDAR*, "DECEMBER"

Yet once more, o ye laurels, and once more,
Ye myrtles brown, with ivy never-sere,
I come to pluck your berries harsh and crude,
And with froc'd fingers rude,
Shatter your leaves before the mellowing year.

—JOHN MILTON, "LYCIDAS"

Oh, a dainty plant is the Ivy green,
That creepeth o'er ruins old.
Of right choice food are his meals I ween,
In his cell so lone and cold…
Creeping where no life is seen,
A rare old plant is the Ivy green.

—CHARLES DICKENS, "THE IVY GREEN," *THE PICKWICK PAPERS*

Bring, bring the madding Bay, the drunken vine;
The creeping, dirty, courtly Ivy join.

—Alexander Pope, *The Dunciad*, Bk. 1

"Pr'y thee, how did the Fool look?"
"Look! Egad, he look'd for all the World like an Owl in an Ivy Bush."

—Jonathan Swift, *Polite Conversation*

Here are cool mosses deep,
And thro 'the moss the ivies creep,
And in the stream the long-leaved flowers weep,
And from the craggy ledge the poppy hangs in sleep.

—Alfred Tennyson, *Lotus-Eaters*: Choric Song, Pt. I.

And then Trystan and Gwalchmai went to Arthur … and there Arthur made peace between him and march ap Merchion. And Arthur spoke with the two of them in turn, but neither of them was willing to be without Esyllt; and then Arthur awarded her to the one of them while the leaves should be on the trees and to the other while the leaves should not be on the trees, the married man to choose. And he chose when the leaves should not be on the trees, because the nights would be longest at that time, and Arthur told that to Esyllt. And she said, 'Blessed be the judgement and he who gave it;', and Esyllt sang this englyn:

There are three trees that are good,
holly and ivy and yew;
they put forth leaves while they last,
And Trystan shall have me as long as he lives.

—from an unknown author of the 15–16th century,
qtd. in Jackson, *A Celtic Miscellany*

LADY'S MANTLE

Name

The name "lady's mantle" refers to the similarity of this herb to a folded cape. The lady in question is not just any gentlewoman, but Our Lady, the Virgin Mary.

The botanical name *Alchemilla* was given to the herb because alchemists once gathered the liquid found in the center of the plants' folded leaves and employed it as "celestial water" in their attempts to create the stone of wisdom. The word "alchemy" itself owes its name to the ancient name for Egypt, where the first alchemists were reported to have lived and worked.

Known botanically as *Alchemilla vulgaris*, lady's mantle is a common perennial plant and a member of the **Rose** family *(Rosaceae)*. There are many species and subspecies of lady's mantle, but the most important are *Alchemilla xanthoclora, Alchemilla mollis, Alchemilla alpina*, and *Aphanes arvensis (Alchemilla arvensis)*, which is an annual.

Folk Names

Lady's mantle is also known as common lady's mantle, Our Lady's mantle, lamb's foot, duck's foot, elfshot, dew cup, lion's foot, bear's foot, nine hooks, and great sanicle. Old herbals mentioned *stellaria, old syndow*, and *leontopodium*. German names are *Frauenmantel, Sintau, Tränenschön, Taublatt*, and *Mäntelichrut*; French names are *alchimille, mantelet*

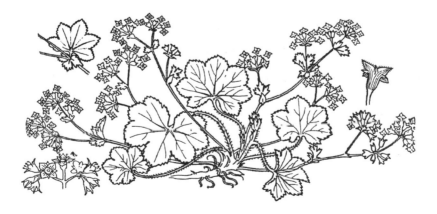

des dames, manteau de Notre-Dame, patte de lapin, and *pied de lion*. In Italian, it is *erba ventaglina* or *erba stella*. The Irish call it *fallaing mhuire*.

Alpine lady's mantle, *Alchemilla alpina*, is also known as *Silbermantel, Alpen-Frauenmantel*, and *Urgebirgsfrauenmantel* in German, and as *alchimille des Alpes* in French.

Aphanes arvensis is called parsley breakstone, parsley piert, parsley piercestone, bowel-hivegrass, colic-wort, percepier, and field lady's mantle. The French call it *perce-pièrre*; the Germans, *Acker-Frauenmantel*; and the Italians, *petricciolo*.

Appearance

Lady's mantle's two most striking features are its accordion-like, cupped, and folded leaves, and the single drop of "dew" almost always found in the center of each of its leaves. The silvery appearance of this droplet led the alchemists to use it in their search for the stone of wisdom. The liquid is actually produced by glands at the tips of the leaves, which combines with dew to form a silver drop.

Lady's mantle plants usually have small rootstocks, although some ancient specimens may be supported by roots as thick as a finger and 1 ft. in length. The rootstock is woody and is usually covered with black bark. In Nicholas Culpeper's words, the plant has

> many leaves rising from the root, standing upon long hairy foot-stalks, being almost round, and a little cut on the edges, into eight or ten [7–11] parts, making it seem like a star, with so many corners and points, and dented round about, of a light green colour.[180]

These leaves are slightly folded, like a fan, and have a mildly astringent and somewhat bitter taste. The plant grows to a maximum height of 18 in., and produces branching flower stalks and masses of greenish-yellow, inconspicuous flowers.

Alpine lady's mantle has much more deeply indented leaves than the common variety. The leaves contain fewer lobes (5–7) and are rounded at the ends, resembling miniature hands. They are dark green in color but are covered on the underside with tiny silken hairs, which give the entire plant a silvery appearance.

Parsley breakstone is much smaller than the two preceding plants, only attaining a height of 6 in. The leaves have 3 lobes and are only ½ in. wide, and gray-green. The plant's flowers are so inconspicuous that they are almost invisible to the untrained eye. They bloom in clusters in early summer.

---

180.   Culpeper, *Culpeper's Complete Herbal* (1653) (London: Foulsham, undated), 208.

Place, Season, and Useful Parts

Lady's mantle is primarily a pasture plant, but can also be found on paths and slopes, in meadows and on riverbanks, in gardens and on damp soil, in open woodland and on rubble. It grows in Europe, North America, Asia, and northern Africa, and blooms from May into the fall. It is replaced in Europe by alpine lady's mantle at altitudes between 3,000 ft. and 9,000 ft.

Alpine lady's mantle will not usually grow on calcareous soil, and is not common in North America. It prefers neither a damp nor a dry position, and appears in pastures and meadows, on rubble and cliffs, on open ground and in copses. It is very common in the Alps, and can be found in the northern Mediterranean area, in Scandinavia, and Scotland. It often forms silvery hummocks, or soft carpets.

Parsley breakstone can be encountered in Europe, northern Africa, and North America to an altitude of 1,500 ft. It grows well on dry soil, barren fields, waste ground, gravel pits, and walls, and will self-seed in an unused, dry corner of the garden.

Gathering, Drying, and Storage

The entire flowering lady's mantle plant, or its leaves and stems, should be gathered in the late spring or summer months when the plant is fresh and green and the leaves dry (it is important not to gather the plant too early in the day). Discolored leaves must be discarded. Swiss herbal authorities recommend addressing the plant politely before gathering it.

Lady's mantle should be laid out in thin layers in an airy but shady place to dry. The plants must be dried quickly, without turning, in order to preserve their green color. Brown leaves are thrown away. The dried drug can be stored for one year in containers with loosely fitting tops.

Seed Saving and Germination

Garden varieties are almost always reproduced through plant division. Wild lady's mantle plants can be propagated by seed, or by encouraging the plants to seed themselves. The seedlings, or large plants, can easily be transplanted.

Gardening Hints

Although lady's mantle is a handsome plant, it is usually accorded a secondary place in gardens as a border herb, or planted as ground cover. It is quite striking in masses, bringing an unusual yellowish-green shade to the garden color scheme. Varieties have been especially developed for this purpose, usually variants of *Alchemilla mollis*. These plants prefer a shaded, somewhat moist position, and respond well to mulching. If the situation is favorable to lady's mantle, it may become invasive. The plants then need to be divided regularly. Alpine lady's mantle is often planted in rockeries because of its silvery leaves.

Culinary Virtues

Both the leaves and the roots of lady's mantle are edible, if not delectable. Young lady's mantle leaves can be added to salads or steamed with other potherbs. Parsley break-stone was once highly valued in the islands of the Hebrides (Scotland) as a scurvy-combating culinary herb. It was added to salads, and pickled for storage like samphire (*Crithmum maritimum*).

Household Applications

A fairly stable yellowish dye for woolens can be prepared from flowering lady's mantle.

Cosmetic Properties

Lady's mantle gently and thoroughly cleanses the skin, bleaching it lightly. It helps to counteract acne and inflammations as well as excessively oily skin, and can help to tighten pores, remove blemishes, and lessen puffiness. The ancient Arabs used this herb extensively. European ladies once bleached unwanted freckles with the juice of the fresh plant or with the secretions exuded by the leaves. Modern cosmeticians add lady's mantle tea or juice to astringent lotions and to creams. Steaming mixtures often contain lady's mantle, and it can be used in eyewashes. An astringent infusion of lady's mantle stiffened with beaten egg white can be applied to a face swollen by crying, pregnancy, or intemperance. Lady's mantle tea, taken regularly for several weeks, can help to eliminate excess water from the body, tightening and toning the skin after birth and regulating excessive perspiration.

May dew was once thought to be an especially effective cleanser for women's skin, and dew gathered on the morning of May Day before sunrise was considered even more effective. May Day dew was believed to possess magical properties and be capable of transforming the plainest woman into a paragon of female beauty. The dew found in the center of lady's mantle leaves is, in truth, not just dew. The plant exudes droplets of a liquid that combines with the dew, rolling toward the center of the leaf. It is of real cosmetic value as a tonic liquid.

> *How to gather and clarifie May-deawe. When there hath fallen no raine the night before, then with a cleane and large sponge, the next morning you may gather the same from sweet hearbs.*
>
> —SIR HUGH PLATT, *DELIGHTES FOR LADIES*

Medicinal Merits

According to one ancient Italian herbal, the easiest way for a woman to tell if her husband is sterile is to drink a tea prepared from alpine lady's mantle for nine days. On the evening of the ninth day, and not before, she should lie down with her husband. If she does not conceive then, then the problem is undoubtedly his. The herb was also considered to be an effective aphrodisiac. Otto Brunfels advised epileptics to swallow lady's mantle juice for three consecutive days to help relieve their ailment, and he also praised its efficacy as an astringent vulnerary herb. Culpeper recommended lady's mantle to "stay bleedings and fluxes," and to help heal ruptures, bruises, wounds, and sores. According to him, women with "over-flagging breasts" should apply compresses of lady's mantle or alpine lady's mantle to tone the skin and make the breasts "grow less and hard."

Modern Medicine

Modern medicine recognizes the use of lady's mantle for female complaints, weaknesses, and disorders. In the early twentieth century, Johann Künzle wrote that if doctors would only have the sense to make their female patients drink lady's mantle tea regularly, then two-thirds of all gynecological operations would become superfluous. Many modern herbalists support Culpeper's assertion that "the distilled water [of lady's mantle] drank for 20 days together helps conception and to retain the birth, if the woman do sometimes sit in a bath made of the decoction of the herb."[181] Lady's mantle is generally administered to strengthen all the female organs, to lessen the chance of internal infection, to normalize menstruation and to lessen the disorders of puberty and menopause, to alleviate the symptoms of morning sickness, to counteract the possibility of miscarriage, to regulate the onset of labor and to make the contractions more effective, and, finally, to counteract excessive bleeding, anemia, and weakness occurring after birth or a menstrual period. Poultices of lady's mantle are applied to hardened or lumpy breasts, or before a period.

Alpine lady's mantle is much more potent than the common herb, and herbalists therefore recommend mixing one part of the alpine herb with two parts of the common plant. The tea should be taken regularly for several weeks or months. Baths of the herb are also effective. A woman wishing to have a child should drink two cups of lady's mantle tea every day before conception and during the first few weeks of pregnancy, and then again at least two weeks before delivery, and for two weeks after birth.

The medicinal merits of this common herb are not limited to its uterine value. It has mildly astringent and softening properties, and helps to heal damaged or infected tissue, to expel excess water from the body, to purify the blood, and to stop bleeding. Children with rickets or weak muscles, as well as the elderly recovering from a heart condition or suffering

---

181.   Culpeper, *Culpeper's Complete Herbal* (1653) (London: Foulsham, undated), 209.

from water retention, can be safely given lady's mantle tea. Lady's mantle is often added to the diuretic tea mixtures given to patients with kidney stones. Glandular disorders and internal infections can be positively influenced with lady's mantle tea, and it is even effective in the treatment of diabetes and in the supplementary treatment of multiple sclerosis. Alpine lady's mantle is given to overweight patients and to those who perspire heavily at night, as well as to women troubled with menopausal symptoms (see the sage chapter).

Lady's mantle is used homeopathically, like the fresh herb, for women's disorders such as menopause, leucorrhea, prolapse, and menstrual complaints, as well as for wound healing.

Lady's mantle is an excellent vulnerary or wound herb. Its action on bruises is similar to that of arnica, although not as pronounced. Fresh lady's mantle leaves can be crushed and then applied to fresh wounds to stop them from bleeding, and to lessen the chance of infection. Excellent results can be obtained by supplementing this first-aid treatment with a tea cure. Lady's mantle tea, taken for a long time, can even have a curative effect on hernias and large internal wounds. It can further hasten the mending of broken ribs and bones. Infected eyes can be rinsed out with a well-strained decoction of the herb, and it also said that Lady's mantle can help ease the pains of an extracted tooth.

Parsley breakstone is taken in tea form for bladder and kidney complaints, and is a folk remedy recommended for patients with kidney gravel and stones.

Special Cures

Digestive Aid: In his herbal, Otto Brunfels recommends a tea for those suffering from mild digestive problems such as constipation. This very gentle tea mixture is composed of two parts elecampane *(Inula helenium)* roots, one part lady's mantle, one part fennel leaves, one part sage, one part parsley, one part hyssop leaves, and one part each of fennel and anise seeds. The tea can be taken in small sips between or after meals.[182]

Tea for Women: A very simple tea with good strengthening and preventive properties for women can be prepared from 4 parts lady's mantle, 2 parts alpine lady's mantle, 4 handfuls of flowering white dead nettles and 2 handfuls of mint leaves, 1 part couch grass *(Agropyron repens)* roots, 1 part horsetail, 1 part marigold flowers, 1 part meadowsweet flowers *(Filipendula ulmaria)*, 1 part nasturtium or Indian cress *(Tropaeolum majus)*, 1 part goose grass leaves *(Potentilla anserina)*, and 1 part of the dried and diced roots of burnet saxifrage *(Pimpinella saxifraga)*. Use 1 tsp. of this mixture to brew ½ pint of tea, and let steep for 10–15 minutes. Take 2–3 times a day for as long as several months at a time.

---

182.   Brunfels, *Contrafayt Kräuterbuch* (1532), facsimile (Munich: Konrad Kölbl, 1964).

Uses in Husbandry

Lady's mantle leaves are eaten by sheep, cattle, and horses, and can be dried as hay with good results. Some farmers encourage it. Cattle will refuse to eat the hairy leaves of the alpine lady's mantle, and it is considered a weed in the Alps.

Veterinary Values

Lady's mantle tea is given to animals in large quantities after parturition. Dried lady's mantle leaves make excellent fodder for cattle suffering from diarrhea, or calves stricken with paralysis.

Miscellaneous Wisdom

In the Scandinavian countries, lady's mantle was once closely associated with the goddess Frigga. In later years, the herb became linked with the Virgin Mary. In the Palatine in Germany, nature spirits are still said to hide between the plant's leaves, and it is rumored that wood women use them as miniature washbowls. In Austria, lady's mantle wreaths are often placed on statues of Jesus at Whitsuntide.

Literary Flowers

One of the most common sights in spring and summer meadows is the reflection of the sun on hundreds of tiny dewdrops. The ladies of the fields spread their pleated mantles overnight on the grass and are rewarded with a single drop of dew, the rejuvenating water of their bath. The alchemists, spiritual scientists, avidly sought these magic drops for their chemical experiments.

Alpine lady's mantle stands even closer to the moon than its lowland counterpart. The underside of the strongly pleated leaves is touched and imbued with silver, the shape of a many-fingered womb.

—SISTER CLARISSA'S UNPUBLISHED BOOK OF NATURAL OBSERVATIONS

Lavender blue, and Rosemary green,
When I am king, you shall be queen.

—FROM *MOTHER GOOSE'S MELODIES*

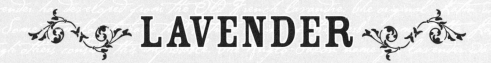

LAVENDER

Name

The name "lavender" has developed from the Old French *lavandre*. The original Latin word was *lavendula* or *livendula*. Some etymologists have tried to trace the origins of this herb's name to *lavare*, the Latin verb "to wash," but others consider this improbable. The Anglo-Saxon name for lavender was *lauendre*.

Lavandula angustifolia (true lavender) is a perennial member of the **Lamiaceae** or **Mint** family. It is also known as *Lavandula officinalis* and *Lavandula vera*, and produces the best oil and the best medicinal herb. *Lavandula pinnata, L. spica,* or *Lavandula latifolia* (spike lavender) is a taller plant with a terminal spike. The essential oil of this plant is much less subtle in aroma than that of true lavender. Among other lavender species and bastard forms, the names of *Lavandula stoechas,* *Lavandula dentata,* and *Lavandula lanata* are most common.

Folk Names

True lavender is also called Dutch or English lavender. Germans have named the herb *Lavendel, Schwindelkraut,* and *Flander;* some French terms are *luvunde, lavande femelle,* and *lavande véritable.* Italian names are lavanda, *lavandula* and *levande,* and Russians call it *lavanda aptečnaja.* Spaniards have named it *langunda;* Turks, *lanvanta;* the Welsh, *lafant;* and the Irish, *labhandar.*

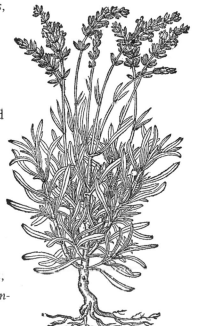

Spike lavender is also called lavender spike, spike, spikenard, lesser lavender, and nardus italica. German names are *deutsche Narde, kleiner Speik,* and *Speik Lavender;* Italian terms are *lavanda spigo, spigo,* and *spigonardo;* French, *aspic* or *spic,* Spanish, *spigo, espliego, alhucena,* and *lavanda;* and Russian, *lanvanda aspik.*

Lavandula stoechas is known as Arabian lavender and French lavender; in German, as *welscher Lavendel* and *Schopflavendel*; in French, as *stoechas arabique*; in Spanish, as *romero santo*; and in Portuguese, as *alfazema*.

Appearance

True lavender is an evergreen, shrublike plant that grows to a height of 3 ft. It has a uniquely pleasant and spicy odor and a somewhat bitter, peppery taste. The stem is short and crooked and covered with flaky, yellowish-gray bark, from which spring many upright stalks with leaves, ending in a flower spike. On older plants, the stem turns woody. Lavender leaves are similar to those of hyssop, rosemary, or tarragon, but are a little blunter and thicker. When young, they are covered with whitish down. Later, the edges roll in and the color changes to a grayish-green. Lavender flowers are elongated, like longish ant eggs, and appear in whorls of 6 to 10 in terminal spikes. They are purple and occasionally white in color.

Spike lavender looks coarse next to true lavender, with its broad rootstock, square woody stems, and broad leaves. The flower spikes are longer and more accentuated, and the flowers are purple or blue in color.

Place, Season, and Useful Parts

Although originally a Mediterranean plant, lavender is now cultivated the world over, to an altitude of 4,500 ft. It can still be found growing wild on sunny Mediterranean mountain slopes.

Gathering, Drying, and Storage

Lavender leaves are picked for kitchen use as needed, but are most fragrant just before the plant blossoms. Lavender flowers or buds are gathered from plants at least two years old, from June to September. It is advisable to gather the flowers before they open completely, after the dew has dried on a clear, sunny morning. The entire blossoming plant is harvested for oil distillation, and the first and third cuttings of the year are said to yield the best lavender oil.

Lavender blossoms should be spread out in thin layers in a dark, airy place and dried quickly. The flowers must retain their purple color on drying, and the dried drug should not contain leaves or stems. Lavender retains its medicinal properties for one year, and its scent for several years. One-year-old lavender flowers should not be used as medicine, but can still be added to potpourri or bath mixtures for household use.

Seed Saving and Germination

Lavender is a polymorph, constantly changing to adapt to local conditions. The plants are usually propagated vegetatively, through plant division, layering, or cuttings. Lavender cuttings root easily, and can be used to maintain valuable varieties. Seed propagation is not generally practiced, but it is advisable to keep plants from forming seeds in warmer climates. If they do, the seeds may fall to the earth, germinate, and produce off-type seedlings. If these are not removed, they will cross into the variety.

Gardening Hints

Lavender can be planted in the herb or flower garden as a perennial border or hedge plant. It was once included in knot-gardens, which were herb gardens, hedged in complicated forms.

Lavender grows best in a loose, well-drained soil in a warm and somewhat moist climate at a slight elevation (1,200–3,600 ft.). The soil should be enriched with humus, and contain some limestone. Lavender must be protected from wind in summer, and from extreme cold in winter. Areas famous for their lavender fields can be found in France and England. Lavender can remain in the same place for five years if the plant is pruned lightly in summer, and given some winter protection. The plants should be cut back every year, but no later than July, or the new shoots will not be hardy enough to withstand frost. In very hot climates they should be cut back earlier in the year, or the cut stems will dry out, causing the plant to die.

Lavender may be raised from seed, although this is often problematic. The herb only produces seeds in the south, and the seedlings do not necessarily come "true" to the mother plant. Furthermore, lavender seeds germinate very slowly, and must be kept evenly moist for a month or even more. In mild climates, they can be sown outdoors in August. In colder areas, they must be sown under glass, indoors, or under a cold frame. The seedlings are then set out in a warm, wind-protected place after all danger of frost has passed with 10–14 in. between plants, or the seedlings can be planted in hedges.

Lavender cuttings should be taken with a heel in the fall, or hardwood cuttings in the spring. Another possibility is softwood cuttings in summer. The cuttings are best placed around the edges of a pot, or in a warm, sheltered, and moist place in the garden in summer. When they are rooted, they should be transplanted into well-drained, sandy soil. Lavender can also be propagated by plant division in fall, or by layering the plants in the spring. It is advisable to take cuttings from locally established plants to ensure maximum hardiness, and also advisable to keep the plant from flowering in its first year for the same reason. Lavender grown for oil and as a cash crop is propagated from one mother plant to ensure uniformity in the final product. *Lavandula x intermedia*, a cross between lavender and spike lavender, is often grown commercially because of its higher yields.

According to Kentish gardening belief, lavender fares best if planted by men. It grows well in the vicinity of sage and St. John's wort, and is sometimes planted next to primroses and yellow crocuses to drive away birds. Carrots can be grown with good results between rows of lavender. Lavender, and especially spike lavender, is sometimes subject to scab infestation.

Culinary Virtues

Lavender is not appreciated enough as a culinary herb. Its fragrant, peppery taste makes it a good substitute for pepper, and it is an important ingredient of some herbal seasoning mixtures. It is bitter, and should always be used sparingly. The famous *"Herbes de Provence"* seasoning mixture contains small amounts of lavender, and would be unthinkable without that herb. Lavender can be added in minute amounts to salads or potherb mixtures, and it can also be prepared as jelly and served with meat. It combines well with other Mediterranean seasonings such as thyme, bay leaves, rosemary, sage, oregano, and basil.

The ancient Romans included lavender among their seasoning herbs, and it was valued in the Middle Ages as a flavoring for medicinal beers. Queen Elizabeth I ate lavender jelly with her lamb, and John Gerard greatly praised the flavor of lavender conserves.

Lavender stalks can be added to barbeque fires, and meat smoked with lavender has a finer flavor. Lavender flowers, without the bitter flower receptacles, can be used to spice custards or cakes. They are also placed in sugar, and the flavored sugar then used to sweeten desserts. A small amount of lavender florets is added to cookie dough, or ice cream and sherbet mixtures. Ginger and lavender complement each other in flavor.

Household Applications

In most people's minds, lavender and linen closets are firmly linked with one another. Lavender-sellers were once a common sight in the major European cities, and herb women can still be seen selling their wares in Munich. Laundry was once dried on lavender bushes, and the sweet-smelling herb was laid between gloves and lace handkerchiefs and underwear, and all the daily accouterments of the gentle life. Ladies also carried lavender smelling salts, or had lavender sewn into their capes to counteract fainting attacks occasioned by a surfeit of emotion, or, more often, a mercilessly tight corset. The herb was strewn to drive away lice, bedbugs, mosquitoes, flies, and moths, and to scent a room on festive occasions. Spanish churches were strewn and adorned with lavender on high festival days.

These days, potpourri, sachets, and sleeping cushions are prepared with lavender, and the herb is sewn into sweetbags placed in cupboards and among linens. Lavender buds are sometimes placed in an open bowl to sweeten and purify the air in a room.

Tiny sacks of lavender, said to exert a relaxing effect, can be hung on sofas or in the bathroom, or tucked underneath pillows. Lavender wood is aromatic and can be burned in an open fireplace, and lavender flowers and leaves can be strewn on an open fire or wood stove to overpower unpleasant odors. Incense is prepared from lavender, and the stalks are sometimes burned as an incense substitute. Lavender oil is used as a scenting agent in oil lamps, which is said to drive away insects. Spike lavender is sometimes added to cleansing mixtures because of its fresh, penetratingly pungent aroma.

Despite its reputation as a moth repellent, lavender buds will actually attract some moths, and lavender sacks have to be checked regularly for moth infestation, or the laundry may be dirtied.

Here's sour sweet Lavender,
Sixteen sprigs a penny,
Which you will find, my ladies,
Will smell as sweet as any.

—AN OLD LONDON STREET CRY OF A LAVENDER WOMAN PRAISING HER WARES

Cosmetic Properties

Lavender oil is an important ingredient of many cosmetic products and perfumes. Unfortunately, cheap synthetic substances are often used in place of true lavender oil, and the herb's cosmetic reputation has suffered as a result. True lavender oil is very volatile, but has a sweet, penetrating, fresh aroma. A good lavender bath oil can be prepared from almond oil and fresh lavender flowers, left to steep for 2–3 weeks. It can be added to baths and footbaths in minute amounts. Lavender water is prepared from the flower buds and can be substituted in cosmetic recipes for rose or orange water, depending on personal preferences. Commercial lavender products include perfumes, shaving lotions, hair lotions, colognes, soaps, and talcum powder.

Lavender has deodorizing, soothing, relaxing, nerve-strengthening, and painkilling properties, which make it an excellent bath herb. The ancient Romans were aware of this, and made extensive use of the herb, as did the Libyans. Lavender water rubbed in after a bath helps to tone the skin and improve the circulation. Fresh lavender leaves, or a lavender mouthwash, can help to cover the traces of bad breath until the next visit to the dentist. The herb was once used in the preparation of the famous Vinegar of the Four Thieves (see sage chapter). Those with dry skin can add lavender to facial steaming mixtures. A simple yet effective steaming mixture can be prepared by mixing equal amounts of chamomile and lavender flowers, preferably direct out of the garden.

Spike lavender is employed by cosmeticians in Germany, but is generally not as highly prized as lavender because of its pungent fragrance. Spike lavender baths are very stimulating, and some commercial firms produce spike lavender soap.

Noteworthy Recipes

Lavender Water: Lavender water is prepared by filling a clean jar one-quarter full with lavender buds, and then filling it to the top with clear, high-proof spirits, such as wine spirits or vodka. Close the jar carefully, and place in a warm spot in the sun. Strain and filter the mixture after 8 weeks (if desired, it can be left in the sun for up to one year), and store in sealed bottles. This water is used as lavender bath water, as a mild deodorant, or as a substitute for rose water.

Medicinal Merits

Lavender has earned the reputation over the centuries of being able to cure "hidden" diseases and complaints for which no medical explanation was forthcoming: sorcery, migraines, headaches caused by ill-spirited black elves, nightmares, catalepsy, melancholy, hypochondria, epilepsy, fainting spells, menstrual cramps, palsy, pantings and passions of the heart, convulsions, and colics. It was also considered a general tonic thought to strengthen the liver, stomach, and spleen. As documented by the German rhyme, "Lavender, thyme and myrtle grow by the garden gate, / Our Nancy is already a bride, and has no time to wait,"[183] lavender has long been employed as an abortifacient medicine, and was once used by midwives to help expel the afterbirth and to ease "still" children from the womb.

Modern Medicine

Modern medicine approves of lavender as a heart (cardiac) and nerve (nervine) medicine. Lavender tea can be given to those afflicted with sleeplessness, neuroses, nervous heart palpitations, neuralgia, dizziness, and migraines. It is also given as a palliative medicine to patients with heart problems. Old people in particular profit from lavender tea: it aids the circulation, strengthens and soothes the heart, helps prevent arteriosclerosis and shaking of the limbs, and is an excellent restorative medicine after strokes, epileptic fits, loss of consciousness, or partial paralysis. Lavender is often used in combination with the roots of burnet saxifrage *(Pimpinella saxifraga)*. Plants found growing at high altitudes are of greater medicinal value than lowland specimens to treat paralysis of the tongue. Lavender can be taken regularly for several months at a time without harmful side effects, but should never be taken in large amounts at one time. Massive dosage

---

183. Gustav Hegi, *Illustrierte Flora von Mittel-Europa*, vol. V/I (Munich: Lehmanns, 1913–1918), 2279.

can cause colic, and inordinately large amounts of lavender oil can result in paralysis or even death.

Lavender, in combination with other herbs, is helpful in the treatment of stomach cramps or upsets, flatulence, loss of appetite, asthma, whooping cough, bronchitis, and influenza. It is said to facilitate birth. British herbalists administer a compound tincture of the herb as a digestive medicine, and it is used as a flavoring agent for other medicines. Strangely enough, it is not often used by homeopaths.

Essential lavender oil can be taken a few drops at a time for all of the above complaints, or it can be added to a sweet oil to produce herbal bath or massage oil for the treatment of rheumatism and paralysis. It can also be used as a counterirritant, or rubbed on the temples to ease persistent headaches. Lavender baths help to strengthen rickety children. Lavender compresses are applied to rheumatic pains, and fresh lavender can be used in inhaling and steaming mixtures to clear the head and lungs. Washing one's head regularly with a lavender infusion is thought to strengthen the nerves, and the juice of the fresh plant is dropped into the ears of a patient suffering from hearing loss. Lavender is a mild antiseptic, and can be applied in various forms to burns, wounds, insect bites, sores, and bruises. Some people develop marked allergic reactions to the herb, and its use should immediately be discontinued if negative reactions occur. It is also not recommended for pregnant or nursing women.

Special Cures

Restorative Tea after Stroke: The four herbs most prized in the Alpine regions as restorative medicines after strokes are lavender buds, burnet saxifrage roots, masterwort roots *(Peucedanum ostruthium)*, and pellitory roots *(Anacyclus officinarum)*. The three root drugs are very potent, and should only be employed in minute quantities as tea, under the supervision of a doctor or experienced herbalist.

Uses in Husbandry

Lavender, and especially spike lavender, is a plant favored by bees, and is also said to have a calming effect on lions and tigers. Because of this, professional lion-tamers sometimes use oil of lavender as a sedative and tranquilizing agent. Chicken farmers have also been known to add a little lavender to their charges' water in May to reduce disease and lice infestation in the hencoop that year. Lavender flowers are dried and included in herbal tobaccos and snuffs. Lavender oil is also employed in the embalming industry, and to denature spirits. Painters prepare porcelain for subsequent painting with the oil of spike lavender.

Veterinary Values

Oil of lavender is an effective aid against parasites and lice. Lavender leaves and flowers act as a mild external anesthetic, and they have, in an emergency, been rubbed onto snakebites. Lavender tea is sometimes used as a disinfecting douche or enema.

Miscellaneous Wisdom

The Tyroleans believed lavender to be blessed by God, and therefore employed it to help them win their battles against the devil and to prevent evil. In Italy, lavender picked on Midsummer's Eve is reputed to be helpful against all black magic, and to keep away the Evil Eye. In Spain, it is burned in midsummer bonfires for the same purposes. In Austria, mothers lay lavender in their children's cradles to keep them safe, and to prevent rashes and convulsions. Unscrupulous women have been known to mix lavender in the foods they serve a man of their desire. The ancient Romans were not as enthusiastic about lavender, for they believed that poisonous asps would always be found in the vicinity of the herb.

Herbal Pastimes

The following nursery rhyme may not be as innocuous as it now appears, given the abortifacient reputation of the two herbs mentioned in the song:

> Lavender blue, and Rosemary green,
> When I am king, you shall be queen,
> Call up my maids at four of the clock,
> Some to the wheel and some to the rock,
> Some to make hay, and some to shell corn,
> And you and I will keep the bed warm.[184]

---

184. *Mother Goose's Melodies*, facsimile of the Monroe and Francis 1833 edition (New York: Dover, 1970) 28.

The several chairs of order look you scour
With juice of balm and every precious flower.

—William Shakespeare, *The Merry Wives of Windsor*

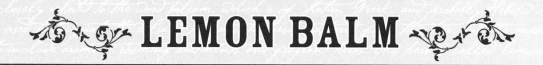

LEMON BALM

Name

"Balm" is closely related to the word "balsam," which is of Latin, Greek, and probably Hebrew origin. The word was originally used to designate the balsam tree and the resin gathered from this tree, but its meaning was later changed to include aromatic soothing ointments and fragrant herbs. The herb is called "lemon" balm because of its fresh and lemony smell.

The botanical name *Melissa* is of Greek origin, and refers to the bees that visit the plant in great numbers. Since it was an officially recognized herbal remedy, the herb is therefore called *Melissa officinalis*. Lemon balm is a perennial member of the **Mint** family.

Folk Names

Lemon balm has been known as apiastrum, bawme, baulm, balme, melissa, balm gentle, smiths bawme, carpenters bawme, iron-wort, sweet balm, garden balm, blue balm, common balm, cure-all, dropsy plant, golden or green balm, and geebalm. In Germany, it is known as *Melisse, Zitronenmelisse, Gartenmelisse, Immenblatt, Hasenohr, Mutterkraut, Herztrost, englische Brennessel*, and *spanischer Salbei*. In France, a few of its current names are *mélisse, citronelle, citronnade, herbe au citron*, and *piment des abeilles*; in Spanish-speaking countries, it is *toronjil*. In Italy, it is called *melissa, apiastro, citraggine, erba cedrata*, and *citronella*. In Danish, it is called *hjertensfryd*; and in Russian, *melissa lekarstvennaja* or *limonnaja mjata*.

A plant with similar properties, also a member of the **Mint** family, is the North American *Monarda didyma*. It is often confused with lemon balm because of the similarity of the plants' names. The American herb is called bee balm, red bee

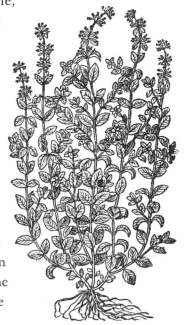

balm, monarda, oswego tea, and scarlet monarda. The herb's German name is *Goldmelisse*.

Appearance

Lemon balm has a perennial rootstock, and forms a thick, medium to light green, leafy and compact bush when well established. A lemon balm plant can grow to be 30 years old and 3 ft. high, although it usually succumbs to hard frosts before then. The entire plant has a strong and sweet lemony smell. Its leaves also taste like lemon, with a spicy, somewhat astringent aftertaste. The many stems are upright, square, branching, and a little hairy, with a pair of heart-shaped leaves at each joint. The leaves are opposite, and either heart-shaped or oval. They are pointed at the ends, serrated at the edge, and wrinkled. They contain oil glands and often have a shiny look, although they will lose this in winter and if the weather is too dry. The leaves are similar to those of catmint, or even nettles, but the smooth, bushy appearance of the plant is its major identifying characteristic. Lemon balm flowers are insignificant and appear in clusters of 3–6. Their color varies from white to yellowish, pink, red, pale blue, or purple. Lemon balm seeds are tiny and black, and fall out easily.

Place, Season, and Useful Parts

Lemon balm is mostly a cultivated plant, and does well up to an altitude of 2,500 ft. It grows wild in some parts of the Orient and southern Europe and can be found as an escapee from cultivation in vineyards and hedges, or even on walls and rubble, or near fences. In abandoned gardens, it is one of the common survivors. It should be treated as an annual in extreme northern latitudes or cold areas, but is perennial in the south. It usually blooms from June through September. Lemon balm leaves are gathered before the plant flowers, or the entire plant is cut before the first frost.

Gathering, Drying, and Storage

For home and kitchen use, it is best to cut lemon balm as needed. Leaves gathered after the plant has flowered are not as aromatic as those gathered before, and dried lemon balm is not as aromatic as the fresh herb. When grown on a commercial scale, the plant is harvested in June with sickles, and then again in September. The plants should not be cut back too severely late in the year, or they may suffer from frost. Like many other herbs, lemon balm plants will go many years without frost damage, but then hard freezes in the early spring with no snow cover can destroy whole stands.

Lemon balm quickly loses its oils on drying and is therefore more effective if used fresh or frozen, or if the medicinal properties of the herb have been preserved in alcohol. If there is a bumper crop, the leaves can be dried. These must be stripped quickly from the stalks and dried in an airy, shady place. The dried leaves should be stored whole, and only crumbled before use. Lemon balm should never be stored in metal containers. Dried lemon balm will only keep for a few months.

Seed Saving and Germination

Several distinct variants of lemon balm exist, including variegated types, and the oil content will also vary widely between varieties. These must be isolated if the varieties are to be kept distinct, for bees love the plant and will cross different strains. It is also difficult to harvest the seeds of lemon balm, for they fall out easily. The best method of gathering seeds is to look at the ripening seeds every day with a magnifying glass. First, the plant flowers, then it forms a yellowish globe, which develops into a seed receptacle. The plants should be cut when a large number of the seeds are almost ripe, and left to ripen on cloths or head down in paper bags. Lemon balm seeds usually retain their fertility for 2–3 years, but can be dried with silica gel and then frozen with good results.

Gardening Hints

Charlemagne recommended lemon balm as a suitable medicinal garden herb. It grows profusely once it has established itself, even becoming a nuisance through its persistent habit of self-seeding. Because of the large numbers of plants produced from one parent plant, it can be used as a border plant to good advantage. In warmer climates, it will form a shrub-like plant in two years' time. Lemon balm is not generally susceptible to frost, but may die back completely in years marked by cycles of alternate thawing and freezing. Lemon balm generally helps to repel garden pests, and aids the growth of plants placed in its vicinity. Lemon balm plants should be renewed every four years if they are to be used for medicinal and culinary purposes.

Lemon balm seeds are sown in April or May, and will sprout in 3–4 weeks. The easiest way to propagate lemon balm is through plant division in spring, or again in fall. Established plants self-seed readily and will tolerate full sun, but prefer moist, humus-rich soil and a shady position. It is advisable to stir up the soil between the plants' roots in fall, and cut down the old stems before the end of summer. In especially cold climates, the plants can be protected with branches, straw, or mulch before killing frosts set in. Some cooks bring a plant indoors for kitchen use in winter. Lemon balm grows well in window boxes during the winter months.

Culinary Virtues

Lemon balm's extraordinary qualities as a seasoning herb are often overlooked. This is probably because the herb does not dry well, and is not often grown in herb gardens anymore. Lemon balm can be substituted for lemon thyme, or even for lemons in most recipes. It has many of the same seasoning properties as mint. Lemon balm loses most of its delicate flavor if cooked or boiled, and tastes best if the small, tender young leaves are chopped and added to food just before serving. Because the leaves are tender and the taste is not overpowering, they can be added in larger amounts than most other herbs.

In the sixteenth century, Otto Brunfels suggested sprinkling meat with the distilled water of lemon balm to discourage maggots. Even in the age of refrigeration and deep freezing, lemon balm tea can be used to wash a piece of meat that is not as fresh as it should be. Chicken or cuts of lamb are often rubbed with lemon balm before roasting. Roast duck stuffed with apples, dried prunes, and chopped lemon balm can be an exciting culinary experience. Fish can also be stuffed with lemon balm before broiling, and eel soup is often flavored with the herb. Chicken is occasionally served with a sherry and lemon balm sauce. Salads, as well as yogurt dressings, can be improved with the addition of a little chopped lemon balm. Olive oil and vinegar are sometimes flavored with lemon balm for winter use. Lemon balm leaves combine well with sweet as well as heartier dishes, and they may be added in small amounts to custards, milk puddings, yogurt, and baked apple dishes.

A few centuries ago, a popular recipe for a medicinal tansy, or pancake, called for eggs, sugar, rose water, and the juice of the lemon balm plant. (A more modern recipe would call for generous amounts of chopped lemon balm added to the pancake batter.) Serve the pancakes with honey or maple syrup. Lemon balm was also valued as a beverage flavoring; according to John Evelyn,

> The tender Leaves are us'd in Composition with other Herbs; and the Sprigs fresh gather'd, put into Wine or other Drinks, during the heat of Summer, give it a marvellous quickness: this noble Plant yields an incomparable Wine, made as is that of Cowslip-Flowers.[185]

In our century, lemon balm's use as in beverages has been restricted to adding the herb to lemonade, sweet wine punches, fruit bowls, and iced tea. Lemon balm spirits or liqueurs are excellent drinks, and can help to combat melancholy on dark and rainy winter days if used in moderation. *Melissengeist* is a medicinal preparation served with boiling water as a warming drink on cold days when the flu is going around.

Lemon balm does not dry well, and is best used fresh. It can be chopped and frozen in small portions in ice trays, and the single cubes then kept in a plastic bag or box in the freezer for winter use.

---

185.   Evelyn, *Acetaria: A Discourse of Sallets* (London: B. Tooke, 1699), 10.

Noteworthy Recipes

Lemon-Yogurt Sauce: This sauce is very simple to prepare, but complements both grain and fruit dishes. It can be served with millet, quinoa, brown rice, bulghur, or couscous, or used to refine desserts made with fresh fruit and fresh fruit salads.

Combine 1 cup of yogurt with 1 heaping Tbsp. of chopped lemon balm leaves. If serving with grain dishes, 1–2 cloves of crushed garlic and a little salt can be added, but if serving with fruits, sweeten with 1–2 Tbsp. of clear honey or pure brown cane sugar.

Household Applications

The fresh lemony scent of lemon balm makes it a delightful potpourri and sachet herb, as well as a pleasant addition to sleeping cushions. It can be used as a strewing herb, or hung in bunches in the kitchen as an air freshener. Lemon balm will help to drive moths out of cupboards and linen closets. A few drops of lemon balm essence or lemon balm spirits can be added to cleansing mixtures and polishes to give them a fresh lemony aroma.

Cosmetic Properties

Lemon balm oil and lemon balm water are added to perfumes and colognes, and used as perfuming agents for cosmetic mixtures. A simple lemon balm water is made by filling a bottle with fresh leaves, covering them with clear, strong spirits, and letting the mixture stand, firmly stoppered, in the sun for one week before straining and filtering through filter paper. The resulting balm spirits can be diluted with distilled water if desired. This water is said to remove freckles.

A strong infusion of lemon balm can be applied to hair to darken it, and to cover the first traces of gray. Lemon balm eye drops or compresses can also ease the pains of tired, sore eyes, and a lemon balm gargle will help to sweeten the breath. A few lemon balm leaves are added to pochettes or bath bags hung over the hot water faucet for a stimulating bath.

Medicinal Merits

The heart-shaped leaves of lemon balm are its medicinal signature. It is one of the best heart and nerve herbs, and was said by earlier herbalists to "strengthen nature much in all its actions,"[186] also banning sadness and melancholy. It was praised profusely by Arab physicians, used by Paracelsus in his *Elixir Vitae*, and taken by monks to aid concentration. It was prescribed to dispel melancholic vapors arising from the heart and arteries,

---

186.   Nicholas Culpeper, *Culpeper's Complete Herbal* (1653) (London: Foulsham, undated), 36.

to counteract hysteria and hypochondria, to cure epilepsy and renew vital spirits, and to strengthen the brain and rejuvenate the body. It was even believed to make the taciturn talkative if laid on their tongues. Lemon balm was occasionally substituted for horehound.

Modern Medicine

Lemon balm's efficacy as a heart and nerve herb has been confirmed by modern medicine. It is one of the few herbs with a strengthening influence on the heart, which at the same time calms the nerves. It can be taken over a long time without harmful side effects as a regular drink for students, elderly patients, invalids, and people with nervous complaints. Its aroma is so exquisitely pleasing and gratifying that even those who categorically refuse herbal teas may be seduced by its fragrance.

Lemon balm can be taken regularly to strengthen the heart and to help prevent coronaries. Homeopaths prescribe the herb for general exhaustion, hysteria, sleeplessness, nervous heart troubles, migraines, and flatulence. Convalescents and those suffering from the aftereffects of too much work or unusual stress can profit by the continued use of lemon balm. Students may find it helpful as a calming drink before exams, and insomniacs should try drinking lemon balm tea regularly as a nightcap ½ hour before retiring. Because of its strengthening effect on the heart and nerves, it is a good herbal follow-up, especially in combination with lavender, for those who have had a heart attack or are suffering from partial paralysis, circulatory troubles, a tendency to faintness, anemia, cramps, and nervous digestive disorders. Lemon balm can help to relieve the symptoms of tobacco poisoning, seasickness, and nervous nausea. Pregnant women can take it to relieve the symptoms of morning sickness, and a tea of lemon balm and goose grass (*Potentilla anserina*) is an excellent relaxant for women plagued with menstrual cramps.

Lemon balm is now being used in the treatment of viral and autoimmune diseases, and has also been shown to have a regulative effect on thyroid imbalances, and consequently on fatigue, chronic fatigue syndrome, and menopausal imbalances. It has also been proven effective in treating acute outbreaks of shingles and herpes. Oil of lemon balm has occasionally been used in the treatment of allergies.

Lemon balm tea is often added to various herbal mixtures to improve their flavor. The best tea is made from the fresh leaves of the green plant. The active principle can also be extracted from the fresh leaves with alcoholic spirits, and this lemon balm water taken a teaspoonful at a time with hot water. Aromatherapy makes extensive use of the herb.

Poultices of bruised fresh lemon balm leaves have a cooling, healing, and soothing effect when applied externally to wounds, bruises, and cuts. The pains of cramps, milk knots, and nervous headaches as well as the symptoms of jet lag can be lessened by rubbing the area or the head with lemon balm water. Baths of marjoram and lemon balm are invaluable for women with nervous female complaints.

Special Cures

Melissa Cordial: Lemon balm water, made as directed in the section on cosmetics, can also be used for medicinal purposes. A lemon balm cordial can be prepared by filling a bottle with the tops of the plant and a few sprigs of betony (*Stachys officinalis*, earlier known as *Betonica officinalis*), a small amount of unsprayed, grated lemon peel, one crushed nutmeg, some coriander seeds, a stick of cinnamon, and a few cloves. Fill the bottle with clear, high-proof spirits, and let stand, well stoppered, in the sun until the mixture darkens. Strain, filter the mixture through cheesecloth or filter paper, and dilute as needed with distilled water. This melissa cordial is said to strengthen the nerves and the heart, while improving the memory and concentration.

A Simple Circulatory Tea: A simple circulatory tea that can be taken as a refreshing drink between meals is mixed from 1 part lemon balm leaves, 1 part European mistletoe, and 1 part whitethorn flowers (*Crataegus laevigata*). Infuse 1 tsp. of the herbs with ½ pint of boiling water, and let stand covered for 10–15 minutes before serving.

Uses in Husbandry

In accordance with its botanical name, *Melissa*, lemon balm is a bee herb. Bees can be fed with lemon balm tea sweetened with honey from another hive, or with sugar. The hives can also be rubbed with lemon balm to discourage bees from swarming. Lemon balm honey, produced by bees kept next to lemon balm fields, is especially aromatic. According to the sixteenth-century German physician Tabernaemontanus, bees will not sting a man if he is carrying lemon balm or wearing a wreath of the herb on his head. As Virgil wrote,

> I urge you, sprinkle round
> Scents of crushed balm leaf and honeywort…
> The bees will settle down on the scented seats,
> And hide in the cradling cells, as ther custom is.[187]

Lemon balm can also be used as fodder, and is said to increase the milk production of dairy cattle. Dried lemon balm leaves are used as flavoring agents for herbal tobacco mixtures.

---

187.   *Virgil's Georgics*, Trans. Smith Palmer Bovie (Chicago: Univ. of Chicago Press, 1956), Bk. IV, l. 82.

Veterinary Values

Lemon balm is administered by veterinarians as a mild animal sedative and to counteract the effects of shock. Cows are given lemon balm and marjoram tea after calving.

Miscellaneous Wisdom

Lemon balm was already recognized as a healing herb by the ancient Greeks, and was used at the Temple of Diana at Ephesus. Dioscurides writes, "ye leaves being drunk with wine, & also applied are good for Scorpion-smitten, & ye Phalangium-bitten, and ye dog-bitten ... "[188] According to Pliny, lemon balm can stop the flow of blood from a wound if the sword that gave the wound can be found, and the herb tied to it.

In more recent times, lemon balm has been used in potions to counteract magic and enchantment, and is hung over the door on Midsummer's Eve to discourage witches and other maleficent influences. German "old wives" suggest wrapping sprigs of lemon balm in babies' diapers to keep away evil spirits, stomachaches, and flatulence.

Literary Flowers

> *Sweet scented herbs her skill contrives*
> *To rub the bramble platted hives*
> *Fennels thread leaves and crimpld balm*
> *To scent the new house of the swarm.*

—JOHN CLARE, *THE SHEPHERD'S CALENDAR*, "MAY"

---

188. Robert T. Gunther, ed., *The Greek Herbal of Dioscurides* (New York: Hafner, 1959), 348.

The brook resumes its summer dresses purling neath grass and water cresses
and mint and flag leaf swording high their blooms to the unheeding eye ...

—JOHN CLARE, THE SHEPHERD'S CALENDER, "MAY"

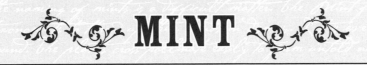

MINT

Name

The naming of mints is a difficult matter. The **Mint** family is one that can cause levelheaded botanists and taxonomists to throw up their hands in dismay, and it is even harder for the layperson to know his or her way around. The plants cross-pollinate easily, forming untold new bastard strains. (Peppermint is actually a bastard produced by a cross between *Mentha aquatica* and *Mentha spicata*.)

All the mints supposedly owe their name, and the botanical term *Mentha*, to Greek legend. Minthe, the daughter of the river god Kokytos, was Hades' lover. She was punished for her fornication by Hades' bride, Persephone, and transformed into a perennial aromatic herb that was given her name. But according to some etymologists, the word has an even more ancient origin—the Sanskrit *manth*.

The following is an incomplete list of some of the recognized mints:

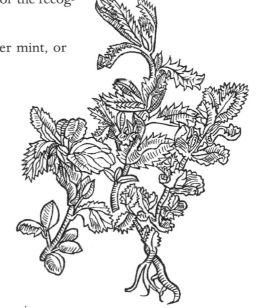

- *Mentha aquatica*—Water mint, wild water mint, or marsh mint
- *Mentha arvensis var. arvensis*—Corn mint
- *Mentha arvensis var. piperascens*—Japanese mint
- *Mentha x gentilis*—American apple mint
- *Mentha longifolia var. longifolia*—Horsemint
- *Mentha x piperita*—Peppermint
- *Mentha x piperita f. pallescens*—White mint
- *Mentha x piperita f. piperita*—Black mint
- *Mentha pulegium*—Pennyroyal

- *Mentha spicata var. crispa*—Curled mint
- *Mentha spicata var. spicata*—Spearmint
- *Mentha citrata*—Bergamot mint, orange mint
- *Mentha rotundifolia*—Apple-scented mint

The sky's the limit with different mints. Dozens of distinct species have been documented, along with countless garden varieties. There are some that smell like cologne or are as biting as Lysol, as pungent as camphor, or as delicate as pineapple. Gardeners have been overdoing themselves for centuries to produce newer and better mint hybrid creations.

> *But if any man can name*
> *The full list of all the kinds and all the properties*
> *Of mint, he must be one who knows how many fish*
> *Swim in the Indian Ocean, how many sparks Vulcan*
> *Sees fly in the air from his vast furnace in Etna.*

—WAHLAFRIDUS STRABO, *HORTULUS*

Folk Names

The best-known mint, peppermint *(Mentha x piperita)* is also known as brandy mint, black peppermint, or lamb mint. Germans call it *Pfefferminze, Edelminze, Hausminze,* and *Pfefferkraut.* French names are *menthe, menthe poivrée,* and *menthe Anglaise.* Italians call it *menta pepe, menta pepecina, mentastro,* and *sisembro*; the Irish, *mismú*; Russians, *mjata perečnaja.* A subspecies, orange mint *(Mentha piperita var. citrata)* is also known as bergamot mint, or, in Spanish, *yerba buena,* a term also used for other local mints.

Spearmint *(Mentha spicata var. crispa)* is also called garden mint, mackerel mint, fish mint, lamb mint, green mint, spire mint, garden spear, sage of Bethlehem, Our Lady's mint, and curled mint. Germans call it *Krauseminze* or *Krausebalsam*; the French, *menthe verte* or *menthe crépue*; and the Russians, *mjata kolosovaja.*

Apple-scented mint *(Mentha rotundifolia, M. suaveolens)* goes by the name of apple mint, round-leaved mint, and Egyptian mint.

Pennyroyal *(Mentha pulegium)* is also known as pudding grass, pennie royall, lurk-in-the-ditch, lurkie-dish, lily-royal, whirl mint, organy (not to be confused with wild oregano!), European pennyroyal, and run-on-the-ground. It was called *pulogium regale* in Latin and *dweorge-dwostle* in Old English, and John Gerard named it *pulegium regium vulgatum.* Germans call it *Poleiminze, Poley,* and *Flohkraut*; the French, *pouliot, herbe aux puces, chasse-puces,* and *herbe de Saint-Laurent*; the Italians, *puleggio, pulezzo, polezzo,* and *mentaccio*; and the Russians, *mjata blošnica.*

Appearance

There is a great deal of variety within this species. The stems range from large and square to thin and red; the leaves can be variegated or large and hoary; the flowers can be tiny and almost hidden or large, open blooms, and the array of scents to be found is truly amazing. But each mint has more or less rounded leaves, in opposite pairs, often tinged with red, and an odor that, despite the variations, is still recognizable as minty.

Peppermint grows to a height of 3 ft. and is, strictly speaking, an annual plant, since it does die back in the winter. However, one plant can produce an incredible number of new plants and runners within that year and literally overrun the garden. Peppermint stalks may be covered with down, depending on the variety, but the leaves are hairless. The flowers are white to purple in color, in panicles 1–3 in. long.

Spearmint grows to a maximum height of 20 in., and also has white, purple, or pink flowers. The flowers of curled mint are of a reddish-purple color. Apple mint has large, grayish-green leaves covered with hairs, similar to water mint. Orange mint has tiny rounded leaves that are extremely aromatic.

Place, Season, and Useful Parts

The mints blossom from June into September. Peppermint is grown in most of Europe, Asia, North and South America, and Africa, and often escapes from cultivated areas. The amount of oil present in the plant varies widely from location to location. It was first grown commercially in Great Britain in 1750.

Spearmint was originally a native of the Mediterranean, and was brought to England by the Romans. It now grows wild in the vicinity of slowly running streams in Europe, Asia, and North America, and is often cultivated. Curled mint and countless other cultivated varieties are to be found in gardens, although they often bastardize with wild mints and may escape beyond the garden gate.

Pennyroyal originally came from the Mediterranean. It was once more widely cultivated than now, especially in the Middle Ages. It can still be found growing wild in damp meadows, flooded places, or on riverbanks in North America, Europe, and the Middle East. Other wild mints can be found in damp places the world over. They are generally perennial.

Gathering, Drying, and Storage

In general, if a mint-like plant has a pleasant taste, it's safe to gather and use it. There are no poisonous, only some unpleasant-tasting, mints. Care should be taken, though, not to gather plants infested by rust, and to remove shriveled and diseased parts of the plant. Mint must never be damp when gathered; the best harvesting time is on a sunny day in the morning, just after the dew has dried.

Peppermint can be cut twice in one year, the first time in July, just when the blossom buds are forming for a leaf crop, and then again in September, for a crop with a high oil content. Peppermint can be cut as needed for home use, or harvested on a large scale with sickles 2–3 in. above ground. Curled mint and spearmint should be gathered before the plant blossoms.

Mint leaves must be stripped from the stalk immediately after harvest, and dried quickly indoors in an airy place to preserve the plants' aromatic oils. Eight lb. of fresh leaves will produce approximately 1 lb. of dried leaves. Mint leaves should be stored in closed containers and will usually not keep their aroma for more than a year.

Seed Saving and Germination

If mints are to be maintained true-to-type, it is necessary to remember that they do set seed, and any seed will produce mixed plants, for there are certainly other mints growing in the vicinity that will cross with the original plants. It is necessary to prevent the plants from going to seed by cutting them down or harvesting them before they blossom. They can be propagated vegetatively if varietal purity is desired. This simply means that new plants are started from a small piece of the mother root, or part of the plant. These plants are then kept from blossoming so that seed is not set, which would produce bastard strains.

Pennyroyal can be very variable, and plants with the desired characteristics should be propagated by plant division. Pennyroyal prefers closely packed or even compacted soil, and may die if planted in loose soil.

In exhibition gardens, mints can be used to illustrate the idea of biological diversity. The visitor is encouraged to smell and sample 10–12 mints, in all their variety. Usually, the reaction is, "I didn't know there were so many mints!" The tour guide can then elaborate on the theme of biological diversity within one plant species.

Gardening Hints

As the Somerset saying goes, "Mint is shy; one should never look at it for a month after planting it; it needs time to settle down." Once it has settled down, though, mint soon makes up for its initial reluctance, and may even attempt to crowd out other plants. This can be prevented by planting mint in old bottomless metal pails or boxes sunk into the ground. Wild mint can also spread and multiply so that it takes over entire meadows. The Swiss say that horse mint can only be eradicated on certain days under the influence of the proper signs. Unfortunately, humans have not been able to discover which days and signs are best for this purpose.

Established mint plants can be walked upon without harming the plants. Because of this characteristic, they are planted in the pathways and borders of formal herbal gardens.

They exude oils that discourage ants and can also help to control aphids and cabbage caterpillars. Mints aid the growth and flavor of cabbages, peas, and tomatoes if grown in their vicinity. Peppermint and chamomile can be planted next to each other to increase the oil content of both herbs, and nettles are also said to exert a positive effect on the oil content of peppermint plants. Potato plants should never be placed next to mint.

Peppermint has been cultivated since ancient times. It was raised in China and Japan thousands of years ago, and the Pharaohs also ordered its cultivation. It is mentioned in the New Testament, and in Dioscurides' *Herbal*, but was first planted on a large scale toward the end of the seventeenth (and in Germany, the end of the eighteenth) century. The present demand for peppermint oil and peppermint tea is so large that is has become one of the most important herbal crops.

Mints prefer loose, humus-rich, damp but well-aerated soil. They will not prosper in standing or stagnant waters, but grow well on moors and in damp, shady places, and will flourish in rich, sandy soil in a southern position. Mints can be grown from seed, but are usually propagated by planting runners or cuttings, or by plant division. Mint seeds should be sown in the spring in a damp, sheltered, and wind-protected spot. The roots and runners are divided in March, or cuttings are taken throughout the summer. Young peppermint plants should be mulched with compost or leaf mold to retain moisture and discourage weeds. Geese may be used to weed mint fields, since they do not like the taste of the plant and will eat everything else in sight (and also manure the fields). Peppermint beds should be fertilized regularly with compost or manure, but not with wood ashes. The beds should be rotated or renewed regularly to prevent the plants from becoming infected with rust. Care must be taken, though, to see that no runners are left in the bed. Some growers renew peppermint plants every 2 years; others wait 3 or even 5 years. Plants spotted with rust should be burned immediately. The bed should not be replanted with mint for several years. Barley is considered a good green manure replacement crop.

The other mints are raised like peppermint, and are usually propagated by root division and runners. Bergamot mint prefers dry soil and does well in rock gardens. It can also be planted as a border. Apple mint is easy to grow and produces large amounts of leaves for tea. Pennyroyal prefers tightly compacted soil and may "wander" away from loose beds into paths. It prefers acid or neutral soil. The seed should be sown in trays and just barely covered with soil.

Culinary Virtues

The mints have a cooling and refreshing taste and are often added to drinks, beverages, and liqueurs. Peppermint and date wine is a Jewish drink from olden times. Peppermint beer was popular in the Middle Ages, and Russian *kvass* is prepared from peppermint, barley, and rye. Mint julep is a favorite American drink in the southern states, and peppermint liqueurs and crème de menthe are known in some form or other throughout the world. Lemonade and iced tea are often flavored with a few sprigs of peppermint, and the herb can also be added to fruit cups and to cranberry and vegetable juices. Peppermint or mint tea is a refreshing tisane, and is served heavily sweetened at all times of the day in Arab countries. After dark, the cocktail bars of the world serve mojitos, prepared with fresh mint, sugar, and rum.

The flavor of mint complements both sweet and salty foods. Mint leaves, fresh or candied, make a pretty garnish. Peppermint is used to flavor soups, sauces, salads, spring rolls, and stuffings. Yogurt salad dressings deserve praise if they are flavored with a few finely chopped fresh mint leaves. Peas, beans, carrots, beets, new potatoes and potato salads, grain dishes, tabouli, cabbage, spinach, and all vegetables with a strong flavor can be flavored with the judicious use of a little mint.

On the sweet side, peppermint can also be added to fruit salads, ice cream, sherbets, milk shakes, and cheesecakes. Peppermint leaves are often candied, and lozenges prepared from sugar and peppermint oil. An excellent mint cake can be made from shortening, sugar, flour, and chopped fresh mint, mixed well together and rolled very thin before baking. Peppermint extract is employed extensively by confectioners for making all kinds of candy. Mint leaves can be crystallized by dipping them first in stiffly beaten egg white and then in sugar, and drying them in a slow oven.

Spearmint and curled mint, and even orange or pineapple mint, have a sweeter taste than peppermint and are therefore often added to drinks, mint sauces, and sweets. Unpasteurized milk keeps better, and does not coagulate as readily, if a sprig of spearmint is floated on it. The ancient Romans used spearmint as a flavoring for wine cups. Mint juleps and mint liqueurs can also be prepared with spearmint. Ginger ale and orange and lemon juice punches can be improved by the addition of the herb. The ancient Romans used it to flavor meat, and spearmint is served today in sauce or jelly form with lamb and mutton. Green peas, new potatoes, pulses, soups, salads, fish, and eggs can also be seasoned with it. An exotic dessert is prepared by dipping sprigs of spearmint in dough, frying them, and serving them with powdered sugar.

Apple-scented mint is often added to mint jellies, and is a complementary seasoning for applesauce and other apple dishes. Some cooks prefer it above all others for mint sauce, although the flavor is not as delicate.

Pennyroyal has a strongly pungent flavor, and is therefore often neglected as a kitchen herb. It once flavored medicinal beers and was added to bag puddings, hog's puddings, and black puddings, and was occasionally used as a condiment.

Water mint can be substituted for peppermint or spearmint, especially in the preparation of drinks. Horse and corn mint are only rarely used because of their strong flavor.

Noteworthy Recipes

Mint Sauce: One of the most famous of all mint recipes is for mint sauce.

> Wash half a handful of nice young fresh-gathered Green Mint (to this some add one third the quantity of Parsley), pick the leaves from the stalk, mince them very fine, and put them into a sauceboat, with a tea-spoonful of moist sugar, and four tablespoonsful of Vinegar.
>
> Obs. This is the usual accompaniment to Hot Lamb; and an equally agreeable relish with Cold Lamb.
>
> If Green Mint cannot be procured, this sauce may be made from Mint Vinegar.[189]

Mint jelly can be used in place of mint sauce with lamb, especially if wine is going to be served with the meal. Mint jelly is prepared in the same manner as basil jelly (see basil chapter). Traditionally, mint jelly is prepared from spearmint.

To Make a Syrup of Mint: The following is an unusual recipe for mint syrup.

> Take the Juyce of ripe Quinces, and of Pomgranates of each a pint and a half: dried Mint half a pound, and of the Leaves (petals) of red Roses two ounces; and let them steep a day and a night in the Liquor; boil it until half is consumed, and add four pound of Sugar to make it into a Syrup.[190]

Two old recipes for pennyroyal may be of interest to adventurous or scholarly cooks, even if they do not please modern tastes.

To Make Sausages the Best Way: Take a Leg of Pork, divide the fat from the lean, and chop the latter small, with Marjorum, Penn-royal, Thyme and Winter Savory, adding Salt, Pepper, and a little Ginger together with half the quantity Of Meat in Beef-Suet; and being very small, fill it in Sheeps-guts with a Whale-bone-fescue, and dry them in a Chimney for your use.[191]

Penny-royal Pudding: Take a pretty Quantity of Penny-royal and Marigold Flower, &c. very well shred, and mingle with the cream (Half a Pint of fresh Cream or New Milk), Eggs (six new laid Eggs, taking out three of the Whites), half a Pound of fresh Butter, near half a pound of Sugar, and a little Salt; some grated Nutmeg and beaten Spice, four spoonfuls of Sack; half a Pint more of Cream, and almost a Pound of Beef-Suet chopt very small, the Gratings of a Two-Penny Loaf, and stirring all well together, put it into a Bag flower'd and

---

189.   William Kitchiner, *The Cook's Oracle* (1817) (London: Samuel Bagster, 1860), 237.

190.   John Shirley, *The Accomplished Ladies Rich Closet of Rarities* (London: N. Bodington, 1688), 30.

191.   Ibid, 115.

tie it fast. It will be boil'd within an Hour: or may be baked in the Pan like Carrot-Pudding. The sauce is for both, a little Rose-water, less Vinegar, with Butter beaten together and poured on it sweetened with the Sugar Caster.

Of this Plant discreetly dried, is made a most wholsom and excellent Tea.[192]

Yogurt Mint Sauce: This comes to us from the Middle East and India, where mint is widely used in cookery. For each cup of plain yogurt, take ½ cup of chopped mint (peppermint is usually used, but orange mint also tastes very good), 2 cloves of garlic, and 1 tsp. of freshly grated ginger root. Thin with fresh lime juice to taste, and add a little salt if desired. Serve fresh with salads and meats, or as a dunking mixture with spicy meals.

Mint Butter: Mint butter is prepared in the same manner as other herbal butters, with creamed butter, half again as much chopped mint, a teaspoon of lemon juice, and salt and pepper to taste. Mix well, and serve on cooked vegetables or grilled meat.

Household Applications

All the mints are used as strewing and garlanding herbs and can also be included in sachet, potpourri, and sleeping cushion mixtures. Freshly strewn mint or mint potpourri can even help to overpower the penetrating odor of cigarette smoke. In Greece, wooden tables are scrubbed with fresh mint and then rinsed with clear water to remove unpleasant odors. Commercial menthol is a common ingredient of household cleansing, waxing, and deodorizing mixtures. Japanese mint contains the high percentage of ethereal oils used to produce menthol.

Water and corn mint are available in such quantities that they are obvious candidates for strewing herbs. Watermint was once considered sacred to Aphrodite, and is still fashioned into bridal garlands by the Greeks. Spearmint and curled mint are preferred for use in sleeping cushions and potpourri because of their very sweet and fragrant odor. In past times, pennyroyal was used as well, but probably more for its insecticidal properties than as a sweet fragrance. Today, it is still used in soaps and in perfumery.

Most of the mints repel insects. All the mints, fresh or dried, as well as commercial menthol, help to protect linens and woolens from moths. Fresh peppermint is widely used in Arab countries to drive away flies. Pennyroyal leaves can be rubbed onto hands and neck to repel midges and mosquitoes. The plant is also, true to its botanical name *pulegium*, a flea repellent when it is burned, and is said to discourage ants and spiders. At a time when polluted or infested waters were called "suspicious," herbalists recommended

---

192.　John Evelyn, *Acetaria: A Discourse of Sallets* (London: B. Tooke, 1699), Appendix.

laying pennyroyal wreaths on these waters to purify them. A similar plant, the American mock pennyroyal, *Hedeoma pulegioides*, is used in commercial insect repellents.

Cosmetic Properties

Commercial, chemically produced menthol is very widely used as a perfuming and refreshing agent for soaps, shaving creams, after-shave lotions, mentholated spirits, toothpastes, and creams. It is also added as a flavoring and perfuming agent to candies, cigarettes, and even paper handkerchiefs. Peppermint and spearmint oils and extracts flavor toothpastes, mouthwashes, chewing gum, cough drops, liniments, muscle rubs, facial lotions, and countless medicinal preparations. Peppermint gives perfumes a fresh aroma, while spearmint oil smells a little like citrus oil. Occasionally, other mints such as ginger mint or eau-de-Cologne mint are used in cosmetic preparations.

Peppermint has antiseptic and disinfectant as well as refreshing and cleansing properties. Peppermint compresses can be applied to oily skin or to blackheads, and skin eruptions or acne are bathed with a peppermint infusion. Peppermint baths were said by the herbalist John Parkinson "to comfort and strengthen the nerve and sinews," and are still considered stimulating, cooling, and refreshing, especially in hot weather. Peppermint oil and menthol are common ingredients of after-bath lotions and skin bracers. At one time, pennyroyal was burnt and applied as powder to bleeding gums.

Medicinal Merits

Peppermint was once considered hot and dry in the third degree, and horse mint even warmer. All the mints were thought to dry out sicknesses, awaken passions and a love of life, and ease digestion. Distilled mint water applied to men's genitals was thought to reawaken their interest in procreation. According to Culpeper, spearmint could "stir up venery or bodily lust"[193] and enable 60-year-old women to conceive. The mints were used to calm hysteria or, as it was then called, the "rising womb," and to lessen cramps. Pennyroyal was believed to ease delivery and the expulsion of the afterbirth. Mint compresses were employed to make a nursing woman's curdled milk flow, and a tea of mint and rue prescribed to stop a mother's milk during weaning. In Dioscurides' opinion, mint was good for many things; mixed with vinegar, it

> kills round worms, & it provokes lust; & two or three little spriggs being drank with ye juice of a sower pomegranate assuageth ye hickets [hiccups], & vomitings, & choler; & being applied with Polenta it dissolveth suppurations, & being laid to ye forehead it pacifyeth headaches, & assuageth ye swelling &

---

193.   Culpeper, *Culpeper's Complete Herbal* (1653) (London: Foulsham, undated), 274.

extension of ye duggs, but with salt it is a cataplasme for ye dog-bitten, but ye juice with melicrate helpeth ye ear paines, but being applied to women before conjunction doth work inconception, & being rubbed on it makes smooth a rough tongue, & it keeps ye milk from curdling, the leaves being seeped in it. And finally it is good for ye stomach, & fitt for sauce.[194]

Even "worms in the womb" were treated with mint. According to the School of Salernum, "The worms that gnawe the womb and never stint, / Are Kil'd, and purg'd, and driven away with mint."[195]

The warming properties of mint were also utilized for their beneficial action on the entire digestive system. Obstructions of the liver and spleen were treated with mint in wine. Worms were expelled by feeding the patient pennyroyal or peppermint salad. The stomach was comforted with mint tea. Melancholy, depressions, and headaches arising from digestive disorders were treated with mint, and mint was also thought to ease constipation and cleanse the kidneys and intestines, as well as combat gout. Spearmint juice in vinegar was used to staunch bleeding and to thin the blood. Too much spearmint was thought to encourage choler; minute doses of pennyroyal were thought to counteract it, and to ease brain fatigue and depression. According to the School of Salernum, "Let them that unto choller much incline / Drinke Penny-royall steeped in their wine."[196]

The mints were used to cleanse sores, to rinse the mouth and gums, and to clear watering or clouded eyes. Water mint was rubbed onto bee and wasp stings. Horse mint, the strongest of the family, was thought to improve hearing if tucked behind the ears and renewed hourly for several days. Ancient herbalists, in contrast to modern medicinal practitioners, considered pennyroyal weaker than other mints and prescribed it to increase the appetite and to treat angina, nausea, fainting spells, epilepsy, and tertian fever. A dangerous abortifacient mixture, which probably killed as many mothers as babies, was prepared from poison hemlock, rue, and pennyroyal.

Modern Medicine

The active ingredient of both peppermint and pennyroyal, menthol, is used by modern pharmacists in a bewildering variety of medicinal products ranging from cough drops to menthol sticks, herbal snuff, nose drops, Vaseline, inhaling mixtures, liniments, salves, mentholated spirits, and throat sprays. Pure peppermint oil is more effective

---

194.   Robert T. Gunther, ed., *The Greek Herbal of Dioscurides* (New York: Hafner, 1959), 274.

195.   Sir John Harrington, trans., *The School of Salernum* (Salerno, Italy: Ente Provinciale per il Turismo, 1953), 52.

196.   Ibid., 60.

than synthetic menthol, but more expensive and therefore seldom used. Peppermint oil is one of the best antispasmodic or cramp-loosening oils, and is added to salves and chest liniments or rubbing mixtures, and also used in inhaling mixtures to treat colds and toothaches.

One of the most interesting aspects of peppermint oil is its effect on the skin: first it works on the nerves to create a cooling sensation, and then it causes the skin to prickle and burn as if it were on fire (as in icy hot preparations). Peppermint oil and peppermint tea also have painkilling properties, and can help to draw out poisons and loosen cramps. A peppermint poultice can often cure a headache, and peppermint compresses can loosen milk knots. Cooled peppermint tea is used for gargling, and for washing bedridden and fevered patients.

Taken internally, peppermint has a warming effect, especially on the digestive organs. It is, contrary to popular belief, quite a strong drug, and should therefore not be taken indefinitely or indiscriminately. Large doses can even exert a harmful effect on the liver. Medical texts speak of peppermint as being antispasmodic, sudorific, febrifugal, and anthelmintic. To put it in plainer language, peppermint tea can be taken after a meal to aid digestion, to settle the stomach, relieve cramps and flatulence, and to discourage intestinal parasites. It can aid those afflicted with nausea, travel sickness, fainting spells, and intestinal colics, and is so soothing for the entire nervous system that it can be recommended for patients troubled with mental strain, overwork, or intellectual exhaustion. It can even alleviate nervous palpitations if taken in large doses (a cautionary note: massive doses can have a paralyzing effect). Two specific medicinal properties of peppermint are that it increases gall bladder secretions, and therefore helps prevent gallstones, and it can thin and finally arrest the milk flow of nursing mothers.

Peppermint is prescribed by homeopaths for stomach pain and flatulence, as well as for dry coughs. In Chinese medicine, peppermint is used to treat inflamation and rashes, sore throats, common colds, fevers, headaches, red eyes, beginning cases of measles, and abdominal distension.

Spearmint oil is less powerful than peppermint oil, for it does not contain menthol. It is usually employed in the treatment of children's respiratory complaints. Fresh spearmint-leaf compresses are applied to aching heads, and to ease the pains of gout and rheumatism. A homeopathic spearmint tincture is used to treat gravel, strangury, and painful hemorrhoids. In Chinese medicine, spearmint warms the stomach and is used to treat indigestion, headaches due to stress, dizziness, the common cold, low spirits, and menstrual pain. It is considered much more warming than peppermint.

The medicinal properties of curled mint are similar to those of spearmint, with one difference: curled mint is even more effective for flatulence.

Pennyroyal is similar in action to peppermint but should be used with caution, for it can, under certain conditions and in large doses, cause poisoning. Pennyroyal oil is applied externally to relieve uterine cramps and bring on a period, or to discourage parasites. It should not be used during pregnancy. Pennyroyal has a homeopathic influence on the right side of the body, especially on the head, eye, shoulder, and hand, as well as on the left kidney.

Special Cures

Tea for Flatulence: Peppermint is an excellent carminative. Those suffering from intestinal distention should drink a tea made of a mixture of peppermint and chamomile. Patients with stomachic complaints can drink a tea prepared from 1 part mugwort, 1 part curled mint, and ⅓ part crushed fennel seeds, taken after a meal.

It is interesting to note, here, how fascinated the English author Aldous Huxley was with the word "carminative." It seems to denote something more pleasant than it does, and his character Denis, in *Chrome Yellow*, expected it to have pleasant etymological connotations, such as enchanting, charming, singing…

Uses in Husbandry

Mint stalks and the residue left over after the extraction of mint oil can be fed to horses, sheep, and cattle. Pliny writes that cattle will begin to low if they eat the plant while it is flowering. Bees are less likely to swarm if their hives are rubbed with mint.

Mice and rats are said to flee from the smell of mint, especially corn mint. A few stalks of the herb placed in a haystack were once thought to adequately protect the crop against rodents. Care must, however, be taken to remove the stalks before feeding the hay to cows, or their milk will be so thinned by the herb that it will not coagulate, and cannot be used for cheesemaking.

Pennyroyal is one of the most effective flea repellents. Sleeping cushions for cats and dogs can be stuffed with the herb, or the animals can be washed with a pennyroyal infusion. Pennyroyal oil can be massaged into fur, or flea collars drenched with it. In Europe, pennyroyal flea collars are widely marketed. The herb has also been found effective in repelling mosquitoes, fleas, ants, and spiders.

Veterinary Values

Virgil reported that wounded deer and stags search for pennyroyal and eat it as healing medicine. The same has been reported about pregnant dogs. The Swiss herbal priest Johann Künzle recommends a tea of juniper berries, caraway seeds, and peppermint for sick cattle. To complete the cure, the sick animal should be placed on a diet of nettle hay. The dog that has lost her puppies, has engorged teats, or has trouble weaning should be given mint tea to stop the flow of milk. The external application of mint leaf compresses will also help. Finely chopped mint leaves can be added to the diet of dogs and cats.

Miscellaneous Wisdom

In ancient Greece, mint was thought capable of arousing love as well as jealousy. Greek women gathered the plants with their hands, but men were supposed to cut it with a wooden knife. Mint was also planted on graves, and dried mint leaves were burned as offerings for the dead.

In the Middle Ages, mint became so notorious for its tonic, arousing properties that soldiers were forbidden to eat it. According to English superstition, a wounded man will never recover if given horsemint. On the other hand, all the mints were thought capable of driving away witches and worms, and curing diseases caused by bewitchment. They were also used to protect young children and their mothers from sorcery.

Legends

As already mentioned, Minthe, the daughter of the river god Kokytos, was Hades' lover. When word of their affair came to Persephone, Persephone was so jealous that she tore the girl to pieces. Hades strewed the remains of his beloved on a sunny slope near Pylos, and fragrant mint plants *(Mentha tomentosa)* sprung up on the hillside. They have grown there ever since.

It is interesting that mint was also the first plant eaten by Demeter after fasting for the loss of Persephone, and that a pennyroyal gruel was given to celebrants before the Elysian mysteries.

Literary Flowers

> *The humble scale of my song will not allow me*
> *To embrace in fleeting verse the many virtues*
> *Of Pennyroyal they say that Eastern doctors*
> *Will pay as much for it as we pay here*
> *For a load of Indian pepper.*

—WAHLAFRIDUS STRABO, *HORTULUS*

> *In our wood blueberries grow:*
> *Come, come, my heart's joy!*
> *If you want, we'll meet there.*
> *Come, lily and columbine,*
> *Come, rose and sage,*

MINT

Come, sweet-smelling curled mint,
Come, come, my heart's joy!
There are flowers and berries in our wood.
But you are dearer to me than all the others.
Come, lily and columbine,
Come, rose and sage,
Come, sweet-smelling curled mint,
Come, come, my heart's joy!

—A 17TH CENTURY SWEDISH SONG,
INCLUDED IN CESAR BRESGEN'S *LIEBESLIEDER*

Drink nettle tea in March, / And Mugwort tea in May
And cowslip wine in June, / To send decline away.
—A Scottish saying

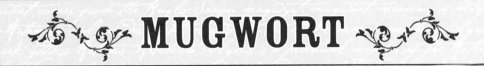

MUGWORT

Name

The name "mugwort" comes from the Anglo-Saxon *mugwyrt* or *mugwurt,* meaning "a midge" or a "fly wort." The botanical name, *Artemisia vulgaris,* designates mugwort as the most common member of a group of plants dedicated to the Greek goddess Artemis.

Artemisia vulgaris is a perennial member of the **Asteraceae** or **Compositae** (**Daisy**) family. Various subspecies of mugwort have been differentiated and classified by botanists.

Folk Names

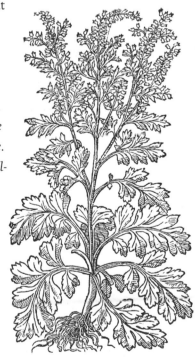

Mugwort is also known as fellon or felon herb, maidenwort, green ginger, apple-pie, dog's ears, smotherwood, fat hen, gall-wood, muggon, old Uncle Harry, bulwand wormwood, midge wormwood, St. John's plant, motherwort, common sagewort, and sailor's tobacco. Germans call the plant *Beifuss, Gewürz-Beifuß, wilder Wermut, Sonnwendgürtel, roter Buck, Muggerk, Besenkraut,* and *Weiberkraut.* French names are *armoise commune, barbotine, herbe aux vers, herbe à cent goûts, couronne de Saint Jean,* and *tabac de Saint Pierre.* In Italy, it is called *artemisia, erba di San Giovanni, assenzio selvatico, amarella,* and *canapaccia;* in Spain, *artemisia común;* in Denmark, *bynke;* in Sweden, *gråbo* or *bunke;* in Wales, *ilysian ieuan;* and in Ireland, *lianthlus.* In Scottish dialect, the plant is often called muggart or muggert. Russian names are *plyn obyknovennaja* and *šernobyl'nik.*

Appearance

Mugwort can grow to be as tall as an adult man. Its root is single, long, and hard, and is covered with many tiny fibers that draw nourishment from the soil. The mugwort stalk is woody and very tough, and of a brownish-red color. The main stalk branches out to support masses of pointed, segmented leaves that somewhat resemble curled claws. These leaves are dark green on top, and are covered with grayish-white felt underneath. The contrast between these two colors is the major identifying characteristic of the mugwort plant, and differentiates it from its close cousin, wormwood. As the year progresses, some of these leaves become discolored and begin to curl, giving the plant an untidy appearance. Mugwort leaves give off an unpleasant odor when crushed, but the smell of the crushed flowers is sweet and aromatic, reminiscent of marjoram. Like marjoram, mugwort flowers are so inconspicuous that they resemble closed buds even when fully opened. The mugwort plant produces great numbers of these tiny flowers at the end of each branch spike. The female flowers are yellowish in color, and the male flowers are often red or reddish-brown.

Place, Season, and Useful Parts

Mugwort grows wild in most temperate regions to an altitude of 5,400 ft., and is cultivated in gardens the world over. It was originally an Eastern plant, but is by now a familiar sight in both North America and Eurasia. It grows profusely on rubble, waste ground, waysides, riverbanks, railroad embankments, walls, and rocky beaches, as well as in hedges and pastures. Mugwort blossoms from July to September. Flowering mugwort tops are usually gathered before they fully open, and mugwort roots are dug in the fall.

Gathering, Drying, and Storage

According to one old Somerset man, "If yew do pick'n right there isn't nothing yew can't wish vor."[197] Picking mugwort "right" usually means harvesting it on Midsummer's Day. Only fresh and healthy roots should be used for medicinal purposes, but for magical purposes, roots with dark spots and "coals" found under the plant (dead and dried roots) are supposed to be especially potent.

Commercial harvesters harvest the upper portion of the plant just before it begins to blossom, once in early summer and once again in fall. Mugwort tops should be stripped from the stems and dried in a shady, airy place. Mugwort roots (young, light-colored roots are preferred by pharmacists) may be dug in the late fall.

The tops of flowering mugwort plants should be bound in sheaves after cutting, and hung up in an airy attic or warm room to dry. As soon as the buds seem dry, strip them from the stems and spread them out once again to dry. Mugwort leaves should

---

197. Ruth Tongue, *Somerset Folklore* (London: The Folk-Lore Society, 1965), 33.

not be included in kitchen mugwort because of their extremely bitter taste. Medicinal mugwort does not have to be sorted as carefully as the culinary herb, and may contain a few leaves.

Fresh mugwort roots should be rinsed quickly under running water to remove the dirt and tiny root fibers. The roots are then spread on sheets in a well-ventilated room to dry for approximately ten days, and turned often. The drying process should be finished near a source of artificial heat to remove the last vestiges of moisture. Dried mugwort roots are brittle, and snap easily.

Seed Saving and Germination

Mugwort flowers are fertilized by wind-borne pollen. Promising plants should be isolated if seed is going to be saved. It is easier to take cuttings of especially good plants, and to propagate them this way.

Gardening Hints

Mugwort is an unusually hardy plant, and very easy to grow. As a matter of fact, it is so large and so persistent that most gardeners will want to banish it to an unused corner of the yard. It needs no particular care once established except for occasional fertilizing, and will usually propagate itself. In large gardens, it may be planted as a windscreen for smaller, more sensitive herbs and vegetables, but should not be allowed to go to seed. In some areas of Japan, it has been planted to help minimize erosion on damaged soil.

Mugwort seeds are sown in April. They germinate best in sunlight, and should not be covered by soil. Cuttings can also be taken in spring, or old plants dug up and divided. Mugwort grows best along a wall, in a sunny, southern, yet somewhat damp position. A space of 18 in. should be allowed between plants.

Culinary Virtues

Mugwort's major virtue as a culinary herb is that it can transform fatty foods into digestible delicacies. The not-quite-opened buds were highly valued in the Middle Ages because of this, and they are still used as a traditional seasoning for heavy foods such as goose, duck, eel, and some cuts of pork. Wild boar and chicken can also be seasoned with mugwort, or it may be added to salads and sauces in minute amounts. Mugwort is a recommended seasoning for foods served to diabetics. Japanese cooks sometimes use the leaves in vegetable mixtures.

In the Middle Ages, hops were only one of a variety of herbs used to spice and preserve beer. One of the most popular medicinal beers was mugwort beer. It is still produced in small amounts in some countries.

Household Applications

Many herbalists list fly-repelling properties among the various virtues of the mugwort plant. The prevalence of this misconception is probably due to the lack of explanatory texts in many herbals. Actually, bunches of mugwort hung upside down in a room tend to attract flies. It was once customary to let flies settle on the hanging herbs in the evening, and then to quickly slip a sack over the herbs and beat the closed sack with a stick, until both flies and the plants were reduced to powder. According to some authorities, the Old German name for the plant, *pipoz*, was derived from the verb *pozan*, meaning "to beat." Other German folk names point to the use of the plant as a broom herb, but this practice has fallen into disuse.

Mugwort leaves are covered with a fine down, similar to coltsfoot leaves. This down can be rubbed off and employed as tinder. Mugwort can be used in herbal moth-repellent mixtures, or in floral bouquets for their unusual green color. Like coltsfoot, the leaves were once used in the Far East as a substitute for tobacco.

Cosmetic Properties

A weak infusion of mugwort can be added to eye-cleansing solutions. Mugwort footbaths are soothing and healing for blistered feet, as well as refreshing for tired limbs. Those who have to stay on their feet many hours every day should make regular use of the herb. According to the herbalist Otto Brunfels, beards grow better if they are washed regularly with mugwort tea.

Medicinal Merits

Mugwort has been used for millennia as a healing herb. It is still employed in China as a counterirritant in a treatment called "moxa." Miniature cones of mugwort are placed on the body meridians, and then lit. The burning mugwort raises small blisters, and the mugwort ash is rubbed into the blisters. Moxa sticks are also used to gently warm cold body areas.

The ancient Mayas and Aztecs also made extensive use of the herb, and the Greeks considered it sacred to Artemis because of its reputation as a gynecological "wonder drug." This reputation was maintained throughout the Middle Ages and on into later centuries. According to Dioscurides,

> "being sodden they are good to be put into womanish insessions for ye driving out of ye menstrua, & ye secondines, & ye Embryo, & ye preclusions, & ye inflammations of ye matrix, & ye breaking of stones, & ye stoppage of urine."[198]

---

198.   Robert T. Gunther, ed., *The Greek Herbal of Dioscurides* (New York: Hafner, 1959).

Mugwort was considered an effective aphrodisiac and, according to old German herbals, could even prolong a woman's fertile span if placed under her pillow or tied to her thighs. Genital pains were cured with mugwort belts; vaginal discharges were treated with mugwort pessaries; and the herb was said to warm and cleanse the uterus, to hasten birth and the expulsion of the afterbirth, and to induce abortions. Tea made from the tops of mugwort plants was supposed to staunch strong menstrual bleeding, but tea made from the lower part of the mugwort plant was though to induce menstruation. A woman having difficulty with childbirth had a mugwort wreath placed on her stomach. When the wreath was removed, the obstruction would, sympathetically, also be removed.

Mugwort gathered on Midsummer's Day was thought more effective than everyday mugwort. It was considered possible to free oneself from illnesses and bodily griefs for an entire year by wearing a mugwort belt and then leaping over the Midsummer fire before relinquishing the wreath to the flames. Those who looked through mugwort at the Midsummer fire were able to improve their eyesight for an entire year. The coals (dead and dried roots, or real coals from charcoal burners' fires) found under the plant while the church bells were striking twelve on Midsummer's Day were also thought effective against fever, plague, ague, carbuncles, cramps, and epilepsy. Mugwort roots dug out of the ground on St. Rosalia's Day and placed under the pillow could cure toothaches. A very early (AD 400) herbal tells of a cure for lumbago: rip out a mugwort plant with the left hand before sunrise, and then tie it to the body. Many ancient herbalists encouraged travellers to carry the herb with them on their journeys: it would protect them against tiredness, wild animals, evil spirits, poison, and sunstroke. Mugwort was further employed to warm "lame" veins and a cold stomach, to cure snake bites, dissolve stones, relieve sciatica, cure consumption, break wind, and loosen knots in one's neck.

> *Forget not, Mugwort, what thou didse reveal,*
> *What thou didst prepare at Regenmeld.*
> *Thou hast strength against three and against thirty,*
> *Thou hast strength against poison and against infection,*
> *Thou hast strength against the foe who fares through the land!*
> —FROM THE ANGLO-SAXON NINE HERB CHARM

Modern Medicine

Modern physicians classify mugwort as a nervine and tonic stimulant. Traditional herbalists prescribe mugwort extract or powdered mugwort roots for epileptics and paralytics, for patients afflicted with nerve pains, and for those struggling against an addiction to opium. Mugwort can also be given as a tonic for a sluggish digestive system, and it helps dispel wind, ease cramps, increase the appetite, cleanse the bowels (and, conversely, ease chronic diarrhea), bring on menstruation, and discourage worms. Mugwort is most effective as a digestive medicine when combined with a bitter herb such as centaury *(Centaurium erythraea)*, marigold, wormwood, or St. John's wort and taken in tea form before every major meal. Mugwort also mildly stimulates the kidneys and the uterus, and can help to dissolve stones and gravel. Since mugwort is usually available in large amounts, it can also be prepared as a bath for women with suppressed menstruation.

It is not recommended for pregnant women.

A homeopathic preparation of the roots is administered to patients suffering from hysteria and epilepsy, and especially those whose attack was precipitated by a blow on the head. Patients suffering from *petit mal* are given mugwort, and it is used to calm unusual excitability.

Mugwort is one of the most important herbs in Chinese medicine. The species most commonly used are *Artemisia vulgaris* and *Artemisia argyi*, called *ai ye* in Chinese, although other species are also employed. Warming moxa preparations are prepared from the wooly plant material of this herb, since it burns evenly and with deep heat, penetrating into the innermost recesses of the body. It warms a uterus damaged by cold, and has also been shown have some antibiotic action if taken internally.

Uses in Husbandry

Mugwort leaves can be added to the diet of chickens and turkey. Sheep will eat the leaves, and even the roots of the plant. Bees will remain in a hive that has been rubbed with fresh mugwort, and poor farmers have been known to manufacture their own brand of homegrown tobacco from the mugwort plant.

Because of its supposed antidemonic properties, mugwort was often employed in barnyard magic. Eggs and milk could be recovered from thieving witches with the help of mugwort. Bewitched animals could also be cured of their ailments by hanging mugwort in their stalls on the days sacred to the memory of St. Phillip and St. Jacob. In Bavaria, some farmers tried to improve the appearance of their horses before market with the help of coals found under the mugwort plant on Midsummer's Day. The animals are rubbed down with the coals, secretly, forty-eight hours before the market is to begin.

Veterinary Values

Cattle with coughs are given mugwort tea. Horses, cattle, and sheep benefit from regular doses of mugwort tea, which will discourage worm infestation.

Miscellaneous Wisdom

Mugwort is reported to be a very strong antidemonic herb. In the fifth century, mugwort was hung up in houses to avert the evil eye, to drive away elves and demons, and to cure magically caused diseases. It is still believed to have an exorcizing effect on demons and even the devil in Denmark, France, Belgium, Japan, and China, to name just a few countries. On the Isle of Man, mugwort was gathered on Midsummer's Eve as protection against witches. In Austria, a bunch of mugwort hung over the door was believed to protect the inmates of the house against pestilence and other dangers. In France and Germany, mugwort hung over the threshold kept lightning and hail from striking the house and destroying the crops. Mugwort also protected its users against fatigue. Pliny advised travellers to place mugwort leaves on their feet; Coles recommended the herb for running footmen. In Dioscurides' words, "If any have ye herb Artemisia with him in ye way, it dissolves weariness, & he that bears it on his feet, drives away venemous beasts & devils." Germans desiring extraordinary strength and power rubbed their feet with mugwort juice. English men wishing to remain young and actively virile wore sprigs of the plant in their buttonholes.

Mugwort is not only used as a preventive herb, but also as a magically potent plant. In ancient Greece, mugwort juice was included in philters and friendship potions. In Germany, marriageable widows carried mugwort to help them find a husband. Prolonged use of mugwort is said to induce clairvoyance, and mixtures of hemp and mugwort were used in England to produce visionary trances. Russian and English love potions sometimes contained the coals (either dead roots, or real coals) found under the mugwort plant on Midsummer's Day. These coals were employed for magical purposes in many countries. The Lithuanians believed that coals found while the bells were striking noon on Midsummer's Day were the best for magic, and that a large black dog guarded the plant at all times. In England, young men placed these coals under their pillows to induce sweet dreams. In Bohemia, it was considered great good luck to find a black worm among the mugwort roots on Good Friday. The worm was picked up and placed in a stoppered bottle, and the finder had to refrain from washing himself or saying his prayers for nine days. He also had to throw a little piece of bread under the table every day for the worm to eat. On the ninth day the worm would begin to talk, revealing fabulous secrets.

Oracular Worth

Anxious relatives of a patient sometimes place a sprig of mugwort under the sick person's pillow without his or her knowledge. If the sick person falls asleep easily, it is taken as a sign of recovery; if the patient has difficulty sleeping, then he may not live to see the mugwort bloom the following year.

Legends

A Scottish girl was once suffering from consumption (tuberculosis), and all the doctors said that she would die. Her disconsolate lover went walking on the seashore one day. He heard a mermaid calling out to him,

> Wad ye let the bonnie May die i' your hand,
> And the mugwort flowering i' the land?[199]

The young man was suddenly filled with new hope. His girl was given the fresh juice of the mugwort plant. In a very short time, she was able to leave her bed and marry her lover.

A similar yet sadder story is also told. A girl had just succumbed to the same disease, and a mermaid could not help but cry out,

> If they wad drink nettles in March,
> And eat muggons in May
> Sae many braw maidens
> Wadna gang to the clay![200]

---

199.   Robert Chambers, *Popular Rhymes of Scotland* (Detroit, MI: Singing Tree Press, 1969), 331.

200.   E. and M. A. Radford, *Encyclopaedia of Superstitions* (London: Rider, 1947), 178.

PLANTAINS

Name

This herb's botanical designation, *plantago*, and its English name, "plantain," both evolved from the Latin word *planta*, meaning the "sole" or "tread" of a foot. The name is an obvious reference to the herb's broad, foot-like shape; and since plantains grow along paths, they are also exposed to the steps of wayfarers.

There are many different plantains. The botanical terms *major*, *media*, and *lanceolata* apply to the size and the shape of the leaves. *Plantago major* (greater or broad plantain) is probably the best known, followed by *Plantago media* (hoary plantain) and then by *Plantago lanceolata* (ribwort plantain). Other plantains include *Plantago maritima* (sea plantain or seaside plantain or sheep's herb), *Plantago arenaria* (sand plantain), *Plantago coronopus* (buck's horn plantain, also known as hart's horn plantain and star of the earth), *Plantago ovata* (the ispaghul plantain), and the annual *Plantago afra* or *Plantago psyllium* (psyllium plantain), to name only a few.

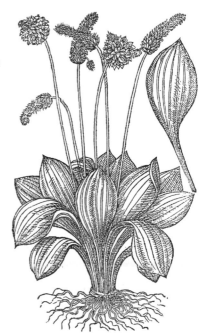

Plantago alpina, alpine plantain, grows at altitudes of 5,400 ft. and higher, and is considered the best plantain for medicinal use. In the southwestern United States, *Plantago wrightiana* and *Plantago rhodosperma* have been cultivated for their seeds. All the plantains are members of the **Plantain** family *(Plantaginaceae)*, and most are perennial.

Plantains should not be confused with the Carribean staple food also named "plantain," which is a starchy banana usually eaten as a vegetable.

Folk Names

The Old English name for the broad-leaved plantains was *wegbráde*. Plantains are now called ribgrass, ripple grass, plantine, land plantaine, cart-track plantain, waybroad, waybread, snakeweed, rat's tail, pony's tail, cuckoo's bread, canary food, birdseed, wayberry, hard heads, healing blade, poverty grass, boots and stockings, scent bottles, ashy pokes, soldiers, fighting cocks, Englishman's foot, lamb's foot, and white man's foot. Germans call them *Wegerich, Breitwegerich, Wegtritt, Sündenkraut, Lügenblat,* and *Heudieb;* the French have given them the simple name *plantain;* the Italians, *piantaggine;* the Russians, *podorožnik bol'šoj;* the Danes, *laegeblad;* the Swedes, *läkeblad;* and the Irish, *slán lus* or *cabbag parick.*

Narrow-leaved plantains are lumped together under the English names ribwort, ribwort-plantain, ribble grass, black plantain, black boys, blackjack, blacksmiths, chimney sweep, sweep's brushes, gypsy, tinker-tailor grass, lords and ladies, swords and spears, conqueror flowers, jack straws, baskets, clock, conkers, carl doddy, long plantain, snake plantain, lamb's tongue, goosetongue, hen plant, wendles, kemps, kempseed, and cocks. German names are *Spitzwegerich, Spitzfederich, Spiesskraut, Schlangenzunge, Katzenstühlche, Hundsrippen,* and *Lügenblattl.* French names are *plantain lancéolé, bonne femme, oreille de lièvre,* and *herbe à cinq cotês;* Spanish call the herbs *llanten.* Some Italian names are *lanciuola, mestolaccio,* and *arnoglossa;* and a Russian name is *podorožnik lancetnyj.*

Buck's horn plantain is also known as hart's horn plantain and star of the earth; in German, *Hirschhornsalat* or *Krähenfuß-Wegerich.* In French, it is known as *corne de cerf;* in Italian, *coronopo;* in Spanish, *cuervo di ciervo* or *estrellamar;* and in Russian, *koronopus.*

Appearance

Greater plantain grows to a maximum height of 1 ft. It has fibrous yellowish roots attached to a short rhizome that looks as if it has been bitten off. Its leaves are gathered into a rosette that is raised above the ground.

Hoary plantain has a leaf rosette that lies flat on the ground. In Culpeper's words, the leaves are "broad, large, and oval, waved at the edges, with 7 [5–11] large nerves running through the whole length of them, and even the broad hollow footstalks into the root."[201] The leaves and roots do not have any particularly noticeable odor, and they taste salty, grassy, and a little astringent. Plantain flowers are clustered together on a single flower stalk that is at least as long as the plant's leaves. These tiny flowers are green, purple, pink, or even brown in color.

The narrow-leaved plantain grows to a maximum height of 1½ ft. It has long, pointed leaves with 3–7 strongly-marked veins that give the leaves the appearance of corduroy. Like corduroy, the leaves become puckered with age. They are rarely wider

---

201. *Culpeper's Complete Herbal* (1653) (London: Foulsham, undated), 273.

than 1 in. across and are of a dark green color. At the base of the rosette, the leaves are woolly. A flower stalk, like that of the broad-leaved plantain, supports a single ear of insignificant-looking flowers of an undefinable color. They produce tiny seeds.

Place, Season, and Useful Parts

The plantains can be found in most of Europe, northern and central Asia, North and South America, Australia, New Zealand, and northern Africa to an altitude of 6,000 ft. They grow on sandy, compacted, or rocky soil as well as on cultivated ground and damp grassland, and can be very persistent weeds. Rumor has it that early settlers brought plantains with them to the New World and it followed in their footsteps, hence the name "white man's footstep." Plantain usually blossoms from April through September.

Gathering, Drying, and Storage

Plantain leaves should be cut above the root just before the seeds form, from April into May and June. Great care must be taken to avoid bruising the plant in any way. Plantain roots can be gathered in the spring, and the seeds harvested as they ripen.

Plantain leaves must be processed or dried immediately after gathering. They are spread out in very thin layers on cloths or screens and dried as quickly as possible, if necessary with artificial heat. Discolored or darkened leaves must be discarded, since they are medicinally worthless. Plantain roots can be dried on a string in an airy place. Plantain syrup keeps well and may be stored for several years in a dark, cool place. Plantain juice will keep for a short time in the refrigerator.

Seed Saving and Germination

Seed savers usually do not maintain plantain varieties, with the exception of a few varieties cultivated for their especially tender and healing leaves. These will cross with other wild plantains of the same species, and must be isolated to maintain varietal purity. The seeds are easy to gather, since they are set in an ear on the stalk, but some will fall off. The resulting plants should be removed to avoid confusion between wild and cultivated varieties. Buck's horn plantain is often cultivated as a winter vegetable. The plant rarely sets seed early in the year, making seed-saving somewhat difficult. It may be necessary to grow it in a greenhouse to gather viable seed.

Gardening Hints

Plantain is almost never grown in gardens because of its reputation as an insistent and pertinacious weed. It usually grows wild in garden paths, and on roadsides and gravel. It is very difficult to control in lawns, especially when the soil has been compacted by machinery, and may often be found growing in the vicinity of red clover.

Culinary Virtues

The young leaves of most plantains are edible and can be cooked or steamed as potherbs. They can also be shredded for use in soups and salads. It is advisable to remove the strings from the leaves before cooking, or to purée and strain the leaves after cooking. Plantain leaves were once widely used as a kitchen vegetable in China. One plantain, buck's horn plantain, was cultivated in Europe as a winter vegetable. The leaves are harvested after the winter, when they are still young and tender. All plaintain leaves become tough, stringy, and unpalatable later in the season. The seeds can be roasted as a survival food, or ground into flour. They are laxative if eaten raw, but lose this quality when cooked. The gelatin-like substance processed from the seeds of ispaghul plantain has been used as an additive for ice cream and medicines. A drink is prepared in India from the seeds.

Household Applications

Narrow-leaved plantains were once used to produce a mucilaginous substance employed for stiffening muslin and linen. The fresh leaves were soaked in water, and the resulting liquid used as starch. Plantain fibers have occasionally been used for household spinning and weaving.

Cosmetic Properties

Infused plantain water can be used as a cleansing mixture with good results. It can also be applied to tighten and tone the skin of women's breasts. As Fynes Moryson once observed in his *Itinerary*:

> "Those of Padoua [are said] to love women with little brests, which makes their women use the juyce of Plantane to keep them from growing."[202]

Medicinal Merits

There is almost no disease that has not been treated with one plantain or another over the years. In ancient times, one book was devoted entirely to the healing properties of the herb, and Pseudo-Apuleius (fifth century) listed twenty-four medicinal merits of the broad-leaved plantain alone. According to Pliny, plantain is so wholesome that it will make meat whole again, even after it has been cut up and is cooking in a pot on the stove. Ancient Chinese herbalists also prized broad-leaved plantains, using them to clear and brighten eyes, ease coughs, cleanse the kidneys, and increase the fertility of both men and women, but especially that of men.

---

202. Moryson, *An Itinerary* (1617), vol. III (Glasgow: James MacLehose and Sons, 1908; original from the New York Public Library; digitized 2007), 457.

Included among the many diseases treated with plantains over the years are the plague, tertian and quartan fever, psychic diseases, chills and headaches, menopausal disorders, hardening of the liver, gout, urinary complaints, thyroid imbalances, tuberculosis, worms, bloody fluxes, and coughs. The leaves are applied to cuts, and early surgeons prepared plantain water to disinfect wounds. Plantain leaves and plantain compresses were applied to gout, podagra, ulcers, burns, boils, fistules, carbuncles, and swollen or sore feet. They were also applied to the bites of mad dogs, scorpions, and serpents, and to ringworm, aching heads, hemorrhoids, stomach pains, earaches, toothaches, numbness of the limbs, and conjunctivitis. The roots of plantain plants were tucked into the cheek to prevent toothache. In England, they were tied around a patient's neck to cure headaches, the thyroid disorders of children, rickets, and fever. Bavarian folk healers told people with recurrent headaches to sew an uneven number of plantain roots into white cloth with white thread, and then to hang the amulet around their necks with a blue ribbon while the moon was rising. The amulet had to be removed the following day during sunrise. Then the patient had to say three Ave Marias and throw the amulet into a swiftly-running stream.

Bavarian girls with the rickets had three plantain roots hung around their necks; boys with the same disease had two roots, worn for three days and then burned. Dioscurides recommended three plantain roots, three glasses of water, and three glasses of wine for the treatment of tertian (three-day) fever; and four roots, four glasses of water, and four glasses of wine for quartan (four-day) fever. In Germany, three roots were tied onto the patient's back, or three plantain leaves were sewn under the bed to treat tertian fever.

According to one folk saying, plantain has ninety-nine roots, and each of them is capable of curing one kind of fever. Hildegard von Bingen recommended tying seven plantain roots, or seven plantain stalks dug before sunup, around one's neck and down one's back to treat fevers. In the Palatine, fever sufferers were given plantain root tea to drink, and five plantain roots were tied under the patient's bed before sunrise. On the first day, the patient had to say five Pater Nosters, on the second day, four, on the third day, three, and so on until the fever disappeared.

> *And thou, Plantain, Mother of herbs,*
> *Open from the East, mighty within,*
> *Over thee chariots creaked, over thee queens rode.*
> *Over thee brides made outcry, over thee bulls gnashed their teeth.*
> *All these thou didst withstand and resist;*
> *So mayest thou withstand poison and infection,*
> *And the foe who fares through the land!*
>
> —from the Anglo-Saxon Nine Herb Charm

Modern Medicine

Although these plantain faith-cures are not taken seriously anymore, the plantains are still held in high regard as medicinal herbs. Ancient authorities thought the broad-leaved plantains to be more efficacious, but modern experts prefer the narrow-leaved and alpine varieties. Narrow-leaved plantain is a strongly cleansing herb, and is often prescribed in tea, juice, or syrup form for spring cures. It helps to flush out the kidneys and to cleanse the stomach, the liver, and above all, the lungs. It also acts to reduce fever, and is therefore invaluable for the treatment of infectious or feverish respiratory complaints. Smokers who are quitting should make use of plantain to cleanse some of the deposits and tars out of the respiratory tract. Only lungwort *(Pulmonaria officinalis)* can compare with plantain as a pulmonary herb.

A homeopathic preparation of the entire narrow-leaved plantain plant is prescribed for neuralgia, scrofula, respiratory troubles, and earaches as well as toothaches. The greater plantain is also used to treat flatulence, skin inflammations, some forms of impotence, bed wetting, and headaches, toothaches, and earaches.

All the plantains are excellent wound herbs. As Sebastian Kneipp, the nineteenth-century herbal priest, once wrote,

> Plantain juice closes gaping wounds as if they were sewn with threads of gold. And no infection or putrefaction will settle on these golden threads, just as rust refuses to settle on gold.[203]

For wound treatment, the leaves should be crushed or bruised, and can then be applied as first-aid "bandages" to cuts, wounds, burns, nettle stings, rheumatic pains, or skin blemishes. Insect bites should be dampened with plantain tincture as soon as possible. The leaves can also be applied to goitrous swellings, eczema, and to infected eyes. Plantain roots, or plantain leaves that have had the strings removed, can be rolled up and tucked into one's cheek next to an aching tooth or used as a loose earplug to ease an earache.

Plantain seeds, and especially psyllium seeds, are used medicinally because of their gelatinous nature when softened in water. They can be taken like flax seeds to ease constipation and to cleanse the intestinal tract. They are mild enough to be administered to children.

An Oriental plantain, *Plantago asiatica*, is used mostly for its seeds, which are prescribed to promote labor in women and well as for prostate disorders, painful urination, edema, coughs, eye problems, and male infertility. Pregnant women are warned against taking the herb.

---

203. *Die deutsche Heilpflanze*, vol. II (Weimar, Germany: Keller, Stollberg/Erzgebirge, 1934), 126.

Special Cures

Plantain Congee: A porridge (*congee*) made of plantain seeds and brown rice is believed to enhance sexual secretions and fertility. 1 oz. of plantain seeds are boiled in 3 cups of water until half of it is consumed, while the rice is soaked in 5 cups of water. Strain the plantain liquid into the rice mixture, and then boil until soft.

Plantain Juice: Fresh plantain leaves can be put through an electric juicer, or the leaves are bruised and then covered with a layer of sugar, and allowed to stand for several hours before pressing. Fresh herb juice should always be used immediately, or poured into sterile bottles, carefully sealed, and stored in the refrigerator Moldy or "off-smelling" juice should under no circumstances be used—it must be discarded. A teaspoon of plantain juice diluted with a glass of water or fruit juice should be taken once or twice daily for several weeks for best results. It is particularly healing for those recovering from pulmonary infections, or for smokers who are trying to kick the habit.

Plantain Tincture: A plantain tincture for the first-aid treatment of cuts, scratches, burns, and insect bites can be prepared by finely chopping or shredding plantain (preferably the leaves of the narrow-leaved varieties) and placing them in a dark glass. Pour in enough clear spirits (any high-proof alcohol fit for consumption can be used) to completely cover the leaves, and then place in a warm, dark room for several days before straining and filtering. This tincture keeps well, and is a useful addition to the home medicine cabinet.

Plantain Syrup: It is wise to always have some plantain syrup at hand. It can be taken whenever colds and influenza seem to be "going around," and can also be administered in the spring as a rejuvenating spring cure, 1–2 tsp. a day on an empty stomach for four weeks.

Plantain syrup is prepared by boiling or fermentation. To prepare the cooked syrup, fill a pan half full with freshly-washed ribwort plantain leaves and, if desired, one or two handfuls of juniper berries. Cover the herbs with water, and cook over a very low flame for 2 hours. Strain, and then add several pounds of sugar to the liquid. Cook gently, stirring often, until a syrupy consistency is reached. Strain the mixture again, pour into cleaned and sterilized bottles, seal, and store in a cool, dark place.

Plantain syrup can also be prepared by alternately packing freshly washed leaves and sugar in a large wide-mouthed jar or crock, and letting the mixture settle for a day. The next morning, and the day after, add more leaves until the jar is filled to within one inch of the top. Carefully seal the jar with several layers of parchment paper, tied tightly with a string. Dig a hole in the garden in a warm place (no deep frost), and lower the jar into the hole. Cover the top of the jar with a board and a heavy stone so that no dirt can get in, and then cover the jar and the board with earth. Part of the stone should remain above ground as a marker and reminder. Let the mixture "work" for 3 months, and then dig the jar out carefully, and bring it indoors. Heat the syrup and bring it to a boil before straining and bottling it in sterilized bottles.

Uses in Husbandry

The plantains are not welcomed when they are found growing in pastures, for they rob space and nutrients from other more profitable hay plants. They also dry poorly, and crumble easily once dried. Their one virtue is as "fire leaves." Husbandmen twist the leaves as a test to see if the hay is dry enough and will not self-combust. The fresh green leaves will cause diarrhea if fed to cattle and horses, although sheep, goats, and pigs can eat them without complaint. Birds are extremely fond of plantain seeds, and they are therefore often added to canary and parakeet food. Some dove-experts say that placing a few plantain spikes in the dovecote will persuade the birds to stay at home; and some beekeepers say that they do not get stung if they keep a plantain leaf under their tongue when working with bees. Broad-leaved plantains are sometimes used as tobacco substitutes.

Veterinary Values

Plantain is an excellent wound herb, for animals as well as humans. The leaves can be bruised and applied directly to wounds to aid healing.

Miscellaneous Wisdom

The classical scholar Erasmus noted in *Colloquia* how a toad once recovered from a spider bite with the help of plantain. Wounded toads supposedly healed themselves by simply creeping under the plant. Another early belief (fourteenth century) was that if a plaintiff carried plantain in court, it would ensure success. Hildegard von Bingen prescribed the herb for those who had been put under a love spell. In Bohemia, hunters, duelists, and soldiers ate plantain roots on an empty stomach to keep from being wounded by a bullet that day. The best plantain for these purposes was said to grow on consecrated soil.

Some Englishmen believe that it is possible to find magical coals under plantain plants on Midsummer's Eve (see mugwort chapter), and dig the roots for use as mandrakes. Mandrakes were originally made from the true mandrake, *Mandragora officinarum*, but substitutes were often used because of the difficulties encountered while harvesting the true mandrake. The true mandrake only grows in the south and could only, according to popular belief, be dug with the help of a completely black dog, who was inevitably killed by the awful, piercing shrieks of the damaged plant. The roots of white briony, iris, gentian, deadly nightshade, plantain, and other herbs were dug and then carved to represent miniature men and women. The figures were worn as amulets or dressed and put in a place of honor, depending on their size. All of them were treated with great respect. Contented mandrakes could bring luck and riches to a house and aid the owners in affairs of the heart, as well as ease births, tell the location of hidden treasures, and positively influence the outcome of lawsuits.

Herbal Pastimes

In France, children are warned not to pick plantain and to never handle it roughly, for it is a plant of God. Children who bring the herb into the house are scolded, for it is believed to cause sickness and even death. But children rarely listen to admonitions, and the temptation to pick the pliable plantain stems is often too great to be resisted. These stems can be braided and bent and woven to make furniture and baskets (hence the name "cat's chair" for the plant in Germany). English children love to slash at each other with plantain "soldiers" or "fighting cocks" until one of the tough stems breaks. German children pair up and rip the leaves apart to study the number of stems protruding from their side of the leaf. The child with the longest threads will be lucky, and the child with an even number of threads will get his wish. In Switzerland and Austria, the child with the most threads is said to have told the most lies, or to have committed the greatest number of sins. In Tyrol, children tell how many decades they have left to live by counting the threads. They also tell how many lovers, or how many children they will have, with the help of the torn leaves: long strings are for boys, and short strings are for girls.

Literary Flowers

Romeo: "Your plantain-leaf is excellent for that."
Benvoglio: "For what, I pray thee?"
Romeo: "For your broken shin."

—WILLIAM SHAKESPEARE, *ROMEO AND JULIET*, I.II

For it was joye for to see him swete!
His foreheed dropped as a stillatorie,
Were ful of plantain and of peritorie.

—GEOFFREY CHAUCER,
"THE CANON YEOMAN'S PROLOGUE," *THE CANTERBURY TALES*

Many insist that the plantain
was once a gentle woman
who is still waiting in pain for her lover.

—FROM HANS VINTLER'S 15TH CENTURY *BLUME DER TUGEND*,

QTD. IN GRIMM'S *TEUTONIC MYTHOLOGY*

He that would live for ay,
Must eat sage in May.

—AN OLD ENGLISH PROVERB

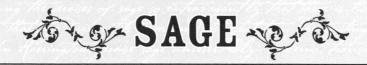

SAGE

Name

The English name "sage" is derived from the Latin word *salvere*, meaning "to be sound," "to be in good health." The Old English form of the name was *sawge*; the Old French forms were *sauge* and *saulje*. This derivation has also led to the Latinate appellation *Salvia salvatrix*, meaning "sage the savioress."

All these names point to the great respect paid to sage as a superb healing herb, as versatile and powerful in its action as any other. Ancient writers have sung the praises of sage so extravagantly that there is little to do but second their acclamations, and to say that sage deserves its name and its reputation. The ninth-century herbal *The School of Salernum* praises sage unreservedly:

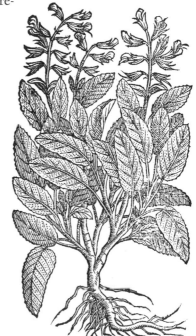

> But who can write thy worth (o soveraigne Sage!)
> Some aske how a man can die, where thou dost grow,
> Oh that there were a medicine curing age,
> Death comes at last,
> though death come ne're so slow:
> Sage strengthens the sinews,
> fevers heat doth swage.
> The Palsy helpes, and rids of mickle woe.
> In Latin [Salvia] takes the name of safety,
> In English [Sage] is rather wise than crafty.
> Sith the name betokens wise and saving,
> We count it nature's friend and worth the having.[204]

---

204. Sir John Harrington, trans., *The School of Salernum* (Salerno, Italy: Ente Provinciale per il Turismo, 1953), 53.

Sage's medicinal merits are indeed so great that the question *"Cur moriatur homo, cui salvia crescit in hortis?"*—"Why do people die, when sage is growing in the garden?"—is not as preposterous as it may sound at first hearing.

Sage is a perennial member of the **Lamiaceae** or **Mint** Family. There are hundreds of sage species including, among others, *Salvia sclarea*, *Salvia pratensis*, and *Salvia coccinea*. Unless otherwise stated, this chapter deals solely with garden sage, *Salvia officinalis*.

Folk Names

Sage, shop-sage, white sage, garden sage, and many other names abound for the countless sage varieties. In French, the herb is known as *sauge* and *serve*; in German, *Salbei*, *Königssalbei*, *Sophie*, and *Altweiberschmecken*; in Spanish, *salvia* and *sarubia*; in Italian, *salvia*, *salvie*, and *erba savia*; and in Russian, *šalfej aptečnyj*.

A related but completely different sage with important medicinal properties is known in English as clary, clary wort, or clear eye. The botanical name is *Salvia sclarea*. It is known in French as *toute bonne* or *sauge sclarée*; in Spanish as *arnaro*; in Russian as *šalfej muskatnyi*; and in German as *Muskatellersalbei*.

Appearance

The most characteristic feature of sage is the rough texture of its leaves, which closely resembles the skin of a tongue, or the warted and knobbly back of a toad. The leaves of sage are greenish-white, tinged in some cases with red. There are hundreds of different sage species, and considerable variation within species. Clary sage *(Salvia sclarea)* and field sage *(Salvia pratensis)* are two of the most common species.

The entire sage plant smells strongly, almost camphor-like, aromatic, and fragrant. The taste of the leaves is warm and slightly astringent. Sage varies greatly in height, and appears as an evergreen shrub in its natural state. The light hairy texture of the leaves and the small purple-lipped flowers are further identifying features.

Place, Season, and Useful Parts

Sage is a perennial herb, flowering (depending on the climactic conditions) from May to August. It grows wild on the mountainous slopes of the western Mediterranean, and the best commercial sage is cultivated in Dalmatia (Croatia). It is grown in gardens throughout most of the temperate world to a fairly high altitude, and raised indoors or in pots in less mild areas in the colder months.

Clary is often grown as an ornamental in gardens, but is also grown commercially in Kenya, in parts of the former Soviet Union, and in southern Europe.

Gathering, Drying, and Storage

Sage leaves are gathered singly by hand, or the top shoots are nipped off just before they blossom, usually in June and July. The plants can be re-harvested two or thee times. The flowers are occasionally gathered singly. In ancient Rome it was customary to hold a celebration at the end of the sage harvest, and it was forbidden to harvest the plant with iron. Because of the fleshy nature of sage's leaves, they should be gathered before the full moon.

Sage leaves are dried in a shady room in which air can circulate freely. The herb should be turned regularly to ensure even drying. Dried sage leaves can be stored in sacks and paper bags, but sage powder must be kept in closed containers. It only keeps for a short time.

Seed Saving and Germination

The seed-saving techniques for sage are very similar to those used for basil, since both belong to the same family. The fairly large sage seeds fall out easily, but can also be difficult to remove from the seed heads. The trick is to find the ideal time to harvest the seeds. Once again, a magnifying glass can be very helpful to discover just when the seeds mature, and when they fall out.

Gardening Hints

Sage is a perennial plant that grows wild in the poor soils of sunny Mediterranean mountain regions. But sage can also be raised easily in most gardens. Some lime must be present in the soil and the plant prefers a sunny position with some shade, but it can also be grown well in areas with little rainfall.

It is quickest to raise sage from bought seedlings, but it is also easy to sow the seeds under glass in spring. Cuttings taken from older plants may be set in spring, or sage may be propagated by a process known as "layering." Branches of the plant are forced down to the ground in the spring or summer and then covered with earth or rocks to keep them in position. As soon as the branches begin to form new rootlets, the branches are cut off and planted separately. Red sage can only be propagated by cuttings or layering.

All sage plants should be renewed at least once every four years, and must be cut back lightly in summer to encourage new growth and make the plants bushier. If the plants are cut too late in the year or into the old wood, their frost-hardiness will suffer. In Swabian folk belief, a sage plant that has been cut back on Good Friday, before dawn, will grow better than any other. Another folk belief says that rue and sage can be planted next to each other to keep toads away, and to keep the sage plant from becoming poisonous. A Warwickshire saying, "Plant your rue and sage together, the sage will thrive in any weather," supports this thesis, but modern authors disagree and say that rue planted next to sage may even poison the plant. Sage and rosemary undisputably stimulate each other to health and growth, and the beneficial effect of sage on cabbage plants has been proven again and again. Spraying with sage infusions is a method employed by organic gardeners to strengthen old or failing plants, and to stimulate them to new growth. A sage spraying mixture has also been employed by organic gardeners to keep pests away from garden plants.

Variegated or golden sage varieties are very decorative in the garden, but may freeze back in the winter. All sages can be kept in pots or window boxes during the winter for kitchen and medicinal use. They transplant well.

Culinary Virtues

A good part of sage's pleasant reputation is due to its culinary virtues. Its flavor and medicinal merits were so highly valued at one time that Dutch businessmen were able to extort three parts of black tea for every part of sage tea from health-conscious Chinese merchants. Even in Europe, sage tea was an accepted substitute for tea or coffee until this century.

Sage is a highly aromatic herb with a strong, warm taste that verges on bitterness. The leaves should be used sparingly. As a seasoning, the leaves are preferable to the powder, which loses its potency quickly. The leaves should be softened in a little water or simmered with the other ingredients to fully bring out the flavor. In many recipes, the flowers can be used instead of the leaves, since they are not as pungent in taste.

The ancient Romans baked sage into sweetmeats served after veal and venison courses to make these heavy foods more digestible. Sage tea served this same purpose in the sixteenth and seventeenth centuries in Europe. At this time, sage was so popular that it was pressed into cheeses, fried in batter, eaten with bread and butter, and added, in some form or another, to half the dishes served at table. The sage and onion stuffings of our day serve a similar function: to make meats such as duck, chicken, goose, pork, or turkey more appetizing and to aid the digestion of fatty foods. Sage, cooked in food, helps to conserve it and makes it keep longer.

Sage's culinary applications are numerous: the leaves are used to season fish, eel, pork and lamb roasts, calves' liver, rabbit, sausages, barley, mushrooms, raw bacon, grilled meats, and buckwheat pancakes. They are added to sauces, dips, bakery products, marinades, forcemeats, apple pastries, peas, broad beans, and sweet fritters. Small birds can be wrapped in sage leaves, and joints are threaded with sage before roasting. Sandwiches are made with sage leaves placed on buttered bread; vinegar is flavored with sage; and young sage shoots are eaten in salads or folded into omelets.

Clary sage was used extensively to flavor beer and to impart a muscatel taste to wine, and has since been employed in the manufacture of vermouth. Sage has also been added on occasion to wormwood wine to lessen its bitterness. Pastry flavored with clary was once a traditional British meal.

The Greeks once candied the small exotic growths similar to oak apples of one sage species, *Salvia pomifera*. This was sold as a great delicacy.

It is possible to ferment wine from sage leaves, but its taste is so overwhelming that it can only be taken as medicine. A tastier and simpler method of preparing sage wine is to pour 1 qt. of red or white wine (a dry white wine complements the taste of sage better) over a generous handful of sage leaves, and then let the mixture stand for 1 week before straining. A small glass with or before meals is the usual dosage, and should not be exceeded.

Noteworthy Recipes

To Roast a Pig: This recipe from the seventeenth century makes good use of sage:

> Take a fat one, cleanse his Belly, put into it minced Sage, Currans [currants], Mace, and grated Nutmeg; roast him indifferently by a soaking fire, then make up a brisk fire to crackle him, and serve him with Currans, Bread, Sage, Butter and Nutmeg, made into a thin Sawce, with Rose-water.[205]

Sage and Onion, or Goose-Stuffing Sauce: Here is a traditional English recipe from the nineteenth century:

> Chop very fine an ounce of Onion and half an ounce of green Sage leaves, put them into a stew-pan with four spoonsful [Tbsp.] of water, simmer gently for ten minutes, then put it in a teaspoonful of pepper and salt, and one ounce of fine bread-crumbs; mix well together;—then pour to it a quarter of a pint of (Broth, or Gravy, or) Melted Butter, stir very well together, and simmer it a few minutes longer.
>
> Observation—This is a very relishing Sauce for Roast Pork, Poultry, Geese, or Ducks; or Green Pease on Maigre Days.[206]

To Make a Sage Cream: And, last, an unusual mixture:

> Take a quart of Cream, boil it well, then add a quarter of a pint of the Juyce of red Sage, half as much Rose-water, and a quarter of a pound of Sugar, and it will be an excellent dish. And thus you may use it with any sweet Herbs, which will render it pleasant and healthful.[207]

---

205. John Shirley, *An Accomplished Ladies Rich Closet of Rarities* (London: N. Bodington, 1688), 108.

206. William Kitchiner, *The Cook's Oracle* (1817) (London: Samuel Bagster, 1860), 237.

207. John Shirley, *An Accomplished Ladies Rich Closet of Rarities* (London: N. Bodington, 1688), 148.

Sage Pesto: Modern cooks will probably prefer a sage pesto to a sweet sauce. Basically, a sage pesto is prepared in the same manner as a basil pesto (see basil chapter), but the sage flowers are used instead of the leaves, because they are much more delicate in taste. Walnut or flax seed oil should be used to create a creamy consistency, and walnuts or piñon nuts to thicken the mixture. Mix well in a blender, and use fresh, or freeze for later use.

Fennel and Sage Salad: Clean and slice 2 fennel "bulbs" very finely on a vegetable slicer, as well as ½ a mild onion. Peel 2 seedless oranges, and cut into thin slices, and then into chunks. Mix well together with ⅓ cup of sage flowers. Season with walnut or hemp oil (olive oil is too strong in taste), cider vinegar, and a little salt. Let stand for at least 30 minutes. Serve on a bed of mixed lettuce greens (red and green head lettuce, arugula, endive).

Roast Chicken with Sage: Clean a roasting chicken, dry the interior, and then salt generously inside and out. Stuff with a small handful of fresh sage leaves, black peppercorns, and 3–4 coarsely chopped cloves of garlic. Roast as usual, and remove the sage before pouring off the excess fat and serving.

Household Applications

Sage, like chamomile, is an excellent disinfectant, and possesses additional aromatic qualities that are displeasing to certain insects and also to mice. Sage was once famous for keeping the bedbugs out of beds. The mouse-repelling properties of sage are supposedly stronger if the plant is gathered at noon on the day devoted to St. Ulrich in the Roman Catholic calender (St. Ulrich being the patron saint of mice). Some herbals suggest burning sage in order to drive away mice. This works in closed rooms, but will result in the most awful hangover if hapless humans decide to stay in the room while it is being smoked.

A yellow-buff dye can be produced with sage tops and alum, a darker yellow with bichromate of potash, a green hue with copper sulphate, and a green-gray with ferrous sulphate.

Cosmetic Properties

Sage's cosmetic properties are closely related to those of chamomile: disinfecting and antiseptic, but more astringent and less gentle than chamomile. Sage is indispensable for oily skin with large pores, and is particularly important in the treatment of facial impurities. Facial steaming mixtures with sage are recommended for people with chronically oily skin (those with very sensitive skin or broken capillaries should avoid steaming altogether). A simple infusion of sage, stored in the refrigerator and preserved for a few days by the addition of a small amount of cider vinegar or benzoin tincture, is an excellent tonic astringent lotion that surpasses many commercial mixtures. Sage compresses help to clear up infections or problem skin. Sage tea or sage vinegar is used externally to lessen the pains of sunburn, and sage-flower vinegar is rubbed on the skin to strengthen the nerves. The essential oil is used commercially in the manufacture of certain perfumes, and sage leaves are often included in potpourri. Sage tea can be added to baths (again, caution: it tends to stain the enamel!) or rubbed in directly as a body lotion. The herb has been added to skin creams and is used in deodorant mixtures. Its mild disinfectant and strengthening action has also made it an important addition to the first bath water of newborn babies.

Sage is justly famous in the area of breath and mouth care. Used either as a tea, a mouthwash, or a gargle, sage helps to cleanse and disinfect the mouth and to sweeten the breath. A single leaf is a good emergency toothbrush, and sage tea is a superb gargle. Sage leaves can be rubbed directly against the teeth and gums, or mixed into a paste for the same purpose, or chewed one at a time. The mouth can also be rinsed with sage mouthwash. Sage is included in almost all commercial toothpastes because of its positive and strengthening influence on gum health: it can stop bleeding and lessen infection.

Sage is also an important hair herb. A neutral shampoo (coconut oil, Castile, or baby shampoo) can be transformed into a shampoo for oily hair by the addition of some strongly brewed sage tea. Sage has the added advantage of strengthening the scalp and the hair roots. It will also darken the hair ever so slightly, which may be an advantage or a disadvantage depending on the user. A mixture of strongly brewed rosemary and sage tea, preserved with vinegar or alcohol, makes an excellent hair tonic for those with dark hair. It should be applied sparingly every second day, and generously before shampooing.

One of the most interesting stories about sage's cosmetic properties is of the Four Thieves of Toulouse and their famous vinegar. In the seventeenth century, the plague was laying waste to the countryside, fear was rampant, and the townspeople were barricading themselves indoors in hopes of escaping from the epidemic. Four thieves learned to overcome their fear, and took advantage of the event. They walked blithely into plague-stricken houses and stole everything in sight. What was so unusual about their activity was that they did not sicken like all the other plunderers. But all good things must come to an end sometime, and the four thieves were caught *in delicto*. The authorities tried to get them to reveal their secret, but they would not comply. Only when promised release and freedom from persecution did they agree to reveal their success formula. They had rubbed their bodies liberally with herbal vinegar before visiting the houses of their victims, and this had kept them from harm. The thieves were allowed to go free, and they lived on their ill-gotten money until their days' end. Those who had acquired the secret of the "Vinegar of the Four Thieves," as it came to be known, had even more luck: the vinegar became a commercial success, business boomed, and all the French people soon bought the Vinegar of the Four Thieves to protect themselves from the plague.

Noteworthy Recipes

The Vinegar of the Four Thieves: Mix 1 handful each of dried peppermint, thyme, sage, and rosemary leaves, 1 handful of dried lavender leaves, and 1 handful of dried lavender flowers in a large ceramic or porcelain bowl. Fresh herbs can also be used, but the amounts must be increased. Add 4 fl. oz. of cider vinegar, and enough soft rainwater (or distilled water) to completely cover the herbs. Cover the bowl, and set in a cool place. Add more distilled water to the herb mixture as needed to replace any water that has evaporated. In a sterile jar with a close-fitting lid, mix 2 fl. oz. of 90% alcohol (or a correspondingly larger amount of lower-proof spirits) with 2 tsp. of pure camphor crystals (note: not mothballs!) and 25 drops of good myrrh tincture. Close the jar tightly, shake well, and let stand in a cool place. After 10 days, strain the herbal mixture through a sieve, mix it with the camphor-myrrh mixture, and filter everything through filter paper. Add a little more vinegar to the mixture if you enjoy the acetic smell. This herbal vinegar can be added to bath waters and used as a rubbing mixture after baths, or simply enjoyed as a refreshing body tonic.

Garlic was once added to the mixture to enhance its medicinal properties, but the penetrating smell hardly makes this advisable. The vinegar odor of the finished mixture is quite strong at first, but is very volatile.

Medicinal Merits

Sage is indeed a wonderful herb, if not a miraculous one. It is one of the herbs longest known to humankind, and has been highly praised by all the great herbalists and healers for the bewildering array of diseases and ailments it treats. Perhaps one of the reasons for its happy reputation is because it was thought to counteract sterility and enhance fertility. Although these beliefs may seem childish to modern readers, they are by no means to be discounted. Scientific research has corroborated the effect of sage on the hormonal balance, and the name *Salvia horminum* has been given to one species. In the Middle Ages, sage was administered to expel a dead body from the womb and was taken in large doses to induce abortions. In the words of Dioscurides, "it is available for all cleansings of a women, but ye most wicked women making a Pessum of it, do apply it, & cast out ye Embrya."[208] Sage essence was given to facilitate birth and combat sterility in women, and the flowers of the white-flowering sage were considered especially effective against strong menstrual bleeding.

---

208.   Robert T. Gunther, ed., *The Greek Herbal of Dioscurides* (New York: Hafner, 1959), 274.

- A closely related medicinal virtue of the herb, recognized by modern medicine, is the ability of sage to reduce the milk flow of nursing mothers who want to wean their babies. Sage tea can be taken internally, and rubbed in externally for 1–2 weeks to slowly dry up the milk.

It is not certain if sage's reputation as an aphrodisiac is due to direct action on the genital organs or on the hormonal glands, or if its influence is mostly magical and suggestive in nature.

Modern Medicine

The medicinal uses to which sage can be put are in fact so varied that some bewilderment on the part of the novice is justified. Sage's possible applications are so numerous because it works effectively in three distinct areas. The first, and most important, area is as a gland drug. Sage works on the hormonal glands in regulatory fashion and can be of great help to adolescents during puberty and women during menopause. It further helps to regulate the production of the perspiratory glands, and to positively influence the digestive system and salivary glands.

The second major area of sage's medicinal importance is an antiseptic, disinfectant drug. Its beneficial influence on a sore throat as a tea or gargling solution is almost proverbial, and it can also be employed with good results as a treatment for sinus infections (as tea or a steaming herb), as well as influenza and a cold in the lungs, stomach, intestines, or bladder.

The third area of sage's medicinal influence is as a generally stimulating and strengthening medicine with positive action on the liver and the digestive system. Its healing effect on the spleen and on (as one German writer once so nicely put it) an "unchaste" liver is gentle, but pronounced. This can have a positive effect on the entire organism, the circulation, the brain, and the nervous system, and has proved especially helpful in treating older people. The smell of sage is particularly exhilarating and heady, especially if combined with vervain or steeped in sweet cider, and can contribute to the cure. The practice of eating bread and butter and sage sandwiches has gone out of practice, but should be revived as a general preventive measure.

To complete the list of sage's medicinal properties, sage is employed externally as a wound herb, and also in warming poultices. Sage leaves have on occasion been smoked as a palliative measure for asthma in Britain. Pregnant women should be extremely careful about the use of sage, even in cooking, because of its not-always-foreseeable effect on the hormonal glands.

Homeopathic sage can act to control night sweats, as well as a tickling cough, bleeding gums, or mouth sores.

Special Cures

Tea to Lessen Perspiration: One of the most effective teas against excessive perspiration is composed of 2 parts sage leaves, 1 part alpine lady's mantle, 1 part figwort (*Scrophularia nodosa*), 1 part mullein flowers, 1 part lovage leaves, and 1 part lovage root. In order to relieve the excessive perspiration and some of the other problems related to menopause, this tea may be added to another, consisting of 3 parts of lady's mantle, 2 parts alpine lady's mantle, 2 parts cowslip flowers, 1 part dandelion leaves, 1 part chicory leaves, 1 part agrimony, ½ part meadowsweet flowers, 2 parts lemon balm, and 2 parts each of woodruff and St. John's wort. The herbs should be mixed well together, and the tea drunk 2–3 times a day over several months for best results.

Uses in Husbandry

Bees visit sage flowers, and sage honey is treasured above all others in Dalmatia, where it grows wild. Sage is a common ingredient in herbal tobaccos and snuff.

Veterinary Values

Sage is just as important for animal health as it is for human health. Animals' coughs, teething, and tooth problems, eye infections, diarrhea, engorged milk , and sterility can all be treated or alleviated with sage tea.

- A combined herbal oil to repel insects such as ticks and fleas can be prepared from equal amounts of southernwood, wormwood, sage, rosemary, vervain, marjoram (or oregano), nasturtium seeds, and pennyroyal. Soak these in olive oil for 1 week, and then carefully strain and filter (if any vegetable matter is included in the herbal oil, it will spoil quickly). A few drops of natural (not synthetic) eucalyptus oil will give the final touch to the oil. Rub the animal's fur with a few drops before going into infested areas or on a walk, and place a few drops on the animal's sleeping place.

Miscellaneous Wisdom

Sage is used just as often to effect magical as medicinal cures. Sage leaves are thought to be so astringent that they will dry up streams, and have been included among burglars' tools because they supposedly ease the task of picking locks. In some areas of Europe, eating a magical number of sage leaves was once recognized as a cure for certain types of fever and mental disease. In Belgium, eating seven sage leaves was believed to cure foot wounds, and in Sussex, it was thought to cure fever. In other areas of Britain and France, it was considered necessary to eat nine leaves on the first day, eight on the second, seven on the third, and so forth to achieve results. A Catholic version of the practice, recorded in Tyrol in the fifteenth century, was to pick three sage leaves from one bush before sunrise, write a prayer on each, read it aloud, and then recite five Pater Nosters and five Ave Marias. If God and Mary were willing, then the fever would leave. In Switzerland, a sympathetic cure against bad breath was to hang a certain number of sage leaves in the chimney so that the source of the bad breath would dry up with the leaves.

Sage has often been brought into association with toads, worms, and serpents, animals figuring heavily in ancient and folk fertility beliefs. John Gerard, the sixteenth-century herbalist, recommended the herb as an antidote to snakebite. Albertus Magnus believed, several centuries earlier, that a worm (or a bird) could be engendered if sage were buried in dung, and that this worm was capable, when thrown on a fire, of causing thunder and lightning. It could also cause a person to lose his reason for a month or more. In powdered form, sage was thought to fill the house with serpents if burned. A northern German witch was accused of making a girl give birth to a toad by feeding her sage-leaf soup. According to an Italian belief, sage can impregnate a woman without the meddling interference of a man: the woman should take a small amount of essence of sage on an empty stomach every morning during one menstrual cycle.

A similar, but more probable, German belief is that sterile women who drink sage tea regularly will become fertile. In Franconia, young women are beaten with "Lebensruten," or sage twigs, on a certain day each year in spring to make them fertile. Sage leaves can also be used to bewitch a reluctant lover if "Adam Eve" is written on one sage leaf and "Jesus Mary" on the next, and the names of the prospective lovers on the last leaf. The leaves are then powdered and mixed with the beloved's food. The magic will begin to work as soon as the person touches the food to his or her lips.

Oracular Worth

In England, sage is definitely associated with women. A Birmingham gardener's saying states this clearly: "If the sage tree thrives and grows, / The master's not the master, and that he knows."[209] This belief is seconded in Buckinghamshire and other English counties. The Welsh version of the belief is that if sage grows tall in the garden, then the pregnant mistress of the house will certainly give birth to a girl. If a sage bush dies in a French or English garden, it is taken as a sign of misfortune for those associated with it (usually the mistress of the house). Norfolk farmers have been said to hang sage up in the house to learn the fates of distant relatives by observing its growth.

A form of love divination is practiced in the northern English counties with red sage. A group of three, five, or seven girls goes into the garden. Each girl gathers a sprig of red sage and then places a stool in the middle of the room, with a basin of rose

---

209. G. F. Northall. *English Folk-Rhymes* (1892) (Detroit, MI: Singing Tree Press, 1968), 492.

water on it, and puts the sage in the water. A clothesline is tied across the middle of the room, and the girls turn their dresses inside out and sit down on the other side of the room on a bench, in total silence. At midnight, the future husband of each girl will appear, pick up her sage, and sprinkle her with rose water.

Legends

The Hessian wild or wood women have a saying that no human has ever been able to understand. When the wood women see farmers hoeing in the fields, they sigh and then call out, "If the farmers only knew how to use the wild white heather, and the wild white sage, then they would be weeding with silver hoes!"[210]

There must be some truth in their statements, for the French Fées have been heard to say much the same thing. After a Fée was captured by a human, some of her companions called out to her from the woods in warning, "Don't betray sage's secret, for if the rich find out about it, then they'll let the poor starve to death!"[211]

Literary Flowers

Sage, moon-friendly; sage, a magic herb if ever there was one; sage, with leaves as warted as toad's skin and as silvery as moonlight; sage, fleshy and felt-skinned to the touch, oily and spicy to the tongue; sage, gentle yet hardy; sage, relentlessly pure, but worldly and magical, her actions as direct, but as veiled, as a woman's body to her lover.

—SISTER CLARISSA'S UNPUBLISHED BOOK OF NATURAL OBSERVATIONS

There are few shrubs which can come close / to Sage
for it is of service to the Doctor / the Cook / the Butler / rich and poor.
It is an exceptionally good herb
for those who don't have to travel to Frankfurt and Venice for it
but should plant it, the noblest German herb, cheaply in their Gardens.

—HIERONYMUS BOCK, KREÜTTERBUCH

---

210. Hanns Bächtold-Stäubli, ed. *Handwörterbuch des deutschen Aberglaubens* (1927–42), vol. VII (Berlin: Walter de Gruyter & Co., 1987), 896.

211. Ibid.

And in his left he held a basket full / Of all sweet herbs that searching eye could cull:
Wild thyme, and valley-lilies whiter still / Than Leda's love, and cresses from the rill.

—KEATS, *ENDYMION*

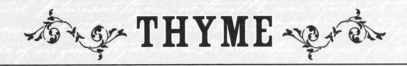

THYME

Name

The name "thyme," and its botanical equivalent, *thymus*, are thought by some etymologists to have originated from the Greek word *thuein*, meaning "burnt offerings." Others believe that it developed from the Egyptian plant called *thm*, a relative of our garden thyme that was used in the preparation of corpses for mummification.

Thyme is a member of the **Mint** family *(Lamiaceae)*. It is usually a perennial plant, but frost hardiness varies between species and varieties. Garden thyme *(Thymus vulgaris)* is a form that is usually more aromatic than the wild thymes (such as *Thymus serpyllum*; *Thymus pulegioides*; or *Thymus x citriodorus*, lemon thyme). Other garden forms are winter or German thyme (a narrow-leaved and strongly aromatic variety) and silver thyme (which has silvery leaves). Gardeners have developed various scented and variegated thymes, and there is a fair amount of confusion among them because wholesalers often use names indiscriminately. Countless bastard and local wild thymes exist, such as Moroccan thyme, Spanish thyme, mastic thyme, and Japanese thyme.

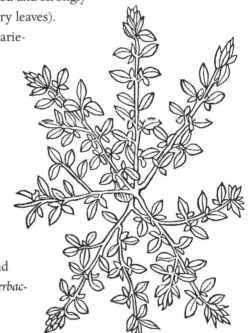

Folk Names

Thyme is also called time, garden thyme, or common thyme. Germans have given it the names *Thymian*, *römischer Quendel*, and *Kuttelkraut*; French call it *thym*, *farigoule*, *frigoule*, and *mignotise des Genevois*. A Russian name is *čebrec*, and Italians address it with the endearing words *timo* or *erbaccia*. The Irish name is *tím*.

Wild thymes have many names. Old herbalists called the plants wild time, running time, creeping time, mother of thyme, mother of time, muske of time, pullial mountaine, and pella mountaine. Wild thymes are now called lemon thyme, Our Lady's bedstraw (not to be confused with the herb with the same name with sweet yellow flowers), mother thyme, creeping thyme, breckland thyme, horse thyme, brotherwort, hillwort, bank thyme, mountain thyme, and shepherd's thyme. Some German names are *Quendel*, *wilder Thymian*, *Karwendel*, *Jungfernzucht*, *Judenmutter*, *Rauschkraut*, *Wohlschmecki*, and *Geismajoran*. French call it *serpolet*; Italians, *serpillo*, *sermollino selvatico*, *serpollino*, *pepolino*, and *timo selvaggio*; and Spanish-speakers, *serpol*. In Denmark, it is called *mutter Mariessengehalm*; in Ireland, *slan-lus*, *lus mna brat*, *lus nan righ bhreatunn*, and *mac righ bhreatunn*; and in Poland, *macierza dusza* (meaning "mother's soul").

Appearance

Garden thyme is usually bushy, and can grow to a height of 12 in. It has a woody and fibrous tap root and an upright, often woody stem that branches repeatedly. The leaves are tiny, numerous, pointed, spear or diamond-shaped, somewhat turned in at the edges, and covered underneath with white down. They grow in pairs and are gray, greenish-gray, or dark green, and occasionally variegated. The leaves are dotted with miniscule oil glands, and the entire plant exudes a strongly aromatic, refreshing smell reminiscent of marjoram. The plant's taste is pungent and slightly bitter. Thyme flowers appear in groups of 3–6 tiny, pink or purple, and occasionally white, blossoms.

According to Culpeper, wild thyme is a plant with

> a small, stringy, creeping root, from which rise a great number of very slender, leaning, woody stalks, having two small, roundish, green leaves, set at a joint, on short footstalks. The flowers grow on the tops of the stalks among the leaves, in small loose spikes of a reddish purple color. The leaves and flowers have a strong pleasant smell.[212]

Wild thyme plants are very small, usually only 10 in. high, but the stems creep along for as much as 2 ft. These stems lie along the ground or hang from banks and cliffs, forming "beds" or "cushions" that give off a very pleasant fragrance when disturbed. Wild thyme flowers are usually lilac, but occasionally white or pale pink.

Place, Season, and Useful Parts

Garden thyme grows wild in some parts of the Mediterranean and in Asia Minor, and may escape from cultivation in warm areas the world over. Despite its susceptibility to

---

212. Culpeper, *Culpeper's Complete Herbal* (1653) (London: Foulsham, undated), 371.

frost, it can be grown in gardens as far north as Iceland. It prefers poor soil on barren hills, stony places, or untilled ground, and can be found wild on hillsides and rocky slopes, and in the *macchia*. It usually blossoms from May to August.

Wild thyme thrives throughout Europe, North America, North Africa, and Asia, from sea level to an altitude of 9,000 ft. It blooms the whole summer through and is not particular about its location. Wild thyme often thrives on anthills, and banks next to paths and roadsides are adorned with tufts of the plant. It grows well on sandy soils, on heaths and dunes, and on rocky mountain hillsides. It will not thrive in salty or very damp soils, where the sun does not shine, or where the air is polluted.

Gathering, Drying, and Storage

Garden thyme can be gathered from May through August, during or shortly before the plant flowers. It is not advisable to cut the plant too late in the year, or it may be harmed by frost. Wild thyme can be gathered from early summer on into September. Only the most aromatic plants are harvested, since there is a great variation in the oil content from plant to plant and in different locations. Mountain varieties are preferable to lowland forms. The plant is cut well above the roots with sharp scissors or a sickle, and the woody stems removed before drying.

Thyme can be hung up in small bundles and dried in an airy, shady, dark place. It dries well, even in damper climates. It is best not to touch or turn the herb until it is completely dry, and then to strip the leaves quickly from the stems. The dried herb must be stored in closed containers to maintain its aroma. Dried thyme keeps well for 1 year, and will begin to lose its strength after that.

Wild thyme is only occasionally dried for medical use, since it can usually be found growing outdoors, even under snow.

Seed Saving and Germination

Thyme seeds retain their fertility under good storage conditions for 2–3 years. There is a lemon-scented form of wild thyme, as well as endless cultivated varieties of garden thyme with different aromas (from caraway to lemon). Most garden varieties are less winter-hardy than wild thyme. All of these differing thyme varieties will bastardize with each other, and must be kept separate if varieties are to be maintained true-to-type. The same is true of the thymes as of the mints: the different thyme varieties should be kept from flowering, and only allowed to flower one at a time to keep bastardization at a minimum. Otherwise, the plants will cross with each other, the seeds will fall to the ground, and it is then almost impossible to recognize the original plants from the crosses. Most cultivated varieties are propagated through plant division or cuttings, and the varieties can be maintained this way. Bushy sprigs about 3 in. long are cut before the plants flower, the lower leaves are stripped and the stem inserted into a rooting medium, and then it is placed in a shaded cold frame, or a pot indoors. Bottom heat can speed the rooting process. Thyme plants can also be layered, and root easily.

Gardening Hints

Thyme grows best in a protected position in full sunlight. It prefers loose or even sandy soil enriched with limestone and not too much fertilizer. It may be grown next to lavender with excellent results. Thyme's miniscule seeds are sown outdoors in April, or somewhat earlier indoors. When sowing outdoors, it is advisable to mix the seeds with sand to ensure even distribution, and to sow them on a dry, warm day. Keep evenly damp. Seedlings should emerge in 3–5 weeks, and can be thinned or transplanted to allow 8–12 in. between plants.

Thyme beds should be replanted or renewed at least every 3 years. Care must be taken to avoid cutting the plants back too late in the year, or they may succumb to a frost. On the other hand, thyme plants that have not been cut back become scraggly and unsightly. The solution seems to be regular harvesting and rigorous cutting back of woody stems in June and July. Many gardeners have puzzled about why thyme succumbs one winter, and easily lives through extreme cold the next.

The major dangers for the plants in winter are drastic day-night temperature changes, especially when there is no snow cover or the soil is dry, as in spring. The plants can be protected with a layer of mulch, put down after a good rain but before the first frost. Or, young thyme plants can be transplanted into window boxes, and brought indoors for winter use.

Old thyme plants are divided as soon as they recover from winter frosts, or cuttings can be taken in early summer. In order to guarantee a continuous supply of thyme, a few plants should be allowed to go to seed every year, or a few branches layered until they form rootlets. New plants should appear the following spring from last year's seed, but they may do it in unexpected places, for ants love to carry the seeds around. Thyme is usually heat and drought-resistant, but requires some cover in winter.

Thyme is especially beneficial to cabbages if grown next to them. Its presence can also help to drive away cabbage root fly and confuse cabbage moths. Thyme is a good plant for containers, quickly forming thick bushes in hanging baskets, window boxes, and terra cotta pots.

Wild thyme is said to grow only where the air is clean and pure and no herbicides are used. It prefers somewhat rocky or sandy, acidic soil. It can be propagated by sowing seeds from established plants in July, or by plant division. The seeds must be tamped down firmly and not covered with soil. Germination may be erratic. It is an excellent plant for planting between the crevices of a garden path, or in a garden border, as a cover plant in rock gardens, on walls, or even on stone seats. Wild lemon thyme is usually raised from cuttings or plant division. Francis Bacon mentioned thyme alleys planted with wild thyme and stonecrop *(Sedum acre)*. Once established, wild thyme beds require little attention beyond hand weeding.

Culinary Virtues

Despite the fact that the French have the highest per capita consumption of wine in the world, their level of general health is surprisingly high. Some authorities maintain that this is due to their wise and discriminate use of onion, garlic, and thyme as seasonings. The ancient Greeks did not make extensive use of thyme, but the ancient Romans employed it as a cheese and liqueur flavoring. Thyme is still used in some warm climates as a food preservative to prevent perishable foods from spoiling. The leaves should always be removed from the woody stalks, and used sparingly as a seasoning.

Thyme can help to stimulate the appetite, and benefits the liver and the gall bladder. Fats are more readily digestible when seasoned with thyme. Because of this, it is added to lamb, mutton, eel, poultry, and sausages. It is used as a spicy seasoning in small amounts for stews, ragouts, marinades, soups, salads, stuffings, sauces, roasts, fish, and seafood. Mayonnaise can be flavored with it, and it is one of the traditional ingredients of the French herb mixture *Herbes de Provence*. A sprig of thyme is included in the *bouquet garni* of French fame, and thyme gives zucchini, carrots, tomatoes, onions, eggplant, guacamole, and pickles a distinctive flavor. Rye, oats, and barley and even soured milk soups can be flavored with thyme, and liqueurs and herbal vinegars are prepared with the herb. Common pork lard is rendered with cherry stems and thyme in order to give it a more delicate flavor, reminiscent of goose fat. Different thyme varieties have a surprising range of aromas, from lemon to caraway to a spicy camphor-like taste.

Thyme jelly is usually prepared with lemon thyme, and can be served with grilled, boiled, or roasted meats and fish. Lemon thyme is also added to cheeses and cream cheeses, and can be used to flavor fruit salads, fruit jellies, and gooseberry dishes. Wild thyme may be substituted for garden or lemon thyme if these are not available. Delicate thyme flowers are used to decorate spicy dishes.

Noteworthy Recipes

Thyme Butter: Beat a stick of softened and unsalted butter in a small bowl, and then mix in several tablespoons of finely-chopped thyme leaves together with a small sprig of French tarragon, chopped fine, and a pinch of hyssop. Add 1 tsp. of fresh lemon juice, drop by drop, beating all the time. Form the butter into a roll, and chill.

Household Applications

Thyme is a strong germicide, and can be used directly in tea form, or combined with cleansing mixtures as a deodorant and disinfectant solution. Thyme and wild thyme have been used for centuries as strewing and fumigating herbs. They are often included in sachets and herbal pillows. Flies are attracted by the herb, but gnats and mosquitoes seem to avoid thyme oil. Thyme pillows are used by some members of the medical profession for their disinfectant qualities. It was once customary to place childbearing women on beds of fresh herbs such as lemon thyme, caraway, or ladies' bedstraw *(Galium verum)* to lessen the risk of infection, and to ease labor.

Cosmetic Properties

Thyme's deodorant and disinfectant qualities make it a valuable cosmetic herb. Wild thyme possesses the same properties in lessened form. Thyme baths are stimulating: they redden, cleanse, and deodorize the skin. To prepare a thyme bath, steep the flowering tops of wild or garden thyme in water for 24 hours, and then strain the liquid into the bath water. Thyme water can also be used as a facial lotion. Powdered thyme is sometimes added to talcum powder or used in the preparation of soap, and thyme oil is an important ingredient of commercial toothpastes and mouthwashes. Essential thyme oil is a recognized germicide. A small amount of thyme water or thyme tea can be added to eye bath solutions, or the leaves included in cosmetic steaming mixtures. Cosmeticians recommend a steaming mixture of equal parts chamomile and lavender flowers and thyme for most skin types. The systematic use of thyme as a seasoning, especially with fatty foods, is reputed to relieve acne.

Medicinal Merits

Thyme was once highly esteemed as a major healing herb. The ancient Romans used both cultivated and wild thyme to treat melancholy and headaches, and it was taken in later years to counteract sleeplessness, nightmares, dizziness, asthma, nervous disorders, and the effects of alcoholic over-indulgence. Pliny reported that burning thyme could drive away poisonous beasts, and it was employed in warming compresses. Hildegard von Bingen wrote about the usefulness of thyme in the treatment of leprosy. Midwives gave thyme to their patients to ease birth, and to help expel the afterbirth and stillborn children. Childbearing women were laid on beds of wild thyme to ease labor pains, and the same beds were thought to inhibit conception and menstruation. Men made use of the herb to treat genital sores. The Anglo-Saxon Nine Herb Charm shows just how much thyme was valued:

Thyme and Fennel, a pair great in power
The wise Lord, holy in heaven,
Wrought these herbs while He hung on the Cross;
He placed and put them in the seven worlds to aid all, poor and rich.[213]

Modern Medicine

Most modern herbalists praise thyme's effective antiseptic qualities. Oil of thyme is an especially potent and effective germicide as well as a mild local anesthetic, and is used in the preparation of a variety of pharmaceutical products. Thyme oil is so potent that it must be diluted with a mild carrier oil when used externally, or it can blister the skin. Syrups, salves, and sterilizing and cleansing solutions often contain thyme oil, and even gauze and bandages are medicated with thyme. Aromatherapy makes extensive use of the herb, especially for the treatment of influenza. Thyme is important for the treatment of influenza because of its germicidal properties, but also because it will cause the patient to break out in a sweat and "sweat off" the disease. The simplest method of flu prevention when the "bug is going around" is to eat foods heavily spiced with aromatic herbs such as thyme and sage, and seasoned with onions and garlic.

Thyme's second major area of medicinal action is as an expectorant, or cough-loosening, preparation. Thyme tea or thyme inhalations are used to ease the mild coughs of children and adults. Essential thyme oil is a powerful medicine, made from garden thyme, that can prove lethal if taken in large doses. But it may be given **under medical supervision** to treat chronic coughs, whooping cough, asthma, tuberculosis, or pulmonary distress.

Thyme is also a stimulating medicine, helpful in the treatment of nervous prostration. It is thought to aid concentration and to counteract mental and nervous exhaustion. People afflicted with anemia or general debility can benefit from a thyme tea (but not a thyme oil) cure. Thyme can also ease cramps and colics, and expel wind from the digestive tract. Oil of thyme is used by physicians to expel hookworms and other intestinal parasites and is usually prepared from a mixture of different thyme species, because they vary in strength. Thyme is considered very warming in Chinese medicine, dispersing colds and counteracting coughs, sore throats, and stomach disorders such as indigestion and vomiting.

Wild thyme can be taken internally as a substitute for garden thyme, although its medicinal action is generally weaker. Wild thyme can be given to those suffering from hangovers and headaches; it is an excellent tea for the long-range treatment of anemia. Since there is little danger of poisoning from wild thyme, it may be given to children or

---

213.   Qtd. in Paul Huson, *Mastering Herbalism* (New York: Stein and Day: 1974), 231.

taken over an extended period. Homeopathic *Thymus serpyllum* is a powerful antibiotic, especially for whooping cough, and has also been used as a sedative.

Both wild and cultivated thymes are used externally for a variety of applications. Thyme baths are considered strengthening, and wild thyme baths are thought particularly effective for bathing children who have rickets. They can also help to strengthen the nerves and ease rheumatic pains. Wild thyme compresses are used as a first-aid measure to treat dislocations and bruising, and sniffing powdered wild thyme is said to still nosebleeds. Wild thyme spirit is a good rubbing mixture for minor pains and cramps, while beds of wild thyme are said to counteract the harmful effects of water currents and earth rays. Injections of thyme oil have been used in the treatment of leprosy. The oil is employed as a painting liquid for certain types of eczema, chilblains, burns, ringworm, and other parasitic skin complaints, as a counterirritant for rheumatic or paralyzed limbs, and in spray mixtures and inhalants for chronic coughs and colds.

Special Cures

Thyme Tea: Because it is so potent medicinally, thyme tea should only be prepared from 1 tsp. of dried garden thyme for every ½ pint of water. Pregnant women and children should avoid using the herb at all, but should especially avoid thyme oil.

Cough Tea for Children: An excellent tea for children's coughs can be prepared from a mixture of 1 part wild thyme leaves, 1 part cherry stems, 1 part chamomile flowers, and 2 parts each of violet and sorrel leaves. One level tsp. of the mixture is brewed with 2 pints of boiling water, and allowed to steep for 10 minutes. This tea, sweetened with honey, can be given a tablespoon at a time as needed throughout the day. It should not be taken for more than 4–6 weeks.

Uses in Husbandry

Thyme is cultivated in large plantations in Spain and France for the production of thyme oil. Dried thyme is an ingredient of commercial herbal tobaccos, and can be added to incense mixtures. It is avidly visited by bees.

Wild thyme is also a bee food, and is greedily gobbled up by sheep and goats. Cats often roll in it and nibble on it, and it is thought to keep chicken lice from the hen coop. In Germany, chickens are given wild thyme water in May as a preventive against disease, and duck and hen eggs are laid on nests of wild thyme so they will hatch more easily. During the twelve days of Christmas, when evil influences are supposedly at their strongest, cows are fed wreaths of wild thyme gathered at Whitsun (the seventh Sunday after Easter). Cows can be protected against disease and encouraged to better milk production by washing their udders with a decoction of wild thyme gathered on Midsummer's Day. Midsummer's Day wild thyme is also used to smoke trees on Christmas Eve so they will produce more fruit the following year. In the Czech Republic and Slovakia, the last few plants of a grain harvest are bound together and decorated with wild thyme. A stone is then placed under this "tent" to produce a winter home for wood women.

Veterinary Values

Animals are often treated with wild thyme instead of garden thyme because of its mild medicinal action and its ready availability. Cattle can be given wild thyme to help cure mild coughs or intestinal disturbances. Very weak newborn animals are rubbed down with an alcoholic extract of wild thyme to strengthen them. Compresses of wild thyme are also applied to ease stomach cramps or colics. Thyme fodder or thyme oil is also used against worms and other intestinal parasites, although care must be taken to get the dosage right, as it will vary with each animal. Thyme oil is used by some veterinary surgeons as an antiseptic and germicidal disinfectant, and it may also be given to induce abortions.

Miscellaneous Wisdom

Wild and cultivated thyme are both believed to have aphrodisiacal properties. They were sacred to the goddess Aphrodite and to Venus. Supplicants presented Venus with offerings of thyme and roses in her temples, and thyme beds played a central part in some Greek fertility rites. The Muses were also partial to offerings of thyme. In the Middle Ages, ladies gave their favored knights sprigs of thyme or cloths embroidered with a sprig of thyme and a visiting bee to increase their courage. Romany men traditionally declare their love with a gift of thyme. In England, country girls wear sprigs of thyme, lavender, and mint when they are intent on attracting the opposite sex, and English boys are convinced of the courage-giving properties of beer soup flavored with thyme. It is traditional for German brides to tuck some blessed thyme into their shoes or blouses before the marriage ceremony. In Brandenburg, a bride may put some thyme in her shoes and then repeat,

> I step, I step on thyme,
> And that will keep your eye,
> Your wanton eye, from wandering.[214]

In the German Middle Ages, it was customary for girls to gather thyme on the holidays sacred to the Virgin Mary, especially August 15th, and to have them blessed in church. Hung over the girls' beds, these sprigs protected them from illness and misfortune. In Austria, France, and Bohemia, girls annoyed by the unwelcome advances of Satan hung

---

214. Hanns Bächtold-Stäubli, ed., *Handwörterbuch des deutschen Aberglaubens* (1927–42), vol. VII (Berlin: Walter de Gruyter & Co., 1987), 418.

bundles of thyme in front of their bedroom windows. Similarly, anyone persecuted by the devil was advised to go and sit on the next tussock of wild thyme. Thyme was also believed to drive away witches and lightning. Pliny wrote that thyme kept dangerous beasts away from workers during their noonday naps. (Maybe it will also keep the boss away during a siesta at the office.)

Southernwood and speedwell (*Veronica officinalis*) are considered especially effective antidemonic herbs in conjunction with wild thyme. In Central Europe, wild thyme and stonecrop (*Sedum acre*) are fashioned into wreaths and carried in the Assumption (August 15th) and Whitsunday (the seventh Sunday after Easter) processions. A Whitsun wreath is reputed to drive witches away from stalls and cellars and help prevent minor household disasters. In one part of Germany, these wreaths are laid on the heads of sick people threatened by the grim reaper, known as the *Bilmesschnitt*. The association of the thyme plant with death is also widespread in Somerset, where people consider it very unlucky to bring thyme into the house, for it may anger the faeries and attract Death. Thyme is often planted on Welsh graves.

An etymologically based German belief is that wild thyme (known as *Quendel*) can be of help in business (*Handel*) and aid a businessman or shopkeeper. All he has to do is swing some wild thyme three times over his head and repeat the words, "Wild time, wild thyme, make it trade time!"[215] In Franconia, the plant is thought to be a quarrelsome plant, for the "mountaine pullail causes us to rail!"[216]

Legends

Wild thyme has long been considered a woman's plant. It was sacred to Freya, who was said to have used it as a bed. It was also associated with Frau Holle (a German mythical figure), and later with the Virgin Mary. The plant is so closely associated with the Virgin Mary that it has been given the local Tyrolean name of Maria Karwendelin ("Mary of the Wild Thyme"). Legend has it that Saint Anne, Mary's mother, softened her bed with wild thyme when she was a child. She was supposedly married wearing a thyme wreath, and is said to have rested on wild thyme during her journey over the mountains. According to Flemish legend, Mary laid the newborn baby Jesus on a bed of sweet-smelling thyme.

Oracular Worth

On the Eve of St. Agnes' Day, January 20th, a girl curious to know the name of her future husband should gather one sprig of rosemary and one sprig of thyme, sprinkle

---

215. Hanns Bächtold-Stäubli, ed., *Handwörterbuch des deutschen Aberglaubens* (1927–42), vol. VII (Berlin: Walter de Gruyter & Co., 1987), 419.

216. Ibid.

them three times with water, and then place each in a shoe. The shoe with the rosemary is put on one side of the bed, and the shoe with the thyme on the other. Before climbing into bed, the girl should repeat the following verse, "St. Agnes that's to lovers kind / Come, ease the troubles of my mind."[217] If St. Agnes is kindly disposed, the girl will dream of her lover that night.

Herbal Pastimes

Children intent on building houses outdoors, designating this clearing as the living room, that as the throne room, will not fail to recognize the place where the wild thyme grows as the bedroom. Adults usually content themselves with savoring the herb's aroma when they sit or step on it by chance.

Literary Flowers

It was a time when silly bees could speak,
And in that time, I was a silly bee
Who fed on thyme until my heart 'gan break
Yet never found the time would favour me.
Of all the swarm I only did not thrive,
Yet brought I wax and honey to the hive.

Then thus I buzz'd when thyme no sap would give,
Why should this blessed thyme to me be dry
Sith by this thyme the lazy drone doth live,
The wasp, the worm, the gnat, the butterfly.
Mated with grief, I kneeled on my knees,
And thus complain'd unto the King of bees:

"My liege, gods grant thy time may never end,
And yet vouchsafe to hear my plaint of thyme,
Which fruitless flies have found to have a friend,
And I cast down when atomies do climb,"
The King replied but thus: "Peace, peevish bee,
Thou'rt bound to serve the Time, the thyme not thee."

—"IT WAS A TIME WHEN SILLY BEES,"
WORDS ATTRIBUTED TO ROBERT, EARL OF ESSEX, MUSIC BY JOHN DOWLAND

---

217. G. F. Northall, *English Folk-Rhymes* (1892) (Detroit, MI: Singing Tree Press, 1968), 112.

Valerian then he crops, and purposely doth stampe,
T'apply unto the place that's hales with the Crampe.

—MICHAEL DRAYTON, *POLY-OLBION*, SONG XIII

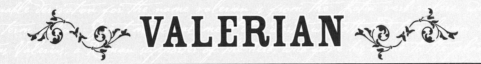

VALERIAN

Name

The most reasonable derivation for the name "valerian" is from the Latin verb *valere*, which has also given us the modern term "value." Others insist that it was Valerius, a Roman supporter of the herb, who gave his name to the plant; and still others believe that Valeria, a town in western Hungary, is the source of the name.

Valeriana officinalis is a perennial member of the **Valerian** family *(Valerianaceae)*. *Valeriana celtica*, or Celtic nard, is another important member of this botanical family. Folk names for this plant are *Speik* and *Alpenbaldrian* in German, and *valériane narde celtique* in French. In Switzerland, the herb is known as *Wildfräulekraut*, or elf-woman herb. Different valerian species vary from each other according to habitat, but most are employed medicinally. *Valeriana phu* used to be a medicinal herb, but is now grown mostly as an ornamental. The European salad green mâche (or corn salad), *Valerianella locusta*, is closely related to valerian and has a very mild smell reminiscent of valerian.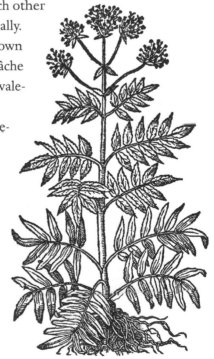

Valerian can easily be confused with American spikenard *(Aralia racemosa)* or, more often, with Indian spikenard *(Nardostachys grandifolia)*, which is used to produce the widely sold essential oil. Valerian is also often confused with catnip *(Nepeta cataria)* because it attracts cats. Similarly, it is sometimes confused with lady's slipper because of its folk name, "American valerian."

Folk Names

Folk names for valerian are cat's valerian, all-heal, heliotrope, setwall, setewale, capon's tail, St. George's herb, vandal root, moon root, and great wild valerian.

Antiquated names for the plant are *phu* (i.e., phew), *theriacaria, marinella, genicularis,* and *amantilla.* Valerian is called *Baldrian, Katzenwurzel, Katzengeil, Tammarg, Arzneibaldrian, Mondwurz,* and *wilder Nardus* in German; *valériane, herbe aux chats,* and *guerit-tout* in French; *valeriana* in Spanish; and *valeriana silvestre* and *amantilla* in Italian. American valerian (lady's slipper) is also called tobacco root.

Appearance

Valerian has been known to grow to a man's height and to tower over all other plants, although its normal height varies between 1 and 4 ft. It has a great number of tiny rootlets balled around a larger tuber, giving the impression of a tangle of nerves or the circulatory system of the brain. The roots are dark brown on the outside and yellow-white inside. While still fresh, the valerian smell is minimal, but it intensifies with drying. The leaves have a peculiar odor when bruised, which some find attractive and others repulsive. The single stalk is hollowed and furrowed, and the paired leaves on foot-long stalks are a dark, somewhat dull, even green color. The leaf form is frond-like, with 6–10 pairs of lance-shaped segments. The flowers are white, pale pink, or a purplish-red and appear in masses at the end of the main stalk. They do not last long, but quickly develop seedheads. The single seed parachutes are disseminated by the wind. New plants then spring up in damp places.

European spikenard, *Valeriana celtica,* is also perennial and grows to a height of 8 in. The leaves are dark green, bald, and shiny, the flowers reddish on the outside and yellowish inside. Spikenard and all mountain forms of valerian have fewer roots, but are more highly prized for their aromatic medicinal merits than lowland varieties. Because of intensive gathering of the wild plants, spikenard has become so rare that it is considered an endangered species in many countries, and the gathering of wild plants is forbidden.

Place, Season, and Useful Parts

Valerian prefers damp places, swampy meadows, marshy thickets, ditches, pits, river banks, or the edges of ponds, and can be found growing among thick underbrush, in hedgerows and light woods, or in the half-shade of trees. It also can be grown on dry ground, on sunny or rocky slopes, and in high pastures and meadows up to an altitude of 7,000 ft. It grows throughout Europe, with the exception of the extreme north and the extreme south. Valerian blossoms from June through August and September. The roots are dug after the plant has died back, in September and October, on into the spring.

European spikenard is found wild in the eastern Alps, and in northern Italy and Switzerland, at an altitude of 6,000–8,500 ft.

Gathering, Drying, and Storage

Two-year-old valerian roots are dug after they blossom in fall, or before the leaves appear in spring. Most ancient instructions for digging the plant maintain that it is safest to ask the plant for permission to harvest it before gathering the roots. They are washed quickly in running water, combed to remove earth particles, and laid out to dry in an airy place.

Some authorities recommend drying the roots outdoors, but this is not advisable if there are any cats in the neighborhood. Their passion for the drug is such that they eat it and roll in it. Tomcats will urinate or even ejaculate on the roots, rendering them unfit for use. Cats should also be kept in mind when storing the herb. Valerian left in an open container is a direct invitation to felines, and herbalists have only themselves to blame if the year's supply is raided. There are also stories of housecats knocking bottles of valerian tablets off the bedside table and then batting the pills around the house. Closed glass, ceramic, or wooden containers will keep the cats out, and the drug fresh.

Seed Saving and Germination

Valerian seeds germinate best if sown directly after they ripen in damp soil. Germination may take up to 1 year once the seeds are in the soil, but a large percentage will eventually sprout. Dried and frozen or stored seeds have notoriously low germination rates. The easiest method of propagating promising valerian strains is through division of established plants. Take a piece of root with a visible crown, and keep the young plants damp until they root.

Gardening Hints

Valerian grown in dry, light, highland soil produces the best roots for medicinal purposes, but valerian grown in the lowlands or in garden soil can also be of value. Wild valerian is found in damp places in the vicinity of water, in poor pastures, or as a garden escape. It requires a large amount of moisture, but also plenty of light and air in order to thrive.

Valerian can be raised from plants found growing wild, or the seeds may be sown directly after they ripen. Best results are obtained by planting root offsets of wild plants at the end of summer. Seeds should be distributed freely on freshly, but not deeply, plowed land as soon as possible after they are harvested in September. The soil must then be stamped down and kept damp. Valerian is self-propagating and its seeds are carried by the wind. The only attention it needs once planted is consequent watering and some weeding.

The advantage of having valerian in the garden is that it benefits the growth of the plants and vegetables planted next to it. It will also increases the phosphorous content of the soil, and its exudations are attractive to earthworms. Experiments conducted with pining vegetable plants have shown that spraying them with valerian tea may stimulate new growth. In case of impending frost, fragile fruit blossoms are sprayed by orchardists with a mixture of water and valerian flower extract to increase their resistance to frost.

The main disadvantage of having valerian in the garden is that the herb, if bruised in any way, will unfailingly attract cats. Anyone with garden experience knows just how much damage these lovesick visitors can make while they roll in the garden and dig unsightly holes.

Culinary Virtues

According to herbalist John Gerard, "They that will have their heale, Must put Setwall in their Keale." In other words, those wishing to avoid disease and epidemics should include valerian in their broths and pottages. But times have changed, and even the suggestion of adding valerian to food provokes more disgust than appreciation from modern cooks.

An African valerian, *Valeriana cornucopiae* or *Fedia cornucopiae,* is still eaten as a salad plant. It is also known as Algerian salad. *Valerianella locusta*, or corn salad, is also known as lamb's lettuce or mâche. It is close relative of valerian, and smells vaguely like valerian when fresh. Its tasty and vitamin-rich leaves can be harvested weeks before normal salads are ready in the spring. The roots of *Valeriana edulis* are edible, and can be eaten after nightlong steaming.

Household Applications

Common valerian's major use in today's household is as a cat luxury item. Pet owners who want to win the approval of their feline companions present them with small amounts of valerian plants or roots. Any cat that turns down such a gift is truly fastidious.

European spikenard was once exported in large quantities to the Orient, and was added to many household and cosmetic items because of its uniquely fresh smell. The aroma of spikenard has gone out of fashion since then and is now termed "exotic," and has been criticized as being too severe. Indian valerian and spikenard are used to perfume exotic-smelling incenses and hair preparations.

Cosmetic Properties

In the Alpine countries, European spikenard soap is still produced commercially by a few companies. Indian spikenard was once used extensively in the perfume industry. Its reputation was so high in Biblical times that Mary used an ointment prepared from the herb to perfume and salve the feet of the Savior. Valerian root tincture may be added in small quantities to massage oil to enhance its relaxant qualities.

Medicinal Merits

Valerian was once a famed eye herb, and was also prescribed against stitches in the side, as a worm medicine, and to warm cold veins and ease paralysis. It was reputed to draw thorns out from damaged flesh, and some believed it capable of healing meat in the kitchen pot. It was widely prescribed as medicine to counteract the "bad vapors" of the plague, and was included in the famous preventive medicine against plague and poison named *theriak*. Valerian was effective in the treatment of the mass hysteria associated with outbreaks of the Black Death. It was also administered during air raids during World War II in Europe as a general sedative.

Modern Medicine

Valerian is one of the most reliable and effective nervine medicines. It is an excellent remedy for nervous disorders and disharmonies, acting as a sedative, strengthening the nerves, and helping to restore equilibrium to the body. It is prescribed to lessen the disturbances and emotional upheavals caused by puberty, menopause, menstruation, pregnancy, coffee and alcohol misuse, hysteria, exhaustion, school and exam fears, unusual emotional stress, cramps, or spasms. It has been specifically employed with varying degrees of success in the treatment of mental derangement and epilepsy, and is used as a sovereign remedy against mild nervous conditions, panic attacks, and floating anxiety. Valerian is the herb of choice for the anxious, hectic, or hypochondriacal patient.

Valerian is further administered as a mild diuretic and to reduce the pressure of nervous intestinal colics and neuralgic pain, as well as to regulate high blood pressure caused by emotional upsets. It is taken to induce sleep, to calm sleepers plagued with nightmares, to prevent sleepwalking, and to calm nervous tics or spasms.

Valerian is an official drug in most countries, and can be administered in a variety of forms: as tea, powder, tincture, wine, extract, distilled water, or syrup. It is most potent fresh, and should never be taken in large amounts, but dosed conservatively.

It is important to keep in mind that too much valerian can stimulate or even excite instead of sedating. Massive doses of valerian in alcoholic form can result in hallucinations and delirium, and extended use of the tea may result in digestive problems or impair the circulation. The patient may also develop a psychological dependency on the drug.

- One tsp. of the dried roots for 1 cup of tea should be considered a maximum dose. Let the roots steep in cold water overnight, and then heat the tea gently before straining and serving. When used to treat sleeplessness, the tea should be taken half an hour before bedtime. A valerian cure should be interrupted after 4–6 weeks of constant use, or only taken occasionally as needed. The constant use of valerian can lead to side-effects.

Special Cures

Tea for Insomniacs: A good nervine tea for insomniacs can be prepared from 1½ parts valerian roots, 3 parts hop flowers, 2 parts each of lemon balm and woodruff leaves, chamomile flowers, heather flowers, and goose grass, 1½ parts each of seedless rosehips, orange blossoms and leaves, and 1 part each of corn poppy flowers *(Papaver rhoeas)*, rose petals, fennel seeds, lavender, and cowslip flowers. Mix the dried herbs together and prepare each cup of tea from 1 level Tbsp. of the fresh, loose herbs for each ½ pint of boiling water. Let steep for 10–15 minutes and drink half an hour before bedtime. If needed, the tea can be filled into a thermos bottle and a second cup taken in the morning or early afternoon.

Uses in Husbandry

Valerian attracts cats, rats, bees, and earthworms. It has been suggested, but not definitely proven, that the Pied Piper of Hamelin had such success with rats because of the valerian that he carried with him.

Veterinary Values

Most animals, with the exception of cats, can be given valerian as a mild sedative. A weak tea of powdered valerian roots is administered to domestic animals to relieve stomach and intestinal cramps, flatulence and nervous digestive disorders, and to increase appetite. Cats are very fond of the roots, but often overindulge. Reactions to the herb vary strongly from animal to animal, producing euphoria in some cats and drunkenness in others.

Miscellaneous Wisdom

Valerian's relaxant influence was once considered to be a side effect of its antidemonic properties against evil and witchcraft. Nervous complaints, nightmares, epilepsy, and various "invisible diseases" were believed to originate from the ill will and envy of sorcerers, devils, elves, and witches. Patients and sickrooms were smoked with valerian as a preventive against "bad" magic. Many believed that witches bent on mischief would be made visible by bundles of the plant hung in the bedroom or stall. Because a witch's main defense is secrecy, it was thought that she would refuse to enter a room protected by valerian. Valerian was especially valued as a witch herb in the Slavic countries.

Valerian is supposed to be more effective when used in combination with other herbs such as organy (wild marjoram). It is also thought to be more magically effective if gathered on the Day of Mary's Ascension, August 15th. In most Germanic countries, it is usually included in the bunch of herbs blessed on Mary's Day, which is prized as a blessed remedy against bewitchment and disease. Cows with red, swollen teats are treated with valerian. Milk that will not turn to butter is poured through a wreath of valerian to counteract the evil influence. Children suffering from magically-induced diseases were given a valerian cure. In Czechoslovakia, newborn children were often bathed in a decoction of valerian as protection against disease, pestilence, and the envy of elves. The Swedes use valerian as a cure for elf-shot (lumbago or sudden back pains). In other countries, the herb was used to cure the ill will of elves and elf-induced nightmares.

According to a fourteenth-century herbal, "Men who begin to fight and when you wish to stop them, give to them the juice of Amantilla id est Valeriana and peace will be made immediately." This statement was seconded in a German herbal from the sixteenth century: valerian "peacefully and happily unites those who drink from the same bowl."[218] Valerian was believed to exorcize the devils of anger and discord, and to temper choleric and irascible natures.

Mention must also be made of valerian's reputed aphrodisiacal powers. It is a powerful muscle relaxant and can help relieve nervous tension, but folk belief attributes its aphrodisiacal properties primarily to its ability to keep maleficent thoughts and beings away. The prospective lovers, both man and woman, should drink valerian wine to each other's health and pleasure. Valerian worn in the girdle or corset of a Welsh lass is also believed to attract lovers. And a man who wears valerian and carline thistle will be hard for women to resist. In Westphalia, the belief was prevalent that the devil will not visit boys and girls who go nutting on Sunday with valerian in their hands. Maybe this was only wishful thinking, taking the notorious reputation of nutting parties into account.

Legends

During outbreaks of the plague, German peasants often reported wood women calling advice from the forest. One of the women told the villagers, "Eat pimpernel and valerian, then the pest won't touch you!"[219]

In other areas, sickly children were smoked with valerian. It was assumed that their disease was caused by elves who sucked the children's vital force from their fingertips. In one case, as soon as the room filled with the pungent smoke, the elves appeared on the floor in the shape of tiny dolls. The elves promised to leave the child alone if a good place could be found for them to live.[220]

---

218.   Otto Brunfels, *Contrafayt Kräuterbuch* (1532), facsimile (Munich: Konrad Kölbl, 1964).

219.   Pimpernel or bimellen is the alpine pimpernel, *Pimpinella saxifraga*. Wilhelm Mannhardt, *Der Baumkultus der Germanen und ihrer Nachbarstämme* (Berlin: Bornträger, 1875), 81.

220.   Wilhelm Mannhardt, *Der Baumkultus der Germanen und ihrer Nachbarstämme* (Berlin: Bornträger, 1875), 62.

Literary Flowers

Few plants can grow peacefully above the roar, against the monotonous mumble of the stream. But a graceful apparition ranges above the others on sodden banks: valerian. Valerian's true power lies in the roots that grip the damp soil determinedly, concentrating the healing powers. These roots can calm a frenzied man, and send the calmest cat into conniptions. The smell of the bruised roots tells of damp banks, of moldy ground, earth, and rotting leaves, and lack of light, but also of pungent rejuvenation, of waters flowing in still channels with turbulent strength.

—SISTER CLARISSA'S UNPUBLISHED BOOK OF NATURAL OBSERVATIONS

A garden inclosed is my sister, my spouse; a spring shut up, a fountain sealed.
Thy plants are an orchard of pomegranates, with pleasant fruits; camphire, with spikenard.
Spikenard and saffron; calamus and cinnamon,
with all trees of frankincense; myrrh and aloes, with all the chief spices:
A fountain of gardens, a well of living waters, and streams from Lebanon.

—SONG OF SOLOMON 4:12–15

VIOLET & PANSY

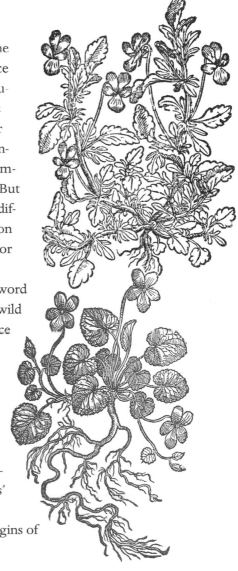

Name

The color violet owes its name to this purple flower. The snowdrop, moonwort, and periwinkle were also once called "violets," and folk botanists still use the term casually for all the wild violets and for wild pansies. *Viola odorata*—the "true," "sweet-smelling," "common," or "March" violet—is derived from the Latin *viola*. A perennial, this violet is only one of many species of the family **Violaceae,** and can be easily confused with them. But while other species may be similar in appearance, they differ in smell or medicinal properties. The most common of these other species is *Viola canina*, the "dog violet" or "heath dog violet."

The term "pansy" is of French origin, from the word pensée, since the herb is a plant of remembrance. The wild pansy is also called "heart's ease." This name was once used indiscriminately for wallflowers or gilliflowers (Cheiranthus cheiri) as well as for the wild pansy, but is now restricted just to the wild pansy. Its botanical name, Viola tricolor, means a "three-colored violet." Heart's ease is an annual or biennial, and occasionally a short-lived perennial. Many colorful and large-blossomed garden pansies have been developed by horticulturalists over the centuries, at the cost of the plants' medicinal properties.

One wishful poet, ruminating on the unknown origins of the charming name "heart's ease," was led to exclaim,

The heart's ease; I could look for half a day
Upon this flower, and shape in fancy out
Full twenty different tales of love and sorrow
That gave this gentle name![221]

One distressing explanation may come from the plant's use as a cure for the so-called French diseases.

Folk Names

The sweet violet and the pansy have countless picturesque folk names. The sweet-smelling violet is also called the common violet, March violet, sweet-scented violet, sweet blue violet, garden violet, English violet, or simply violet. In German, *Veilchen* also go by the names *wohlriechendes Veilchen, Märzveilchen, Mariennägelein,* and *Violaten.* The French call the herb *violette odorante, violette de Mars, violette de carême, fleur de Mars,* and *violette des haies.* The Italians name it *viola mammola, violetta,* and *viola zopa.* In Spain and Portugal, it is *violeta;* in Iceland, *tyrsfiola;* in Wales, *gwiolydd;* in Russia, *fialka.*

Heart's ease has excited the naming fancy of folk botanists. It is called heartsease, lovers' thoughts, wild pansy, herb constancy, herb trinitatis, love-in-idleness, love-and-idle, live-in-idleness, love-lies-bleeding, love-in-vain, love-true, loving idol, two faces in a hood, call-me-to-you, jack-jump-up-and-kiss-me, johnny-jump-up, look-up-and-kiss me, kiss-me-quick, kiss-her-in-the-buttery, jack-behind-the garden-gate, kit-run-in-the-fields, kit-run-about, kitty-run-the-street, cull me, cuddle me, tittle-my-fancy, meet-me-in-the-entry, pinkeney john, pink-eyed john, pink-o'-the-eye, pink o' my john, flower o' luce, flamy, bird's eye, lark's eye, biddy's eyes, bouncing bet (also used as a name for soapwort), gentleman-tailor, stepfathers and stepmothers, stepmother, godfathers and godmothers, banewort, pussy-face, monkey's face, cat's face, coach-horse, and bullweed. German names are *Stiefmütterchen, Feldstiefmütterchen, Freisamkraut, Dreifaltigkeitskraut, Samtveilchen, Schöngesicht, Mädchenauge,* and *unnütze Sorge.* Some French names are *pensée, fleur de la trinité,* and *herbe de la trinité.* In Italy, wild pansies are called *viola del pensiero, viola di tre colori, erba della trinitá, viola farfalla,* and *suocera e nuora.* Spaniards call them *pensiamento* and *trinitaria;* Danes, *stedmorsblomst;* Swedes, *styfmorsfiol;* Irish, *goirmín;* and Russians, *anjutiny glazki.*

The dog violet is also known as blue violet, pig violet, snake violet, summer violet, hypocrites, hedge violet, horse violet, blue mice, shoes and stockings, cuckoo's shoes, and cuckoo's stockings.

---

221.   Mary Howitt, "Philip of Maine," *The Seven Temptations* (London: Richard Bentley, 1834; original from Oxford University; digitized 2006), 275.

Appearance

The sweet-smelling March violets produce small leaves and showy flowers in March or April. Later in the year, the flowers are small and insignificant-looking (but fertile), and the leaves are large. The blossoms may vary in color from deep purple to blue, pink, or even white. The leaves form a rosette and are downy on the underside, and this plant can easily be recognized by its unmistakable fragrance. Dioscurides described it:

> Viola hath a leaf less than Ivy, & thinner, but blacker, and not unlike, a little stalk in ye midst from ye root, on which a little flower very sweet, of a purple: it grows in shady and rough places.[222]

Nicholas Culpeper's description is more detailed:

> The root is perennial; it is long, slender, crooked, and fibrous; they [the leaves] are supported on long slender leafstalks, of a roundish figure, heart-shaped at the base, slightly notched at the edges, and of a dark green colour, several slender creeping stems rise from among them, which take root at the joints, and so propagate the plant. The flowers are supported singly on long, slender, fruit-stalks, which rise direct from the root; they are large, of a beautiful deep blue or purple, and extremely fragrant. The seeds are egg-shaped, numerous, and firnished with appendages.[223]

The wild pansy resembles its biennial garden cousins, but it has a longer flower stalk and much smaller flowers. It grows to a maximum height of 1 ft., and the blossoms are usually no more than 1 in. in diameter. Its head droops at night and during rainy spells, and its roots smell suggestively of peach kernels. The stem is triangular and hollow, and it branches more than the stems of other violets. Lower pansy leaves are heart-shaped, and the upper ones are divided into serrated and rounded lobes. Pansy blossoms have a grassy taste and no distinguishable odor, and are divided into 5 petals. Each petal is colored purple, white, and yellow. Pansies growing in a damp place, and marked by predominately purple blossoms, are thought to be especially valuable as medicine. All wild pansy flowers have a bottom petal striped with dark honey lines, to guide bees to the nectar and pollen. Pansy seeds are yellow and pear-shaped.

Place, Season, and Useful Parts

The sweet March violet is one of the first flowers to blossom in the spring, and is soon followed by the scentless violets. The March violet prefers a damp position and rich

---

222. Robert T. Gunther, ed., *The Greek Herbal of Dioscurides* (New York: Hafner, 1959), 513.

223. Culpeper, *Culpeper's Complete Herbal* (1653) (London: Foulsham, undated), 380.

soil in a cold, shady, and uncultivated place. It grows well under underbrush, in grassy borders, or on the edges of paths and woods, in hedges and on stream banks, on sloping meadows, and next to ruined walls. Violets sometimes escape from cultivated areas and can be found growing next to gardens, orchards, and graveyards. The home of the wild violet is the south and west of Europe. It has become naturalized in other areas, and grows to an altitude of 2,500 ft. in Europe, Asia, India, some parts of Africa, and occasionally in North America. Violet leaves are gathered singly or together with the flowers, violet flowers are gathered singly, and violet roots are dug when the plant is dormant.

Pansies are found growing wild in most of the Northern Hemisphere, especially in Eurasia and eastward into India, in fields, meadows, gardens, cultivated ground, riverbanks, sandy hills, mountainsides, dunes, and grain fields. Pansies are one of the first "weeds" to appear on fallow ground, and their massive presence can be taken as a sign of lime deficiency in the soil. Pansies bloom off and on for most of the year, and can be annual, biennial, or even perennial. Herbalists usually harvest the entire blossoming plant, without roots.

Gathering, Drying, and Storage

The first March violets can be gathered in large numbers without endangering the plants or their capacity to reproduce themselves—the plants are actually stimulated to new flower production if the first flowers are picked. Seed-bearing flowers are only produced later in the year, carefully hidden under the plants' leaves. Keep in mind that garden violets do not possess the same medicinal properties as wild violets.

Violet flowers should be gathered on a sunny morning, just before they open fully, and placed, without bruising or crushing, in large, flat baskets. Violet leaves are gathered before the plants flower, and violet roots are dug from September on into November. Violets must be dried as quickly as possible in a dry, airy place or with the help of artificial heat, for their fragrance is volatile. They should be spread out singly on sheets of paper, screens, or cloths, and turned often. Discard the papers or change the cloths if they become damp, for the flowers must retain their color throughout the drying process. Pale or discolored flowers are medicinally worthless. Dried violets weigh only a fifth of what the fresh herb weighs. The roots should be washed quickly, and hung up to dry on strings.

Wild pansies gathered from unsprayed rye fields are said to be medicinally more potent than other pansies, especially for the treatment of grain allergies, skin diseases, and rashes. They should be gathered on the morning of a sunny day, and dried carefully to avoid mildew.

Seed Saving and Germination

If medicinally potent violet varieties, or varieties with unusual flowers, are to be maintained, they must be carefully isolated from other varieties. Ants love to drag violet seeds around, which is the reason why they spring up again and again in the most unexpected parts of the garden. According to natural observation, the best time to sow seeds is directly after they ripen, in damp soils, and then to cover them with leaf mold. Because of ants' activities, different violets will inevitably become intertwined if special care is not taken to keep the varieties separate.

Violet seeds are hard to find and often overlooked by the novice because they are close to the ground, hidden by leaves, and develop late in the year. A bit of hunting is necessary to find them, and they should be observed for several days to determine when they ripen fully. They can be sown immediately, or the seed capsules dried carefully in an airy, dark place.

Wild pansies will not usually bastardize with garden varieties, and produce seed the same season in large amounts. Seed-bearing pansy plants can be gathered without roots, and the seeds allowed to ripen onto paper, cloths, or thin-meshed screens placed in the sun. Potential seed savers should remember that garden pansy varieties usually produce seeds in the second year if they are not sterile. Many well-meaning gardeners clean up their gardens too thoroughly in the fall and don't give biennial plants such as pansies, dame's rocket, foxglove, or evening primrose a chance to develop the rosette that will guarantee next year's blossoms and seeds.

Gardening Hints

The sweet-smelling violet is cultivated on a commercial scale for the production of violet oil, but is also a common sight in many gardens because of its early blossom. Larger-blossom garden varieties and hybrids have been developed by horticulturalists since the seventeenth century. Violet plants usually produce flowers in the spring of their second year, and should be replanted or renewed after every flowering season for optimum flower display. Violets demand warm and moist, but not clayey, somewhat alkaline soil. They prefer partial shade in the summer, and full sun in the fall months. Violets are liable to attack by red spider mites (the leaves turn suddenly and unexpectedly yellow) if subjected to too much sun. They may also deteriorate if grown in total shade. Violets thrive in somewhat sandy, deeply worked soil that has been fertilized with decayed manure, compost, or leaf mold. They respond well to clean, fresh air, and may be harmed by noxious fumes. Violets may also be grown indoors on sunny windowsills.

Most gardeners prefer to divide the plants, or to set runners instead of starting plants from seed. Violet seeds germinate very slowly, and may be carted off by busy ants before sprouting. They should be stratified, or sown before a winter cold spell. Violets planted in April should bloom in September, and those set in October blossom the following spring. Violets grow well between sweet peas, and benefit from a mulch of ripe manure or leaf mold. They should be set on an overcast, humid day, allowing 1 ft. of space between plants. The plants can be kept moist by covering them with an inverted flowerpot until well rooted, if ants are not a menace in the garden. The bed should be hoed or weeded regularly, and runners removed. Some gardeners like to train their violets to grow into a "tree." Several strong plants are bound to a stake firmly placed in the earth, and the plants are well-fertilized for two or three years. During that time, all the flowers and runners are removed. As soon as the tree is established, the plants are allowed to blossom.

Ants spread the seeds of wild pansies, and the plants will spring up persistently year after year. They germinate best in the vicinity of rye, and do not do well next to wheat. Wild pansies are sometimes used in gardens as bedding plants, and large-petaled garden varieties are planted as ornamentals. Annual wild pansies should be sown in the spring, garden and biennial varieties in the fall for an early spring crop. Pansies should not be fertilized with lime or dolomitic limestone, and will not do well in soils with high lime content.

Culinary Virtues
Very young violet greens make acceptable salad greens, and can be cooked as a spring vegetable. Violet leaves are considered to be a good seasoning for string bean salads, and are rich in vitamin C and carotin. One of the wild violets, *Viola verecunda*, was once cultivated in China as a vegetable plant.

Violet blossoms are highly prized by confectioners because of their coloring properties and their sweet odor, despite the somewhat sour taste. Even violet blossom tea has a pleasant purple color, as does the violet vinegar so highly recommended by Francis Bacon. The ancient Romans prepared a violet-colored wine from fresh violets. Violet jelly, violet marmalade, violet sherbet, violet syrup, violet ice cream, violet candies, violet pastes, violet sugar, and violet liqueurs can all be prepared from the dainty flowers. Young violet flowers and flower buds are candied whole as garnishes and sweets, and used to decorate cakes, pastries, and puddings. "Violet plate" was a famous violet confection taken to strengthen the heart and to fortify the innards.

Heart's ease flowers can be used to prepare an excellent cordial syrup, and the flowers are good garnishes for dishes like potato salad, cottage cheese, avocado dips, poached salmon, and green or fruit salads. Even garden pansies can be used as garnishes and in the preparation of syrups.

Noteworthy Recipes

Syrup of Violets: A fine syrup of violets used for sherbets, confections, or tea can be prepared by taking

> the Flowers of the blew Violets, clipping off the Whites, and to a pound of them add a quart of boiling-water, and four pound of white Sugar; stirring them together, and stopping them close in an Earthen Vessel four days; then strain them, pressing out the liquid part; which being moderately heated on a gentle fire, will thicken into a Syrup.[224]

The whites mentioned in this recipe are the flower calyxes, which should be removed. Some authors recommend letting the syrup stand in a closed pewter container for a more distinctive flavor and color, and then adding a few drops of lemon juice at the last minute.

Candied Violet Flowers and other Recipes: Candied violet flowers are a delight to the eye as well as the tongue. According to an old recipe, one should

> take your various sorts of Flowers, cut the stalks, if they are extraordinarily long, somewhat shorter; and having added about eight spoonsfuls of Rose-water to a pound of white Sugar, boil it to a clearness; and as it begins to grow stiff and cool, dip your Flowers into it; and taking them out presently, lay them one by one in a Sieve, and hold it over a Chafing-dish of Coles (Coals), and they will dry and harden.[225]

Modern cooks who own a candy thermometer should heat the rose water syrup to a temperature of 240° F and maintain it for a full minute while dipping the flowers. A baking sheet in a warm oven is a good substitute for a chafing dish.

Yet another easy method is to beat an egg white until stiff and then add a few drops of high-proof spirits such as vodka. Choose very fresh and unblemished flowers, and then paint them with the egg white, using a kitchen brush. Then dip the flowers in a bowl of sugar, making sure to cover all parts of the flower. Carefully put the flowers on a piece of baking parchment or butter paper on a cake rack to dry. When completely dry, place in an airtight container. If you are candying a large amount they can be frozen in an airtight container, but they will not taste as good as the fresh flowers.

Violet Jelly and Violet Marmalade: To prepare violet jelly and violet marmalade, steep violet blossoms in boiling water. Strain, add approximately the same amount of

---

224. John Shirley, *The Accomplished Ladies Rich Closet of Rarities* (London: N. Bodington, 1688), 22.

225. Ibid., 38.

sugar to the liquid, as well as some apple juice, and heat carefully until the mixture boils. Cook until it reaches the jellying point, and fill into sterilized jars.

Violet Paste: Violet paste can be made by heating a very thick sugar syrup made with two pounds of sugar and a little water until the thread stage (219° F) is reached. Then add one pound of crushed violet blossoms and one pound of apple jelly, and cook over a very low flame for 10 minutes only, before filling into sterilized jars.

Violet Candies: Violet candies are produced by mixing ½ pound of crushed violet blossoms with one pound of sugar, and just enough water to dissolve the sugar. Heat to the soufflé stage (230° F). Then immediately fold in a stiffly beaten egg white sweetened with some confectioner's sugar, and pour the mixture into a buttered form. Dry very slowly in a warm (lukewarm) oven.

Violet Ice Cream: Beat 1¾ cups of sugar and 8 egg yolks until they form a ribbon, and then blend in 1½ pints of boiling milk, a few tablespoons at a time. Add ½ pint of fresh cream, and a few tablespoons of violet syrup, and heat gently, stirring all the while, until the mixture sticks to a spoon (but not to the bottom of the pan!). Do not let the mixture come to a boil, or it will curdle. Freeze the mixture in salt and ice in an ice-cream maker, or pour it into a tray and freeze it at the highest freezer setting.

Violet Vinegar: Remove the stems from 3 handfuls of fresh violet blossoms, and place in a quart bottle. Cover with good clear cider or white wine vinegar. Let the closed bottle stand 2 weeks in the sun or in a warm place. Then strain, filter through filter paper, and pour into decorative, scrupulously cleaned bottles. Cork well for later use.

Household Applications

Queen Victoria was one of the most enthusiastic supporters of the violet, and had her gardeners grow the flowers in great quantities for posies, wreaths, and garlands. Primroses, violets, and the flowers known as maiden's blushes were often strewn at English weddings as symbols of the bride's purity and modesty. To the Greeks, the violet was a symbol of beauty and the transitory nature of life. In Lincolnshire, it is customary to wear white violets in one's buttonhole on Good Friday. The inhabitants of Gloucestershire do not bring violets into the house for fear of bringing in fleas. The ancient Romans had other uses for the violet: flower wreaths were said to counteract the effects of inebriety.

All violets, especially the sweet-scented common violet, may be added to potpourri. All the violets may be woven into wreaths and garlands. The violet roots (orris root) traditionally used in perfumery, crafts, or as teething roots for children are not violets at all but an iris root *(Iris germanica var. florentina)* with a violet-like odor.

Cosmetic Properties

Most commercial "violet" products have never seen a violet, and are prepared from synthetic but inexpensive essences. True violet oil is volatile, exquisitely scented, and prohibitively expensive. It is made from fresh violet blossoms, and violet leaves gathered just before the plant flowers. Violet oil temporarily paralyzes the olfactory nerves. An inexpensive but authentic violet bath oil can be made by steeping violet blossoms for several weeks in fresh almond or jojoba oil. Violet leaves are applied as compresses to freshen tired eyes, and violet flowers steeped in goat's milk are employed as a washing lotion. A healing salve prepared with white wax, rose oil, and violet oil can be applied to chapped lips and work-roughened hands.

A tea cure of heart's ease leaves and flowers can help to cleanse the skin from the inside out and counteract blemishes. Heart's ease flowers are added to facial lotions for sensitive skin.

Noteworthy Recipes

Toilette Water: A sweet-smelling toilette water can be prepared from a combination of scented flowers such as roses, violets, and lavender, together with other fragrant flowers and herbs such as whitethorn blossoms, orange blossoms, lemon thyme, orange mint, apple blossoms, or lemon balm. Fill a glass with the flowers and herbs, and cover with a mixture of 1 part wine spirits and 2 parts distilled water. Let stand, covered tightly, for at least 3 weeks in a cool place, and then strain, and filter through filter paper. Add a little distilled water if necessary, pour into decorative small bottles, and stopper.

Medicinal Merits

As Nicholas Culpeper writes in his herbal, the violet is "a fine, pleasing plant of Venus, of a mild nature, and no way hurtful." The herb is so mild that it can be given to children to treat their sore throats and coughs. Violet flowers have mild expectorant qualities, and have been recommended by herbalists for centuries to ease coughs, colds, angina, whooping cough, asthma, and inflammation of the lungs as well as consumption, and to strengthen singers' voices. The Athenians prepared a violet cordial to moderate anger and cure sleeplessness, and the Salernian herbal authorities considered the plant effective against the results of alcohol overindulgence and abuse. Violets were thought to strengthen the heart and to ease pains, to drive out the poisons of cholera, and to relieve thirst and feverish sensations. In Germany, Denmark, France, and Pennsylvania, the belief was widespread that a person who swallowed the first three spring violets would be protected from cold fever for a year. In Silesia in Germany, swallowing the first three violets was expected to guarantee "good blood" for that year. The

Thuringians (Germany) believed that touching one's eyes with the first three spring violets would bring good health. The first violets were also woven into a wreath to cure headaches and a "damp head."

Violet leaves have been used for centuries as poultice herbs to treat swellings and bruises. Hippocrates recommended violet plasters as a cure for headaches and melancholy. Pliny prescribed a liniment prepared from vinegar and violet roots as an external remedy for gout and splenetic disorders. According to another ancient herbal, a good cure for headache was to stroke the aching head with fresh violet leaves, and then to repeat a spell. Hildegard von Bingen applied violet-leaf plasters to cloudy eyes. The botanist Otto Brunfels seconded this suggestion, and also recommended violet water to help cool fevers, feverish growths, the heat of a swollen liver or of the bubonic plague, and to dispel ragings of the brain, stabbing sensations in the heart, and stomach aches. Hildegard von Bingen extolled the external and internal use of violets as a treatment for cancer. Nicholas Culpeper was of the opinion that the violet is

> cold and moist while fresh and green, and is used to cool any heat or distemperature of the body, either inwardly or outwardly ... It eases pains in the head, caused through want of sleep; or any pains arising from heat, if applied in the same manner, or with oil of roses.[226]

The wild pansy was primarily employed in ancient times as a children's herb, but it was also used for the treatment of venereal and skin diseases, and occasionally administered as an aphrodisiac. An infusion of wild pansy was added to the bath water of newborn babies, or the child was given a few drops of distilled pansy water to prevent an allergic reaction to milk and grains. The lung complaints, asthma, fevers, and epilepsy of young children were also treated with wild pansy tea or the distilled herbal water.

> *Though Violets smell sweete, Nettles offensive,*
> *Yet each in severall Kind much good procures,*
> *The first dot (doth) purge the heavy head and pensive,*
> *Recovers surfets, falling sickness cures.*
>
> —THE SCHOOL OF SALERNUM

Modern Medicine

During the last centuries, the reputation of the violet as a medicinal herb has suffered considerably. Until recently, it was demoted to the rank of a smelling-salt herb. But now it has enjoyed something of a comeback. A tea prepared from equal amounts of violet

---

226. Culpeper, *Culpeper's Complete Herbal* (1653) (London: Foulsham, undated), 380.

leaves, red clover flowers, and sorrel leaves is now thought by some herbalists to be an effective preventive medicine against cancer of the throat, tongue, uterus, and lungs, to ease some of the pains of malignant growths, and, in some cases, to even stop the spread of the cancer. Internal treatment can be supported by the external application of violet-leaf poultices, violet-leaf footbaths, or violet liniments, by eating violet leaves, or by gargling with them.

Those who are worried about contracting cancer, or who are at a high risk because of family history or their working environment, or are prone to allergies, can try a preventive tea-drinking regimen. The violet-clover-sorrel mixture should be taken 2–3 times a day for 4 weeks, and then substituted for the next 4 weeks with a marigold-flower tea, which is also reputed to have a preventive effect, especially against cancer of the stomach, liver and spleen. Another possibility is a tea of European mistletoe. The herbs are very mild, and can be taken for several months at a time with no ill effects.

Violet roots are richer in saponines than the leaves or the flowers, and are also strongly purgative. Violet roots can be taken under medical supervision to expel a persistent cough or the poison of contaminated foods, to ease constipation, and to help pass kidney stones. Violet seeds also have a strongly purgative effect, and are administered to patients with kidney gravel and kidney stones. Violet leaves are gentle laxatives, and violet flowers are even gentler. Teas of violet leaves and violet flowers can safely be given to constipated children. They can also induce perspiration and help to "break" childhood fevers. Young and old alike value them for the treatment of colds, coughs, and sore throats.

Viola odorata is a homeopathic remedy for right wrist tension and pain in the finger joints, as well as spasmodic coughs and eye and ear pains. Violets *(Viola yedoensis)* are used in Chinese medicine to clear heat and heated swellings as well as for swollen eyes, throat, and ears. They are also used to treat mumps.

Poultices of fresh young violet leaves can be applied to growths, wounds, and rashes. Violet oil is rubbed, like rose oil, onto temples to ease a headache or a fever. Violet vinegars, cold compresses, and violet tinctures are employed for the same purpose, and also applied to swellings and rheumatic pains. Swollen tonsils and sore throats are soothed with violet-leaf gargle.

The medicinal action of the wild pansy is similar to that of the violet, although the plant has more pronounced blood-cleansing properties than its sweet-scented relative. Pansy root or pansy seed tea can be taken as an emetic and strong purgative. A tea of the flowering plant helps to induce perspiration, expel stones and gravel, and cleanse the kidneys. Colds, coughs, catarrhs, and rheumatic complaints can all be relieved with wild pansy tea. It is also helpful in the treatment of acne, rashes, and scrofula, as well as allergic digestive and skin disorders. Pansy tea can safely be given to children, but a wild pansy tincture should only be given to children a drop at a time. Pansies are employed homeopathically, like the fresh herb, for children's skin complaints such as eczema and milk crusts. They are especially indicated if the urine smells strong, like cat's urine. The efficacy of the plant in the treatment of milk and grain allergies as well as neurodermitis needs to be better researched, since it is one of the few herbs that has proved effective in this area and is mild enough for children.

The fresh herb, or the powdered dry herb mixed with honey, can be placed on wounds and rashes, and the tincture of the blossoming plant applied to cutaneous eruptions. The adult dose for a tea is ½–1 oz. of wild pansy leaves and flower to 1 pint of boiling water. Two or three cups of tea can be drunk daily for a maximum of 3–4 weeks.

Special Cures

Children's Cough Tea: A mild tea mixture to mitigate children's coughs caused by a tickling throat can be made from a mixture of the following herbs: 1 part wild cherry stems, 1 part thyme leaves, 2 parts sorrel leaves, 1 part chamomile flowers, and 2 parts of sweet violet leaves. 1 tsp. of the herbs are brewed in ½ pint of boiling water, allowed to steep for 10 minutes, strained, sweetened with honey (optional), and given to the child a teaspoonful at a time as needed. This mixture can be made more potent, but less pleasant in taste, by the addition of a pinch of sundew *(Drosera rotundifolia)*, 3 parts lungwort *(Pulmonaria officinalis)*, 2 parts ribwort plantain leaves, and 1 part finely-chopped licorice roots *(Glycyrrhiza glabra)*.

Preventive Tea for Skin Disorders: Those with a tendency to develop rashes, eczema, or acne can try to prevent outbreaks by drinking a tea composed of walnut *(Juglans regia)* leaves, mixed with equal parts of fumitory *(Fumaria officinalis)* and heart's ease. Take 2–3 times a day for 2–3 weeks at a time, 2 or 3 times a year.

Uses in Husbandry

Violet flowers contain a large amount of nectar and are eagerly visited by bees. Butterflies are also attracted to violets, and sometimes lay so many eggs in a violet stem that it bursts. Both violets and wild pansies are used in technical tests to determine the acidity or alkalinity of substances. Massive presence of heart's ease in a field can be taken as a sure indication of lime deficiency in the soil.

According to agricultural superstition, bringing the first violets, or less than a full handful of violets, indoors may be the cause of bad luck and misfortune. In Worcestershire, bringing less than a full handful of violets into the house will cause all the "duckens and ducklings" to die. In Bavaria, violets are placed under broody geese to make the goslings hatch faster.

Veterinary Values

Heart's ease tea or tincture may prove harmful to cats, but can be given in small doses to dogs suffering from heart problems. Horses, greyhounds, and pigeons suffering from racing stress respond well to the herb, either in infusion form or as honey syrup.

Miscellaneous Wisdom

In ancient Greece, the violet was considered sacred to Persephone and the flowers were strewn on the graves of virgins and boys who died after the age of three. Since that time, the violet has been associated with the death of the very young and the very innocent. Magicians use violet roots as a scrying incense to facilitate entry into the spirit world. Violets are still thought to grow best on the graves of virgins, and the Wends believe that the violet is actually an enchanted maiden. Every ten years on Walpurgis Night (the eve of May 1st), the flower turns back into a virgin. A man who manages to pluck the flower in the right manner at the right moment will win the maiden, together with her treasure.

The violet was cultivated in Athens long before the birth of Christ and at one time symbolized that city. Romans also venerated violets. In Arabia, it is literary tradition to speak of one's beloved as having eyes like a violet. For, as John Gerard put it, violets

> bring to a liberall and gentle manly minde, the remembrance of honestie, comlinesse, and all kinds of virtues: for it would be an unseemly and filthy thing (as a certain wise man saith) for him that doth looke upon faire and beautiful things, to have his mind not faire, but filthy and deformed.[227]

The symbolic importance of the violet has not diminished since then. It is widely used in heraldry, and modern gypsies consider it to be a symbol of uncertainty and restlessness.

At the turn of the thirteenth century, a Viennese Duke ordered his subjects to search the banks of the Danube for the first violet. The "chasest" maiden in his realm was then sent to pick the flower and bring it to Court with great ceremony. In Bohemia, the Whitsun Queen was crowned with a garland of the first violet flowers and daises. A tenth-century herbal described these first violets as particularly effective against "wykked sperytis."

In Germany, the wild pansy, also known as Herb Trinitatis, is carried into church together with other herbs to be blessed on Trinity Sunday (the Sunday following Whitsunday, the fiftieth day after Easter). These Trinity herbs are believed to possess great power to cure the diseases of both humans and animals. Love philters were once prepared with the herb, and magical cures for tuberculosis were concocted from heart's

---

227. Gerard, *Gerard's Herball* [1597]: *The essence thereof distilled by Marcus Woodward from the edition of Th. Johnson, 1636.* Ed. Marcus Woodward (London: Gerald How, 1927), 198.

ease picked between eleven and noon on Midsummer's Day (June 24th). In Transylvania, newborn babies were bathed in a wild pansy bath to protect them against disease and evil influence.

Oracular Worth

In popular imagination, violets are closely associated with spring, and are carefully observed when they appear as omens about the coming year. In Bavaria, people say that the harvest will come early if the violets blossom before March 19th, St. Joseph's Day. If the violets have long stalks, then the flax will also grow to a good height. If violets are still blossoming on June 8th, then the grain will be subject to disease, and the second hay harvest will be meager. According to British belief, a plague or epidemic will invariably follow if both roses and violets flower in the fall.

Bohemians believe that violets lose their sweet scent after the first thunderstorm of the year. This observation is correct, for sweet-smelling violets stop blooming before summer, and the various scentless violets follow later. Similarly, the Bavarian belief that smelling the first violets will cause freckles is due to the fact that the March sun causes the skin to freckle easily. People who find the first violet have probably spent so much time outdoors that they are already freckled. Tasting the first violet is thought to impair one's sense of taste, or to impart bad breath. The French have given the flower the name *Violette folle*, and Germans call it *Dulle Vyoliken* because they believe that anyone who smells the first spring violets will get spring fever, or turn into a lunatic. In Saxony, children never bring wild pansies into the house for fear of harming or killing their mothers (similar to the fear of stepping on cracks in the sidewalk).

Herbal Pastimes

It was once customary in England to present female servants with their pay and a gift of gloves on Easter Day. Out of this business transaction grew the custom of asking for gloves on Valentine's Day. In Oxfordshire, a young woman would address a young man on Valentine's Day with the words,

> The rose is red, the violet's blue,
> The gilly-flower's sweet, and so are you;
> Those are the words you bade me say
> For a pair of new gloves on Easter-Day.[228]

This rhyme was included in an American Mother Goose collection, out of context, and then gave rise to countless "roses are red, violets are blue" Valentine rhymes.

In Switzerland, the servants' pay was also due in spring when the violets bloomed. Children still chant a verse today, a remembrance of this custom:

---

228. G. F. Northall, *English Folk-Rhymes* (1892) (Detroit, MI: Singing Tree Press, 1968), 199.

Violet, violet gay, put it on the table,
Let the Master pay, let him pay this very day![229]

Legends

The violet has at various times been considered sacred to Persephone, to Pan, to Aphrodite, to Priapus, to Saturn, and to the Icelandic god of war. Greek house gods were honored with the flowers, and they were woven into garlands during Saturnalia. One of the ancient Greek names for the violet was Priapeion. According to the herbalist John Gerard, the nymphs of Ionia presented violets to Jupiter. Another version is that Zeus transformed his lover Io into a cow to escape Hera's jealousy, and the earth brought forth violets for her to eat. Since that day, the purple flowers have carried her name. According to yet another legend, it was Apollo who transformed the daughter of Atlas into a violet when she tried to hide from him.

There is a tale behind each of the many folk names with which the wild pansy is graced. Because of its cordial, aphrodisiac, and pleasing properties, it is thought to ease the heart. Robert Herrick gives us the low-down on "How Pansies or Heartsease came first":

Frollick Virgins once these were,
Over-loving, (living here:)
Being here their ends deny'd
Ranne for Sweet-hearts mad, and dy'd.
Love in pitie of their teares,
And their losse in blooming yeares;
For their restlesse here-spent houres,
Gave them Hearts-ease turn'd to Flow'rs.[230]

Another term for the wild pansy, "herb trinitatis," comes from the plant's three-colored blossoms and their subsequent use on Trinity Sunday. A Palatine legend further explains the origins of the name: the wild pansy once smelled as sweet as March violets, and so people always picked it even if they had to trample through grain fields to get it. The wild pansy prayed to the Holy Trinity, begging to be relieved of its sweet odor so that the grain would be spared. The prayer was granted, and the plant was from then on blessed with the name of the Trinity.

The color-blotched pansy flower is also compared to the ugly face of a stepmother, or to the face of a cat. According to another tradition, the plant is called "stepfathers" and "stepmothers," or "godfathers" and "godmothers," or simply "stepmother" because of the number of the flower petals. While the common violet has three upper and three

---

229. Gustav Hegi, *Illustrierte Flora von Mittel-Europa*, vol. VII (Munich: Lehmanns, 1913–1918), 652.

230. Herrick, *The Complete Poetry of Robert Herrick* (New York: NYU Press, 1963).

lower petals, the wild pansy has four upper petals and one lower one. The two middle petals, or "chairs," are supposed to belong to the stepmother. Each of her daughters has one of the two remaining upper petals, but her two stepdaughters have to content themselves with the single bottom petal.

In the Ukraine, the plant is known as "brother" and "sister." The legend goes that a brother and sister once got married, unaware of their common ancestry. When they discovered the truth, they were so terrified that God took pity on them and turned them into a pansy.

The derogatory use of the word "pansy" to refer to homosexuals is relatively new, dating from the end of the nineteenth century. It may have developed from the use of the pansy as an aphrodisiac, or as a fanciful version of the derogatory term "Nancy-boy."

Literary Flowers

The rose is fragrant, but it fades in time:
The violet sweet, but quickly past the prime:
White lilies hang their heads, and soon decay,
And white snow in minutes melts away.

—THEOCRITUS (TRANS. DRYDEN), "THE DESPAIRING LOVER"

Ah, cruell Love! must I endure
Thy many scorns, and find no cure?
Say, are thy medicines made to be
Helps to all others, but to me?
Ile leave thee, and to Pansies come;
Comforts you'll afford me some:
You can ease my heart, and doe
What love co'd ne'r be brought unto.

—ROBERT HERRICK, "TO PANSIES"

Remembering mine affliction and my misery, the wormwood and the gall.
My soul hath them still in remembrance, and is humbled in me.
This I recall to my mind, therefore have I hope.

—LAMENTATIONS 3:19–21

WORMWOOD

Name

The name "wormwood" conjures up a vision of wormy wood, worm-gnawed lumber, and worm infested furniture. This is due to etymological confusion. Wormwood was *wermód* in Old English, and *Wermouta* or *Weramote* in Old High German. The precise meaning of these ancient terms is not clear, but it can be assumed that they were in some way associated with the word for intestinal worms. Our present-day term "wormwood" is, very simply, the name for a plant used medicinally to expel worms; in other words, a plant taken as a vermifuge. "Wood" here denotes a stout, sturdy herb with a woody stalk.

Wormwood's botanical name is *Artemisia absinthium*. The Latin term *Artemisia* originated from the Greek goddess Artemis (the Roman Diana). Myth relates that she disclosed the medicinal virtues of the plant to the healing centaur, Chiron. In keeping with this association, wormwood was highly prized in ancient times as a woman's herb. It was used as an aphrodisiac, to "provoke the courses," and to induce abortions. The origin of *absinthium* is uncertain. It may be traced back to a Greek word meaning either "unpleasant" or "undrinkable." Since wormwood has such an unpleasant taste, "undrinkable" may well be the proper interpretation.

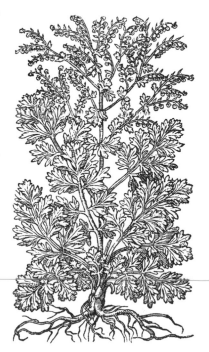

Wormwood is a perennial member of the **Daisy (Asteraceae)** family. The genus *Artemisia* contains many healing or culinary herbs, including mugwort, tarragon, southernwood, European and Mexican wormwood, and maritime wormwood. Most of the *Artemisias* are employed in the preparation of alcoholic drinks or in perfumery, but are also used to cultivate barren land.

Folk Names

Some of the English folk names for wormwood are absinth, absinthe, warmot, mugwort, green ginger, and old woman (the counterpart of southernwood, which is known as old man). German variants are *Wermut, Alsem, Grabkraut, Wiegenkraut, Kampferkraut,* and *Wurmtod.* The French call the herb *absinth, absinthe,* and *aluine*; the Spaniards, *ajenjo* and *agenjo*; the Italians, *assenzio, assinz,* and *assenzio romano.* Scandinavian names are *malurt, malört,* and *bartholomaeisblomster*; Welsh, *wermod*; Russian, *polyn gor'kaja.* An ancient Latin name was *aloxinum,* and an old German one was *Alahsam.*

Appearance

The entire wormwood plant is shrubby and weedy in nature, and the stems are firm, branched, and leafy, forming a woody rosette at the base. The leaves are hairy on both sides and have a silver sheen. They are broader and more splayed than the leaves of southernwood, and contain oil glands. The flowers are inconspicuous, and yellowish or greenish-yellow. The distinctly pungent and aromatic odor of the plant when the leaves are crushed is its most remarkable characteristic. The taste is extremely bitter, spicy, almost burning.

Nicholas Culpeper describes wormwood as a "useful plant" that

> grows about a yard high; the stalk is pale green, tough, upright, and divided wildly into many branches: the leaves of a pale green on both sides, divided into many parts, soft to the touch, but make the fingers bitter. The flowers are numerous, small, chaffy, hang down, and of a pale olive colour at first; but, after standing a while, they grow brownish.[231]

Place, Season, and Useful Parts

Wormwood prefers dry, lime-containing soil, although it has been known to grow under an amazing variety of conditions. It is a common perennial plant in most of Europe and Eurasia, and has been brought from the Old World to the American continent. It grows to an altitude of 6,000 ft. and can be found on cliffs and riverbanks, in gardens, vineyards, abandoned quarries, rubble heaps, stony paths, driveways, and waste areas, along garden fences, hedges, and walls, in meadows and stony pastures, and beside roads. It will not thrive in swampy situations, and prefers half-shade. Wormwood flowers from July through October or even November, and the entire blossoming plant is gathered

---

231.   Culpeper, *Culpeper's Complete Herbal* (1653) (London: Foulsham, undated), 393.

without the roots in July or August, before the flowers have started to turn brown. In Westphalia (Germany), the best wormwood is considered to be that picked after August 15th, the Day of Mary's Ascension. According to the saying, "you should gather the wormwood from the garden as soon as Mary has traveled to Heaven."[232]

Gathering, Drying, and Storage

Wormwood is cultivated in the United States, Brazil, southern Siberia, and in some areas of Europe. Wild wormwood is gathered in Russia and in the areas around the Black Sea. It should be gathered on dry, sunny days from insect-free plants. The first cut can already be made after one winter, but it is best to wait with a major harvest until the plant begins to flower. The tops are cut with a large knife or heavy shears just as they begin to bloom, and the fresh green leaves stripped from the stalks and dried on cloth or paper. The cut stems can also be tied together in small bundles or in a fan shape and dried quickly in an airy place. According to Piemontese (Italian) tradition, wormwood used for magical purposes must be ripped from the ground with an ungloved left hand.

Wormwood is usually dried commercially outdoors on large wooden platforms in a shady place, or hung on strings across a not-too-sunny field. It will only dry properly if the weather is warm and dry, about 70° F. The plants can also be hung on strings in an airy shed or attic. If the plants are still not dry after several days or if the weather is especially damp, then artificial heat must be used to finish the drying process.

The dried herb should be stripped from the stems and cut to size. A fine product can be obtained by crushing the leaves through a coarse sieve. Dried wormwood should be stored in airtight boxes, since its felty leaves tend to absorb moisture.

Seed Saving and Germination

There is considerable variation in the oil content of wormwood plants grown in different locations, as well as differences in growth habit. Many different botanical species of *Artemisias*, with widely varying medicinal properties, exist in almost all corners of the globe.

Wormwood is usually propagated by the division of existing plants. It is possible to save seed from ripe plants, but germination is erratic after storage. Plant or root division is easier and guarantees varietal purity.

A sprig of wormwood placed in bean seed containers before storing can help to discourage bean beetles, but it is wiser to dry the beans and then freeze them to destroy the beetles. Some of the insects can survive freezing temperatures, and will crawl out after thawing to eat their way through new seeds. They usually succumb after another round

---

232. Hanns Bächtold-Stäubli, *Handwörterbuch des deutschen Aberglaubens* (1927–42), vol. IX (Berlin: Walter de Gruyter & Co., 1987), 501.

in the freezer. Bean beetles are more dangerous than pea beetles, because they can eat more than one bean and therefore systematically destroy an entire jar of seeds.

Gardening Hints

Wormwood was common in prehistoric Europe, and was cultivated in the cloister gardens of southern Germany as early as the ninth century AD. It will grow on most soils, although it prefers rich, dry, calcareous earth and a dry climate. The root is perennial, and the plant self-propagating and requires little attention beyond occasional watering and weeding. It may be propagated by seed, plant division, or cuttings. It is now planted in moon gardens because of its silvery leaves, but that is not always advisable because of its quarrelsome nature.

Wormwood exerts a negative influence on most plants grown next to it. Fennel, sage, caraway, and anise will be overpowered by wormwood, and may die as a result. But this negative effect is also extended to garden pests: most of them do not like wormwood. The plants may be grown next to currants with excellent results to keep away insects, or a brew can be prepared from the herb and sprayed on endangered plants. Some experts recommend a mixture of wormwood extract and the juice of the fresh tomato plant set out in a saucer to keep flies out of the house. It is a safer alternative to the traditional but poisonous mixture of fly agaric and milk.

Occasionally, wormwood is subject to insect damage: aphids descend on wormwood in such numbers that the stalks turn black from the infestation. The stalks should be cut back, and only the younger, healthy leaves used for medicinal purposes. Organic gardeners may want to leave the aphids on the leaves so that natural enemies of these pests, such as ladybugs and earwigs, can gorge themselves. The beneficial insects will then reproduce, and help to combat aphids naturally during the rest of the season and the following year.

Culinary Virtues

Wormwood seeds help to denature or rectify spirits, and the plant has been added in minute quantities to kitchen sauces on rare occasions. The bitter aromatic and thirst-quenching properties of wormwood make it an ideal herb for liquor manufacturers. Cinzano, absinthe, vermouth, absinth wine, and most compound bitters contain wormwood. It is occasionally added to must, or hard cider. Wormwood also helped to flavor beer in the Middle Ages. The resulting drink was taken for medicinal reasons, but did not keep as well as other beers. Because of this, and changing tastes, hops were soon substituted for wormwood as a beer additive.

The notoriety that absinthe has obtained since its introduction into France from Algiers in the nineteenth century was not only due to the inferior quality of some absinthes, but also to the high wormwood content of the drink. Wormwood can be very dangerous if taken in large amounts over an extended period. The mixture of a potentially dangerous drug, high-proof spirits, and the unhealthy lifestyle that usually accompanies alcoholism can be lethal. Dizziness, cramps, nausea, blackouts, or fits similar to epilepsy may be the result. Because of this, absinthe was forbidden in Switzerland in 1908, and many countries have followed that government's example. Absinthe (known in France as *muse verte, verte, apéro*) can be green or colorless. Some of the herb and spices traditionally added to the drink to give it is unique color and flavor include Chinese or star anise, anise, hyssop, fennel, angelica, marjoram, and lemon balm.

Beverages made from a combination of herbs with the addition of wormwood are not necessarily dangerous, and can, on the contrary, have a tonic and beneficial effect if taken occasionally as an aperitif or bitter. The flavor of wormwood drinks can be very pleasant, one to treasure if enjoyed in moderation and not on a regular basis.

Household Applications

When fleas, lice, and bedbugs were common even in well-kept households, wormwood was often strewn on the floors and hung on the walls to discourage the vermin. Bed linen was stored in cupboards with wormwood placed between the sheets. Hatbands had sprigs of wormwood tucked in them to keep away flies and other insects. Furs and woolens were laid in chests cushioned with wormwood. Housekeepers kept wormwood in the library to prevent bookworms from burying into the expensive volumes, and mixed wormwood with ink to keep mice from the written pages.

Flower bouquets can be made more striking with the addition of a few silvery wormwood stalks. Some incenses are prepared with the addition of a little wormwood, and it is also used as a dye plant. A simple decoction of the herb produces a yellow tint. With the addition of salt, a green-blue hue results, and the addition of green vitriol produces an olive-green dye. Grimy, oily hands can also be cleaned by rubbing them underwater with fresh wormwood.

While wormwood hath seed, get a bundle or twain
to save against March, to make flea to refrain:
Where chamber is swept, and wormwood is strewn,
no flea, for his life, dare abide to be known.

—THOMAS TUSSER, *FIVE HUNDRED POINTES OF GOOD HUSBANDRIE*

Cosmetic Properties

Wormwood is not a generally accepted cosmetic herb. An infusion of wormwood can be helpful to poultice dark circles under the eyes or to lessen the pains of rheumatism, swellings, sprains, or fallen arches. A wormwood infusion diluted with a little vinegar has on occasion been employed as a blemish-controlling facial lotion.

Medicinal Merits

Wormwood is said to be one of the two bitterest herbs known to humankind (the other is rue). As Dioscurides assures us, it was familiar to the Egyptians under the name of *somi* as early as 1600 BC. It is mentioned repeatedly in the Old Testament, and the ancient Celts valued its medicinal worth. The Greeks gave it the name "mother of herbs" and used it primarily to treat female diseases. It was also employed by the Greeks as an antidote against hemlock and mushroom poisoning and the venomous bite of the sea dragon. Dioscurides wrote that "it hath a warming, binding digestive facultie, & of taking away ye cholerick matter sticking to ye stomach & ye belly." He further goes on to insist that "it is good for the strangulations that come from mush-rumps, being with Acetum. But with wine for ye poison of Ixia & hemlock & ye bitings of ye shrew mouse and ye dragon of ye sea." [233]

The ancient Greek physician Theophrastus observed that sheep force-fed with wormwood lost the content of their gall bladders. As a direct consequence of this observation, Tabernaemontanus, the sixteenth-century physician, recommended wormwood to quiet "spiteful women too full of gall."[234] The ninth-century herbal *The School of Salernum* prescribed it against seasickness; Hildegard von Bingen recommended it against headache, podagra, melancholy, toothache, and incontinence. Otto Brunfels believed that it was capable of freeing the body of all choleric vapors through the intestines and the bladder. It was applied externally as a poultice for the treatment of exhaustion, worms, and evil winds. Wormwood juice was rubbed into the sores of the black pox (bubonic plague) to keep scars from forming. One macabre Italian cure, which preceded the discovery of vaccination, called for wormwood soaked in water, then stroked onto the sores of the pox, boiled in water, and finally drunk as tea.

Modern Medicine

Wormwood is now considered to be one of the most effective herbs against worms and intestinal parasites, especially when used in conjunction with garlic (or other *Alliums* such as ramsons), thyme, and a laxative herb.

The second major area of wormwood's medicinal action is as a bitter stomachic and liver drug with a stimulating effect on the intestines. It should only be taken by those with *weak* stomachs and *weak* digestions, and not by those with gastritis, ulcers, or

---

233. Robert T. Gunther, ed., *The Greek Herbal of Dioscurides* (New York: Hafner, 1959), 259.

234. Gustav Hegi, *Illustrierte Flora von Mittel-Europa*, vol. VI/2 (Munich: Lehmanns, 1913–1918), 655.

internal bleeding, or when fever or stomach pains are present. Wormwood can help to increase the appetite, and to relieve flatulence and a full stomach while easing elimination. It stimulates the liver and gall bladder to better function, and is an ideal drink for patients after gall bladder operations. It is effective in the treatment of anemia and is occasionally employed as an antidote for some poisons. Wormwood's medicinal action is often quite individual and idiopathic: some find it astringent and others laxative, and there are often unexplained interactions with other herbs or drugs. A wormwood cure should be interrupted immediately if negative reactions occur, and it should never be given to pregnant women. Some patients will experience better results with homeopathic preparations of the herb.

Wormwood also acts as an emmenagogue: it helps to bring on menstruation and to ease delivery, and has been used in massive doses to induce abortions. Unfortunately, this has also resulted in many cases of wormwood poisoning.

Wormwoods acts as a mild diuretic and has been employed to reduce minor fevers. Folk medicine still believes in its efficacy in the treatment of epilepsy. This may have something to do with the fact that large doses of the herb have been known to produce a temporary condition very similar to epilepsy.

Caution is the word that should be associated with wormwood. It should by no means be used indiscriminately. Regular use of large doses of wormwood can be as harmful as self-medication with absinthe. Pregnant or nursing women, and people with ulcers or internal bleeding, should think of wormwood as a poison. It is best to test individual reactions to wormwood two or three times before taking it as a medicinal herb, even if prescribed by a naturopath or herbalist. It is not advisable to take the herb longer than 8 weeks in small amounts. For best results, take wormwood tea made from 1 tsp. of leaves for every ½ pint of water ½ hour before meals. Wormwood tincture or extract should only be taken in minute doses for short periods. Wormwood oil is also available in some countries on prescription as a digestive tonic and vermifuge.

Artemisia maritima is used homeopathically as a worm remedy. Wormwood is prescribed by Chinese physicians to clear deficient fevers and low-grade summer fevers, to cool the blood, and to stop bleeding caused by heat.

Special Cures

Gripe Oil: "Gripe oil" was once a proven folk remedy against children's colics and stomachaches. The recipe calls for a large handful each of chamomile and peppermint, and a small pinch each of wormwood and rue brewed with 2 pints of water, strained, and administered one teaspoon at a time. No more than 3 tsp. should be given in one day. Keep the mixture in a cool place, and renew every second day.

Uses in Husbandry

Wormwood is employed in the storeroom and in the house to keep mice, beetle, weevils, and other pests from pilfering. It can also be grown in the corners of grain fields for this purpose. It discourages mice if placed strategically in the barn or granary. Pantries and storerooms are sprayed with wormwood infusions against insect predators, and it is used by beekeepers to protect themselves when approaching their charges. Animal salts are denatured with wormwood.

Veterinary Values

Wormwood is employed in magical, household, and also official veterinary medicine. Bunches of the plant are hung in the house or stall as a precautionary measure against magical diseases. Flea-ridden cats, dogs, and other household pets are washed in wormwood baths, or sprayed with wormwood infusions. Wormwood can cause negative reactions in sensitive animals if given internally and should always be used with caution. If problems occur, southernwood can be substituted for the herb. Wormwood is a strong antiseptic, insectifuge, and vermicide, and is helpful in the treatment of mange. Most herbal worm mixtures, especially those prepared for horses, contain wormwood or its Mexican cousin, *epazote*. Veterinarians sometimes include wormwood in mixtures used to treat animal epidemic diseases.

Miscellaneous Wisdom

Wormwood is often used as protection against "bad" magic at weddings, burials, and processions. Women who take care of corpses carry wormwood. It is laid in open coffins, burnt at cremations, and thrown into graves. In Switzerland, the bride and groom wear the plant in their pockets to protect themselves against evil influences. The Mexican festival of the Goddess of Salt was once celebrated by dancing women ornamented with wormwood garlands. In 1483 in Erfurt, 2,136 virgins wreathed in bitter wormwood paraded through the streets in an attempt to ban the bitter aspects of drought and poverty from that town.

Wormwood owes its magical reputation to its bitter principles. Death, illness, and misfortune are often personified in folk belief, or directly attributed to the machinations of witches, spirits, devils, sorcerers, or other malicious beings. These creatures are believed to dislike wormwood's bitter taste as much as any human does. According to the Roman scholar Pliny, wormwood laid under the pillow protects the sleeper from evil spirits of the night. Martin Luther wrote of people who drove away changelings by smoking them with the "cradle herb" wormwood. A bitter mixture of rue and wormwood was used in Switzerland to protect sleepers against the night folk. "Evil people" were prevented from harming animals if wormwood and other antidemonic herbs were buried under the stall door. In northern Germany, a bunch of wormwood is hung on the stall wall. In northern Italy, believers hold wormwood and garlic in their mouths during exorcisms to keep the Evil One from taking their immortal souls. Lovers in all of Europe wear wormwood to protect themselves against the envy of witches. In some areas, the plant is also believed to counteract any evil magical influence on a gun or musket. In Russia, it is worn as an amulet, or tucked under an armpit against water spirits. In the week following the seventh Saturday after Easter, it is advisable to throw wormwood into the water if bathing at night. In the southern Slavic countries, women lay wormwood, laurel leaves, and blessed oil on the kitchen fire to keep hail from destroying house and crops, and to stop storms caused by witches and "bad" priests. If witches are responsible for the storm, the women fill pieces of pottery with burning coals and throw wormwood onto the embers. The smoke is supposed to make the witches so drunk that they fall out of their storm clouds.

Wormwood is also believed to be magically effective in curing diseases. The Lithuanians believe that it could cure the "fright" responsible for so many serious children's illnesses. It is also worn on the body, like mugwort, to ward off exhaustion. In Germany, sick or bewitched people are still occasionally beaten with wormwood branches to drive away disease and the evil spirits responsible for the illness. A century ago, Italians from the Abruzzi treated smallpox by beating patients with wormwood and filling their mattresses with the herb. Austrian peasants, until not very long ago, used wormwood to beat the ungodliness out of children who had turned violent against their parents.

Oracular Worth

If wormwood grows to a great height in the fall, there will be heavy snow in winter. A uniquely British belief is that dreaming of wormwood will signify luck in everyday life. The Slavs consult the herb as an oracle about the recovery chances of sick relatives: the patient has to bite into a fresh wormwood stalk every morning. If the wormwood dies, then the patient has a good chance of recovery; if not, then there is little ground for hope.

Literary Flowers

Wormwood is a herb as bitter as love, as bitter as life: it is known as the herb of sadness, the herb of trials, and tribulations, and lamentations. But even this most feared herb, this herb most bitter, shines soft with the powers given it by virgins, the moon, and lunatics.

—*SISTER CLARISSA'S UNPUBLISHED BOOK OF NATURAL OBSERVATIONS*

Wormwood

For the lips of a strange woman drop as an honeycomb, and her mouth is smoother than oil;
But her end is bitter as wormwood, sharp as a two-edged sword.
Her feet go down to death; her steps take hold on hell.

—Proverbs 5:3–5

Where chamber is sweeped and Wormwood is strowne,
What saver is better (if physick be true)
For places infected than Wormwood and Rue?
It is a comfort for hart and the braine,
And therefore to have it is not in vaine.

—Thomas Tusser, *Five Hundred Pointes of Good Husbandrie*

✤ BIBLIOGRAPHY ✤

Abbildungen der Heilkräuter. Ed. Deutscher Kräuterhaus. Carola-Verlag, Demantsfürth, Germany, 1937.

Albertus Magnus. *The Boke of Secrets* (1200s). Amsterdam: Columbia Univ. Press, 1969.

Androsko, Rita J. *Natural Dyes and Home Dying*. New York: Dover, 1971.

Angier, Bradford. *Feasting Free on Wild Edibles*. Harrisburg, PA: Stackpole Books, 1972.

Arber, Agnes. *Herbals: Their Origin and Evolution* (1918). Cambridge, MA: Cambridge Univ. Press, 1953.

Arrowsmith, Nancy. *A Field Guide to the Little People*. New York: Hill & Wang, 1977.

Artusi, Pellegrino. *La Scienza in Cucina e l'Arte di Mangiare Bene*. Turin, Italy: Einaudi Editore, 1974.

Ashworth, Suzanne. *Seed to Seed*. Decorah, IA: Seed Savers Exchange, 1991.

———. *Saatgutgewinnung im Hausgarten* [translation of *Seed to Seed*]. Trans. Nancy Arrowsmith. Krems, Austria: Arche Noah Verein, 1996.

Auda, Domenico. *Breve Compendio di Maravigliosi Segreti*. Rome: Nicolo Germano, 1663.

Aylett, Mary. *Country Wines*. London: Odhams, 1953.

Babudri, F. *Fonti Vive dei Veneto Giuliani*. Milan: Trevisini, 1926.

Back, Phillipa. *Herbs around the House*. London: Pan Books, 1977.

Bächtold-Stäubli, Hanns, ed. *Handwörterbuch des deutschen Aberglaubens* (1927–1942). 10 vol. Berlin: Walter de Gruyter & Co., 1987.

Baker, Charles H. *The Gentleman's Companion*. New York: Crown Publishers, 1944.

Barash, Cathy Wilkinson. *Edible Flowers: from Garden to Palate*. Golden, CO: Fulcrum, 1995.

Bastanzi, Giambattista. *Le Superstizioni delle Alpi Venete*. Treviso, Italy: Zoppelli, 1888.

Bedevian, Armenag K. *Illustrated Polyglottic Dictionary of Plant Names*. Cairo: Argus and Papazian Presses, 1936.

Beeton, Mrs. Isabella. *The Book of Household Management* (1861). New York: Farrar, Straus & Giroux, 1977.

Bellman, Carl Michael. *Der Lieb zu Gefallen*. Munich: Heimeran, 1976.

Bensky, Dan, and Andrew Gamble. *Chinese Herbal Medicine Materia Medica*. Seattle: Eastland Press, 1993.

Bernus, Alexander von. *Alchymie und Heilkunst*. Nuremberg, Germany: Hans Carl, 1969.

Bertoldi, Vittorio. *Un Ribelle nel Regno de' Fiori*. Geneva: Leo S. Olschki, 1923.

Besler, Basilius. *Hortus Eyestettensis* (1613). Facsimile of the 1713 edition.

Bingen, Hildegard von. *Heilkunde*. Salzburg, Austria: Otto Müller Verlag, 1957.

―――. *Naturkunde*. Salzburg, Austria: Otto Müller Verlag, 1959.

Bitterkraut, Christoph. *Artzney-Kunst* (1677). Karlsruhe, Germany: Antiqua, 1971.

Boccaccio, Govanni. *Das Dekameron* (1353). Munich: Winkler, 1952.

Bock, Gisela Reineking von. *Bäder, Duft und Seife*. Cologne, Germany: Kunstgewerbemuseum der Stadt Köln, 1976.

Bock, Hieronymus H. *Kreütterbuch* (1565). Facsimile (Konrad Kölbl, Munich, 1964).

Boland, Maureen, and Bridget Boland. *Old Wives' Lore for Gardeners*. New York: Farrar, Straus & Giroux, 1976.

Boksch, Manfred, Irmgard Bott, and Herbert Zucchi. *Das Ökokräutergartenbuch*. Frankfurt: Krueger W., 1983.

Bose, Sir J. C. *Life Movements in Plants*. Calcutta, India: Bose Research Institute, Longmans, Green & Co., 1918.

―――. *The Motor Mechanism of Plants*. London: Longmans, Green & Co., 1928.

―――. *The Nervous Mechanism of Plants*. London: Longmans, Green & Co., 1926.

Boulestin, Marcel. *Boulestin's Round-the-Year Cookbook*. New York: Dover, 1975.

Brand, John, and Sir Henry Ellis. *Observations on the Popular Antiquities of Great Britain* (1849). 3 vol. Detroit, MI: Singing Tree Press, 1969.

Braun, Hans. *Heilpflanzen-Lexikon für Ärzte und Apotheker*. Stuttgart: Fischer, 1974.

Bronzini, Giovanni B. *Vita Tradizionale in Basilicata*. Matera, Italy: F.lli Montemurro Editori, 1964.

Browne, Sir Thomas. *The Works of Sir Thomas Browne*. 4 vol. London: Faber & Faber, 1965.

Brunfels, Otto. *Contrafayt Kräuterbuch* (1532). Fascimile (Munich: Konrad Kölbl, 1964).

Buchman, Dian Dincin. *Feed Your Face*. London: Duckworth, 1973.

Budd, Charles, trans. *Chinese Poems*. London: Oxford Univ. Press, 1912.

Budge, E. A. Wallis. *Amulets and Superstitions*. New York: Dover, 1978.

Buffler, Martha, and Willi Reich. *Gemüse im Garten*. Stuttgart: Ulmer, 1967.

Burbank, Luther. *The Harvest of the Years*. New York: Houghton Mifflin, 1927.

———. *My Beliefs*. New York: Houghton Mifflin, 1927.

———. *Partner of Nature*. London: Heath Cranton Ltd., 1940.

Burgess, W. V. *Birds and Flowers in Fact and Fancy*. London: Sherratt and Hughes, 1907.

Burne, Charlotte Sophia, ed. *Shropshire Folk-Lore* (1883). 2 vol. Wakefield, England: E. P. Publishing, 1973.

Burns, Robert. *Poems and Songs*. Oxford: Oxford Univ. Press, 1969.

Burton, Robert. *The Anatomy of Melancholy* (1621). London: Tudor, 1977.

Castiglioni, Arturo. *Storia della Medicina*. Milan: Unitas, 1927.

Cerruti [family]. *Von der gesunden Lebensweise*. Facsimile (Munich: BLV, 1983).

Chambers, Robert. *Popular Rhymes of Scotland*. Detroit, MI: Singing Tree Press, 1969.

Chaucer, Geoffrey. *The Complete Works*. London: Oxford Univ. Press, 1947.

Cherfas, Jeremy, Michel Fanton, and Jude Fanton. *The Seeds Savers' Handbook*. Bristol, England: Grover Books, 1996.

Child, Francis James. *The English and Scottish Popular Ballads*. 5 vol. New York: Dover, 1965.

Choice Notes from Notes and Queries. London: The Folk-Lore Society, 1859.

Clair, Colin. *Of Herbs and Spices*. London: Abelard-Schuman, 1961.

Clare, John. *The Shepherd's Calendar* (1827). London: Oxford Univ. Press, 1964.

Cobbett, William. *Cottage Economy*. London: P. Davies, 1926.

Cockayne, Rev. Oswald. *Leechdoms, Wortcunning and Starcraft* (1864–66). 3 vol. London: Holland Press, 1961.

Coles, William. *Adam in Eden, or Nature's Paradise*. London: J. Streater, 1657.

———. *The Art of Simpling*. London: J. Streater, 1656.

Colum, Padraic. *A Treasury of Irish Folklore*. New York: Crown Publishers, 1967.

Coon, Nelson. *Using Wayside Plants*. New York: Hearthside Press, 1969.

Cortese, Isabella. *I Segreti della Signora Isabella Cortese*. Venice, Italy: 1588.

Crow, W. B. *The Occult Properties of Herbs*. Wellingborough, England: The Aquarian Press, 1969.

Culpeper, Nicholas. *Culpeper's Complete Herbal* (1653). London: Foulsham, undated. [Reprint of a nineteenth-century edition, also undated.]

———. *English Physician*. Arranged by Mrs. Leyel. London: Herbert Joseph Ltd., 1947.

———. *English Physician and Complete Herbal*. London: 1653.

———. *The English Physician*. London: Peter Cole, 1652.

Dähnhardt, Oskar. *Natursagen*. 4 vol. Leipzig, Germany: Teubner, 1909.

de Bhaldraithe, Tomás, ed. *English-Irish Dictionary*. Dublin: Oifig An tSoláthair, Baile Átha Cliath, 1959.

de Gubernatis, Angelo. *La Mythologie des Plantes*. 2 vol. Paris: C. Reinwald, 1882.

Delatte, A. *Herbarius, Recherches sur le cérémonial usité les Anciens*. Liége, Belgium: Faculté de Philosophie et Lettres, Librairie E. Droz, 1938.

Delfino, Giuseppe, and Aidano Schmuckher. *Stregoneria Magia Credenze e Superstizioni a Genova e in Liguria*, vol. 39. Biblioteca Lares. Florence: Leo S. Olschki, 1973.

de Nino, Antonio. *Usi e Costumi Abruzzesi*. 6 vol. Florence, Italy: Barbera, 1883.

Densmore, Frances. *How Indians Use Wild Plants for Food, Medicine & Crafts* (1928). New York: Dover, 1974.

Dent, Alan. *World of Shakespeare: Plants*. New York: Osprey, 1971.

de Renzi, Salvatore. *Storia documentata della Scuola Medica di Salerno*. Naples: Gaetano Nobile, 1857.

Deutsche Heilpflanze, Die. Weimar, Germany: Keller, Stollberg/Erzgebirge, 1934.

Dinand, August Paul. *Handbuch der Heilpflanzenkunde*. Munich: I. F. Schreiber, 1921.

Dragendorff, Georg. *Die Heilpflanzen der verschiedenen Völker und Zeiten*. Stuttgart: Ferdinand Enke, 1898.

Drayton, Michael. *Poly-Olbion* (1622). Oxford: Oxford Univ. Press, 1961.

Dunmire, William W., and Gail D. Tierney. *Wild Plants of the Pueblo Province*. Santa Fe, NM: Museum of New Mexico Press, 1995.

Dye Plants and Dyeing—a Handbook. Brooklyn, NY: Brooklyn Botanic Garden, 1973.

Dyer, Rev. T. F. Thiselton. *British Popular Customs*. London: George Bell & Sons, 1876.

———. *Domestic Folk-Lore*. London: George Bell & Sons, 1881.

———. *The Folk-Lore of Plants*. London: George Bell & Sons, 1889.

———. *Folk-Lore of Shakespeare* (1883). New York: Dover, 1966.

Eberhardt, P. *Les Plantes Médicinales*. Paris: Paul Lechevalier, 1927.

Elsevier's Dictionary of Pharmaceutical Science and Techniques. Amsterdam: Elsevier, 1968.

Emboden, William. *Narcotic Plants*. London: Studio Vista, 1972.

Encke, Fritz, Buchheim, et al., eds. *Zander Handwörterbuch der Pflanzennamen*. Stuttgart: Ulmer, 1984–present.

Englert, Dr. Ludwig. *Von altdeutscher Heilkunst*. Leipzig, Germany: Bibliographisches Institut, 1935.

Evelyn, John. *Acetaria: A Discourse of Sallets*. London: B. Tooke, 1699.

Faber, Stefanie. *Das Rezeptbuch für Naturkosmetik*. Munich: Molden, 1974.

——— . *Kräuter-Kosmetik*. Munich: Molden, 1979.

Fahrenkamp, Hans J. *Wie man eyn teutsches Mannsbild bey Kräfften hält*. Munich: Heimeran, 1975.

Farmer, Fannie. *The Fannie Farmer Cookbook*. 12th edition. New York: Knopf, 1980.

Ferguson, John. *Bibliographical Notes on the Histories of Inventions and Books of Secrets*. London: Holland Press, 1959.

Finamore, Gennaro. *Tradizioni popolari Abruzzesi*. Turin, Italy: Clausen, 1894.

Fischer, Eugen. *Heilpflanzen*. Bern, Switzerland: 1975.

Fischer, Hermann. "Die Heilige Hildegard von Bingen." *Münchener Beiträge zur Geschichte und Literatur der Naturwissenschaften und Medizin*, vol. 7/8 (1927).

Fitter, Richard, and Alistair Fitter. *The Wild Flowers of Britain and Northern Europe*. London: Collins, 1974.

Flaws, Bob. *The Tao of Healthy Eating*. Boulder, CO: Blue Poppy Press, 2005.

Fletcher, William. *Superstition in Review*. London: 1933. [self-published]

The Folk-Lore Journal. 7 vols. London: The Folk-Lore Society, 1883–89.

Folk Lore Quarterly. 6 vols. (1890–1895). Paris: 1948.

Fossel, Annemarie. *Das Jahr der Blumen*. Innsbruck, Austria: Deutscher Alpenverlag, 1940.

Foster, Gertrude B., and Rosemary F. Loude. *Park's Success with Herbs*. Greenwood, SC: Geo. W. Park Seed Co., 1980.

Fournier, P. *Le Livre des Plantes Médicinales et Vénéneuses de France*. 2 vol. Paris: Paul Lechevalier, 1948.

Francé, Raoul. *Harmonie in der Natur*. Stuttgart: Frankh'sche Verlagshandlung, 1926.

——— . *Die Seele der Pflanze*. Berlin: Ullstein, 1924.

——— . *Die technischen Leistungen der Pflanzen*. Leipzig, Germany: Veit & Comp., 1919.

——— . *Die Welt der Pflanze*. Berlin: Ullstein, 1912.

Frazer, Sir James George. *The Golden Bough* (1890-1915). 13 vol. New York: Macmillan, 1966.

Freeman, Margaret B. *Herbs for the Medieval Household*. New York: Metropolitan Museum of Art, 1943.

Fuchs, Leonhardt. *Alt Kreüterbüchlein* [1500s]. Heilbronn, Germany: Eugen Salzer, 1951.

———. *Neu Kreüterbuch* (1543). Facsimile (Munich: Konrad Kölbl, 1964).

———. *The New Herbal of 1543, New Kreüterbuch*. Cologne, Germany: Taschen, 2001.

Galen. *On the Natural Faculties*. Trans. Arthur John Brock. London: Heinemann, 1952.

Ganzenmüller, Wilhelm. *Die Alchemie im Mittelalter*. Paderborn, Germany: Bonifacius Druckerei, 1938.

———. *Das Naturgefühl im Mittlealter*, vol. 18 of *Beiträge zur Kulturgeschichte des Mittelalters und der Renaissance*. Berlin: Teubner, 1914.

Garland, Sarah. *The Complete Book of Herbs and Spices*. London: Francis Lincoln, 1979.

———. *Der duftende Kräutergarten*. Munich: Mosaik, 1988.

Genders, Roy. *The Wild Flower Garden*. London: Ward Lock, 1976.

Gerard, John. *Gerard's Herball:* [1597] *The essence thereof distilled by Marcus Woodward from the edition of Th. Johnson, 1636*. Ed. Marcus Woodward. London: Gerald How, 1927.

———. *Catalogus Arborum, Fructicum ac Plantarum* (1599). Facsimile (Weilheim, Germany, 1962).

Gessner, Otto, and Gerhard Orzechowski. *Gift- und Arzneipflanzen von Mitteleuropa*. Heidelberg: Carl Winter Universitätsverlag, 1974.

Geuter, Maria. *Kräuter in der Ernährung*. Schaffhausen, Switzerland: Novalis, 1976.

Gianci, Sergio. *Le Piante Medicinali delle Isole Eolie*. Pungitopo Editore, 1978.

Gibbons, Euell. *Stalking the Healthful Herbs*. New York: David McKay, 1966.

———. *Stalking the Wild Asparagus*. New York: David McKay, 1970.

Gilbertie, Sal. *Herb Gardening at its Best*. New York: Macmillan, 1984.

Gill, W. W. *A Second Manx Scrapbook*. Bristol, England: Arrowsmith, 1932.

Gladstar, Rosemary. *Herbal Healing for Women*. New York: Simon and Schuster, 1993.

Glasse, Hannah. *The Art of Cookery Made Plain and Easy*. London: Millar, Tonsan, et al., 1760.

Goethe, J. W. *Die Metamorphose der Pflanzen*. Bern, Switzerland: Francke, 1947.

———. *Die Natur*. Munich: Beck, 1962.

Golowin, Sergius. *Die Magie der verbotenen Märchen*. Hamburg: Merlin, 1973.

Goodwin, Jill. *A Dyer's Manual*. London: Pelham Books, 1982.

Graubard, Mark. *Astrology and Alchemy*. New York: Philosophical Library, 1953.

Gray, Asa. *New Manual of Botany*. New York: American Book Co., 1908.

Greene, Richard Leighton. *The Early English Carols*. Oxford: Clarendon Press, 1977.

Gregory, Lady Augusta. *Visions and Beliefs in the West of Ireland*. London: Colin Smythe, 1970.

Grieve, Mrs. Maude. *A Modern Herbal* (1931). London: Penguin, 1976.

———. *Culinary Herbs & Condiments* (1934). New York: Dover, 1971.

Grigson, Geoffrey. *The Englishman's Flora*. London: Granada / Paladin, 1955.

Grimm, Jacob. *Deutsche Mythologie* (1835). 3 vol. Berlin: Ferdinand Dümmlers Verlagsbuchhandlung, 1875–78.

———. *Teutonic Mythology*. New York: Dover, 1966.

Grimmelshausen, H. J. Chr. *Der abenteurliche Simplicissimus*. Munich: Winkler, 1956.

Gunther, Robert T., ed. *The Greek Herbal of Dioscurides*. New York: Hafner, 1959.

Hagger, Conrad. *Neues Saltzburgisches Koch-Buch* (1719). Facsimile (Salzburg, Austria: Residenz, 1976).

Hahn, Mary. *Praktisches Kochbuch*. Berlin: Mary Hahns Kochbuchverlag, 1952.

Hall, Dorothy. *The Book of Herbs*. London: Pan Books, 1976.

Hansen, Harold A. *The Witch's Garden*. Trans. Muriel Crofts. Santa Cruz, CA: Unity Press, 1978.

Holy Bible: Authorized King James Version. London: HarperCollins UK, 2001.

Harrington, Sir John, trans. *The School of Salernum*. Salerno, Italy: Ente Provinciale per il Turismo, 1953.

Hazlitt, W. Carew. *Old Cookery Books and Ancient Cuisine*. London: Elliot Stock, 1902.

Hegi, Gustav. *Illustrierte Flora von Mittel-Europa*. 13 vol. Munich: Lehmanns, 1913–1918.

Heilmann, Karl Eugen. *Kräuterbücher in Bild und Geschichte*. Munich: Konrad Kölbl, 1973.

Helm, Eva Marie. *Feld-, Wald- und Wiesenkochbuch*. Munich: Heimeran, 1978.

Henderson, William. *Notes on the Folk-Lore of the Northern Counties of England and the Borders*. London: The Folk-Lore Society, 1897.

Hendrick, U. P., ed. *Sturtevants's Edible Plants of the World* (1919). New York: Dover, 1972.

Henggeler, S., and O. Schmid. *Biologischer Pflanzenschutz im Garten*. Aarau, Switzerland: Wirz, 1980.

Henglein, Martin. *Die heilende Kraft der Wohlgerüche und Essenzen*. Munich: Droemer Knaur, 1988.

The Herbal Review, and *Herbs: The Journal of the Herb Society*. London: The Herb Society, 1976–present.

Herrick, Robert. *The Complete Poetry of Robert Herrick*. New York: NYU Press, 1963.

Hewitt, Jean. *The New York Times Natural Foods Cookbook*. New York: Quadrangle Books, 1971.

Hippocratic Writings. Trans. Francis Adams (1849). London: Watts, 1952.

Hobday, E. *Cottage Gardening*. London: Macmillan, 1877.

Hodgart, Matthew. *The Faber Book of Ballads*. London: Faber & Faber, 1965.

Höfler, M. *Deutsches Krankheitsnamen-Buch*. Munich: Piloti & Loehele, 1899.

Horace. *Satires, Epistles, and Ars Poetica*. Trans. H. Rushton Fairclough. Cambridge, MA: Loeb Classical Library, 1926.

Howarth, Sheila. *Herbs with Everything*. New York: Holt, Rinehart and Winston, 1976.

Howitt, Mary. "Philip of Maine." *The Seven Temptations*. London: Richard Bentley, 1834 (original from Oxford University; digitized 2006).

Hübner, Barbara. *Die Zubereitung von Getreidegerichten*. Bad Liebenzell-Unterleugenhardt, Germany: Arbeitskreis für Ernährungsforschung, e. V., 1974.

Hunnius, Curt. *Pharmazeutisches Wörterbuch*. Berlin: Walter de Gruyter, 1966.

Huson, Paul. *Mastering Herbalism*. New York: Stein and Day, 1974.

Hutchinson, J. *Wild Flowers in Colour*. Middlesex, England: Penguin, 1974.

Huxley, Alyson. *Natural Beauty with Herbs*. London: Darton Longman and Todd, 1977.

Hyatt, Richard. *Chinese Herbal Medicine*. New York: Schocken Books, 1978.

Hyott, J. K. *The Cyclopedia of Practical Quotations*. New York: Funk and Wagnalls, 1896 (original from Univ. of Wisconsin; digitized 2007).

Jackson, Kenneth Hurlstone, ed. and trans. *A Celtic Miscellany*. London: Penguin, 1976.

Jacobs, Betty E. M. *Growing Herbs and Plants for Dyeing*. Mountain View, MO: Select Books, 1977.

Jäger, Gerhard. *Die Rezepturen der königlich-bayerischen Leib- und Hof-Apotheke*. Bayreuth, Germany: Hestia, 1984.

Jahrbuch für Volkskunde. Würzburg, Germany: Echter, 1965.

Johnson, Ben. *The New Inn, or The Light Heart*. (1631) Ed. George Bremner Tennant. New York: Henry Holt, 1908.

Jung, C. Gustav. *Mysterium Coniunctionis*. Zurich, Switzerland: Rascher, 1955.

Kaiser, Ernst. *Paracelsus*. Reinbek bei Hamburg, Germany: Rowohlt, 1969.

Kamphoeven, Elsa Sophia von. *An Nachtfeuern der Karawan-Serail*. Hamburg: Christina Wegner, 1970.

Keats, John. *The Poetical Works of John Keats*. Ed. W. Garrod. London: Oxford Univ. Press, 1962.

Kirk, Donald R. *Wild Edible Plants of Western North America*. Happy Camp, CA: Naturegraph Publishers, 1975.

Kitchiner, William. *The Cook's Oracle* (1817). London: Samuel Bagster, 1860.

Knap, Alyson Hart. *Wild Harvest*. Toronto: Pagurian Press, 1975.

Kneipp, Sebastian. *Heilkräuter nach Kneipp*. Munich: Josef Kösel & F. Pustet, 1936.

———. *So sollt ihr Leben* (1897). 4 vol. Facsimile (Munich: Ehrenwirth Verlag, 1976).

Koschtschejew. *Wildwachsende Pflanzen in unserer Ernährung*. Leipzig, Germany: Fachbuchverlag, 1986.

Kranich, Ernst Michael. *Die Formen-Sprache der Pflanze*. Stuttgart: Freies Geistesleben, 1976.

Krauss, Friedrich S. "Südslavische Hexensagen." *Mitteilungen der Anthropologischen Gesellschaft in Wien*, vol. XIV (1884).

———. "Südslavische Pestsagen," *Mitteilungen der Anthropologischen Gesellschaft in Wien*, vol. XIII (1883).

Krayer, E. Hoffmann, and Hanns Bächtold-Stäubli, eds. *Handwörterbuch des deutschen Aberglaubens*. 10 vol. Berlin: Walter de Gruyter, 1932.

Kremer, Bruno P. *Duft- und Aromapflanzen*. Stuttgart: Kosmos, 1988.

Kreuter, Marie-Luise. *Kräuter und Gewürze aus dem eigenen Garten*. Munich: BLV, 1979.

———. *Der Bio-Garten*. Munich: BLV, 1988.

———. *Wunderkräfte der Natur*. Geneva: Ariston, 1978.

Kroeber, Ludwig. *Zur Geschichte, Herkunft und Physologie der Würz- und Duftstoffe*. Munich: Lang, 1949.

Künzle, Johann. *Chrut und Unchrut*. Munich: Kräuterhaus Alpina, 1915.

Kulturpflanze, Die. Periodical published by the Institute for Plant Genetics and Crop Plant research, Gatersleben, Germany (1952–1990).

Lankester, Edwin. *Vegetable Substances used for the Food of Man*. London: Charles Knight, 1832.

Läufer, Otto. *Farbensymbolik im deutschen Volksbrauch*. Hamburg: Hansischer Gilden, 1948.

Lauter, Dr. Werner. *Hildegard-Bibliogrfie*. Alzey, Germany: Rheinhessische Druckwerk-stätte, 1970.

Leese, Otto. *Pflanzliche Arzneistoffe in Lehrbuch der Homöopathie*. Heidelberg: K. F. Haug-Verlag, 1973.

Levy, Juliette de Baïracli. *The Complete Herbal Handbook for the Dog and Cat*. London: Faber & Faber, 1992.

Leyel, Mrs. C. F. *Herbal Delights*. London, Faber & Faber, 1937.

Liebster, Günther. *Heilkraft aus dem Garten*. Munich: BLV, 1985.

Lieutaghi, Pierre. *Il Libro delle Erbe*. Milan: Gruppo Editoriale Electa, 1981.

Lilienkron, Rochus von. *Deutsches Leben im Volkslied um 1530*. Hildesheim, Germany: Georg Olms, 1966.

Linnaei, Caroli. *Systema Naturae* (1748). Facsimile (Leipzig, Germany: Teubner, 1914).

Lippert, F. *Zur Praxis des Heilpflanzenanbaus*. Planegg, Germany: Müllersche, 1939.

Loewenfeld, Claire, and Phillipa Back. *Herbs for Health and Cookery*. London: Pan Books, 1965.

Low-Fat Mexican Cook Book. Menlo Park, CA: Sunset Publishing, 1994.

Lu, Henry C. *Chinese System of Food Cures*. New York: Sterling, 1986.

Lumbroso, Matizia Maroni. *El mal del moc*. Rome: Fondazione Ernesto Besso, 1968.

Lupton, Thomas. *A Thousand Notable Things*. London: James Ridgway, 1791.

Lyly, John. *The Complete Works*. 3 vol. Oxford: Oxford Univ. Press, 1973.

Mabey, Richard. *Das neue BLV Buch der Kräuter*. Munich: BLV, 1989.

Machado y Álvarez, Antonio. *Biblioteca de las tradiciones populares españolas*. 11 vol. Seville, Spain: Francisco Alverez, 1883–86.

MacNicol, Mary. *Flower Cookery*. New York: Fleet, 1967.

Mann, H. *Die Moderne Parfümerie*. Augsburg, Germany: Verlag für Chemische Indu-strie, 1912.

——— . *Die Schule des modernen Parfümeurs*. Augsburg, Germany: Verlag für Chemische Industrie, 1912.

Mannhardt, Wilhelm. *Der Baumkultus der Germanen und ihrer Nachbarstämme*. Berlin: Bornträger, 1875.

Mansfeld, Rudolf. *Kulturpflanzen-Verzeichnis*. 4 vol. Ed. Jürgen Schultze-Motel. Berlin: Akademie Verlag, 1986.

Markham, Gervase. *A Way to Get Wealth*. London: John Harison, 1625.

———. *Cheape and Good Husbandry* (1614). Facsimile (New York: Da Capo Press, 1969).

Marzell, Heinrich. *Bayerische Volksbotanik*. Nuremberg, Germany: Lorenz Spindler, undated.

———. *Geschichte und Volkskunde der deutschen Heilpflanzen*. Stuttgart: Hippokrates, 1938.

———. *Die Pflanzenwelt der Alpen*. Stuttgart: Hippokrates, 1933.

———. *Volksbotanik*. Berlin: Verlag Enckehaus, 1935.

———. *Wörterbuch der deutschen Pflanzennamen*. 5 vol. Leipzig, Germany: Hirzel, 1951.

Matthiolus, Pierandrea. *Kräuterbuch* (1626). Facsimile (Munich: Konrad Kölbl).

Mauerhofer, Walter. *Heimische Gewürzkräuter*. Saalfelden, Austria. [self-published, no date.]

Meeks, Wayne A., ed. *The Harper Collins Study Bible, New Revised Standard Version*. New York: HarperCollins, 1993.

Mercatante, Anthony S. *The Magic Garden*. London: Harper & Row, 1976.

Mességué, Didier. *Die Kräuter meines Vaters*. Munich: Molden, 1974.

Mességué, Maurice. *Von Menschen und Pflanzen*. Munich: Molden, 1972.

———. *Das Mességué Heilkräuter-Lexikon*. Munich: Molden, 1976.

———. *Die Natur hat immer Recht*. Munich: Molden, 1973.

Meyer, Th. *Arzneipflanzenkultur und Kräuterhandel*. Berlin: Springer, 1934.

Meyer-Berkhot, Edda. *Würzige Kräuterküche*. Munich: Heimeran, 1972.

Millspaugh, Charles F. *American Medicinal Plants* (1892). New York: Dover, 1974.

Milne, A. A. *When We Were Very Young*. New York: Dutton, 1950.

Miloradovich, Milo. *Growing and Using Herbs and Spices*. New York: Doubleday, 1952.

Montagné, Prosper. *Larousse Gastronomique*. New York: Crown Publishers, 1965.

Montez, Lola. *The Arts of Beauty*. New York: Dick & Fitzgerald, 1858.

Moore, Michael. *Medicinal Plants of the Desert and Canyon West*. Santa Fe, NM: Museum of New Mexico Press, 1989.

———. *Medicinal Plants of the Mountain West*. Santa Fe, NM: Museum of New Mexico Press, 1979.

———. *Los Remedios. Traditional Herbal Remedies of the Southwest*. Santa Fe, NM: Red Crane Books, 1990.

Moryson, Fynes. *An Itinerary*, vol. III. Glasgow: James MacLehose and Sons, 1908 (original from the New York Public Library; digitized 2007).

Mother Goose's Melodies. Facsimile of the Monroe and Francis 1833 edition (New York: Dover, 1970).

Muenscher, Walter A., and Myron A. Rice. *Garden Spice and Wild Pot-Herbs*. Ithaca, NY: Comstock, 1955.

Mühle, E. *Die Krankheiten und Schädlinge der Arznei-, Gewürz-, und Duftpflanzen*. Berlin: Akademie Verlag, 1956.

Murr, Josef. *Die Pflanzenwelt in der Griechische Mythologie*. Innsbruck: Wagner, 1890.

Murray, Margaret. *The Witch Cult in Western Europe*. Oxford: Oxford Univ. Press, 1962.

Nares, Robert, James O. Halliwell, and Thomas Wright. *A Glossary: Or, Collection of Words, Phrases, Names, and Allusions to Customs, Proverbs, Etc.*, vol. I. London: Gibbings, 1901 (digitized).

Nielsen, Esther. *Natürlich färben*. Haldenwang, Germany: 1985.

Northall, G. F. *English Folk-Rhymes* (1892). Detroit, MI: Singing Tree Press, 1968.

Oertel-Bauer. *Lexikon der Naturheilkunde*. Cologne, Germany: Lingren, 1976.

Ohrbach, Barbara Milo. *Kräuter und Blumendüfte im Haus*. Cologne, Germany: DuMont, 1988.

Ohrt, F. *Herba, Gratia Plena*, vol. 28, nr. 82. Helsinki: F.F. Communications, 1929.

Orient-Cluj, Julius. *Die Arzneimittel des Volkes und dessen Mystizismus*. Mittenwald/Bayern, Germany: Arthur Nemayer, 1931.

Ostermann, V. *La Vita in Friuli*. Udine, Italy: Domenico del Bianco, 1894.

Owen, Elias. *Welsh Folk-Lore*. Owestry, England: Owestry & Wexham, 1887.

The Oxford Dictionary of Quotations. London: Oxford Univ. Press, 1968.

Paracelsus. *Von der rechten Heilkunst*. Stuttgart: Hippokrates, 1939.

Parkinson, John. *A Fragment from Theatrum Bontanicum* [1640], *"or An Herball of a Large Extent."* Falls Village, CT: Herb Grower Press, 1967.

———. *Paradisi in Sole, etc.* Facsimile of the 1629 edition (New York: Dover, 1976).

Partridge, Eric. *Usage and Abusage*. London: Hamish Hamilton, 1969.

Payne, Joseph Frank. *English Medicine in the Anglo-Saxon Times*. Oxford: Oxford Univ. Press, 1904.

Pegge, Samuel. *The Forme of Cury*. London: J. Nichols, 1780.

Pepys, Samuel. *The Diary of Samuel Pepys*. 2 vol. Ed. Henry B. Wheatley. New York: Random House, undated.

Perger, H. Ritter von. *Deutsche Pflanzensagen*. Stuttgart: Verlag von August Schaber, 1864.

Perring, F. H., and S. M. Walters. *Atlas of the British Flora*. London: Thomas Nelson & Sons, 1962.

Peterson, Roger Tory, and Margaret McKenny. *A Field Guide to Wildflowers of Northeastern and Northcentral North America*. Boston: Houghton Mifflin, 1968.

Philbrick, Helen, and Richard B. Gregg. *Companion Plants*. London: Stuart & Watkins, 1967.

Phillips, Harry R. *Growing and Propagating Wild Flowers*. Chapel Hill, NC: Univ. of North Carolina Press, 1985.

Phillips, Roger. *Wild Flowers of Britain*. London: Pan Books, 1977.

Pickering, Charles. *Chronological History of Plants*. Boston: Little, Brown & Co., 1879.

Piemontese, Alessio (pseud. for Girolamo Ruscelli). *The Secrets of Alessio*. London: Ihon Day, 1559–66.

Pitré, Giuseppe. *Medicina Popolare Siciliana*. Florence, Italy: Barbera, 1949.

Planta Medica. Stuttgart: Hippokrates, 1952.

Platt, Sir Hugh. *Delightes for Ladies* (1594). London: Penguin, 1948.

Pomini, Luigi. *Il Campo Sperimentale delle Piante Medicinali Aromatiche die Varallo Sesia*. Vercelli, Italy: Camera di Commercio Industria Agricoltura Vercelli, 1953.

———. *Erboristeria Pedemontana*. 2 vol. Vercelli, Italy: Camera di Commercio Industria Agricoltura Vercelli, 1953.

Pope, Alexander. *The Poetical Works of Alexander Pope*, vol 1. Ed. Robert Carruthers. London: Ingram, Cooke, and Co., 1853.

Porta, Joh. Baptistae. *De Miraculis Rerum Naturalium*. Naples: Mattio Cancer, 1558.

———. *Magia Naturalis*. Leyden, Italy: 1644.

Porter, Enid. *Cambridgeshire Customs and Folklore*. London: Routledge, Keagan, Paul, 1969.

Prato, Katharina. *Die Süddeutsche Küche* (1885). Graz, Austria: Styria, 1903.

Pritzel, G., and C. Jessen. *Die deutschen Volksnamen der Pflanzen*. Hannover, Germany: Verlag von Philipp Cohen, 1884.

Radford, E., and M. A. Radford. *Encyclopaedia of Superstitions*. London: Rider, 1947.

Ralston, W. R. S. *The Songs of the Russian People*. London: Ellis & Green, 1872.

Rantasale, A. V. *Einige Zaubersteine und Zauberpflanzen im Volksglauben der Finnen*, vol. 712. Helsinki: F.F. Communications, 1959.

Reid, Daniel. *A Handbook of Chinese Healing Herbs*. New York: Barnes and Noble / Shambhala, 1999.

Reiser, Karl. *Sagen, Gebräuche, und Sprichwörter des Allgäus*. 2 vol. Kempten, Germany: J. Kosers, 1895.

Relics of Popular Antiquities. Publication of the Folk-Lore Society. London: Nichols & Sons, 1878.

Riccardi, Paolo. *Pregiudizi e Superstizioni del popolo Modenese* (1891). Rome: Il Fiorino, 1969.

Ricci, Franco Maria. *Herbarium, natural remedies from a medieval manuscript*. Milan: Rizzoli Editore, 1980.

Richardson, Rosamond. *Hedgerow Cookery*. Middlesex, England: Penguin, 1980.

Rodale, J. I. *How to grow Vegetables and Fruits by the Organic Method*. Emmaus, PA: Rodale Press, 1970.

Rogers, Julia Ellen. *The Book of Useful Plants*. New York: Doubleday, 1913.

Rogler, August. *Kräutersegen*. Munich: Hippolyt, 1971.

Rohde, Eleanour Sinclair. *A Garden of Herbs* (1936). New York: Dover, 1969.

Rothenberg, Jerome. *Technicians of the Sacred*. New York: Doubleday, 1968.

Sanecki, Kay N. *The Complete Book of Herbs*. London: Macdonald and Jane's, 1974.

Sappho. *Greek Lyric*, vol. 1. Trans. David A. Campbell. Cambridge, MA: Harvard Univ. Press, 1982.

Scherzer, Conrad. *Die Flora alter Bauerngärten und Friedhöfe*. Nuremberg, Germany: 1922.

Scherzer, Hans. *Erd- und Pflanzengeschichtliche Wanderungen durchs Frankenland*. Kaufbeuren, Germany: I. Wunsiedel, 1920.

Schrödter, Willy. *Pflanzen-Geheimnisse*. Eschwege, Germany: G. E. Schroeder, 1968.

Schuppli, Ida, and Betty Hinterer. *Grabnerhof-Kochbuch*. Vienna: Franz Deuticke, 1918.

Schwarz, Hedwig. *Pharmaziegeschichtliche Pflanzenstudien*. Mittenwald/Bayern, Germany: Arthur Nemayer, 1931.

Schweizerisches Archiv für Volkskunde. 20 vol. Zurich: Société Suisse des Traditions Populaires, 1897–present.

Shakespeare, William. *Historical Plays, Poems, and Sonnets*. London: Dent, 1950.

Sheperd, Renee. *Recipes from a Kitchen Garden*. Berkeley, CA: Ten Speed Press, 1993.

Shirley, John. *The Accomplished Ladies Rich Closet of Rarities*. London: N. Bodington, 1688.

Simonis, Werner-Christian. *Taschenbuch der Heil- und Gewürzkräuter*. Frankfurt: Klostermann, 1976.

Singer, Charles. *Early English Magic and Medicine*. Proceedings of the British Academy. London: Humphrey Milford/Oxford Univ. Press, 1924.

———. *From Magic to Science* (1928). New York: Dover, 1958.

Sister Clarissa's Unpublished Book of Natural Observations. Personal papers, 1980-2000.

Smith, John. A *Dictionary of Popular Names of the Plants*. London: Macmillan, 1882.

Söhns, Franz. "Unsere Pflanzen." *Zeitschrift für den deutschen Unterricht*. Leipzig, Germany: Teubner, 1897.

Spenser, Edmund. *The Works*. 7 vol. Baltimore, MD: John Hopkins Univ. Press, 1943.

Starkie, Walter. *Auf Zigeunerspuren* [*In Sara's Tents*]. Munich: Carl Hanser, 1957.

Stearn, William. *Botanical Latin*. Newton Abbot, England: David & Charles, 1973.

Steinbichler, Eveline. *Steinbichlers Lexikon*. Frankfurt: Govi-Verlag, 1963.

Steinmetz, E. F. *Vocabularium Botanicum*. Amsterdam: Steinmetz, 1947.

Stevens, John. *The National Trust Book of Wild Flower Gardening*. London: Dorling Kindersley, 1987.

Stevenson, Burton. *Stevenson's Book of Quotations*. New York: Cassel, 1967.

Strabo, Wahlafridus. *Hortulus* (c. 840). Trans. Raef Payne. Pittsburg, PA: Hunt Botanical Library, 1966.

Strunz, Franz. *Geschichte der Naturwissenschaften im Mittelalter*. Stuttgart: Ferdinand Enke, 1910.

Thompson, William A. R., et al. *Healing Plants, a Modern Herbal*. London: Macmillan, 1978.

Thorpe, Benjamin. *Northern Mythology*. 3 vol. London: Edward Lumley, 1851.

Tillyard, E. M. W. *The Elizabethan World Picture*. London: Penguin, 1970.

Tomkins, Peter, and Christopher Bird. *The Secret Life of Plants*. New York: Avon, 1973.

Tongue, Ruth L. *Somerset Folklore*. London: The Folk-Lore Society, 1965.

Treben, Maria. *Gesundheit aus der Apotheke Gottes*. Waidhofen, Austria: 1978. [self-published]

Tusser, Thomas. *Five Hundred Pointes of Good Husbandrie* (1573–75). London: English Dialect Society, 1878.

UNESCO. *Medicinal Plants of the Arid Zones*. Arid Zone Research–XIII. Paris: United Nations Educational, Scientific and Cultural Organization, 1960.

Valnet, Jean. *Aroma-Therapie*. Munich: Heyne, 1986.

Virgil. *The Aeneid*. Trans. Patrick Dickinson. New York: New American Library, 1961.

———. *Virgil's Georgics*. Trans. Smith Palmer Bovie. Chicago: Univ. of Chicago Press, 1956.

Vogel, Virgil J. *American Indian Medicine*. Norman, OK: Oklahoma Univ. Press, 1970.

Walters, W. D. *Wonderful Herbal Remedies*. Swansea, Wales: Domino Books, 1973.

Warnke, Fr. *Pflanzen in Sitte, Sage, und Geschichte*. Leipzig, Germany: 1878.

Watts, Alan W. *Nature, Man and Woman*. New York: Vintage Books, 1970.

Weckerin, F. Anna. *Ein köstlich new Kochbuch* (1598). Facsimile (Munich: Heimeran Verlag, 1977).

Wiesener, Julius von. *Die Rohstoffe des Pflanzenreichs*. 6 vol. Weinheim, Germany: Cramer, 1962.

Wilde, Lady. *Ancient Cures, Charms and Usages of Ireland*. Detroit, MI: Singing Tree Press, 1970.

Willfort, Richard. *Gesundheit durch Heilkräuter*. Linz, Austria: Rudolf Trauner, 1973.

Winkelmann, H. C. W. *Die Wirkstoffe unserer Heilpflanzen*. Freiburg, Germany: Otto Walter, 1951.

Winter, Fred. *Technik der modernen Kosmetik*. Vienna: A. Hartleben, 1921.

Withalm, Berthold. *Naturgemässes Volksheilbuch* (1842). Graz, Austria: Leopold Stocker, 1955.

Wittstein, G. C. *Etymologisch-botanisches Handwörterbuch* (1856). Niederwalluf bei Wiesbaden, Germany: Saendig, 1971.

Woodman, Mary. *Home-Made Wines*. London: Foulsham, undated.

Wordsworth, William. *Wordsworth's Poems*. 3 vol. London: Dent, 1955.

Wright, Joseph, ed. *The English Dialect Dictionary*. London: Oxford Univ. Press, 1898.

Wright, Michael, ed. *The Complete Indoor Gardener*. London: Pan Books, 1974.

Zimmermann, Walter. *Geschichte der Pflanzen*. Stuttgart: Thieme, 1969.

Zingerle, Ignaz. *Sagen aus Tirol*. Graz, Austria: Verlag für Sammler, 1969.

HERBAL USE CHART

Most Common Methods of Using Herbs

	What part used?	Amount	Used with	Container	Method of preparation	Remarks
Tea: infusion	Leaves, stems, flowers, occasionally fruits, all delicate parts, cut or shredded.	1 heaping Tbsp. fresh herb, 2 tsp. dried herb.	1 cup boiling water.	Glass, ceramic or enamel with cover, teapot or thermos bottle.	Pour boiling water over herbs, let steep 10–15 minutes, strain, drink lukewarm. If drinking for taste, let steep a shorter time. Can be drunk chilled.	The same results are obtained if the herbs and water are brought just to a boil, then steeped and strained.
Tea: cold infusion	Sensitive tea herbs that may be harmed by too much heat.	Same as above.	1 cup cold water.	Same as above.	Pour water over herbs in tea strainer bag, or tea egg, or over loose tea. Heat to body temperature before drinking or using, strain.	When using tea as eyewash or to sniff up into sinuses, be sure to strain through filter paper, and dissolve ca. ¼ tsp. salt in 1 cup warm tea.
Tea: decoction	Roots, seeds, woody stems, all sturdy parts of herb, cut small or shredded.	1–2 tsp. dried or fresh herbs, depending on species.	1 cup water.	Same as above, cook in enameled, glass or stainless steel pot with cover.	Boil herbs and water 10–15 minutes (according to herb used and how small it is shredded). Let steep, covered, 10–15 minutes, strain, drink lukewarm.	Can also be left to macerate overnight, brought just to a boil the next day, strained and served.
Tea: cold decoction	Same as above, heat-sensitive herbs.	Same as above.	Same as above.	Same as above, do not boil.	Steep overnight in cold water, heat the following morning to body temperature and no higher, use within the day.	

Most Common Methods of Using Herbs

	What part used?	Amount	Used with	Container	Method of preparation	Remarks
Medicinal Bath	Same as above, all parts of the plant.	1 handful herbs for 5 qt. of water, use proportionally less for roots.	Same as above.	Use large pot for boiling, no Teflon or aluminum. Be sure to clean out tub immediately, or will stain.	Leafy herbs are heated to the boiling point, roots are boiled for a few minutes and allowed to steep, and strained. Or hang sack on faucet and let hot water pour over it. Dry yourself after bath carefully, rest for 30–90 minutes afterwards.	Too strong or too hot baths may strain the heart. Best taken in morning because of possible stimulant effect.
Hip Bath	Same as above, all parts of the plant.	Same as above.	Thick decoction added to warm bath.	Same as above, can also use bidet, small tub.	Place herbs in muslin sack, tie ends together tightly with long string. Place in pot with water, boil and simmer gently for 10 minutes. Let steep 20 minutes, pour water into bath. Add hot water as necessary.	Dry yourself well, rest in warmed bed for 30 minutes. Don't take more than 1–2 times a week.
Foot Bath	Infusion of whole herb, leaves, flowers, decoction of roots, stems, seeds.	One handful of herbs for each gallon of water. Use less for roots.	Usually, 2–3 gal. of water.	Herbs boiled in non-aluminum pot with cover. Footbath container is enameled, or heat-resistant plastic.	Bring herbs and water in pot to a boil. Steep for 15–20 minutes. Strain into footbath, dilute with cool water. Remain in footbath until water begins to cool, or add more hot water. Don't use for more than 30 minutes.	Always dry yourself fully after bath, rest if necessary. Can be repeated once daily.
Douches and Enemas	Same as above.	Same as for tea.		Strain well, and filter through filter paper to remove particles.		Use only under supervision, since intestinal and vaginal flora can be damaged.
Steaming Mixture	Same as for foot bath.	Same as foot bath.	½ gal. usually enough for face, larger amounts for body.	Herbs are cooked in pot with cover, no aluminum.	Heat as for footbath, steep with cover 15–20 minutes. Cover face and pot with towel, remove cover carefully to avoid burns on face and hands, and remain under towel for 15 minutes or until cooler, stirring occasionally. Whole body is steamed with chair and blanket "tent" propped up with broomstick.	Do not use on face more than 1 time a day, on body more than 1–2 times a week.

Most Common Methods of Using Herbs

	What part used?	Amount	Used with	Container	Method of preparation	Remarks
Poultice	Fresh leaves, fruits, whole herbs, mashed to a pulp. Ground seeds, roots. Occasionally, fresh whole bruised leaves/roots.	Enough to cover damaged area.	Herbal pulp or powder mixed to a thick consistency with water.	Herbs are crushed with mortar and pestle or ground with coffee grinder, applied to skin with sterilized gauze.	Lay damp herb pulp or powder on cloth, either warm or cold, and cover damaged area, fasten with bandage, and leave on until dried or cooled off.	Hot poultices can be kept warm with hot water bottle. Damp steamed herbal cushions can also be applied as poultices.
Hot Pillow and Cushion	Flowers, leaves, whole herb.	Fill linen, muslin or cotton sack loosely with herbs.	Hot water bottle laid on hot herbal pillow keeps it warm.	Cooking pot with flat cover.	Boil water in pan, cover loosely, place herb pillow or cushion on top of pot until warm, pillows can also be steamed effectively on canning rack or steaming sieve in pot.	Do not use on face more than once a day, or may cause thread veins.
Salve	Any part of herb, usually powdered.		Use only the finest quality lard or oils with good keeping qualities.	Ceramic or glass pots for storage, occasionally plastic.	The simplest method, used by farmers, is to heat the herbs with lard and then strain through cheesecloth into pots.	See marigold chapter. Plant parts are extracted in alcohol or directly in oil and then mixed into a salve.
Oil	Whole shredded plant, leaves, fruits, flowers. Extract, essence, or powdered seeds, roots.		Fresh olive, sesame, jojoba, avocado, or almond oils.	Clean and dark glass bottle.	Proceed as for alcoholic tincture, the oil should take on the characteristic smell. Filter through filter paper to remove herb residue. Discard if the oil goes rancid.	Used for herbs such as St. John's wort flowers that can be extracted in oil.
Essence	Essential oil, usually commercially produced.		Alone, or mixed with alcohol or oil.	Clear glass bottles, dark bottles if light sensitive.	Essential oils are taken internally few drops at a time, usually on sugar cubes or bread, or combined with oils for external use. Rooms may be smoked or aromatized with them.	Synthetic oils usually smell very strongly if rubbed on the skin. Natural oils take longer to give off aroma.
Powder	Roots, also whole herb, leaves, seeds, or fruits.		Usually mixed with honey/syr up to form electuary, or dissolved in alcohol, but also to make salves.	Mortar and pestle or coffee or meat grinder or grain mill used only for herbs, or strong blender. Store in airtight containers.	Grind manually, or pulverize dried leaves and whole herbs. Commercial powder is often extracted with solvents, dried, and then ground to powder.	

Most Common Methods of Using Herbs

	What part used?	Amount	Used with	Container	Method of preparation	Remarks
Tincture	Usually fresh plant parts, occasionally dried.	1 part of fresh herb in 2 parts grain alcohol or wine spirits.	High-proof clear spirits such as Everclear. Good vodka or clear fruit schnapps will also do if available.	Dark glass bottles with tops that close tightly to prevent evaporation.	Steep for 1–2 weeks in a warm place out of direct sunlight. Press out the herb residue with cheesecloth, strain through filter paper (coffee filter) to obtain clear tincture. Procedures will vary with different herbs. Store in dark glass bottles, close well.	People sensitive to alcohol should avoid the use of tinctures altogether. The correct dosage can be difficult for the novice to determine.
Alcoholic Solution or Extract	Any part of herb, crushed or powdered.	Varies with herb. Usually 1 handful fresh herbs for 1 qt. alcohol.	Enough 95% alcohol to cover herbs. Dilute for external use. For internal use, use vodka or clear spirits.	Herbs are usually steeped in a clear glass bottle, stored in a dark glass bottle.	Pour alcohol over herbs in bottle, cork and let stand in the sun until mixture has taken on characteristic odor and taste of herbs (from 2 days to months). Strain and then filter through filter paper into clear bottles. Store away from sun.	In a solution, the herbs will dissolve completely in the alcohol.
Medicinal Wine	Same as above.	Same as above.	White wine is usually used, as in rosemary wine, sometimes red wine.	Same as above.	Same as above.	Often used for its fine taste, and only secondarily as medicine.
Distilled Herbal Water	Any part of herb.				Must be distilled, fairly material intensive.	Was once widely used, has now gone out of fashion.
Extracted Juice	Any part of the herb, usually juicy leaves and fruits.			Store in sterilized jars, vacuum sealed and refrigerated.	Remove juice by pressure or in a juicer, or grind herb in mortar and leach off the juice with distilled water.	Commercially extracted juices are expensive, but are usually extracted with state-of-the-art techniques, and keep well.

Most Common Methods of Using Herbs

	What part used?	Amount	Used with	Container	Method of preparation	Remarks
Syrup	Fruit pulp, extracted juice, juicy leaves, plant infusion or decoction.	Add just enough herbal mixture to the syrup so that it stays syrupy, or cook down.	Boiled-down water and sugar.	Same as above, store in jars with seals.	Mix sugar syrup and herbal pulp or concentrated tea together, boil briefly until syrup consistency is reached, strain if necessary through filter paper.	There are many individual recipes —see chapter listings such as plantains.
Seasoning	Powdered roots, finely cut leaves and flowering tops, seeds, fruits, or fresh plant, whole or part.	According to recipe and taste. Don't overuse.	Most foods, sauces, salads, in drinks and bakery goods.	Stored in tightly closing wood, glass or ceramic containers, no metal.	Use according to recipe. Some herbs can be cooked with food; others lose their taste and are always added at the end of the cooking process.	There is no comparison between dried and fresh herbs. Use fresh whenever possible.
Medicinal Biscuit	Herbal powder, fresh crushed leaves, or fruits.		Dough made of flour, water, eggs, baking powder, salt, spices.	Bake on cookie sheet or casserole pan, or bake on stones in front of open fire.	Precise recipes are a matter of experience and taste. Make a fairly stiff dough, spread on baking sheet and bake at low temperature until mixture is somewhat dry.	Unusual, but pleasant method of taking medicine, especially for children.
Wine and Beer	Any part of herb, fresh juice, or crushed fruits.		Sugar, yeast, sometimes cream of tartar.	Never use metal containers for making wines and beer. Store in sterilized glass bottles, cork well.	Procedures vary from plant to plant. For herbal wines, see dandelion chapter. For herbal beers, see stinging nettle chapter.	
Candied Herb	Roots, seeds, fruits, occasionally stems, leaves, and flowers.	Only use fresh, undamaged, juicy plants.	Sugar, sugar syrup.	Enamel or earthenware pot. Store in glass, crockery, earthenware.	Fairly large pieces of root or stem are cooked in syrup until the candying point is reached. The pieces are then dried in the air or a warm oven.	Delicate flowers are dipped in egg white and sugar and then dried.
Conserve	Roots, seeds, fruits. Occasionally extracted juice, leaves, stems.	Same as above.	Sweetened with sugar, a little water. Wild apple jelly or pectin will make the mixture "jell."	Cook in an enamel or stainless steel pot, store in glass.	Cook herb in syrup until the jellying point is reached, add wild apple jelly or commercial pectin. Strain through cheesecloth for clear jelly, or pour directly into sterilized jars for thick jam. Seal.	

Illustrations are used with the permission of Dover Publications;
specifically, from the following:

1001 Plant and Floral Illustrations from Early Herbals by Richard G Hatton;
200 Illustrations from Gerard's Herbal by John Gerard;
Decorative Floral Woodcuts of the Sixteenth Century by Henri Louis Duhamel du Monceau;
Medieval Herb, Plant and Flower Illustrations by Carol Belanger Grafton;
Plants and Flowers: 1761 Illustrations for Artists & Designers
by Alan E. Bessette and William K. Chapman

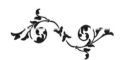